MODERN PERSPECTIVES IN PSYCHIATRY

Edited by John G. Howells

4

MODERN PERSPECTIVES
IN
ADOLESCENT PSYCHIATRY

MODERN PERSPECTIVES IN PSYCHIATRY

Edited by John G. Howells

MODERN PERSPECTIVES
IN
ADOLESCENT PSYCHIATRY

Edited by
JOHN G. HOWELLS
M.D., D.P.M.

Director, The Institute of Family Psychiatry
The Ipswich Hospital
England

Introduction to the American Edition by
GRAHAM B. BLAINE, JR.
M.D.

BRUNNER/MAZEL *Publishers* · New York

Library of Congress Catalog Card No. 76–177253

SBN 87630–040–9

Originally published in United Kingdom by Oliver & Boyd, Edinburgh

CONTENTS

★   ★   ★

PART ONE

SCIENTIFIC

Part Two

CLINICAL

INTRODUCTION TO THE AMERICAN EDITION

GRAHAM B. BLAINE, JR.
M.D.

Chief of Psychiatry, Harvard University Health Services
Assistant Psychiatrist, Adolescent Unit,
Children's Hospital Medical Center,
Boston, Massachusetts

This volume takes a giant step in the direction of increasing our understanding of the diagnosis and treatment of adolescents. More than twenty authors of international eminence have contributed their research findings and personal experience, and have also given wise suggestions for the implementation of both toward the improvement of our understanding and treatment of emotional illness in the adolescent.

Adolescent psychiatry has captured the attention of clinicians throughout the world. There are many reasons for this, but among the principal factors have been the pioneer work of Erik Erikson and the unexpected explosion of youth activity along with varied manifestations of underlying psychopathology which have frightened and mystified the adult generation. Erikson's eight stages in the development of human personality originally projected in his early volume, *Childhood and Society*, discussed conflicts normally encountered by an individual during his entire life cycle. It was the adolescent struggle to achieve identity, however, which struck the most responsive chord in his readers. Encouraged by this response, the author soon expanded his concept of the identity crisis in further writings, including his sensitive psychobiographies of Martin Luther and Gandhi.

These writings inspired other psychiatrists and behavioral scientists to think more extensively and in greater depth about this crucial period of development. A further impetus to such thought came from the challenge presented by the Russian development of their space program. Suddenly we began to look more than ever before to our young men and women for help in meeting what then seemed to us a dangerous threat to our national welfare. Much thought went into trying to help adolescents achieve their intellectual potential by understanding them better and in this way knowing how to provide them with the most stimulating and nurturant climate for growth and performance.

A decade or so later adolescents throughout the world began to draw attention to themselves in extremely dramatic ways. There is no doubt that since the first campus demonstrations erupted during the last decade, the adult world has had to cope with a more demanding, unruly, and dissatisfied group of adolescents than probably has existed in recorded history. The gap between generations has never been wider. While it appears that the most violent phase of this explosive era has passed, we are too close to it to have been able to achieve any real understanding of its true meaning. *Modern Perspectives in Adolescent Psychiatry* provides an excellent guideline for where we are today in our concepts regarding adolescents.

Psychiatrists who deal with disturbed adolescents have increasingly been asked to explain as well as to contend with the distressingly self-destructive behavior of the young. It is true that not all of these disturbing youngsters should be called "disturbed" but it is also true that psychopathology among this age group has increased over the past decade. Hospitalization of the young adolescent has gone up almost 400 percent and of the late adolescent by over 100 percent. This is far beyond the rise proportional to the population growth. Many feel that adolescent psychiatry should be a subspecialty and perhaps such an innovation would help researchers focus more fruitfully on this unique and largely unexplored area.

Although the title of the book is *Modern Perspectives in Adolescent Psychiatry*, far more than just the psychiatric aspects of adolescence is dealt with. The first section of this book, labeled *Scientific*, primarily discusses normal adolescence. The chapter by Daniel and Judith Offer discusses the conflict areas common to all adolescents—those involved with sex, parents, inner turmoil, and identity formation. It also contains encouraging words about the number of "silent" young people who do not cause distress to the world around them. One senses that perhaps it might be possible to develop a climate in which all our children could grow without suffering through a period of unhappiness and alienation. A few chapters later, Dr. Szurek lucidly delineates Erikson's and Josselyn's theories of adolescent development and offers specific and wise advice to parents about dealing with the problems this period of development may bring. Dr. Mays in another chapter discusses the need to form groups as a help to identity formation and distinguishes these groups from gangs. Dr. Schofield discusses the innovations in sexual morality brought to us by this new generation and evaluates its impact on our present and future society objectively and to my mind accurately. Dr. Howells himself closes this section with suggestions for an up-to-date nosology which is refreshingly simple.

The second section of this book is labeled *Clinical* and is devoted to the psychopathology of adolescence. Each disease is discussed thoroughly and suggestions for therapy are clearly given. Dr. Harris discusses psychosomatic illness, organ system by organ system, and mixes psychoanalytic theory in explaining dynamics with hard-nosed common sense in his discussion of therapy. Hilde Bruch deals in depth with obesity. She states it represents a "deficit in perceptual and conceptual awareness of 'hunger' [which] is a prerequisite for the misuse of the eating function in the service of various non-nutritional needs with widely different symbolic meanings." She goes on to demonstrate these various symbolic meanings in a series of fascinating case histories. Dr. Ushakov contributes an equally enlightening chapter on Anorexia Nervosa, a topic which has recently drawn increased interest.

The complicated subject of drug abuse is well-handled by Dr. Boyd, who lists the various drugs abused with their effects and then makes suggestions about legal and parental attitudes toward this troubled area which are neither alarmist nor permissive in nature. Dr. Toolan suggests that adolescents experience depression in the same way that adults do and then discusses the dynamics and treatment of this illness in a most helpful way.

There are other chapters on adolescent psychosis, institutional care, derealization, family therapy, problems of university students and community health, all of which are well written and informative. This volume cannot help but broaden the knowledge and understanding of adolescent psychiatry for any reader no matter how experienced he may be.

Cambridge, Massachusetts
1971

EDITOR'S PREFACE

This Fourth volume in the 'Modern Perspectives in Psychiatry' Series is devoted to *Adolescent Psychiatry* and, like all the volumes in the Series, aims to bring the facts from the growing points in a particular field of psychiatry to the clinician at as early a stage as possible. Thus, a single volume in this Series is not a textbook; a psychiatric textbook has the double disadvantage of rapidly becoming out of date and of restricting to one, or at best to a few, authors the coverage of a field as large as psychiatry. However, the eventual scope of the volumes in the whole Series is such as to constitute a complete international system in the theory and practice of psychiatry.

Contributions likely to be significant in the development of international psychiatry are selected from all over the world. It is hoped that the Series will be a factor in effecting integration of world psychiatry and that it will supply a forum for the expression of creative opinion wherever it may arise.

The present volume has benefited from the contribution of authorities from Australia, Germany, the Netherlands, the United Kingdom, the United States of America and the Union of Soviet Socialist Republics. Each chapter is written by an acknowledged expert, often the leading authority in his field. He was entrusted with the task of selecting, appraising and explaining his special subject for the benefit of colleagues who may be less well acquainted with it. Each chapter is not an exhaustive review of the literature on the subject, but contains what the contributor regards as relevant to clinical practice in that field. The volume will be valuable to the psychiatrist in training.

The place of the Series as a major work of reference is assured by the appearance of cumulative indices in each volume.

Volumes in 'Modern Perspectives in Psychiatry' are complementary. Readers of this volume will find especial interest in the already published volume 1, *Modern Perspectives in Child Psychiatry*, and volume 3, *Modern Perspectives in International Child Psychiatry*. *Modern Perspectives in World Psychiatry*, volume 2, also contains relevant material to Adolescent Psychiatry, as does volume 5, *Modern Perspectives in Psycho-Obstetrics*, about to be published. The list of contents of the volumes already published will be found at the back of this volume.

As in the previous volumes, the cumulative indices of this volume have been prepared by my Editorial Assistant, Mrs Maria-Livia Osborn. My grateful thanks are due to her for her valuable work and for her expert help with many matters of preparation, presentation and editing.

Grateful acknowledgement is also made to the following publishers and editors of journals, and to the Authors concerned for kind permission to reproduce the material mentioned:

W. B. Saunders Company, Philadelphia and Professors J. M. Tanner and Lytt I. Gardner, Ch. 1, Figs. 8 and 10 (from *Endocrine and Genetic Diseases of Childhood*); Pergamon Press Ltd., Oxford, Ch. 1, Fig. 11; Mr Christopher Gathercole, Ch. IV, Table IV (from *Assessment in Clinical Psychology*); *World Medicine*, for the photograph in Ch. XVII.

PART ONE

SCIENTIFIC

I

THE PHYSIOLOGY OF ADOLESCENCE (INCLUDING PUBERTY AND GROWTH)

H. Boutourline Young

M.D., F.R.C.P.

Associate Professor of Clinical Pediatrics and Public Health, Yale University formerly Assistant Professor of Physiology and Research Associate in Human Growth and Development, Harvard University
U.S.A.

1

Introduction

Imperfect knowledge of growth and physiological changes in the second decade of life may lead to errors in interpretation of major aspects of the life situation of a person.

Important is an awareness of sometimes neglected sex differences. It is still surprising to find well-prepared medical practitioners who take little account of the fact that, on the average, girls begin puberty two years ahead of boys. There is a fair amount of individual variation, so that at the extremes of the distribution one may find some boys even more precocious than girls. Nevertheless, at this vital point in human development average girls commence well ahead of average boys and complete their physical development correspondingly earlier.

This same earlier commencement of the puberal growth spurt, which is a self-limiting phenomenon, explains much of the adult sex differences in linear measurements. Additional major contributory factors are that in boys peak velocity is somewhat higher and the growth spurt is longer.

Of fundamental importance for the physician meeting adolescents is awareness of the great age range when puberty may commence. At the age of 14 or 15 one may find an early developed boy who is already a man with fully developed sex characteristics and destined to grow but little more in height. At approximately the same age, and therefore adjacent in many social settings, may be a later-developing boy who is just about to begin his growth spurt and who is little more than a child in his physical characteristics; this is illustrated in Fig. 1. The late developer at this time will usually be much shorter and lighter than his advanced companion but frequently he may eventually well surpass him in body height. The same differences may occur in girls.

Important therefore in the appraisal of a teenager is to establish his biological age or puberal maturity. Fortunately there are established methods for doing this[14,30,48,50,56,60,61] and the phase of development may be quickly and precisely determined by any observant physician without any special experience in the field of adolescence (see page 8).

(see page 8).

2

Some General Aspects of Data Collection and of Growth at Adolescence

The Origins of Data

Data available are from two kinds of study: (*a*) cross-sectional, in which each subject is examined only once, and (*b*) longitudinal, in which a subject is examined repeatedly over time. As there is always some loss of subjects in a longitudinal study, there may be subjects examined on only two occasions and others many times. Such data may be termed 'mixed longitudinal'.

In growth terms cross-sectional studies are suited to acquisition of knowledge of the distance curve of any variable, but in order to obtain

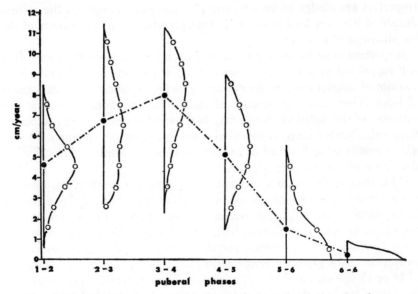

FIG. 2. Growth velocity of total body height in males during the phases of puberty.

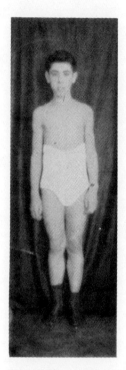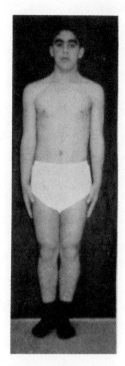

FIG. 1. Physically retarded and advanced boys of the same age.

equivalent knowledge of the velocity curve, first derivative of the distance curve, about twenty times as many observations are required as in a longitudinal study. When it is necessary to obtain knowledge of the variation in the velocity curve, i.e. the acceleration or second derivative, then there is no substitute for the longitudinal method.

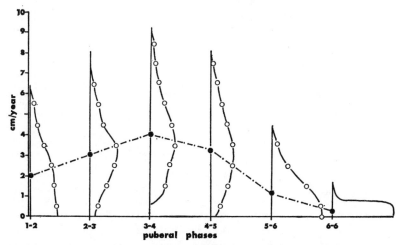

FIG. 3. Growth velocity of sitting body height in males.

It is a pity that much longitudinal data has been analysed in a cross-sectional manner, thus throwing away much of the advantage which this costly kind of research might have conferred.

Somatic Growth

There are differences between the velocities of different variables, and I am presenting in Figs 2, 3, 4 and 5 velocity curves for selected variables from our own longitudinal study of 343 male adolescents of Southern Italian

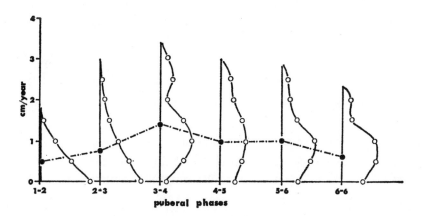

FIG. 4. Growth velocity of bone muscle (arm) in males.

origin. These data have the advantage in being presented by phases of puberal maturity, thus eliminating the 'flattening' effect caused by variation of age at time of maturity.

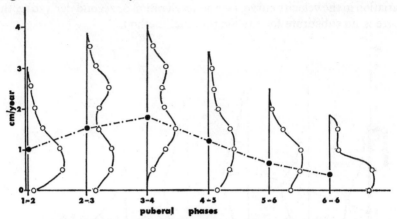

FIG. 5. Growth velocity of bone muscle (leg) in males.

The curves for total body height and sitting height (Figs 2 and 3) show that total body height and sitting height both have peak velocities at mid-puberty, although sitting height velocity is more sustained than total height velocity through to full maturity.

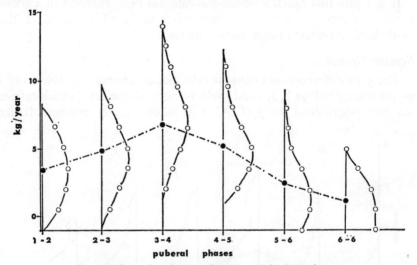

FIG. 6. Growth velocity of body weight in males.

The curves for bone muscle, that is fat-free circumference of arm and leg (Figs 4 and 5) also show their peak velocities at mid-puberty (phases 3 and 4), but relative to linear growth the velocities are sustained at a higher level through to maturity.

The curve for body weight (Fig. 6), as expected, is more similar to the bone muscle velocity curve. The peak in strength appears to occur about a year after the peaks in bone muscle (see Fig. 13).

Practically all tissues, except the brain, seem involved in the adolescent growth period. In most cases the growth is positive, that is, there is a *spurt* but in a few cases, such as limb subcutaneous fat in boys and lymphatic tissue in both sexes, there is a decrease.

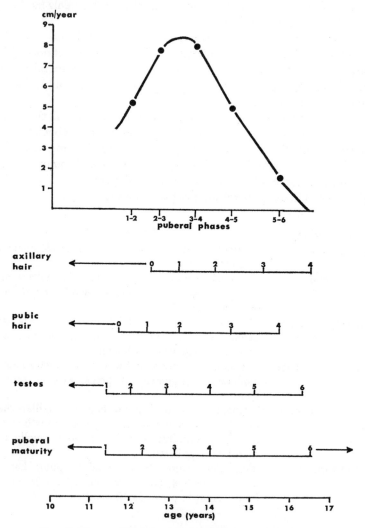

FIG. 7. Some of the physical events of puberty in males.

Physical Development in Boys

Puberty, shown graphically in Fig. 7, usually begins in boys with increase in the size of the testis. At the time there may be some increase of non-pigmented downy pubic hair. Usually about a year after, there follows the growth spurt; pubic hair, curly and usually pigmented, appears and increases steadily. When, after $1\frac{1}{2}$ to 2 years it has reached a moderate quantity, axillary hair usually appears. At this point the peak of the growth spurt has already passed and as pubic and axillary hair develop to their adult levels so the velocity of growth steadily falls to zero level. In up to 50 per cent of boys there may be swelling of one or both breasts during mid-puberty. This may last more than a year. The skin of the areola has become darker and the areola itself larger.

This is a description of the most frequent order of events; individual cases may show variation in the pattern. The above-mentioned Fig. 7 illustrates the development of an average boy, and how puberal maturity may be measured. Fig. 8 illustrates the development of pubic hair and genitalia in males and females.

Facial hair increases with the appearance of axillary hair, and the enlargement of the larynx with deepening of the voice also occurs about this time. Also at this time the axillary sweat glands enlarge, giving rise to the characteristic adult odour. The first ejaculation in well-nourished boys appears to be at about 14 years in average developers.

We have classified[14] puberal maturity as follows:

Classification	*Characteristics*
1. As a child	Testicular volume 1, generally no development of secondary characteristics
2. Pre-puberal	Testicular volume 2, pubic hair 1, axillary and body hair 0, slight increase penile length and diameter, voice 1
3. Puberty 1st stage	Testicular volume 3, pubic hair 2, no axillary hair, definite enlargement of penis, hair on face and body 1–2, evident growth spurt
4. Puberty 2nd stage	Testicular volume 4, pubic hair 3, axillary hair 2, moderate enlargement of penis, evident growth spurt
5. Puberty 3rd stage	Testicular volume 5, pubic hair 3–4, axillary hair 2–3, further enlargement of penis, growth spurt tailing off rapidly: annual increment usually less than before puberty
6. Adult form	Testicular volume 6, voice adult, pubic hair 6, axillary hair 3–4, not more than 2·0 cm growth in body height in previous 12 months

Axillary and pubic hair are rated as:

0. No visible hair.
1. Downy straight hair in small quantity.
2. Curly pigmented coarse hair in small quantity.
3. Curly pigmented coarse hair in moderate quantity.
4. Curly pigmented coarse hair in large quantity.

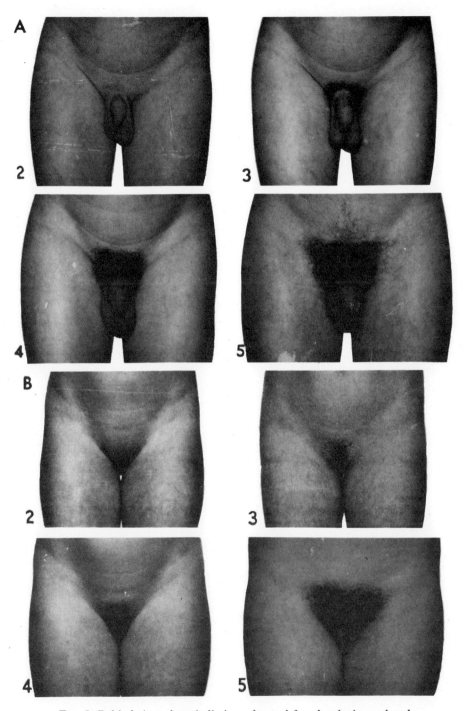

FIG. 8. Pubic hair and genitalia in males and females during puberal development.

Puberal Assessment

Hair:	Face	0	1	2	3	4
Hair:	Axillary	0	1	2	3	4
Hair:	Body	0	1	2	3	4
Hair:	Pubic	0	1	2	3	4
Test.	Volume	1 (1·5 cc) 2 (3·0 cc) 3 (6·5cc) 4 (10·5 cc) 5 (15·5 cc)				

6 (21·5 cc). (By comparison with wooden models varying from 1·5 cc (1) to 21·5 cc (6))

Voice: Childish, Transit, Adult

Maturity in boys may be calculated by the equation:

0·5 (pubic hair rating) + 0·4 (testicular vol. rating) + 0·3 (axillary hair rating) + 0·5 (constant).[14]

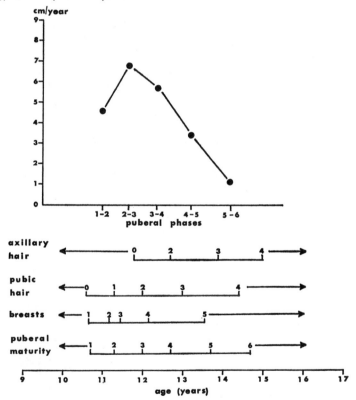

FIG. 9. Some of the physical events of puberty in females.

Physical Development in Girls

Fig. 9 presents the events in girls. Budding of the breast is usually the first indication. Fig. 10 presents the phases of breast development. The physical growth spurt begins at about the time of the breast bud. The pubic hair at this time is usually longer and downy, and the presence of a small amount of dark coarse curly hair (stage 2) is most often about a year later. This is close to the peak of the growth spurt and menarche occurs on the downward slope of the velocity curve, usually 6–12 months following peak velocity. At this time the pubic hair has reached, or is approaching, stage 3 and the appearance of axillary hair is imminent. It is believed that frequently the first menstrual cycles are anovulatory.

We have classified[15] puberal maturity in girls as follows:

Classification	Characteristics
1. As a child	No growth of puberal hair, no growth spurt
2. Pre-puberal	Downy pubic hair; little if any growth spurt, elevation breast papilla; perhaps early budding
3. Puberty 1st stage	Pubic hair, pigmented, coarse and curly in small quantity; budding of breasts, areola enlargement; marked growth spurt; enlargement of labia
4. Puberty 2nd stage	Pubic hair as described above in moderate quantity; filling out of breasts, sometimes projection of areola and papilla to form a secondary mound; axillary hair in small quantity; menarche usual in this phase; growth spurt marked, but already falling away; further growth of labia
5. Puberty 3rd stage	Pubic hair further increased and approaching or reaching adult quantity and distribution; moderate quantity axillary hair; breasts approaching or reaching adult-type configuration with recession of areola to level of the breast; labia approaching or reaching adult type; annual growth less than before puberty; menstruation usually well established
6. Adult	Further growth axillary and perhaps pubic hair to adult type and distribution; breasts adult; labia adult; growth in height less than 1·5 cm in previous 12 months

Sex Differences in Somatic Development

Although there are some differences, such as the presence of the penis and vagina, which are already determined *in utero* and others which are established steadily during childhood, e.g. forearm growth, most of the evident sex differences arise at puberty. These differences at puberty are due not only to the effects of different hormones but also possible tissue susceptibility and also the differences in timing previously described.

Size: there are only small sex differences before puberty, but by the time growth is finished the male is 10 per cent greater in weight, and there are considerable differences in most body measurements, including the head and face. Very evident are the differences in shoulder and hip width, leg and arm length.

Shape: females have rather more subcutaneous fat before adolescence and a great deal more after growth is completed. Fig. 11 presents sex differences in subcutaneous measurements found in our own work. This is

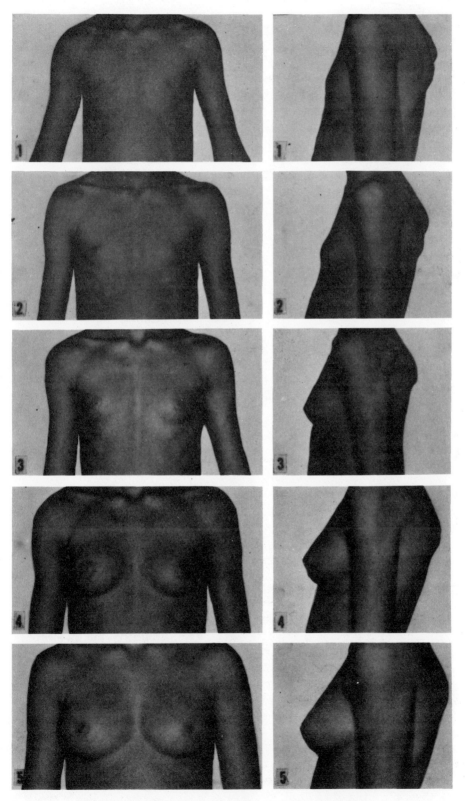

Fig. 10. Development of the breast in females in puberty.

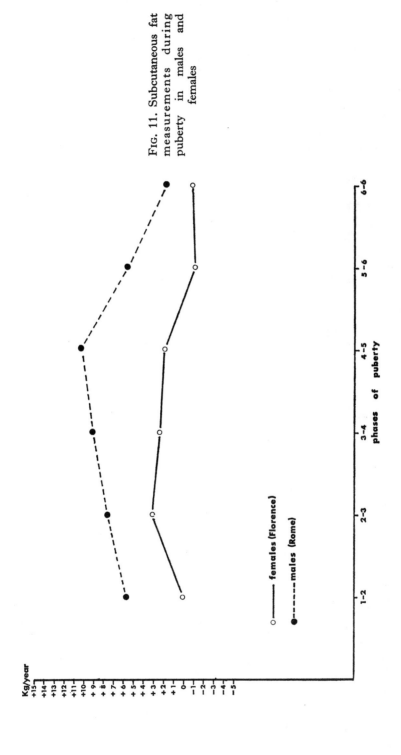

FIG. 11. Subcutaneous fat measurements during puberty in males and females

presented by distance curves. Similarly there is little difference in bone and muscle mass before puberty, but in males there is a large adolescent spurt in bone and muscle mass accounting for the large differences found when somatic growth is completed. Fig. 12 presents some of our data to illustrate this (velocity curves).

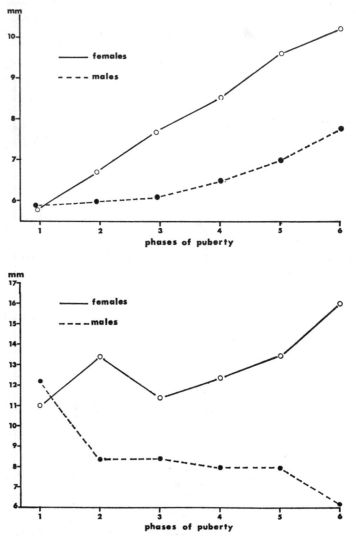

FIG. 12. Velocities of bone muscle circumferences of arm and leg in males and females.

Strength: similarly physical strength, in so far as it may be measured by the hand dynamometer, follows the velocity of growth of bone muscle. At this time the considerable divergence in physical strength becomes steadily more evident.

3
Influences Upon Growth and Maturation

Body Shape

In both boys and girls there is a clear relationship between endomorphy (plumpness) and a tendency to mature early.[11,15,60,71] In boys there appears to be a relationship between mesomorphy (muscularity) and a tendency to mature early.[61]

Socio-economic Factors

There is substantial evidence that adverse economic circumstances, mediated possibly by nutrition, may retard the appearance of puberty. This view is supported by documented socio-economic differences within societies[10,43,70] and by natural changes during periods of adversity such as wars. In general, during the past 100 years in Western-type societies, the age of puberty has been decreasing 3–4 months every decade, but it seems that in those social classes which have remained at a stable and satisfactory economic level from one generation to the next there is little, if any, difference between mothers and daughters in recorded age of menarche.[15,41] On the other hand, there is evident change when a family has been strongly upward-mobile.[15]

There is an inverse relationship between family size and both body size and physical maturation.[51,53,61] The reason for this is not yet clear, but it is likely that it is explained, at least partly, by economic influences upon nutrition and hygiene.

Climate and Race

Climate seems to have negligible effects upon rate of development. With regard to race, there is evidence[35] of effects upon growth and maturation which may not be accounted for by economic circumstances—economically privileged Nigerian girls[22] reach menarche later than 14 years and therefore much later than similarly privileged girls in Europe[15]—but it is not easy as far as maturation is concerned to separate out the effects of body shape which may be associated with race.

Seasonal Variation

Both girls and boys grow more in height in the spring and more in weight in the autumn, but there are wide individual differences, some children and adolescents fluctuating very little with season and others not corresponding to the general pattern. We have found an increase of 100 per cent in height velocity in economically deprived children when the springtime is compared with winter. There is evidence, at least for body weight, that the seasonal effect is reduced in well-nourished children.[16,17]

Sex Differences in Respect of Adverse Circumstances

It appears that at all ages the growth process of girls is more resistant to malnutrition and other environmental insults including the effects of atomic energy.[28,][29,][32] It has been demonstrated that the male is more susceptible to a variety of diseases, and this has been ascribed to biological differences rather than socio-cultural effects.[67]

Published mortality figures also favour girls in that the rates are lower for almost all forms of mortality. Similarly there is greater expectation of life for females. Widdowson and McCance, in observation of undernourished children in orphanages in Germany during the famine period 1947–1948, found the girls less retarded before supplementation and quicker than boys to return to normal growth levels following supplementation.[69]

Emotional Deprivation and Growth

There is some evidence that emotional deprivation may be associated with physical growth disorders,[12,18,49] although there is still some controversy here.[12] Patton and Gardner[49] have analysed six case histories where maternal deprivation appeared to be related to growth failure. Widdowson,[68] in orphanage studies in Germany in 1948, noted a clear effect of absence of love and affection upon children who failed to thrive as expected despite adequate supplementation. Similarly in certain English boarding schools, the rate of physical growth has been shown to be less in term time than in the holidays.[24,25]

As there appears to be a relationship between early growth failure and delay in arriving at puberty, further observations are called for to confirm and amplify these findings in well-planned longitudinal studies which may also attend to the question of reversibility and take better note of the many non-maternal variables.

Illness and Growth

Minor illnesses appear mostly to have no long-lasting effect,[39, 59] although there do appear to be effects in the less privileged.[32] Severe illness may slow up growth in any child. The most grossly retarded may not survive,[4] while those who recover may experience a period of 'catch-up' growth.

4

Physiological Changes at Adolescence

Blood pressure: in mid-childhood there is no sex difference, but with the advent of puberty the systolic pressure rises from a mean of about 100 to 106–108; at this point the female pressure stabilizes, while that of boys increases to the male level of 114–118 by the age of 17.[54]

Pulse rate: this falls steadily during childhood, but without sex differences until just before puberty, when in girls the fall becomes markedly less, leading to the adult sex difference of about 10/minute.[34]

Haemoglobin: both sexes enter puberty with a level of 13–14 grams. In girls no change occurs but in the boys the level steadily rises during the course of development until the adult level of approximately 16 g/100 ml is reached.[44,45] Table I presents some of our data in males, illustrating this rise and also showing that it is related to the process of development itself and not to the chronological age. It is important to be aware of this, as a

TABLE I

Haemoglobin (gm) during Puberal Development in Males

Chronological age		Puberal maturity					
		1	2	3	4	5	6
11	x̄	13·5	13·4	(13·5)			
	n	52	27	6			
12	x̄	13·3	13·6	13·8	(14·4)		
	n	12	44	25	3		
13	x̄		13·8	13·9	14·7		
	n		26	46	20		
14	x̄		(14·2)	13·9	14·5	15·1	
	n		10	21	35	16	
15	x̄			(14·6)	14·3	15·0	(15·2)
	n			4	24	35	4
16	x̄			(14·1)	(14·9)	14·8	15·6
	n			2	6	32	31
17	x̄				(13·8)	15·0	15·7
	n				2	11	37
18	x̄						15·7
	n						9

The values in parenthesis have been obtained from groups too small for differences to be significant.

fully developed boy of 15 with a haemoglobin level of 13 g/100 ml needs iron therapy for his anaemia, while in the late developer of similar age the level is perfectly normal. The physiological changes, just as the growth changes, are related to the maturity level rather than the chronological age. The haemoglobin level reflects the difference of red blood cell counts, i.e. 4·6 million/mm in both sexes immediately before puberty, with no subsequent change in the girls but a climb to 5·4 million/mm in boys. It is thought that the difference is mediated by testosterone which can increase the level of red blood cells/cu. mm in both women and eunuchs.

Metabolism: the basic metabolic rate in relation to surface area is consistently higher in males throughout childhood and these differences become greater during puberty.[37]

There are also sex differences in total body water, extracellular water,

B

intracellular water and exchangeable potassium where men have more than women, presumably reflecting the differing proportions and composition of muscle, fat and bone.[38] These differences do not appear to be present in childhood.

Sex differences in respiration also occur at puberty. During childhood there is little sex difference, with the rate of breathing coming steadily down. However, at puberty there occurs the sex difference in alveolar pCO_2 with men finally stabilized at 40–41 mm Hg, while women descend to a mean of 38 mm Hg reflecting a greater effective alveolar minute volume. There appears to be a fluctuation in pCO_2 during the menstrual cycle and, as well documented, during pregnancy; the level then falls progressively to 31–32 mm Hg.[13]

Another difference in sex patterns is in gastric acidity.[66] At puberty, in boys, there is a much larger increase in free HCl secreted in response to a test meal. The difference persists into late middle age.

The mouth temperature of girls departs abruptly from the male trend at the time of puberty.[34] The male temperature continues to fall steadily until late adolescence until the differences are about 0·7° F. The fluctuation in temperature with the menstrual cycle presumably commences with ovulation.

There is a change in the physiologic response to exercise at puberty, much more marked in boys. The total ventilation required for each litre of oxygen metabolized decreases steadily throughout childhood and at puberty falls markedly lower in boys.[3] The better athletic performance of boys results from both this and the difference in muscle size and strength.

Also at about mid-puberty and presumably reflecting the sex differences in muscle mass developing at that time, possibly in relation to male sex hormones, the male urine creatinine excretion becomes markedly larger than in girls.[19]

The muscles increase not only in size but also in strength. Fig. 13 gives the performance of the right-hand grip in boys and girls from our Florence and Rome studies. The point of greatest acceleration in boys appears to be between stages 4 and 5 of puberty. It is important to remember that motivation enters considerably into performance on this test and that here there may be considerable sex differential. The negative velocity in females at the end of the puberal growth phase is presumably due to changes in motivation.

5

Growth Disorders

Patterns of growth and development depend a great deal on heredity and a first step in the assessment of apparent linear growth deficiency is a careful family history with time of arrival at puberty of parents and siblings, parents' height and a prediction of the adolescent's height from the mid-

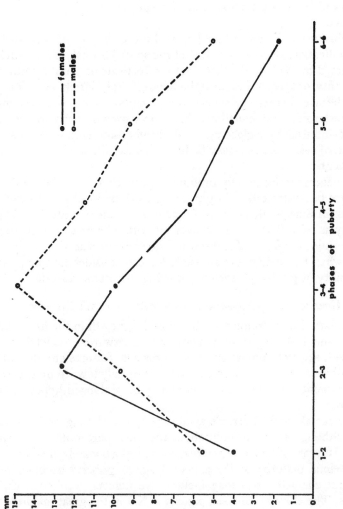

Fig. 13. Hand dynamometer scores in males and females during puberty

parental height.[27] It is important to bear in mind that such prediction tables are based upon the assumption of adequate environmental circumstances during growth for both generations. At the extremes of environmental pressure, mature body height may be reduced by more than 15 per cent.[8, 42] Further investigations of apparent growth failure will include observation of growth increments and a medical examination which will give special attention to presence of congenital defects, chronic infection or the long-term results of previous infection, and nutritional disorders. An X-ray of the hand and wrist, and possibly other centers, for skeletal age is part of this examination. Endocrine disorders, such as hypothyroidism, need to be excluded.

Exclusion of the above factors, in the presence of marked retardation, is an indication for referral to one of the special growth clinics, such as that conducted by Prof. J. M. Tanner at the Institute of Child Health, London University, or Prof. A. Prader at the Kinderspital, Zürich. Here it is possible to undertake further specialized investigations, such as determination of 17-ketosteroids and gonadotrophins, and growth hormone response to insulin-induced hypoglycemia, and chromosome studies. In a small proportion of cases, patients may be identified as suitable for growth hormone treatment.

Teenagers are frequently brought to physicians with the complaint that they are backward either in physical growth or in physical development. At least in Europe, this request for advice may stem as much from parental anxiety as from that of the teenager himself. The first investigating step is to determine the phase of maturation and compare this with family patterns. Only when familial factors are excluded can consideration be given to the possibility of pituitary deficiency or of chromosome disorder.

Some Genetically or Congenitally Determined Growth Disorders

Pituitary dwarfs frequently show normal growth in the first 1 or 2 years of life and begin to show deficits only afterwards. Skeletal maturity is retarded, skeletal proportions normal for age, features childlike and gonadotrophins and 17-ketosteroids levels are usually low. In most cases sexual development does not occur. There may be prolonged hypoglycemia with insulin.

The female with Turner's syndrome (gonadal dysgenesis) grows fairly well, although most are only about the third percentile of velocity, until about 10 years of age but then becomes proportionately smaller in stature; the skeletal maturity at the expected age of puberty becomes retarded.[2] Physical characteristics may include eye defects, webbed neck, cubitus valgus. The chromosome sex pattern is XO in the great majority of cases. There are infantile female organs, although some pubic and axillary hair may be present. Urinary gonadotrophins are at a high level, thus demonstrating that there is no ovary to stimulate. The excretion of 17-ketosteroids is low.

Another chromosome disorder is the Klinefelter syndrome in boys, where the patients remain sterile because of testicular tubular deficiency, but have low normal interstitial cell function. Bilateral gynecomastia may be prominent. The chromosome pattern is XXY. The urinary output of gonadotrophins is elevated. The skeletal age follows that of the normal male in contrast to Turner's syndrome which follows that of the normal female until the onset of puberty, when retardation commences. It has been shown[62] that the sex difference in skeletal development depends on the retarding effect of genes on the Y chromosome. Frequently there is mild mental retardation.

As already mentioned, hypothyroidism may also produce considerable dwarfing. Here there is a normal birth weight, marked retardation in skeletal maturation, infantile skeletal proportions, 'cretinoid' features, late sexual development, epiphysial dysgenesis, high serum cholesterol and low protein-bound iodine. Mental retardation is characteristic.

In Western societies, the majority of cases of growth failure will have been identified during childhood.

Growth of hair on the face and body may be a reason for seeking the advice of a gynecologist. Tanner[61] states that hair on the face may have a relatively high threshold to adrenal androgens and is more influenced by testosterone. Women in the child-bearing period with increased facial hair have a greater production of 17-ketosteroids and a more masculine body build.

Skeletal Age

This important biological indicator is used widely in clinical investigations of growth disturbance and in epidemiological studies. Different standards have been created for boys and girls because girls are consistently more mature.[31, 64, 65]

It is now possible to predict, fairly accurately from the age of 8 on, the adult height of a person and such predictions are of potential value where height is attached to an occupation involving long training (e.g. ballerinas). Bayley's prediction tables[7] involve consideration of actual height, actual age and skeletal age. If practicable methods were available for slowing down height, the methods would be of considerable value in dealing with the problem of very tall girls.

Attempts to Suppress Excessive Growth in Girls

Oestrogens have been used for this purpose,[6] but it has been questioned whether there is significant difference between mature height after treatment and that previously predicted.

Growth-related Disorders in Adolescents

Obesity is also a common problem in girls. Height and weight tables should be interpreted with care as some mesomorphic girls may have excess weight due to muscle and bone. Fat may be satisfactorily measured by skin calipers.[63] Obesity occurs when intake of calories systematically exceeds body requirements. Appetite is regulated by a number of factors, and it is important to remember that excess eating may not only be a bad habit but also may protect against many stresses. Many fat girls exercise little and motion-picture studies of obese subjects at camps have confirmed habitual economy of movement in many of them.[40] Before initiating treatment with diet and exercise it is important to exclude metabolic defects, and we should remember that fatness occurs in some families and here there may be limits to what may be achieved by diet and exercise.

Acne is a cause of concern amongst adolescents. The prevalence rises from zero in the pre-puberal period to a peak of 30 per cent in American boys in the final phase of puberty. Due to oestrogen–androgen imbalance, it is more common in males than females and may continue for several years. The treatment has been discussed by Gallagher[25a] who also deals with other disorders such as defects of posture and the common orthopaedic disorders. Flat feet are frequently seen, but few of them are painful; these must be treated. Gallagher has found that self inspection in the nude by means of a long mirror will encourage an adolescent to ask for measures which may improve his posture. Improved posture and exercises for the pectoral muscles may also improve the figure, a desire of many adolescent girls. It is also important to distinguish functional from structural scoliosis to bring important early treatment to the latter.

Fatigue is another common complaint to be dealt with by a thorough physical examination with special attention to possible anaemia, after-effects of acute disease, such as mononucleosis or hepatitis, and poor habits such as going to bed late. With medical and hygienic causes excluded, many cases will be found to have psychological origins.

There is a striking incidence of myopia at adolescence,[57] and also an increase in the severity of existing myopia.[26] Regular vision testing is therefore particularly indicated at this time.

6

Menstrual Symptoms, Socio-cultural Factors and Age of Arrival at Menarche

It has been hypothesized that socio-cultural factors may so affect attitudes as to lead to markedly differing prevalence of dysmenorrhea in different environments. Our own unpublished observations have failed to support this, but instead show an increased prevalence of dysmenorrhea in the precocious girls. At least in the two cultures of Italy and the United States, the late developers appear to accept menarche as a gift, while those who arrive early demonstrate a tendency to attach symptoms to the function. If this work is confirmed, it may be helpful in indicating to school health educators where one of their investments should be.

Following menarche it may take some time for the pituitary–ovarian mechanism to establish itself with optimum feed-back mechanisms. Menarche starts with release of gonadotrophins from the pituitary, and the ovaries respond with follicle development and release of oestrogens. Before the pituitary releases luteinizing hormone (LH) to produce ovulation there may be sufficient fluctuation in the oestrogen level to cause endometrial breakdown and bleeding. Severe and irregular bleedings may lead to anaemia which should be treated. It may be useful to perform serum iron estimations as well as haemoglobin and haematocrits as a low level of serum iron will indicate a depletion of iron stores in a subject with a relatively normal haemoglobin and therefore preventive iron therapy will already be indicated.

Control of the cycles may be achieved by giving an oestrogen (such as ethinyl oestradiol 0·05 mg twice a day) for ten days beginning on the 5th day of the bleeding. This should be followed by administration of a progestogen such as norethisterone (Primolut N) 5 mg, three times a day, or dydrogesterone (Duphaston) 5 mg, three times a day, for ten days, making 20 days treatment in all. This will produce 'normal menstruation' with shedding of a secretory endometrium.

It is wise to complete three cycles of this treatment and then discontinue it, to see if spontaneous ovulation will occur. If irregular bleeding persists, treatment should be continued for three cycles at a time until spontaneous ovulation occurs. This may take time, varying from a few months to one or two years, to achieve.

7

Iatrogenic Disorders

Whenever growth is rapid there is a possibility for excessive reaction to therapeutic weapons, and adolescence is no exception. We have observed some 100 male adolescents who were given by their private physicians varying amounts of chorionic gonadotrophin. The reasons for consultation varied from concern about growth and maturation to enuresis. Anxiety of the mother appeared a prominent factor.

Some of the boys could be diagnosed as delayed familial-type adolescence, but most of them lay within the normal range and were treated because the physician either was not aware of the width of the normal distribution curve of maturation or else was not able to convince the mother of this.

Table II summarizes the results. It does not seem possible that the growth potential of the subjects may have been increased by the therapy. The trend is in the opposite direction. A planned follow-up will investigate the fertility of these subjects and their final body height in relation to that which might be predicted from their parents' height.

TABLE II

Increments (cm) in Growth in Adolescents Who Received Varying Doses of Hormone Therapy and a Comparison with Those Who did Not Receive Such Therapy

Type of Group	Puberal Phases					Total height increments
	1–2	2–3	3–4	4–5	5–6	
Normal without therapy	5·2	7·6	8·0	5·0	1·7	27·5
Small quantity or recommended and did not follow treatment	4·9 (15)	7·5 (23)	8·2 (22)	4·3 (21)	0·6 (4)	25·5
Medium quantity 10–30 injections	5·0 (20)	6·5 (29)	7·4 (24)	5·0 (19)	1·2 (3)	25·1
Considerable quantity >30 injections	4·3 (12)	6·6 (16)	6·8 (14)	4·7 (8)	1·5 (6)	23·9

Between the four groups there was no significant difference in the chronological age at each puberal phase from one through six; nor were there significant differences in total body height by chronological age in early puberty.

8

Early and Late Physical Maturation and Personality

Various studies[46,47] have reported a relationship in boys between physique and rate of physical development and personality structure. In general, in the American studies, late maturers have been perceived by trained observers as less physically attractive, less well-groomed and more unrealistic. The late maturers were rated higher in sociability, social initiative (often immature) and eagerness. Their peers saw them as more attention-seeking, restless and bossy, but less grown-up and less good-looking.

TAT tests[47] showed late maturers as more likely to have negative self concepts, feelings of inadequacy, strong feelings of being rejected and dominated, prolonged dependence needs and rebellious attitudes towards parents. Instead the early maturers showed a more favourable psychological picture. More of them appeared to be self-confident, independent and capable of playing an adult role in interpersonal relationships.[47] Some personality differences between early and late maturers seem to persist into adult life.

However, it has been shown in our own studies upon adolescents in Italy and those of Italian origin in the United States[46] that Italian early maturing boys do not have more positive self-concepts. On the other hand, the Italian American early maturers resemble the Americans in self-confidence but they are rebellious and view their parents as restrictive, controlling and lacking nurturance. These negative attitudes may be the result of their exposure to conflicting cultural values. One sees from these studies the danger in extrapolating well-designed studies without taking account of differing environmental influences and cultural milieu.

9

The Growth of Mental Abilities

During adolescence, growth in mental abilities continues, but it is still not clear if a spurt occurs. The balance of evidence is against such a view.[5,33,58] There is a paucity of longitudinal data: the tests used were changed in certain items; sometimes different, and not fully comparable, tests were used and there is the learning effect which makes longitudinal analysis difficult. A further difficulty in interpretation is the presence of probable strong changes in motivation during the course of puberty and adolescence. Another difficulty is the built-in linearity of IQ scores. If all children matured at the same time it would be impossible to detect a spurt from standardized scores. It may be that more work needs to be done with early and late maturers.

There is one interesting fact. In both sexes early maturers appear to perform better on tests of mental ability than do late maturers; that is, they performed better both before, during and after puberty. There is also a relationship between size and intelligence; that is larger children perform better.[9,21,23,36,53,55]

As children are becoming larger because of the secular trend, one might expect there to be a secular trend in intelligence test performance. One of the objects of the Scottish survey of 1947,[53] following that of 1932,[52] was to ascertain if average IQ was dropping, as it was thought that adults of low IQ were producing more children than those with high IQ. In fact, no change was seen in performance on the Binet, and in the Moray House test there was an actual rise of just more than two points. Obviously a great deal more research work needs to be done here in order to establish the facts. Now, all one can say is that the balance of the evidence suggests that the average level of adult intelligence remains constant, although the rate of growth of intelligence in children may be increasing.

Acknowledgment

I am indebted to my colleagues for the greater part of the new work which has been presented here. We thank Mr William Grant and the Grant Foundation of New York who gave to Harvard University the financial support for our cross-cultural longitudinal study of adolescents. I thank Dr James L. Whittenberger for his encouragement and critical reviews of this and other publications. I thank Miss Fiona Mallett for her careful preparation of the chapter and its bibliography.

I thank Miss Josephine Barnes, D.M., F.R.C.S., F.R.C.O.G., F.R.C.P., Professor André Prader and Professor J. M. Tanner for reviewing sections of this chapter.

REFERENCES

1. ACHESON, R. M. and HEWITT, D. 1954. Oxford Child Health Survey. Stature and skeletal maturation in the pre-school child. *Brit. J. prev. soc. Med.*, **8**, 59.
2. ACHESON, R. M. and ZAMPA, G. A. 1961. Skeletal maturation in ovarian dysgenesis and Turner's syndrome. *Lancet*, **i**, 917.
3. ASTRAND, P. O. 1952. *Experimental studies of physical working capacity in relation to sex and age*. Copenhagen: Munksgaard.
4. BAUER, H. 1954. Nephrosesyndrom und Körperwachstum. *Helv. paediat. acta*, **9**, 127.
5. BAYLEY, N. 1949. Consistency and variability in the growth of intelligence from birth to 18 years. *J. genet. Psychol.*, **75**, 165.
6. BAYLEY, N., GORDON, G. S., BAYER, L. M., GOLDBERG, M. B. and STORMENT, A. 1962. Attempt to suppress excessive growth in girls by oestrogen treatment: statistical evaluation. *J. clin. Endocr.*, **22**, 1127.
7. BAYLEY, N. and PINNEAU, S. R. 1952. Tables for predicting adult height from skeletal age: revised for use with the Greulich–Pyle hand standards. *J. Pediat.*, **40**, 423. (Erratum corrected *J. Pediat.*, **41**, 371.)
8. BLOOM, B. S. 1964. *Stability and change in human characteristics*. New York: Wiley.
9. BOAS, F. 1941. The relation between physical and mental development. *Science*, **93**, 339.
10. BOJLÉN, K. W., RASCH, G. and WEIS-BENTZON, M. 1954. The age incidence of the menarche in Copenhagen. *Acta obstet. gynec. Scand.*, **33**, 405.
11. BOOTHBY, E. J., GUY, M. A. and DAVIES, T. A. L. 1952. The growth of adolescents. *Mon. Bull. Minist. Hlth., Lab. Serv.*, **11**, 208.
12. BOUTOURLINE YOUNG, H. 1963. Deprivation of maternal care. *Develpm. Med. Child Neurol.*, **5**, 520.
13. BOUTOURLINE YOUNG, H. and BOUTOURLINE YOUNG, E. 1956. Alveolar carbon dioxide levels in pregnant, parturient and lactating subjects. *J. obstet. gynaec. Brit. Emp.*, **63**, 509.
14. BOUTOURLINE YOUNG, H., GREULICH, W. W., GALLAGHER, J. R., CONE, T. and HEALD, F. 1968. Evaluation of physical maturity at adolescence. *Develpm. Med. Child Neurol.*, **10**, 338.
15. BOUTOURLINE YOUNG, H., ZOLI, A. and GALLAGHER, J. R. 1963. Events of puberty in a group of 111 Florentine girls. *Amer. J. dis. Child.*, **106**, 568.
16. BRANSBY, E. R. 1945. The seasonal growth of children. *Med. Offr.*, **73**, 149, 157, 165.
17. BRANSBY, E. R. 1945. Further note on the seasonal growth of children. *Med. Offr.*, **74**, 95.
18. CASLER, L. 1963. Maternal deprivation: a critical review of the literature. *Monogr. Soc. Child Develpm.*, **26**, 2.
19. CLARK, L. C., THOMPSON, H. L., BECK, E. L. and JACOBSON, W. 1951. Excretion of creatine and creatinine by children. *Amer. J. dis. Child.*, **81**, 774.
20. DOUGLAS, J. W. B. and BLOMFIELD, J. M. 1958. *Children under five*. London: Allen & Unwin.

21. Douglas, J. W. B., Ross, J. M. and Simpson, H. R. 1965. The relation between height and measured educational ability in school children of the same social class, family size and stage of sexual development. *Hum. Biol.*, **37**, 178.
22. Ellis, R. W. B. 1950. Age of puberty in the tropics. *Brit. med. J.*, **1**, 85.
23. Franzblau, R. N. 1935. Race differences in mental and physical traits: studied in different environments. *Arch. Psychol.*, 177.
24. Friend, G. E. 1935. *The schoolboy*. Cambridge: Heffer.
25. Friend, G. E. and Bransby, E. R. 1947. Physique and growth of schoolboys. *Lancet*, **ii**, 677–81.
25a. Gallagher, J. R. 1960. *Medical care of the adolescent*. New York: Appleton Century Crofts.
26. Gardiner, P. A. 1954. The relation of myopia to growth. *Lancet*, **i**, 476.
27. Garn, S. M. and Rohmann, C. G. 1966. Interaction of nutrition and genetics in the timing of growth and development. *Ped. Clin. N. Amer.*, **13**, 353.
28. Greulich, W. W. 1951. The growth and development status of Guamanian school children in 1947. *Amer. J. phys. Anthrop.*, N.S., **9**, 55.
29. Greulich, W. W., Crismon, C. S. and Turner, M. L. 1953. The physical growth and development of children who survived the atomic bombing of Hiroshima or Nagasaki. *J. Pediat.*, **43**, 121.
30. Greulich, W. W., Dorfman, R. I., Catchpole, H. R., Solomon, C. I. and Culotta, C. S. 1942. Somatic and endocrine studies of puberal and adolescent boys. *Monogr. Soc. Res. Child Develpm.*, **7**, 85.
31. Greulich, W. W. and Pyle, S. I. 1959. *Radiographic atlas of skeletal development of the hand and wrist*. Second edition. Stanford, California: Stanford University Press.
32. Hewitt, D., Westropp, C. K. and Acheson, R. M. 1955. Oxford Child Health Survey: effect of childish ailments on skeletal development. *Brit. J. prev. soc. Med.*, **9**, 179.
33. Honzik, M. P., MacFarlane, J. W. and Allen, L. I. 1948. The stability of mental test performance between two and eighteen years. *J. exper. Educ.*, **17**, 309.
34. Iliff, A. and Lee, V. A. 1952. Pulse rate, respiratory rate, and body temperature of children between two months and eighteen years of age. *Child Develpm.*, **23**, 237.
35. Ito, P. K. 1942. Comparative biometrical study of physique of Japanese women born and reared under different environments. *Hum. Biol.*, **14**, 279.
36. Klausmeier, H. J., Lehmann, I. J. and Beeman, A. 1959. Relationships among physical, mental and achievement measures in children of low, average and high intelligence. *Amer. J. ment. Defic.*, **63**, 647.
37. Lewis, R. C., Duval, A. M. and Iliff, A. 1943. Standards for the basal metabolism of children from 2–15 years of age, inclusive. *J. Pediat.*, **23**, 1.
38. Ljunggren, H., Ikkos, D. and Luft, R. 1957. Studies on body composition: I. Body fluid compartments and exchangeable potassium in normal males and females. *Acta endocr. (Copenhagen)*, **25**, 187.
39. Martens, E. J. and Meredith, H. V. 1942. Illness history and physical growth. I. Correlation in junior primary children followed from fall to spring. *Amer. J. dis. Child.*, **64**, 618.
40. Mayer, J. and Bullen, B. 1964. *Nutrition and athletics: nutrition*. Eds C. F. Mills and R. Passmore. Edinburgh: E. & S. Livingstone.
41. McCammon, R. W. 1965. Are boys and girls maturing physically at earlier ages? *Amer. J. pub. Hlth.*, **55**, 1.
42. Meredith, H. V. 1968. Body size of contemporary groups of pre-school children studied in different parts of the world. *Child Develpm.*, **39**, 335.

43. MICHELSON, N. 1944. Studies in physical development of Negroes. IV. Onset of puberty. *Amer. J. phys. Anthrop.*, N.S., **2**, 151.
44. MUGRAGE, E. R. and ANDRESEN, M. I. 1936. Values for red blood cells of average infants and children. *Amer. J. dis. Child.*, **51**, 775.
45. MUGRAGE, E. R. and ANDRESEN, M. I. 1938. Red blood cell values in adolescence. *Amer. J. dis. Child.*, **56**, 997.
46. MUSSEN, P. and BOUTOURLINE YOUNG, H. 1964. Relationships between rate of physical maturing and personality among boys of Italian descent. *Vita humana*, **7**, 186.
47. MUSSEN, P. and JONES, M. C. 1957. Self-conceptions, motivations and interpersonal attitudes of late and early maturing boys. *Child Develpm.*, **28**, 243.
48. NICOLSON, A. B. and HANLEY, C. 1953. Indices of physiological maturity: derivation and inter-relationships. *Child Develpm.*, **24**, 3.
49. PATTON, R. G. and GARDNER, L. J. 1962. Influence of family environment on growth: the syndrome of 'maternal deprivation'. *Pediatrics*, **130**, 957.
50. REYNOLDS, E. L. and WINES, J. V. 1951. Physical changes associated with adolescence in boys. *Amer. J. dis. Child.*, **82**, 529.
51. SCOTT, J. A. 1961. *Report on the heights and weights (and other measurements) of school pupils in the County of London in 1959.* London: County Council.
52. Scottish Council for Research in Education. 1949. *The trend of Scottish intelligence: a comparison of the 1947 and 1932 surveys of the intelligence of eleven-year-old pupils.* London University Press.
53. Scottish Council for Research in Education. 1953. *Social implications of the 1947 Scottish Mental Survey.* London University Press.
54. SHOCK, N. W. 1944. Basal blood pressure and pulse rate in adolescents. *Amer. J. dis. Child.*, **68**, 16.
55. SHUTTLEWORTH, F. K. 1939. The physical and mental growth of girls and boys age six to nineteen in relation to age at maximum growth. *Monogr. Soc. Res. Child. Develpm.*, **4**, No. 3.
56. SIMMONS, K. and GREULICH, W. W. 1943. Menarcheal age and the height, weight and skeletal age of girls aged 7 to 17 years. *J. Pediat.*, **22**, 518.
57. SLATAPER, F. J. 1950. Age norms of refraction and vision. *Arch. Ophthal. (N.Y.)*, N.S., **43**, 466.
58. SONTAG, L. W., BAKER, C. T. and NELSON, V. L. 1958. Mental growth and personality development: a longitudinal study. *Monogr. Soc. Res. Child Develpm.*, **23**, No. 2.
59. SONTAG, L. W. and LIPFORD, J. 1943. The effect of illness and other factors on the appearance pattern of skeletal epiphyses. *J. Pediat.*, **23**, 391.
60. STOLZ, H. R. and STOLZ, L. M. 1951. *Somatic development of adolescent boys. A study of the growth of boys during the second decade of life.* New York: Macmillan.
61. TANNER, J. M. 1962. *Growth at adolescence* (second edition). Oxford: Blackwell Scientific Publication.
62. TANNER, J. M., PRADER, A., HABICH, H. and FERGUSON-SMITH, M. A. 1959. Genes of the Y chromosome influencing rate of maturation in man: skeletal age studies in children with Klinefelter's (XXY) and Turner's (XO) syndromes. *Lancet*, **ii**, 141.
63. TANNER, J. M. and WHITEHOUSE, R. H. 1955. The Harpenden skinfold caliper. *Amer. J. phys. Anthrop.*, N.S., **13**, 743.
64. TANNER, J. M. and WHITEHOUSE, R. H. 1959. *Standards for skeletal maturity based on a study of 3000 British children.* Inst. Child Hlth., London University, M.S.

65. TANNER, J. M., WHITEHOUSE, R. H. and HEALY, M. J. R. 1961. *Standards for skeletal maturity based on a study of 3000 British children*. II. The scoring system for all 28 bones of hand and wrist. Inst. Child Hlth., London University, M.S.

66. VANZANT, F. R., ALVAREZ, W. C., EUSTERMAN, G. B., DUNN, H. L. and BERKSON, J. 1932. The normal range of gastric acidity from youth to old age. *Arch. intern. Med.*, **49**, 345.

67. WASHBURN, T. C., MEDEARIS, D. N. and CHILDS, B. 1965. Sex differences in susceptibility to infections. *Pediatrics*, **35**, 57–65.

68. WIDDOWSON, E. M. 1951. Mental contentment and physical growth. *Lancet*, **i**, 1316–18.

69. WIDDOWSON, E. M. and McCANCE, R. A. 1954. Studies on the nutritive value of bread and on the effect of variations in the extraction rate of flour on the growth of undernourished children. *Med. Res. Council Spec. Rep. Ser. No. 287*.

70. WOFINDEN, R. C. and SMALLWOOD, A. L. 1958. *School Health Service. Annual Report of the Principal School Medical Officer to City and County of Bristol Education Committee*. Bristol.

71. WOLFF, O. H. 1955. Obesity in childhood: a study of the birth weight, the height and the onset of puberty. *Quart. J. Med. N.S.*, **24**, 109.

II

FOUR ISSUES IN THE DEVELOPMENTAL PSYCHOLOGY OF ADOLESCENTS

DANIEL OFFER
M.D.

Associate Director
Institute for Psychosomatic and
Psychiatric Research and Training
Michael Reese Hospital
Chicago, U.S.A.

JUDITH OFFER

Research Associate
Institute for Psychosomatic and
Psychiatric Research and Training
Michael Reese Hospital
Chicago, U.S.A.

1

Introduction

Adolescence has often been characterized as the 'in-between stage', when the boy is not quite a man or the girl has so many childish qualities. A conceptualization of adolescence as a transitional stage characterizes it as a unique period of disruption and change. This theoretical framework focuses subsequent observations onto personality changes and defensive maneuvers of the adolescent. The continuities of individual patterns of development and the qualities demarcating a relative stability of functioning within adolescence have already been discredited by the initial characterization. In contrast to the above, it is our thesis that adolescence should be understood *as a stage in itself*, and comparisons can be meaningful when one adolescent population is contrasted with another. Each cycle in life will bring new challenges and opportunities, but the changes will be incorporated into the basic personality structure.

Our working definition of adolescence is as the stage of life that starts with puberty and ends at the time when the individual's independence from his parents has attained a reasonable degree of psychological congruence. The beginning phase is obviously easier to define, although there is some difference of opinion as to which of the pubertal changes should be utilized to mark the beginning of adolescence. The end of adolescence is much more difficult to describe. Each new dissertation on late adolescence suggests ways of defining 'reasonable' independence or utilizes other criteria which are equally difficult to define for delineating an end to adolescence.

The span of years devoted to adolescent development will vary in different cultures, and with different definitions. The term 'adolescence' is no longer equivalent to 'pubescence'. The former is seen as the psychological developments which are related to the biological growth, which the latter term is utilized to depict. In the last fifty years within Western cultures, adolescence has become a progressively longer stage. The concept of reasonable independence has been translated into financial independence and/or marriage. If these behavioral criteria are accepted, a high-school student who upon graduation begins work in a factory and marries at 19 experiences a shorter period of parental dependence than the individual who continues his education, attending college and graduate school, and is supported by his parents until the age of 26, marrying at 28.

In the United States, adolescents are conspicuously grouped by their presence in a school setting. Twelve- to fourteen-year-olds are in junior high school. Most 14- to 18-year-olds are in high school. The term 'teenager' is often used to refer to the high-school-age adolescent. The 18- to 21-year-old either begins full-time work, marries, or enters a university or professional school. He has been described as the 'young adult', the 'late adolescent', or the 'post-adolescent'. Individual variances as well as the specification of developmental tasks, the accomplishment of which predicate an ideal and the measurement of which require the ideal tool, reveal the use of age limits as only arbitrary devices. We use them as aids for communication.

In order to limit tne scope of this chapter we have decided to concentrate on the years from 12 through 21. We discuss the reactions of adolescents to pubertal changes. The necessity for the adolescent to habituate himself to his changing body and to his changing needs is the one common denominator of all discussions on adolescence. The adolescent will also be reacting to the attitudes of the parent generation and to the cultural biases.

Certain developmental theories of adolescence are to be found repeatedly in comprehensive collections of essays. One author choses an Eriksonian frame of reference. Another stresses Piaget's cognitive development while a third describes adolescence in terms of 'object-loss' and 'object-seeking' maneuvers. The language is different, thus obscuring important differences between the various systematizations. Furthermore, the data available from empirical studies seems to be far too limited to be able to list, for example, four developmental tasks. There are too many populations as yet unsampled for us to be able to make generalizations about the whole. We shall evaluate what is written now, summarize data on one group of adolescents, and examine the issues which such evaluations have shown to be central to the clinician's understanding of the developmental psychology of adolescence. We discuss certain aspects of developmental psychology while emphasizing the importance of considering the theoretical positions as tentative and population-specific.

The conceptualization of the normative developmental psychology of adolescents has, to a large extent, depended upon the clinical experiences of psychiatrists and psychoanalysts with disturbed adolescents or juvenile delinquents. Thus, in the process of extrapolating from psychopathology to normative theory, it has been difficult for psychiatrists to focus upon the adaptive in human behavior. Despite the above, psychiatrists do engage in discussions about typical, average, or normal patterns of development. Their data, however, has been minimal.

In order to avoid such obvious methodological pitfalls, we began, in 1962, a longitudinal follow-up study on a group of nonpatient adolescents in two Chicago suburbs (see Offer[17]). We intentionally selected a group of teenagers whose adaptation to their environment was not seen as deviant by parents, teachers, or our initial selection instruments. Subjects were selected on the basis of the *normality as average* perspective. (See Offer and Sabshin,[20] for a detailed theoretical discussion of concepts of normality and mental health.) A typical or normal student was defined as one whose answers on our self-image questionnaire fell within one standard deviation from the mean in nine out of ten scales which described various aspects of adolescent functioning. The questionnaires were given to 326 entering freshmen boys in the two suburban high schools.

Two psychiatrists, Drs Offer and Marcus, have been interviewing the seventy-three males selected. The project is in its eighth year. The subjects are now four years post-high school. In addition to the psychiatric interviews of the adolescents, the subjects were given psychological testing twice (at the ages of 16 and 20). Parents were also interviewed. Teachers completed rating scales on the adjustment of the students. The same interdisciplinary team of researchers studied the development of thirty female adolescents (Offer and Offer[19]).

In this chapter we will utilize our data on the developmental psychology of our normal subjects as an example of how one group of adolescents passes through adolescence. It should not be construed to mean that we are unaware of the limitations of our data. There are many other samples of normal adolescents in other socio-cultural, ethnic, and religious settings.

However, we believe that generalizations about development are meaningless if the specifics from which the generalizations were made are not identifiable. Thus, our data will identify the reasons for our positions.

The chapter is concerned with four issues: (1) sexual behavior; (2) the adolescent and his parents; (3) adolescent turmoil; and (4) identity.

2

Sexual Behavior

Developmental Issue

After the physical changes of puberty have taken place, the individual is biologically a sexually mature adult. Biological development and emotional readiness for heterosexual relationships do not proceed at the same pace. Though the sexual impulses are present with increasing strength, there exist psycho-social blocks which do not allow for discharge of these urges. What happens to the sexual impulses and when is the 'correct' time for their expression is a question which has plagued many investigators and theoreticians in the field of adolescent psychiatry and psychology.

Normal Adolescent Project Findings

The high-school students participating in our research projects were free to discuss sexual feelings during any of the interviews. However, the male adolescents rarely spoke about sexual incidents when asked in one of their sophomore year interviews when they had experienced feelings of shame, guilt, depression, and anxiety. The sixth interview which occurred during the teenager's junior year at high school was devoted to questions about heterosexual relationships. The adolescent males might blush and then answer our questions, adding questions of their own. In discussing heterosexual behavior more than in any other area of discussion, the subjects would ask what others had told us.

The cardinal findings are that there was a discrepancy of several years between the time our adolescent subject was biologically able to produce children and the time the adolescent engaged in intensive heterosexual activities. In this sense, the male adolescent subject was 'slow' in becoming involved sexually with a female. Ten per cent of our study population had sexual intercourse by the end of high school (18 years). The rate rises to 30 per cent by the end of the first post-high-school year (19 years), and 50 per cent by the end of their third post-high-school year (21 years).

Although the teenager was uncomfortable when he talked about his own sexual feelings and impulses, he liked to appear 'liberal' when talking about such issues as premarital sex. The high-school student generally thought that sexual intercourse was 'okay' after high school. Interviewer: 'Why not sooner?' Student: 'The girl might become pregnant.' Interviewer: 'There are contraceptive methods available.' Student, flushing: 'Well, we're just not mature enough to handle "it" yet, and teenagers should wait until they are old enough.'

The adolescent male in early and mid-adolescence was not as worried about his participation, or lack of it, in heterosexual activities as were our female subjects in the concomitant study which we undertook. For the male, learning to curb his aggressive impulses is more important than learning to handle his sexual impulses. When he acts out, it is most often aggressively, in delinquent or violent behavior. In contrast, the adolescent female is more preoccupied with sex, and the girl who does act out is likely to utilize the sexual route.

Many questions during our interviews would elicit blushing or seductive behavior, but the female adolescent, particularly, wanted to talk about her sexual attitudes and fears. Her fantasy life is vivid, and kissing a boy for the first time may be equivalent unconsciously to becoming pregnant. Gratification from fantasy life aids the female in handling her sexual impulses and in experimenting in thought with her changing and eroticized body without the massive guilt feelings which are as yet associated with heterosexual activities.

Dating was considered as part of the social format. The adolescent wanted to do the right thing. The female's concern with her place in the social field gave rise to questions like, 'Am I popular?' or 'Am I attractive?' much more than, for example, 'What kind of feelings do I have toward a specific girl or boy?' Though the action is often limited, whatever does occur attains significance for the adolescent and her self-image. We asked a 15-year-old girl when she had experienced shame. Answer: 'When I did something terrible with a boy.' She had told only her best girlfriend about what she had done and she would tell us no more. In another interview two years later, she revealed that the 'terrible thing' had been kissing a boy. Apparently for this subject at age 17, to kiss a boy was no longer as great a sin.

Implications for Theory

Have new cultural mores revolutionized today's sexual practices?

Recent empirical studies on adolescents and young adults do not support claims of increased sexual experiences for today's adolescents as compared to past generations. Our data on heterosexual behavior is consistent with our results from our questionnaire which has been given to 800 boys and 400 girls. Our results are also consistent with those of Reiss,[21] Douvan and Adelson,[6] and Simon, Cagnon, and Carns.[22] For the teenagers studied, adolescent sexuality remained an emotional taboo as well as an environmental one. Even a complete revamping of sexual codes might not necessarily lead to earlier, less inhibited, and 'healthier' sexual adjustments. It would take a more global shift in environmental and psychological conditioning of these adolescents.

What does seem to be changing more than the practices is the openness of discussing sex. Interviews of adolescents conducted within the context of studies on non-patient populations indicate that adolescents welcome the opportunity to talk about sexual feelings and experiences. Could this be another way of handling the impulses which were formerly reported as a subject of conversation of peer groupings on street corners?

The inexperienced adolescent must formulate new rationale which will aid him in proceeding at his own pace toward heterosexuality. Since the advent of modern contraceptive methods, the adolescent who feared that intercourse would lead to pregnancy must develop other reasons for postponing sexual intercourse. In addition, prevalent cultural mores can exaggerate or ameliorate the adolescent's responses to his changing self. Newspaper and television reporting, as well as classroom discussions and theoretical dissertations on the freedom of today's youth to engage in sexual activities, may accentuate the abstaining teenager's belief that he/she is abnormal or, at least, inferior in comparison with his peers. His choice of defenses, be they adaptive or maladaptive, will be at least partially determined by cultural factors, of his own and his parents' generations.

Perhaps as a reaction to the glorification of 'free sex' as an answer to our neuroses, theoreticians of adolescent development have been underscoring the dangers of proceeding toward heterosexuality when biological readiness is not matched by emotional readiness.

H. Deutsch tells us of a seminar in which Freud suggested the value of delayed sexual activities (H. Deutsch,[5,12] p. 24): 'Years ago, Freud, in a meeting that was limited to a small number of participants, expressed his opposition to Wilhelm Reich's insistence that sexual activity should begin in adolescence—that is, as soon as the biological readiness is manifested. Freud regarded the postponement of gratification as an important element in the process of sublimation and thereby essential to development.'

H. Deutsch[5] confirms the importance of the early same sex relationships and warns of the disadvantages of early sexual gratification replacing too rapidly the homosexual friendships. In a discussion on female adolescents, she states: 'I consider those girls who are involved prematurely in "free love" as not the victors but the victims of the rebellious adolescent society. A great number of them are still involved in their earlier relationships with girlfriends. They "fool around" as the saying goes, with boys—but it is still with a side glance at the girls, and the heterosexual activity actually shows very little inner participation.'

H. Deutsch later describes the case of Nora who could not decide which of three boys she preferred: 'All three of the boys concerned were directly connected with her high school past; two of them were brothers of her old girlfriends; the third had had a mild affair with another of her friends from back home. This information was sufficient for me to understand that the homosexual attachments of her earlier adolescence had not yet been fully resolved and had in fact continued into her present pseudoheterosexual relationships.'

Blos[3] describes a type of frantic heterosexual activity which is defensive. For the female, he explains this in terms of the preoedipal attachment to the mother which is now revived. 'The pseudoheterosexuality of this type of delinquent girl serves as a defense against the regressive pull to the pre-oedipal mother, that is, against homosexuality.'

Erikson[7] believes that sexual experimentation will provide a necessary part of identity-formation but sexual pleasure need be preceded by a sense of one's own identity. The individual lacking a clear sense of who he is will be threatened by intimate relationships. In early and mid-adolescence, the teenager can concentrate his energies on less dangerous terrains, such as the football field or the classroom exam. There his emotional investments can be less intense and his disappointments be more easily reversed.

3

The Adolescent and His Parents

Developmental Issue

During adolescence, the individual must separate from his parent emotionally and intellectually. He must begin to know his own limitations and to utilize this knowledge in caring for himself. Ideally, the dependency characteristic of childhood should be relinquished. During adolescence, the former parent–child relationship should be changed sufficiently to allow the adolescent to proceed into a generational dyad in which he will be a primarily independent figure.

Normal Adolescent Project Findings

Profile of Jim: a normal middle-class suburban American adolescent

At 11 years of age, Jim became increasingly argumentative. He disliked taking the garbage out every evening. The problem for him was that he would feel guilty, when he promised his mother he would empty the garbage and then would neglect to do it or when he would argue with his mother about why the job had to be his. He would also argue with his two brothers about which television program to watch or whose turn it was to do the dishes. Jim felt ashamed when his mother had to do things for him—like the time when he had a bad knee and mother drove him to school, even though dad disapproved of her chauffering. Jim was an average student, considering a future in engineering. He was on his school's basketball team and very involved with the team members, the coach, practice sessions, and the big games. He began dating toward the end of his junior year in high school. His first date was for a party after the last basketball game of the season.

After high school, Jim went to a college two hundred miles from his home. He thought all students should leave home after high school in order to learn to be on their own. During his freshman year, he was lonesome, missing his mother's cooking and weekends with the family. He added: 'It's not my parents that I need, but a girlfriend.' During summer vacations, he returned home. He had his hair cut a little shorter than was fashionable at his school in order to be able to secure a good summer job, working for a friend of his father's. He now enjoyed talking with his father more than previously. His father would invite Jim to join him for a drink. In general, Jim believed that both his parents treated him more like an adult since he had begun college. It did bother him when his mother questioned him about his activities. He tended to reply in monosyllables (or less) and 'get away' as soon as possible if she became 'too prying'.

Two years post-high school, he brought his girlfriend home to meet his parents and once brought her along to wait outside while the psychiatrist interviewed him. During his junior year in college, he had sexual intercourse for the first time with a girl who was known to be 'easy'. He never dated her again, and felt that he had taken advantage of her.

At present, Jim is planning to go to graduate school in engineering or go into the army. He wants to spend next summer traveling.

As illustrated by Jim's behavior and the affect elicited within the interviews, Jim wanted to be accepted by his parents and admitted into their way of life but he wanted to do this with a feeling that he was acting as his own free agent. Jim was separating from his parents but without alienating them. During both Jim's high school and college years, his parents expressed a pride in their son and his activities. The letting-go period was a gradual one. Conflicts were present but did not spiral out of control.

For the majority of students whom we studied, independence could be achieved without a total devaluation of parents. The adolescents studied in our normal population rarely rejected important patental values. Similarily, studies of student protesters and cvil rights workers (Solomon and Fishman,[23] Haan et al.[15]) have shown a congruence of parent–adolescent values.

The struggle for emotional disengagement was enacted in areas which could be seen as trivial to the adult eye. When the parent could keep the issue in perspective, the adolescent could achieve the victory needed for his sense of self-esteem. These 'battles' could be won without a risk for the adolescent of having to jeopardize parental support. Even the issues chosen for the arguments were dependent upon parental preferences, but in a negative way. This has been conceptualized by Baittle and Offer:[2] 'When the adolescent rebels, he often expresses his intentions in a manner resembling negation. He defines what he does in terms of what his parents do not want him to do. If his parents want him to turn off the radio and study, this is the precise time he keeps the radio on and claims he cannot study. If they want him to buy new clothes, the old ones are good enough. In periods like this, it becomes obvious that the adolescents' decisions are in reality based on the negative of the parents' wishes, rather than on their own positive desires. What they do, and the judgments they make, are, in fact, dependent on the parents' opinions and suggestions, but in a negative way. This may be termed a stage of "negative dependence". Thus, while the oppositional behavior and protest against the parents are indeed a manifestation of rebellion and in the service of emancipation from the parents, at the same time they reveal that the passive dependent longings are still in force. The adolescent is in conflict over desires to emancipate, and the rebellious behavior is a compromise formation which supports his efforts to give up the parental object and, at the same time, gratifies his dependent longings on them.'

Our data also document the gradual shifts away from reliance on the parents. When the sport activities of high school terminate and the intensive home life of the younger adolescent dissipates, the adolescents must find substitute satisfactions. In follow-up interviews, the father of the male adolescent was mentioned much more frequently than had been true during early and mid-adolescence. Fewer, too, are the incidents of boys telling us that their mothers are beautiful or the unconscious shifting of the conversations to discussions about mothers directly after the males were asked questions about their female peers. For certain males, the next stage was the period of taking out a girl in order to test the reactions of his parents. Finally, several of our subjects have begun to tell us for the first time of specific characteristics of their girlfriends.

The subjects are also relating to us the opinions and reactions of their peers more frequently in the post-high-school interviews. One male at age 16 told us that he agreed with his parents on the subject of the war in Viet Nam: 'The Communists must be stopped or they will take over everything.' Three years later he was at the conservative college of his choice. His political sentiments were unchanged except that replacing the comparison with the parental point of view was: 'And I'm the most liberal guy on my campus.' Meanwhile a more liberal former classmate at the radical college of his choice was berating himself for not having the 'guts' to act on his principles and burn his draft card as certain of his more radical peers had done.

By the content of the subjects' responses, we could see the changes in interpersonal relationships. The adolescents were seeking out non-family members with whom they could share emotional experiences. There were some adolescents whose dependence upon parental figures had not altered significantly. For those adolescents whose development was delayed, the theoretical demarcation of an end to adolescence will be additionally complicated. Perhaps, it will be marked by a rigidity of the earlier adolescent patterns, never transcended.

Implications for Theory

Anna Freud[10] writes: 'There are few situations in life which are more difficult to cope with than an adolescent son or daughter during the attempt to liberate themselves.' (See also A. Freud.[11])

Without erring in underestimating the conflicts which exist during adolescence, it is of importance to refrain from expecting momentous battles to characterize parent–adolescent relationships. In our study, parents and adolescents reported 'bickering' during the early adolescent years. For the vast majority of our subjects, later difficulties failed to produce sustained feelings of misery or doom in either parent or adolescent.

The conflicts which do exist may be further encouraged by our own theoretical conceptualizations of relationships between the generations. Anthony[1] writes: 'The adult in our Western culture has apparently learned to expect a state of acute disequilibrium and anticipates the "storm and stress" in his adolescent child as he once anticipated the negativism of his two-year-old. The expectation has seemingly been incorporated into the literature of psychological development, and it may take methodical research and many years of endeavor to remove it from the textbooks. There is, however, growing support for the concept that society gets the type of adolescent it expects and deserves, and this is true of even those members who come into daily contact with the ordinary teenager.'

In addition to the observation Anthony has made, it seems to us that the stereotype also has another effect. We have seen the parent (as well as the psychiatrist) who, expecting difficulties with adolescents, will minimize the importance of the problems which do exist, labeling them 'normal' for the development of all adolescents. From parents who were interviewed while their sons were in high school, we heard frequent variations of the following sentiment: 'We have some problems but our son is far better than most boys his age.' The same parents had reacted more strongly to the negativism of their son when he was 11 and 12 years old. During their offspring's early adolescence, parents believed that precedents must be established for handling future conflicts, and they worried about what the future would bring if they were 'already' having disagreements with their youngster. This outlook may contribute to the reporting by our subjects and their parents of greater disagreements during early adolescence than in the ensuing years. To a certain extent rebellion has been sanctioned, institutionalized, and encouraged for the later adolescent years. The interplay between cultural expectations and behavioral patterns constantly complicates the formation of neat stage-specific psychological generalizations concerning behavioral patterns.

Are parental–adolescent conflicts inevitable? The adolescent must disengage himself from parental domination. He can do this without total renunciation of parental values, but rather through conflicts on minor issues which have been endowed with major importance for the adolescent's own growth and development. Battling between the generations need not characterize adolescence, as apart from other life stages when developmental tasks require infant, child, or adult to assert his independence from parental pressures. Adolescence, though, should be characterized by a significant emotional disengagement of the adolescent from the parent and a development of emotional relationships with others outside of the nuclear family complex. The emotional transfer to non-family members will, of course, never be complete; most importantly, the transfer of emotions must be accompanied by an emotional growth toward independence. Successful adaptation requires that the original preoedipal and oedipal conflicts be resolved sufficiently, so that adult interpersonal relationships will not be a repeat of the former child–parent or adolescent–parent psychological patterns. As the biological and cultural situation changes, so should the psychological variables retain their transactional role in the complex. If psychological stagnation occurs, the effects will be manifested throughout the entire system.

4

Adolescent Turmoil

Developmental Issue

Psychoanalytic literature describes adolescence as a time of psychological imbalance when the functioning of ego and superego are severely strained. Instinctual impulses disrupt the homeostatic arrangements achieved during latency and inner turmoil results. Unresolved preoedipal and oedipal conflicts are revived; the repression characteristic of latency will no longer be sufficient to restore a psychological equilibrium. The adolescent's intensive aggressive and erotic strivings are focused primarily upon parents and parent-figures. The physical, muscular, and hormonal growth of the adolescent endows the re-aroused drives with a potency denied to the former child and frightening to the developing adolescent.

According to psychoanalytic theory, the strength of these aggressive and sexual impulses revived during adolescence necessitates an emotional disengagement from the nuclear family. However, the adolescents' value systems and self-esteem have been structured by internalizations of parental attitudes and behavior or, according to Grinker,[13] by the experiences of the infant in reaction to an influx of stimuli emanating from parents or parent-substitutes. To devaluate parents is to discredit also one's own internalizations gained from interactions with the parents. The adolescent's inner controls are loosened and his self-esteem is fluctuating as he challenges the 'truths' of his childhood. The re-evaluation occurs at the same time as the adolescent's judgment and coping abilities are being weakened by demands of increased instinctual impulses.

The adolescent who now needs the support of strong, loving parents can least afford to accept that support. The loss of the parents as the supportive pillars of the individual's development has been conceptualized as 'object-loss'. According to Blos,[3] the primary theme of adolescence is the object-loss and the subsequent object-seeking. The adolescent depleted by his necessary rejection of dependency upon his parents must strive for narcissistic gratifications from deceptive magnifications of his own powers and from temporary identifications with peers and parental figures outside of the home. These defensive maneuvers are first steps in replenishing his strength.

This brief psychoanalytic conceptualization of early and mid-adolescence has been presented because we believe that psychoanalytic theory still provides the most comprehensive theoretical framework which we have today. If we accept it, the question arises as to how the adolescent manages to function during a period of such inner turmoil? Will he be likely to display behavioral contradictions? Will his psychological state match that of the 'as if' patient described by H. Deutsch (see Anna Freud[9])? Will we be able to distinguish the symptoms of adolescence from symptoms displayed by the adult who has been diagnosed as suffering from a psychiatric disorder?

Given circumstances creating disequilibrium, the tendency of the living organism is to mobilize its forces toward a restoration of its equilibrium. Defensive maneuvers will be instituted in the service of adaptation to disquieting elements in the internal and external environment. Our question now concerns the affect experienced by adolescents and the character of the coping devices utilized. Additionally, through an examination of the organism's observable behavior, we can also gain information about the developmental requirements to which, it is postulated, the organism is reacting. Theory must be susceptible to revision from empirical examinations of the populations the theory attempts to describe. Although our data from our normal adolescent project may lack the depth of psychoanalytic patient data, they have the attribute of being collected from one segment of the non-patient population whose psychological development the above theory is designed to describe.

Normal Adolescent Project Findings

To cope is to seek and utilize information under a variety of conditions in order to regulate behavior. Adolescence offers the individual an opportunity to test his defensive structure and/or his ability to cope. Our normal adolescent sample usually managed to cope with even severe stresses through their particular individual defensive structures and their action-orientation. When an unusual situation occurred, such as the death of a father, the adolescent would first deny the full emotional impact of the event. Then, he would cope with the stressful situation as well as the affect aroused by it through doing something. He would involve himself in time-consuming activities; often these activities were ones which would be necessitated by practical realities. Only slowly would he let himself experience the loss and mourn.

The stresses produced by the changes in body, in body image, and in emotional states were managed by these adolescents with little evidence of total personality upheavals or ascetic renunciations of all bodily desires. As stated earlier, the male adolescent experienced the most difficulty with controlling his impulses during early adolescence. In mid-adolescence the involvement in sports, in cars, in hobbies, or on debating teams channeled his energies quite effectively. The girls, for whom culturally provided aggressive outlets were more limited, tended to handle these stresses in a more passive way by employing introspection or turning to close girlfriends with whom they could gain emotional satisfactions from hours of intimate discussions. For both sexes during late adolescence, there was a decrease in these types of sublimatory activities and an increase in heterosexual experiences.

Our normal subjects' action-orientation was coupled with a good sense of reality. Their overall pattern of behavior was goal-directed toward a future which they could envision and for which they were making mental time-schedules. Although they had questions concerning their vocational choices, most of these adolescents have been following their original plans with surprisingly few obstacles.

Psychological patterns of coping have retained an underlying similarity as different problems to be mastered have emerged. We see variations on a theme rather than extreme shifts in behavioral patterns. For example, at 11 years old, George was fighting for his rights in reaction to a boy scout master's false accusation that he had started a fight; at 20 years old George was being accused of taking drugs, even though, he reports, he was an innocent bystander, in no way involved in any illegal activities. His interest in painting, the family avocation, had remained constant, and he retained a good grade average. He associated with many of his peers but never had any particularly close friends.

Implications for Theory

Research on this group of normal adolescents does not validate psychological conceptualizations of extreme turmoil characterizing adolescent development (see also Masterson[16] and Grinker[14] for similar findings). We base this judgment upon observations of patterns of behavior of adolescents and the meaning of these patterns to the individuals participating in our project. The nature of turmoil is not such as to be able to keep itself hidden from the world, while presenting a picture of flexibility and good control over reality. In the segment of the adolescent population which we studied, behavior which might be considered as radically deviant by general American middle-class cultural standards was the exception rather than the rule. In home and school the majority of these adolescents displayed an overall pattern of consistency. Our follow-up studies on the adolescents have revealed a continuity of individual personality structures throughout the stages of adolescence (Offer, Marcus, and Offer[18]).

This being the case, we challenge the concept of great inner turmoil, swift mood swings, or other seemingly pathological symptomotology as being a *necessary* part of adolescence. The turmoil experienced by our subjects is quantitatively different from the turmoil experienced by patient and delinquent populations seen in our hospital clinics and described in psychiatric case reports. The rebellion which we see in our research subjects and the emotional conflicts and crises that are both seen and postulated, point toward theoretical conceptualizations of at least one type of normal adolescent with a lower level of turmoil than indicated in much of accepted psychiatric theory. We have studied our subjects for eight years now, and have found no evidence to suggest that they are withdrawn, underdeveloped, or inhibited adolescents.

Interestingly, investigators who have spent most of their professional lives studying disturbed adolescents stress the importance of a period of turmoil for the developmental growth of the individual, while investigators who, like us, have studied normal adolescent populations find a minimal amount of turmoil displayed during the growth processes of many members of their research samples. We believe that the development of many adolescents can be better characterized by a concept of gradual shifts than by volcanic eruptions. Possibly, their clasp onto their parents was not so tight as to require a quick, total withdrawal for success in development.

Data on non-patient populations suggest that adolescents can meet the requirements of emotional disengagement from internalized parental imagos and of pubertal growth spurts without displaying gross behavioral aberrations. In fact, the latter would, in adolescence as well as in other life stages, indicate a need for psychiatric evaluation and treatment. Neurotic symptomatology during adolescence should not be regarded as something the adolescent will 'grow out of'. According to Masterson,[16] diagnostic problems for the psychiatrist evaluating the adolescent relate to difficulties in classifying the sickness, not to determining its presence or its durability.

Once again, though, we must be sure to define adolescent behavior by norms for adolescents within cultural contexts and stages of biological maturity. An explanation of the adolescent's behavior by comparisons with the child's or the adult's ignores the particular context of the tasks of adolescence and will result in more theories which regard the adolescent's normal behavior as being abnormal.

5

Identity

Developmental Issue

The crystalization of identity is one of the developmental issues of adolescence. As conceptualized by Erikson,[7] it is not one specific process but rather the culmination of many events which lead to: (1) a conscious sense of one's own individual identity; (2) an unconscious striving for a continuity of personal character; (3) a criterion for the silent doings of ego synthesis; (4) a maintenance of an inner solidarity with the groups' ideals. It has never been stated specifically when in adolescence identity conflicts either arise or should be resolved, though it has often been assumed that the answer to the question: 'Who am I?' has to come in late adolescence.

Normal Adolescent Project Findings

Within our subject population, Jack is an example of a subject who had some identity conflicts. He revealed an array of contradictory plans and goals, but the contradictions did not appear especially disturbing to him. At 20 years old, he thought he might become a history professor, a social worker, or an athletic coach. When the psychiatrist indicated that Jack's plans were not too concrete, Jack momentarily retreated: 'Well, I might not even finish college.' Immediately afterwards, though, he presented still other alternatives. He even suggested living a couple of years in Alaska after telling us that he had left the Northern college which he had first attended because of his aversion to cold weather.

Andy, on the other hand, had planned his future long in advance. He was inclined towards introspection, depression, and a certain degree of rebelliousness. He retained consistent control over his life so that he was able to compensate for his disappointments through experiences which were highly satisfactory to him. An accurate self-appraisal allowed Andy to proceed according to his plans.

Our emphasis in our book, *The psychological world of the teen-ager*,[17] has been on the recognition of more than one route through adolescence. At present we can see three groups within our subject population. Subjects who, like Andy, tended toward introspection and depression are now adapting themselves to the demands of young adulthood. Others remain dependent upon their parents, or may be gradually shifting the dependency to male or female peers. For them, a sense of their identity may be delayed or never experienced. A third group belong to the category described by Erikson as young people in whom the identity crisis is a noiseless one (Erikson[8]). For those subjects the tasks of adolescence are being met without overt self-dissatisfaction or excessive narcissism. Of necessity, further definition of routes through adolescence must await further evidence of the development of our subjects.

The identity conflicts experienced by the vast majority of our subjects range from mild to moderate. We have seen only a few subjects who manifested the Eriksonian type of identity crisis in which neurotic symptomatology becomes a temporary condition of normal development. The resiliency of the earlier self-confidence has continued for the majority of our subjects who feel satisfied with their choices and opportunities.

Implications for Theory

Our subjects can be understood in terms of Blos's[4] concept of adolescence as the second stage of individuation, the first having been completed toward the end of the third year of life which was marked by rapid developmental progress toward the attainment of object constancy. He writes: 'Not until the termination of adolescence do self- and object-representation acquire stability and firm boundaries.' Working within this framework which is, unfortunately, extremely difficult to measure empirically, we believe our subjects can be seen as approaching the end of the second stage of individuation. To what extent individuals ever completely separate from their internalized parental imagos and become firmly established in their own worlds of mature object representations is a variation of the question which we asked earlier when describing the difficulties of determining when adolescence terminates.

Late adolescence is portrayed as a time of delimitation in order to gain organization. The adolescent assumes adult responsibilities which are seen as limitations upon the scope of his activities and the freedom of his movement. However, the young adult who has successfully adapted to the biological, psychological, and sociological requirements of earlier stages of development will now be freer from the emotional conflicts which previously limited his world. Optimally, he is finding satisfactory ways of expressing himself, patterns for handling unresolved conflicts, which enable him to widen his horizons in ways which were impossible for him earlier when changing developmental tasks absorbed and restricted his energies to a greater degree. Thus, to conceive of adolescence as a stage of psychological expansion to be terminated by the choices and limitations that proceed with the defining of oneself, is not to present a complete picture. The process of defining oneself does not terminate with the termination of adolescence; what does happen is that the areas of focus and the meaningful interpersonal relationships of the future become manifest. If the passage through adolescence has been accomplished successfully, this focusing becomes as much a freedom to express oneself as it is a limitation to the mode for expression.

6

Summary

In this chapter, we have utilized our data on the developmental psychology of our normal subjects as an example of how one group of adolescents passes through adolescence. The chapter is concerned with four issues: (1) sexual behavior; (2) the adolescent and his parents; (3) adolescent turmoil; and (4) identity.

REFERENCES

1. ANTHONY, E. J. 1969. The reactions of adults to adolescents and their behavior. In *Adolescence*. Eds G. Caplan and S. Lebovici. New York: Basic Books.
2. BAITTLE, B. and OFFER, D. 1971. On the nature of adolescent rebellion. In *Annals of adolescent psychiatry*. Eds S. Feinstein, P. Giovacchini and A. Miller. New York: Basic Books.
3. BLOS, P. 1962. *On adolescence*. New York: The Free Press of Glencoe.

4. BLOS, P. 1967. The second individuation process of adolescence, *Psychoanalytic Study of the Child*, **22**, 162–187.
5. DEUTSCH, H. 1967. *Selected problems of adolescence*. New York: International Universities Press.
6. DOUVAN, E. and ADELSON, Y. 1966. *The adolescent experience*. New York: John Wiley.
7. ERIKSON, E. H. 1968. *Identity: youth and crisis*. New York: W. W. Norton.
8. ERIKSON, E. H. 1968. Identity: psychosocial. *International Encyclop. of the Soc. Sc.*, **7**, 61–65. New York: Macmillan Company and Free Press.
9. FREUD, A. 1936. *The ego and the mechanisms of defense*. New York: International University Press.
10. FREUD, A. 1958. Adolescence. *Psychoanalytical Study of the Child*, **13**, 225–273.
11. FREUD, A. 1969. Adolescence as a developmental disturbance. In *Adolescence*. Eds G. Caplan and S. Lebovici. New York: Basic Books.
12. FREUD, S. 1967. As quoted by H. Deutsch in *Selected problems of adolescence*. New York: International University Press.
13. GRINKER, R. R. 1953. *Psychosomatic Research*. New York: W. W. Norton.
14. GRINKER, R. R. 1962. Mentally healthy young males (Homoclites). *AMA Arch. gen. Psychiat.*, **6**, 405–453.
15. HAAN, N., SMITH, M. B. and BLOCK, J. 1968. Moral reasoning of young adults: political–social behavior, family background and personality correlates. *Journal of Personality and Social Psychology*, **10**. 3, 183–201.
16. MASTERSON, J. F., JR., 1967. *The psychiatric dilemma of adolescence*. Boston: Little, Brown.
17. OFFER, D. 1969. *The psychological world of the teen-ager: a study of normal adolescent boys*. New York: Basic Books.
18. OFFER, D., MARCUS, D. and OFFER, J. L. 1970. A longitudinal study of normal adolescent boys. *Amer. J. Psychiat.*, **126**, 917–924.
19. OFFER, D. and OFFER, J. L. 1968. Profiles of normal adolescent girls. *AMA Arch. gen. Psychiat.*, **19**, 513–522.
20. OFFER, D. and SABSHIN, M. 1966. *Normality: theoretical and clinical concepts of mental health*. New York: Basic Books.
21. REISS, I. L. 1961. Sexual codes in teen-age culture. *Annals Am. Acad. Pol. & Soc. Sci.*, **338**, 53–63.
22. SIMON, W., CAGNON, J. and CARNS, D. 1968. Sexual behavior of the college student. *Paper read at The Academy of Psychoanalysis*, New Orleans, Louisiana.
23. SOLOMON, F. and FISHMAN, J. R. 1964. Youth and Race. *J. Social Issues*, **20**, 54–73.

III

NORMAL SEXUALITY IN ADOLESCENCE

MICHAEL SCHOFIELD

Social Psychologist
London, England

1

Normality

Adolescents who visit a psychiatrist have problems, and quite often these are sexual problems. Of course it is possible that the young patient thinks he has a sexual problem which turns out to be just a part of growing up and if it is a problem at all, it is one that most of us have known at some period of our lives.

But it is worth remembering that the only adolescents that a psychiatrist meets in his professional life are boys and girls who have been unable to resolve their problems. To this extent their patients are abnormal: they are not typical adolescents. Psychiatrists may be misled if they make generalisations about sexual behaviour which are based on knowledge acquired from their clinical work. In order to understand an abnormal sexual situation, it is necessary to know something about the normal situation and this can only be done by studying the non-psychiatric population.

This is not the moment to provoke an argument about what is normal. It must be recognised that there are very wide variations of behaviour among adolescents. Furthermore, it is particularly difficult to find out what are the sexual norms of a particular group or society. But it is valuable to have some base with which comparisons can be made, and the object of the researches I have been carrying out have been to provide the factual information about normal adolescent sexual behaviour without in any way equating normal activities with the desirable behaviour.

The following data are the result of a study undertaken in the United Kingdom.[5]

2

Sexual Intercourse

Incidence

More than one in five (21 per cent) of the teenage boys and over one in ten (11 per cent) of the girls (aged fifteen to nineteen) that we interviewed had experienced sexual intercourse. But these figures by themselves may give the wrong impression. For this is the period when adolescents start to take a serious interest in the opposite sex and set out upon their first early sexual adventures.

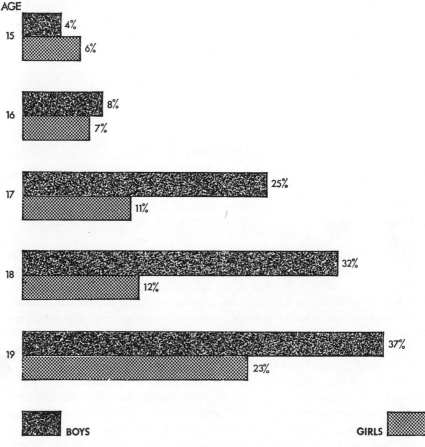

AGE

15   4% 6%

16   8% 7%

17   25% 11%

18   32% 12%

19   37% 23%

BOYS   GIRLS

FIG. 1. Boys and girls with experience of sexual intercourse (in percentages).

By the age of fifteen most boys have taken a girl out for a date and most girls have started dating a year or two earlier. In quite a large number of these dates there is no sexual element beyond a goodnight kiss—an almost obligatory end to the evening in some teenage circles. As they get older, the dates may involve some fairly intimate sexual experiments, especially if the couple have been out together on several occasions. On a few dates sexual intercourse takes place, but this is most likely to happen when the couples are 'going steady' and perhaps formally engaged.

Therefore age is a very important factor, and a better indication of the situation is given when we examine the extent of sexual intercourse at each age. Before the age of fourteen it is quite rare. Less than one in a hundred boys (0·9 per cent) and one in a thousand girls (0·1 per cent) have had experience of sexual intercourse. Even at fourteen the figures are not much higher. About one in fifty boys (2·3 per cent) and less than one in two hundred girls (0·4 per cent) have had premarital intercourse. Although reports about unmarried mothers of thirteen and fourteen are distressing, it should be noted that such cases are very exceptional.

Fig. 1 shows how more and more teenagers go on to experience sexual intercourse as they get older. At the ages of fifteen and sixteen the figures are still less than one in ten for both boys and girls. This suggests that the fears often expressed about the extensive sexual activities between school-boys and schoolgirls may be exaggerated. Although every secondary school probably contains a few boys and girls who are sexually experienced, it is unlikely that they are more than a small minority.

It is at seventeen that there is a sudden increase in the percentage for boys, but not for girls. At this age a quarter of all boys have experience of sexual intercourse, but this applies to less than an eighth of the girls. At nineteen one in three of the boys and nearly a quarter of the girls are sexually experienced. So premarital intercourse among teenagers is not uncommon, but it is not universal or even an activity in which the majority take part.

Validity

How can we be sure that these figures accurately reflect the true situation? The answer to this very relevant question is that exact measurement of human behaviour is rarely possible, but the precautions taken in this research to ensure veracity make it unlikely that these percentages are very far out.

Problems of validation are common to all social surveys, and are particularly pertinent in a research into sexual behaviour. No topic is more personal and private than the sexual activities of the individual, and a person who gives truthful and straightforward answers about his shopping habits or voting intentions may well hesitate before he decides to be equally frank about his sex experience. This may seem obvious, but it is surprising how many questionnaires on sexual behaviour assume that people will answer all questions with equal candour.

We did not assume that reliable information about sex activities could be easily obtained just for the asking. It does not require much skill or cost much money to make up a questionnaire on sex, and then send it out to thousands of people in the hope that a few hundred will reply. This has

c

been done by newspapers, college magazines and advertising agencies. The results are unlikely to be of much value. The number who do not answer the questions is often so large that they form a sizeable proportion of the population under consideration; nor is this a method that is likely to elicit the truth on such a personal matter.

No other research on sexual behaviour has based its results on such a representative sample. This is not a boastful claim of assiduousness or skill, but simply the result of being provided with enough money and time to do the sampling thoroughly.

All the adolescents were seen alone in conditions which encouraged them to talk freely and in complete confidence. Often it was quite difficult to make arrangements to see the adolescent alone, away from parents and friends. Sometimes parents would make remarks like: 'You don't have to see her alone. She tells us everything. There are no secrets in this family.' But on many occasions our interviewers found that the confidence of the parents was misplaced.

Once it was possible to settle down to talk quietly and privately, it was not very difficult to win the confidence of the teenager, especially as all our interviewers were young and sympathetic to the teenage point of view.

As a result of experience during a pilot research and after intensive training, we found it was possible to reach the point where the interviewers could be reasonably sure they were getting truthful answers. Of course it is impossible to make a teenager tell the truth if he does not feel inclined to cooperate, but by this time the interviewers had learnt enough to avoid being deceived or misled. In any case this rarely happened. One of the most pleasing advantages of studying this particular age group is that young people of today are more frank and open about sex than is the case with older people.

The First Sexual Partner

Information was obtained about the age of the other person at the time of the first experience of sexual intercourse. It was found that over half (56 per cent) of the sexually experienced boys had intercourse with a girl of about the same age, and over a third (36 per cent) with the older girls. Among the experienced girls a third had intercourse with a boy of the same age and two-thirds with someone who was older. In quite a large number (38 per cent) of cases, the girl was introduced to sexual intercourse by a man aged twenty-one or over. The number of female adults who have introduced boys to intercourse is very small (2 per cent)—the proselytising older woman in search of virgin boys is either a myth, or very unsuccessful.

The teenagers were asked if they thought it was also the first time for their partners. Fig. 2 shows their replies. Only a minority thought it was the first experience of sexual intercourse for both of them. Considering that an experienced boy might be tempted to tell the girl that this was also the first time for him, and an experienced girl might be reluctant to volunteer the information that she was not a virgin, these results show a remarkably high number of cases where the partner was more experienced at the time of the teenager's first experience of intercourse.

Several other questions were asked about the first experience of sexual intercourse. For example, nearly all the girls (81 per cent) maintained that the boy on this first occasion was a 'steady'; 16 per cent described the

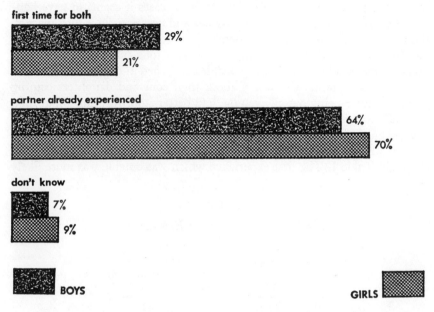

FIG. 2. The experience of the other person when the teenager first had sexual intercourse.

first partner as an acquaintance, and only 3 per cent said the boy was a pick-up, i.e. someone they had met on the same day that intercourse took place. The figures for the boys are more equally spread over these three categories, probably because their idea of a 'steady' is quite different from the definition the girls would give. In fact 45 per cent of the boys described their first partner as a steady, 34 per cent as an acquaintance, and 16 per cent as a pick-up. Although the girls may have been over-defensive when answering this question, even allowing for this, it seems likely that the first experience for boys as well as girls was usually with a friend, and often with someone they knew very well.

Location

When those who had experienced sexual intercourse were asked where they had met their first partner, all sorts of places were mentioned. Some met at a dance, others at a party, club, cinema, school or outdoors, while others said they had grown up together. Boys occasionally go out in groups to look for girls, and this seems to be the way some of them met their first sexual partner. But in general there seems to be no particular place where teenagers go to find sexual partners, and in the vast majority of cases they met their future sexual partners during the ordinary intercommunication among young people.

But the answers to the question on where the first experience actually took place are much more revealing. In most cases it seems to have happened in the parental home of the partner and occasionally it took place in the home of the boy or girl experiencing intercourse for the first time. In fact the first experience of sexual intercourse took place in the parental home of one or other of the young people concerned in more than half of all the cases. So parents who worry about their sons and daughters coming home late after being out all evening, had better stop worrying about that, and start wondering what is happening in their own front room when *they* (the parents) go out in the evening.

The other places where boys and girls had their first experience are shown in Table I. The first experience which was outside was more likely

TABLE I

The Location of the First Experience
of Sexual Intercourse

Place	Boys %	Girls %
Partner's house	50	43
Own house	13	15
Flat, digs	1	12
Party	7	9
Park, rural	10	3
Car	3	7
Others	16	11
TOTAL	100	100

to be in an urban park or the rural countryside for a boy, and more likely to be in a car for a girl. This reflects the much larger number of girls whose first experience was with an adult who was more likely to have a car.

The Reason Why

We were surprised to find that the first sexual intercourse was nearly always unpremeditated. Very few of them (14 per cent) had set out with the intention of having intercourse on that particular evening.

This point was pursued still further when the sexually experienced teenagers were asked: 'Have you any idea why it happened.' This would be a difficult question for anyone to answer and naturally many of the replies were vague and inarticulate. But it was a good question, because it forced the teenager to look back on this first episode, and the answers can be classified fairly easily into six main categories, as shown in Table II.

The replies reveal the big difference in attitude between the two sexes. The boys were more likely to reply that they were impelled by sexual desire, whereas the girls were more likely to say they were in love. This would confirm the suspicions of those who see the male as essentially a predatory animal whereas the female is amative and romantic.

TABLE II

The Reason for the First Experience of Sexual Intercourse

Reason given	Boys %	Girls %
Sexual appetite	46	16
In love	10	42
Curiosity	25	13
Drunk	3	9
Others	4	8
Don't know	12	12
TOTAL	100	100

A large number of boys and quite a few girls were driven towards their first experience for reasons that can best be summed up by the word *curiosity*. Admonitory articles in the press and hand-wringing by important people have given some adolescents the impression that most teenagers are sexually experienced, and some of the boys and girls must have wondered why they were exceptional. Perhaps they thought they were missing something, or that something was missing in them.

A few boys and more girls said they were drunk at the time, and two girls said they had their first experience because they were bored. No one gave drugs as a reason and indeed amphetamines and cannabis, the drugs usually associated with teenagers, do not appear to be aphrodisiacs.

Reactions to First Experience

But this first adventure was not always an unqualified success, and did not always result in sexual gratification. Less than half the boys (48 per cent) and less than a third of the girls (30 per cent) said they liked it when they were asked for their reactions to this first experience of sexual intercourse. On the other hand some of them said they actively disliked it, while others said they were disappointed. The answers to this question are classified in Table III.

The boys were more likely to express their feelings in terms of pleasure and enjoyment, or the lack of it. The girls were more inclined to describe their later reactions after the sexual excitement was over.

TABLE III

The Reactions to the First Experience of
Sexual Intercourse

Reaction	Boys %	Girls %
Liked	48	30
Disliked	7	7
Disappointed	14	7
Ashamed	10	25
Afraid	5	15
Unworried	2	9
No reaction	14	7
TOTAL	100	100

Rather pleased with myself. Swaggering, in fact. It's only natural, isn't it? (boy, aged seventeen).

I didn't know what had happened actually. I was quite enthralled by it all (boy, aged eighteen).

I felt a bit older, that was about all. Everybody had been talking about it and now I'd done it. Something to tell my mates. You don't feel much of a person yourself afterwards; at least I didn't (boy, aged seventeen).

Well, I wouldn't say it was anything fantastic (boy, aged nineteen).

Tears. Up until then I'd thought of it as something I'd wanted to save until marriage. It seemed so silly that I'd lost it all in one night (girl, aged sixteen).

I wasn't actually disappointed. I didn't feel it was wrong, but it just didn't seem to have worked out right. I must have been worried about having a baby (girl, aged eighteen).

Hell, what's all the fuss about (girl, aged eighteen).

Leaving aside those who did not express a strong opinion either way, it still leaves over a third (36 per cent) of the boys for whom the first experience of sexual intercourse was not a success—that is, nearly half of all those boys who expressed an opinion. In the case of the girls, 54 per cent—that is, two-thirds of all those who expressed an opinion—were disenchanted with their first experience. These are unexpectedly high figures, especially for the boys who might have been reluctant to admit to the interviewer that they did not immediately take to sexual intercourse like a duck to water.

As so many of them did not enjoy their first sexual intercouse, one is prompted to ask why they should continue to repeat the experience if it was such a disappointment the first time. A few of them (6 per cent boys, 11 per cent girls) had not tried again, and there was an interval of over six months before some of the others (7 per cent boys, 6 per cent girls) had their second experience. But the disillusioned ones were in a minority, as Table IV shows. Most of them, girls as well as boys, were ready to try again, and within a month 54 per cent of the boys and 63 per cent of the girls had experienced sexual intercourse more than once; 7 per cent of the boys and 2 per cent of the girls had their second experience within twenty-four hours of the first.

TABLE IV

The Interval Between the First and Second
Experience of Sexual Intercourse

Interval	Boys %	Girls %
One day	7	2
Up to a week	19	33
Up to 2 weeks	12	13
2–4 weeks	16	15
1–6 months	33	20
Longer	7	6
No more sex	6	11
TOTAL	100	100

More girls (35 per cent) than boys (26 per cent) had sexual intercourse again within a week of their first experience. The girls may start later than the boys, and be more reluctant at first, but once they have crossed this barrier, they are not more inhibited than the boys.

Promiscuity

The teenagers were asked if they had intercourse with their first partner on more than one occasion. Over half the boys (54 per cent) and three-quarters of the girls (76 per cent) repeated the experience with the same person. The relationship continued for quite a long time in many cases, for a fifth of the boys and more than a third of the girls had sexual intercourse with their first partner on more than five occasions.

The boys, who in general were more likely to enjoy their first experience, were also more likely to move on to fresh fields and new conquests. Although the girls often felt unhappy about the first experience, they were prepared to try again with the same boy, sometimes for a considerable period. It is clear that, in some circumstances at least, the first sexual intercourse did not weaken or strain the relationship between the girl and the boy, and it may even have deepened and strengthened their association.

A large number of the sexually experienced teenagers have premarital intercourse with very close friends, and often with the person they will eventually marry. This is confirmed by the fact that a third of the experienced boys and three-quarters of the experienced girls had sexual intercourse with one partner only during the year before they were interviewed.

In addition to the engaged couples who decide to have sexual intercourse before their wedding day, there are also courting couples who decide to get married when the girl discovers that she is pregnant. This further increases the number of experienced teenagers who only have premarital intercourse with the person they will marry. It seems likely that much of the premarital activities of teenagers is not promiscuous behaviour.

Sometimes the newspapers seem to use the word 'promiscuity' as if it meant the same thing as premarital sexual intercourse. The *Oxford Dictionary* definition of promiscuity uses the words 'indiscriminate mixture' and it is usually taken to mean sexual intercourse with several partners over a period of time. Our results indicate that promiscuity is not a prominent feature of teenage sexual behaviour. Those who were most active sexually tended to have intercourse with only one person, while those who had many sexual partners tended to have intercourse less often. People often equate promiscuity with debauchery, but it appears that the promiscuous teenagers either do not want much sex, or else are not very successful at finding willing partners.

3

Other Sexual Behaviour

Inceptive Activities

Of course sexual intercourse is not the most important sexual activity for teenagers. Well over half the teenagers take part in activities which are often referred to as 'petting'. This is an American expression used to cover a wide variety of activities from a simple caress to a situation closely resembling sexual intercourse. We found this was rather too wide a term and so we used the word *inceptive* to cover three specific forms of sexual behaviour, namely: stimulating breasts under clothes, genital stimulation and genital apposition.

We found that just about a half (49 per cent) of our sample of nearly 2000 teenagers had inceptive experience, but did not have experience of sexual intercourse. It is just possible that a boy may be under the impression that he has had sexual intercourse when he has not in fact penetrated the girl. This is rare, but it does happen. Much less rare are the boys who have experienced genital apposition, but tell their friends that they have had full sexual intercourse.

It is significant that inceptive activities are likely to occur in the same sort of place and in the same sort of circumstances where intercourse could have occurred. So there are a large number of cases when the teenagers chose to have inceptive experience when they could have had intercourse.

About a quarter (17 per cent boys, 28 per cent girls) of all those with experience of genital apposition said they would prefer this to sexual intercourse. Some said they prefer it because it removes anxiety about pregnancy and venereal disease—although it is possible to catch VD during genital apposition, it is much less likely. Others (17 per cent boys, 26 per cent girls) agreed to genital apposition but disallowed sexual intercourse for moral reasons. According to their way of looking at things, intercourse troubled the conscience, whereas genital apposition did not. These arbitrary lines between what is morally permissible vary quite a lot. One boy said that anything is allowed so long as it is above the belt.

Then there are others who deliberately use these inceptive activities as a form of birth control. The girl may encourage the boy to reach orgasm before full intercourse can occur.

The other very interesting thing is that inceptive activities are much more acceptable behaviour to middle-class teenagers than to working-class boys and girls. We found—very much to our surprise—that there was practically no class difference between those who had intercourse and those who did not. Working-class boys and girls were neither more nor less likely to have experienced sexual intercourse than middle-class teenagers. But for some reason middle-class teenagers were much more likely to get satisfaction from inceptive activities.

Homosexuality

About a fifth (21 per cent) of all the boys said they knew of homosexual activities among their school friends, and 5 per cent admitted they took part themselves. These figures are probably under-estimates. Westwood[6] found that sexual play between boys aged thirteen to fifteen was usually a form of curiosity, and was not recognised or acknowledged as homosexuality by the boys themselves. After a phase of experimentation there was usually a latent period even for the boys who would eventually become adult homosexuals. Between sixteen and nineteen those with homosexual tendencies went through a period of shame and guilt combined with a strong determination to combat these inclinations. Only at a later age, usually in the early twenties, can the homosexual begin to accept himself and find his way to the homosexual coteries.

Therefore it can be seen that boys aged fifteen to nineteen will not readily answer questions about homosexuality, and information about these activities is more easily obtained by asking older people to look back to the time when they were teenagers.

Just under 2 per cent of the boys admitted to homosexual experience with adults, although 35 per cent said that at least one man had made sexual advances to them. In an attitude inventory, 47 per cent of the boys agreed that homosexuals should be severely punished and 35 per cent disagreed with this statement. So many of the men who were alleged to have made sexual advances to these boys risked being rudely repulsed. But it is not unknown for manifestations of friendship towards a boy to be mistaken for signs of homosexuality (Schofield[4]).

Among the boys who had homosexual experiences with other boys there is little difference between the social classes. Homosexuality was slightly more prevalent at boarding schools. Among the boys 23 per cent said they knew of homosexual activities which had occurred at their segregated school (4 per cent admitted taking part themselves), compared with 17 per cent who said homosexual activities occurred at their coeducational school (5 per cent admitted taking part). At the boarding schools 44 per cent said homosexual activities between the boys were not unknown (28 per cent admitted taking part), whereas at the day schools 18 per cent said homosexual activities went on between the boys (only 3 per cent admitted taking part).

A similar trend was found in the girls' schools although the figures are smaller; homosexual activities occurred in 13 per cent of the segregated schools, 10 per cent of the coeducational schools; it was also reported in 39 per cent of the boarding schools and 11 per cent of the day schools. Kinsey[3] found less homosexuality among the females he interviewed. We found 12 per cent who said there were homosexual activities at school and 2 per cent who admitted taking part.

Slightly less than 1 per cent of the girls admitted homosexual activities with an adult, and 9 per cent said that a woman had made sexual advances to them. If these figures are credible, then it seems as if about one in ten girls to whom homosexual advances are made is likely to succumb, and about one in seven boys to whom homosexual advances are made may submit. But attitudes to homosexuality have changed so much in the last few years, especially since the change in the law, that changes in behaviour are now taking place. The new generation of young people take a far less solemn view of this problem and they cannot see what all the fuss is about. If a boy or a girl does have sexual experience with someone of the same sex, they are far less likely to feel guilty about it, or jump to the conclusion that they must be homosexual. Young men are also more affectionate to each other and are less afraid of touching and embracing other males.

This new attitude may mean that casual homosexual acts are more frequent, but it will also mean that far fewer young men and girls are likely to be plagued with a homosexual 'problem'.

4

Learning About Sex

Knowledge and Conception

When do children find out about sex? We found that girls learnt about 'the facts of life' before boys; the average age for girls was 12·2 and for boys 12·5.

About a quarter of the boys and a third of the girls said they knew about the facts of life at the age of eleven or earlier. By thirteen two-thirds of the boys and three-quarters of the girls knew about conception. Whether or not their information was accurate is not relevant in this context; the important point is that most adolescents have heard at least one version of how babies are born soon after entering secondary school, if not before.

Fig. 3 shows that most boys (62 per cent) and many of the girls (44 per cent) learnt about conception from their friends, usually through jokes which are quite often smutty and obscene. In over a quarter (27 per cent) of the cases the girls obtained this information from their mothers. Fathers seem to have no role at all at this stage of their daughter's education and sons do not fare much better. Only 7 per cent of the boys learnt about conception from their fathers and the same number obtained this information from books. Girls are still less likely to learn from books and it appears that the many thousands of books published on this subject for adolescents are read after they have heard about conception from other sources, if they are read at all. Teachers appear to fulfil a more important role for both sexes, and are the second most frequent source for boys—but a long way behind school friends; 12 per cent of the boys and 18 per cent of the girls first heard about conception from teachers. For both sexes they are probably the most important source of accurate information.

But the significance of the part teachers play can be better understood when we combine the source of information with the age when they first learnt about the facts of life. Those who learn from friends or from parents tend to get the information early, while those who learn from teachers are more likely to get the information at fourteen or later, as shown in Fig. 4.

The younger the boy learns the facts of life, the more likely he is to learn from friends. As he gets older, the influence of the teacher increases and the influence of the parent decreases. Those who feel that the parents are the right people to give sex instruction should note that there seems to be a maximum age when parents will do this. If the parents have not instructed the child by twelve or thirteen, it becomes more and more unlikely that they will ever do so.

There is also a social class factor here. The middle-class adolescents learn about conception before the working-class children. I know that some people have the impression that sex is talked about more simply and naturally in working-class homes, and it is the middle-class parents who are reluctant to discuss sexual matters with their children. But this is not what we found.

The most likely explanation is that some middle-class mothers feel that it is necessary to warn their daughters before their first menstruation and this in turn leads to an explanation of conception. It is possible, of course, that working-class mothers are equally anxious to forewarn their daughters, but find it more difficult to put this into words. Sociological research on the use of language has shown that there are wide social class differences in the way people make use of abstract terms and generic notions, something which middle-class teachers and youth leaders do not always take into account (Bernstein).[1]

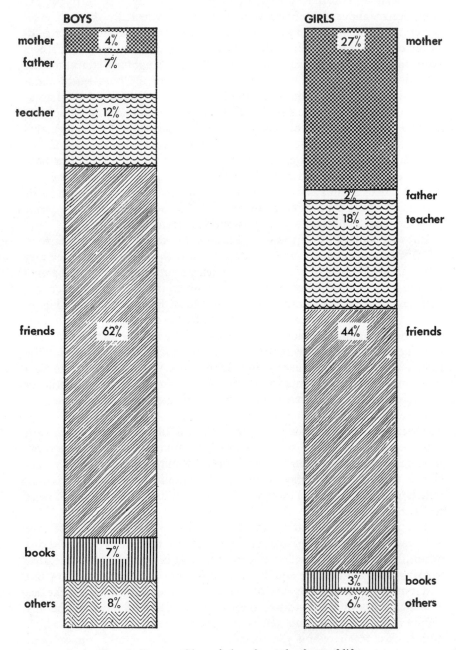

FIG. 3. Source of knowledge about the facts of life.

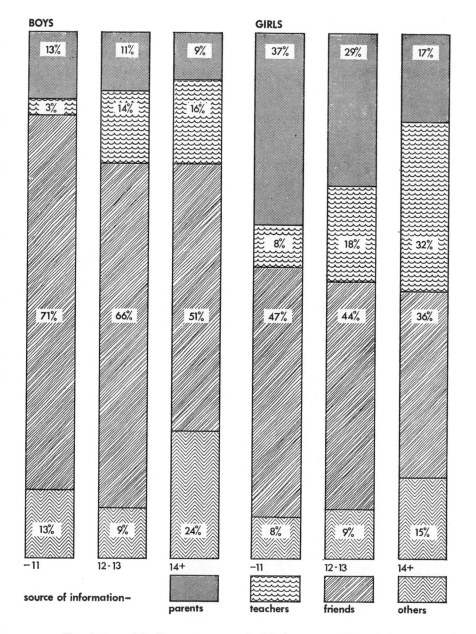

FIG. 4. Age of finding out compared with the source of knowledge.

Fig. 5 shows that the middle-class mother is much more likely to have talked to her daughter about the facts of life; indeed, middle-class girls are the only group who are more likely to have heard about conception from parents than from friends.

The schoolteacher is more likely to be the source of information for working-class girls, but not for the boys. Only 13 per cent of working-class

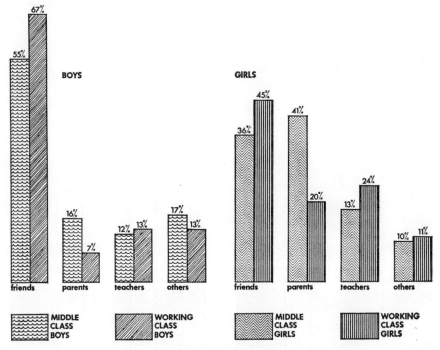

FIG. 5. Source of knowledge about conception by social class.

boys learnt the facts of life from a teacher, and this compares with 12 per cent middle-class boys. But 24 per cent of working-class girls learnt from a teacher, and this compares with 13 per cent of the middle-class girls. So for a quarter of the working-class girls the teacher is an important influence.

By far the most important source amongst working-class boys is their friends; about two-thirds of the boys learn the facts of life from people of their own age. It is clear that the working-class boy is the one who most needs sex education, and he is also the one who is least likely to get it.

Advice from Parents

We have seen that parents are only rarely the initiators of sex knowledge. But parents can play a continuing role as sex educators, and many people have suggested that this is the best method: the parents should avoid a lecture on sex, but should continue to inform the child as the need arises.

We tried to find out how far this worked out in practice. In fact, we found that 67 per cent of the boys and 29 per cent of the girls said they never at any time had any advice about sex from their parents.

It is possible that some of these adolescents were advised by their parents, but they did not listen, or perhaps found the advice so unacceptable that they dismissed it from their minds. Even so, it is remarkable that over two-thirds of the boys and a quarter of the girls felt that neither of their parents had helped them to deal with the problem of sex.

Sex Education

In view of all the discussions about sex education in recent years, it was surprising to find that over half the boys said they had never received any kind of sex education at school. Girls are much more likely to be given some kind of formal education about sex and the extent does not seem to vary among the different types of schools. Whether they go to private or state schools, eight out of ten girls will receive sex education. Seven out of ten boys going to private schools are likely to receive sex education; but less than half the boys going to state schools receive sex education, and this was just as true of those at grammar schools as for those at secondary modern, technical or comprehensive. The lack of sex education is exactly where it is most needed; it is the working-class boys who are least likely to learn about sex from their parents, and are least likely to receive sex education at school.

There were signs of a lack of frankness in the teaching. Sex education, when it occurred, seemed to concentrate on biological and physiological matters, and seemed to be unrelated to human affairs, except when it was wholly concerned with putting across a particular moral point of view.

Nearly half the boys (47 per cent) and girls (43 per cent) felt they should have been told more about sex at school. The teenagers were dissatisfied with the amount of sex education they received, and with its quality. Of course, the difficulties of providing viable education about sex are immense; much of the moral code is based upon religious thinking which the teenagers do not accept and many of the arguments against premarital intercourse, when unsupported by moral exhortations, sound rather weak to many young people. In addition we have found a strong inclination among a large number of teenagers to reject adult advice of all kinds. But there is also plenty of evidence from this research that teenagers are anxious to be informed about sex and want sex education, providing it is given with an assurance which is backed by knowledge and with a proper understanding of their particular problems.

Advice for Teenagers

Most boys and girls know about sexual intercourse before the age of thirteen. So it is clear that most attempts at sex education are given too late. Even fewer teenagers get advice on sexual matters from their parents. Over two-thirds of the boys and a quarter of the girls said that neither of their parents had given them any advice about sex. But of course one can assume that by the time these boys and girls are eighteen and nineteen they know quite a lot about sex. Most of their information would not have been obtained from books, or teachers or parents, so one must assume that they also possess a large amount of misinformation as well.

It is worth remembering that if someone misses out on an important fact about sex, it is almost impossible for that person to ask his friends for information—he would not want to look so naïve to his friends. So even at the late age of eighteen there are some teenagers with quite surprising gaps in their knowledge.

Incidentally one of the gaps is what to do about crab lice, a not uncommon infection among some groups. I was surprised to find how distressed many young people are when they get the crabs and find that these lice cannot be killed or removed by washing. Some of the teenagers we met had been trying desperately for weeks to cleanse themselves; one was taking a near-boiling bath twice a day; another used a garden insecticide; another shaved his entire body. All because they did not know they could be rid of the crabs with one single application of Gamma Benzene Hexachloride.

A more serious gap in young people's knowledge is about the venereal diseases. We had some very strange replies when we asked them what they knew about VD; the most disturbing reply was: 'I don't know anything about it and I don't want to know.' There were quite a few who replied in this way, a situation where ignorance is a greater menace than the disease itself.

People who comment on teenage morality often bracket illegitimacy and venereal disease as equal scourges of society. But this is a mistake. There is no doubt that the risks of illegitimacy are far greater and the consequences are more serious. I think it should be stated in a straightforward way that VD can always be completely cured, providing it is detected and properly treated in the early stages.

In the field of venereal diseases medicine has had some of its greatest success. They are no longer a great social menace. However, deep down in many people there still remains the superstition that they are different from other diseases, that they are punishment for sin. There are still some doctors who are reluctant to make clear the medical fact that VD is quite curable, providing it is properly treated. They seem to prefer to look upon VD as a kind of retribution—a punishment for those who indulge in premarital sexual intercourse. I consider this attitude to be quite unethical.

On the other hand it would be wrong to ignore the whole subject. The disease is only curable if it is detected early, and it will only be detected early if those at risk know the symptoms. In fact we found that only a few boys (14 per cent) and still fewer girls (11 per cent) can really be said to know the symptoms of the venereal diseases.

It appears to me as if the educational campaign about venereal disease has been misdirected. It has been used to scare people off sex. The important thing is to make sure that people who have been infected are not scared to come to a clinic where they can be cured easily and quickly.

Contraception

At one time rubber contraceptives for males could only be sold in some States of America on condition that they were used solely and specifically for the prevention of disease. This was a kind of compromise between those who felt that people should be helped before they risked catching VD and those who thought they should be helped only after they had caught the diseases. The same sort of attitude can be seen today between people who are for and against giving the contraceptive pill to unmarried girls.

We found that a large number of boys and girls having sexual intercourse were not using any kind of contraceptive device. We asked all the teenagers with experience of sexual intercourse if they always took precautions. Less than half of the boys always used some form of birth control and a quarter of the boys having sexual intercourse had never used any kind of birth-control method.

Even fewer girls used any birth-control methods. Many girls still feel that birth control is the man's business, and so all the experienced girls were asked if they insisted that their sexual partner took precautions. About a third (35 per cent) always insisted, but nearly a half (45 per cent) did not insist. Although the girls must bear nearly all the consequences of an unwanted pregnancy, the majority neither took precautions themselves, nor insisted upon their partners using any contraceptive method. And yet they are the ones that have to deal with the problem and have to face up to the embarrassment and difficulties of conception before marriage, an illegitimate birth or an abortion.

Of course it is easy for us to imply that young people are careless and irresponsible because they do not use contraceptives. In fact it is still quite difficult for teenagers to get contraceptives despite the policies of some student health departments and family-planning clinics. Furthermore, the circumstances in which intercourse is likely to take place make it difficult for many young people to use contraceptives. As sexual intercourse within marriage is socially accepted, it is not too difficult to make preparations and have contraceptives available. But premarital intercourse is discouraged, and therefore when it does take place, it is often unpremeditated and furtive; in these circumstances birth control is less likely to be practised. Unfortunately the consequences of an unwanted pregnancy are far more serious for the unmarried than for the married.

An advisory youth service can be most helpful to an engaged couple who are regularly sleeping together, but for many young people sexual intercourse is an impulsive act. The contraceptive pill is of no value unless it is taken regularly and therefore cannot protect the girl who is persuaded at the moment of sexual excitement to agree to have intercourse with a boy.

The very success of the student health services has created the curious situation that advisory centres have become the social work cliché of the moment. But students are not representative of other young people who are less articulate, less able to analyse their situation and verbalise their problem, and are less likely to seek help and advice. The person who sits in his room waiting for adolescents to come to him with their problems is going to miss those who most need help. The adolescents who are most likely to be misinformed about sex would not think of going to an advisory centre, and probably do not even admit that they have got any problems.

5

The Sexual Revolution

Comparisons with the Past

People always ask if there is more sexual activity now than before, as if there were something inviolable in the standards of the past. We talk about a sexual revolution, but it is more likely to be a gradual trend. Kinsey[2] showed that changes in sexual behaviour vary only slightly over the years. Attitudes, of course, change much faster than actual behaviour. It is much easier to express an opinion than to put it into practice. I would say that twenty years ago adolescents probably had more sex than they would admit to, whereas today adolescents almost certainly have less sex than they say they have.

Attitudes influence behaviour and clearly a change in attitudes will eventually cause a change in behaviour. This can be illustrated with a simple diagram.

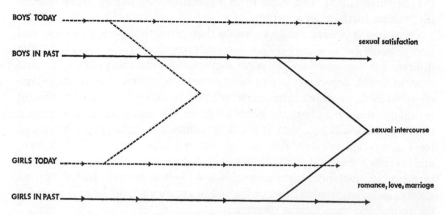

In general the boy's goal is sexual satisfaction, whereas the girl's goal is romance, love and marriage. When the boy modifies his attitude and starts to think in terms of love and marriage, and when the girl modifies her attitude and is aroused sexually, then intercourse is more likely to occur. Attitudes today have changed. The boy's attitude against early marriage has hardened, but only slightly. The girl's attitude to sexual satisfaction has become more permissive; so the two attitudes are closer than before, and therefore it is easier for the two attitudes to be modified sufficiently to allow intercourse to take place.

The Future

My view of the future is no more acute than anyone else's. It seems probable that more young people will accept premarital sexual intercourse as a normal prelude to marriage, and there is less opposition to this from adults who advise adolescents. The idea seems to have got around that if you are unmarried and want contraceptives, you have got to convince the doctor at the local clinic that you are really in love. The so-called permissive radicals have emphasised so much that premarital sexual intercourse is acceptable when it is a lasting mature relationship with one partner, that there is a danger that the first time in bed for two young people will become more binding than an engagement ring. This would be a great pity, for it remains true that people who marry young tend to have less stable marriages, and one is more likely to make a better choice if one has a wider choice.

It is not completely inconceivable that in the future psychiatrists will be saying that we need more promiscuity, not less. At all events it is time we all agreed that most people find sexual intercourse very enjoyable. It follows from this that there are a lot of people who enjoy their sexual activities so much that they want more of them with more people. You may wish to call these people hedonistic or immoral, but I would hesitate before I called them disturbed or maladjusted.

REFERENCES

1. BERNSTEIN, B. 1961. Social structure, language and learning. *Educ. Res.*, 3, 3, 163.
2. KINSEY, A. C., POMEROY, W. B. and MARTIN, C. E. 1948. *Sexual behaviour in the human male*. Philadelphia: Saunders.
3. KINSEY, A. C., POMEROY, W. B., MARTIN, C. E. and GEBHARD, P. H. 1953. *Sexual behaviour in the human female*. Philadelphia: Saunders.
4. SCHOFIELD, M. 1965. *Sociological aspects of homosexuality*. London: Longmans.
5. SCHOFIELD, M. 1968. *The sexual behaviour of young people*. Harmondsworth: Penguin Books.
6. WESTWOOD, G. 1960. *A minority: a report on the life of the male homosexual in Great Britain*. London: Longmans.

IV

THE SIGNIFICANCE OF INTELLIGENCE RATINGS IN ADOLESCENCE

JOHN R. LICKORISH

B.D., B.A., DIP.ED., A.B.PS.S.

Principal Clinical Psychologist
The Institute of Family Psychiatry
The Ipswich Hospital
Ipswich, England

1

Introduction

The Intellectual Importance of Adolescence

Adolescence is the developmental phase between childhood and adulthood. According to Tanner[24] it may extend from the age of nine to eighteen years. Its duration varies not only with the individual but also according to the criteria used to define it. During adolescence the individual may undergo more changes than in any other comparable phase of development; except the first five years. Adolescence is a time when many decisions are taken which have far-reaching effects upon the individual's future welfare. Prominent among them are decisions regarding education and vocation. These in turn are largely influenced by the individual's intellectual ability. Late adolescence is usually considered to be the period during which the individual's intelligence attains its maximum development. Intelligence ratings are therefore of particular importance to the adolescent and a discussion of them is appropriate in a volume devoted to the psychiatry of adolescence.

Scope of the Discussion

A full discussion of intelligence would obviously require a volume to itself. In one chapter, only a few selected aspects of this important topic can be discussed. Accordingly, the present discussion is concerned with some of the more important notions of intelligence and its assessment and with the application of intelligence ratings in day-to-day clinical work. In order to distinguish between theory and application, this chapter is divided into three parts. The first part discusses salient concepts of intelligence; the second, methods of assessing it; whilst the third part describes the relevance of these assessments to the problems and decisions of the adolescent.

Since adolescence is such an attenuated phase of development, it seemed advisable to relate this discussion to the latter part of the period, when major decisions are frequently made. The discussion is highly selective. No attempt is made to review all the problems, or to survey the extensive literature in this field. Nor is there much discussion of the main tests of intelligence, since they are well known and their general usefulness is not in dispute.

Terminology

In the present discussion of intelligence ratings and assessments, references are frequently made to experimental and advisory procedures. In these contexts the term 'patient' is hardly appropriate, and so the terms 'client' and 'subject' are often employed. 'Subject' is denoted by **S** in the conventional manner (plural **Ss**, and apostrophe **S's Ss'**). Also the term experimenter, or examiner, **E**, is more suitable in some contexts than the professional designations of psychiatrist, or psychologist.

2

Theoretical Aspects of Intelligence

The Semantic Problem of Definition

There is still considerable controversy about the exact nature of intelligence, and no one definition is acceptable to all authorities. The difficulty of defining intelligence arises from two sources. First, there is a *semantic difficulty*, due to the fact that ordinary language is frequently misleading when used to describe scientific concepts. Secondly, intelligence is a concept which is difficult to define in simple terms. A brief theoretical consideration of these two difficulties may enable a clearer understanding of the nature of intelligence to be obtained.

The *semantic difficulty* may be illustrated by the use of three pairs of simple questions. Consider the two questions:

1. Where is his heart?   2. Where is his intelligence?

Both these questions have the same simple structure and are precisely alike in grammatical form. They could both be regarded as rhetorical questions. But considered as scientific questions, there is a clear, precise answer to question 1; whereas there is no such answer to question 2. The word 'intelligence' is an abstract noun and refers to a concept only. The word does not refer to any 'thing' which a person possesses, in the sense that he possesses a heart.

Next consider the questions:

1. What is his blood-pressure?   2. What is his I.Q.?

To both of these questions it is possible to give a numerical answer. But there the similarity between them ends. Blood pressure is measured in terms of the pressure exerted by a column of mercury and is expressed in physical units, which are part of the general scientific system of physical measurements. (The c.g.s. system.) But the numerical answer to the second question is not related to any kind of physical measurement. It is either a ratio, as the term intelligence *quotient* (I.Q.) indicates, or it denotes the person's *ordinal position* with respect to the other members of a certain class. Whichever view of the 'I.Q.' is accepted, it is a *number*, which derives its significance from other numbers and not from c.g.s. units. A person's 'intelligence' cannot therefore be measured in the ordinary sense of the word 'measure'. For measure implies a *unit* of measurement, and no such unit of intelligence exists. It follows that it is correct to speak of the *assessment* of intelligence, but not of its measurement. The widely used term 'psychometrics' is therefore a misnomer and should be abandoned.

The third pair of questions brings us to the crucial issue of defining intelligence. We ask:

1. What is a heart?   2. What is intelligence?

Again the first question has a precise answer in terms of the material structure and functioning of nerve cells, muscle fibres and so on. The second question has no such precise answer, since intelligence is not a 'thing', but simply a name for whatever it is 'that enables a person to carry out effectively, a specified set of operations'. By referring to intelligence in this way, it is possible to define it in terms of the actions that S performs. This is an *operational definition* of intelligence, which stands in contrast to the *open* or *descriptive* type of definition.

Open and Operational Definitions

There are broadly two distinct ways of defining intelligence. They are known as the *open* and the *operational* types of definition. The former conceives of intelligence along popular, common-sense lines and judges intelligence in terms of success in a variety of real-life situations. It is a *descriptive* rather than a definitive view. The *operational* viewpoint on the other hand demands precise, scientific definition. If strictly adhered to, this view would result in an impoverishment of the concept of intelligence. It would exclude the higher ranges of ability and the more interesting and unusual human achievements. At present, an operational definition must be specifically related to the scores obtained in some kind of test. Yet, so far no test has been devised which would do justice to the diverse intellectual abilities of an Einstein, a Churchill or a Sibelius. For all practical purposes, it may be that an operational definition, with a relatively low 'ceiling' of ability, is all that is needed. Whether the full range of the human intellect can ever be comprehended within its own definition is at least doubtful. It is by no means certain that the study of intelligence cannot form 'an integral part of scientific enquiry' unless the 'open' concept is replaced by 'an agreed and measurable dimension or set of dimensions' (Butcher[6]). There is of course no objection to limiting intelligence to a 'set of dimensions', so long as it is remembered that the dimensions may exclude some of the statistically infrequent, but immensely important, aspects of intelligence. The most significant aspects of intelligence may not be those which are common to everybody. Far more important may be the characteristics possessed by relatively few people which elude an operational definition. Behind this demand for the all-embracing definition lurks the belief that scientific psychology is unable to deal with what is unique, but can deal only with typical examples of a general law. This is part of the behaviourist fallacy and is of diminishing importance in current psychological theory.

Whatever criticisms may be levelled against current concepts of intelligence the general idea of intelligence is, according to Butcher,[6] 'no less satisfactory than other psychological abstractions and a great deal more useful than many of them'.

Intelligence as an Intervening Variable

Discussion of the fundamental nature of intelligence can be sidetracked if intelligence is regarded as an *intervening variable*. The nature of this concept is clarified by reference to Fig. 1. This is a simple, input–process–

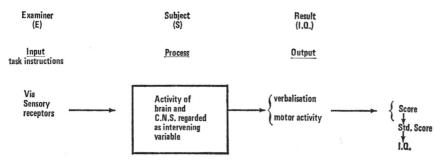

FIG. 1. Diagram to illustrate the concept of intelligence as an intervening variable.

output diagram. So far as the concept of intelligence is concerned, the *input* consists of task instructions given by **E**, about the materials which have to be manipulated. As a result of this *sensory input*, certain unspecified *processes* occur within **S**'s brain and CNS. The *output* consists of verbal answers and/or materials which have been arranged in an appropriate manner. The *output* is scored, and these *raw scores* are converted into standard scores and so into an I.Q. Provided that the information on the *input* side is always presented in a *standardised manner* and provided that the *output* is always assessed in a *standardised manner*, then it is possible, if inadvisible, to forget about the actual nature of intelligence for practical purposes. The output of each individual is assessed by his standard score, which, in turn, gives the value of his I.Q. The standard score locates his position on the curve of normal distribution, Fig. 2. It also places him within a given range of intellectual ability, as shown on the linear scale below the curve in Fig. 2.

Innate Cognitive Ability

The current concept of intelligence arose from the work of Spencer and Galton in the nineteenth century. They both believed in a *general ability*, underlying, but distinct from, *special abilities*. The well-known physiologists Hughlings Jackson and Sherrington supported this idea and it was accepted by many psychologists, including Burt[4] and Spearman.[22] The latter writer popularised the concept of 'g', the *general factor* in mental ability. This *general factor* was thought to depend upon the number of cells in the cerebral cortex and the complexity of the nervous pathways between them. This view is still held by many neurologists and psychologists.

Burt defined intelligence as 'innate general cognitive ability'. However, it is known that scores on intelligence tests are influenced by environmental factors. It follows therefore that 'intelligence' as defined by Burt[4] is not necessarily the same as the 'intelligence' assessed by tests. The evidence for an *innate* ability is fairly impressive and is derived from three different types of investigations: (1) the study of pedigree records of families; (2) the correlation of data taken from family groups; (3) the study of the resemblances between twins.

Genetic Factors

Whilst the general case for the hereditary factor in intellectual endowment is quite strong, very little is known about its genetic transmission. Consequently there are a number of hypotheses about the hereditary transmission of intelligence. None of them is entirely satisfactory, but according to Thomson[26] any adequate theory must account for the following facts. (*i*) Intelligence is a quantitative character with a wide dispersion. (*ii*) The fact that the intelligence of offspring does not increase, or decrease consistently from generation to generation, but that it tends to revert towards the mean value of the intelligence of the population as a whole. (*iii*) The variation of intelligence between siblings tends to be greatest within the middle range of intelligence and not at the extreme ranges. (*iv*) The correlation of intelligence between parents and children has often been found to be equal to, or greater than, the correlation between siblings. The second of these points would seem to require that 'normal intelligence' should exert

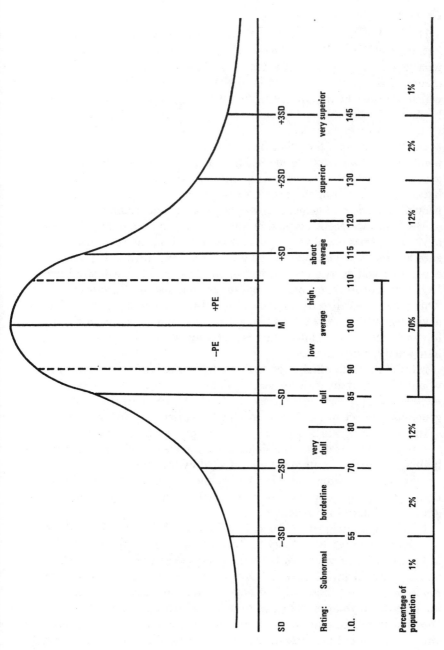

FIG. 2. The curve of normal distribution and linear scale of categories of ability.

a dominant genetic effect, but points (*iii*) and (*iv*) are not consistent with this requirement.

Intelligence A *and Intelligence* B

Hebb[14] put forward the view that there were two basic types of intelligence which he called *intelligence A* and *intelligence B*. Intelligence *A* he regarded as innate potential, which is the individual's *capacity* for development. This concept corresponds to the geneticist's idea of the *genotype*, which refers to the inherited qualities of the individual. These qualities can be neither observed nor measured; they are inferred from the ways in which individuals behave.

Intelligence *B* on the other hand is not an inherited quality. It corresponds to the *phenotype*, and depends upon the *interaction* between the genes and the pre- and post-natal environment of the individual. Intelligence *B* is not simply learned, or acquired ability, but the result of a person's natural endowment *interacting* with the environment.

Much of the recent discussion about intelligence concerns the relation of *A* to *B*. It has not always been realised that if the effects of early experience are more or less generalised and permanent, then it is possible that experience will exert a major effect upon the I.Q. But it will still leave the I.Q. with its constancy and its validity as an index of future performance. This view leads directly to the opinion that an enriching and adequate environment may raise the I.Q. but that it will not rise above a given limit for each individual. This limit is determined by the *capacity* of each individual for development.

Most of the facts which suggest that intelligence is genetically determined would be consistent with the assumptions: (1) that heredity sets a *limit* to intelligence; (2) that early learning tends to be permanent and has a generalised effect, which is not specific to particular situations.

Intelligence *A* will not develop to the limit set by genetic endowment unless the brain itself as a physiological organ also develops properly. The brain of the foetus in utero may be affected by the mother's illness, anxiety or other stressful situations. Hence the child may be born with a brain that does not develop properly, and hence it is incapable of realising its full *genetically* determined potential.

In later life, intelligence *B* may be affected if the brain is injured, or if it deteriorates so that its capacity for further learning is impaired. Variations in the intelligence ratings of the same person over a period of time are due to variations in intelligence *B*. On the other hand, a person reared in a *stable environment* shows little if any variation in successive ratings of his intelligence. It follows from this that *B* is affected by cultural conditions, and that it will be assessed in terms of the criteria which are acceptable within a given culture. In western-type societies these criteria are mainly concerned with problem-solving, the grasping of relationships and the manipulation of symbols, especially verbal symbols.

Vernon[28] points out that 'an intelligence test is no more than a sample of the kinds of skills we regard as intelligent'. So far as school children are concerned, these skills are often sampled by the Stanford–Binet type of test, which assesses intelligence B fairly accurately in western cultures. However, other tests do not give identical estimates of B, since presumably they sample rather different abilities. As children grow older, the traditional type of intelligence test becomes less useful as a means of sampling the qualities that are generally held to indicate intelligence. The more sophisticated popular view judges intelligence on the basis of success, cleverness, quickness of thought and action, 'understanding of life', and general information and 'know-how'. These qualities may well differentiate between the more and the less intelligent, but they are not always represented in orthodox intelligence tests.

Moreover, most tests do not adequately differentiate between the mediocre and the outstandingly able person in high-grade secondary schools or universities. Members of these groups would all score fairly highly in a test, yet some are obviously more 'intelligent' than others. As a means of distinguishing the ability denoted by a test score from other intelligent ability, Vernon[28] proposes the use of the term 'intelligence C'. In this usage 'intelligence C' is related directly to the score obtained in a test. It may, or may not, be an accurate assessment of intelligence A or B.

Factor Theories of Intelligence

The first theory of specific factors of intelligence was put forward by Spearman as long ago as 1904. He suggested that the performance of any given intellectual task depended upon a general factor 'g', together with a specific factor 's', which was applicable to that task only. Moreover, different tasks depended upon 'g' and 's' in varying degrees. For some tasks the relative value of 'g' might be high and 's' low, and for others, vice versa. He thus developed a two-factor theory of intellectual ability.

Other types of theories are:

Monarchic—ability depends on only *one* factor. *Oligarchic*—ability depends upon several factors, all of which are approximately equal in importance. *Anarchic*—each task requires a specific ability. Spearman's *two-factor theory* lies between the monarchic and the oligarchic types.

Although Spearman's theory has been subjected to very searching criticism, it has withstood the attacks remarkably well. It is perhaps too simple a view of the complexity of human ability, and it can logically be superseded by the *four-factor theory* propounded by Burt.[4] This theory is based upon a logical analysis of what the factors must account for and resolves itself into four categories as follows:

A factor in *all* activity	g
A factor present in *some* activities	p
A factor present in *a particular activity*	s
A factor present *on a particular occasion*	e

The total effect (T) of the various factors in any one test is therefore, $T = g + p + s + e$. But the influence of each factor varies from test to test, and therefore each factor has a *loading* which indicates how much it contributes to the result in a given test. Thus if M stands for the total measured output of a person in a given test, on a given occasion then:

$$M = n \cdot g + \Sigma(m \cdot p) + \Sigma(q \cdot s) + \Sigma(r \cdot e)$$

In this equation the sign Σ stands for 'the sum of' and the letters n, m, q, r are the *factor loadings* which are always decimal fractions. There may be several of each of the factors p, s and e, each with its own appropriate loading. It is therefore necessary to determine the sum of the values of these various factors; hence the use of the sign Σ. There is of course only one value for g on each occasion, but the *factor loading* for g may vary from test to test.

The Distribution of Intelligence

It is frequently assumed that intelligence is *normally distributed* throughout the general population. In practice, this implies that the scores on an intelligence test gained by a large population would, when plotted, form a curve very similar to the Gaussian curve of normal distribution, Fig. 2. Many other human traits are assumed to be normally distributed, especially those to which many genes contribute. There is clear evidence for a large genetic component in intelligence, and it is also a fair assumption that the genetic influence is multifactorial. On these assumptions Lewis[17] points out that each factor which influences intelligence may be regarded as one allele in a pair of genes, say Aa, where A is the factor contributing to intelligence. If the number of pairs is large (Aa, Bb, Cc . . . Nn), and if each allele always has an equal chance of being present in the zygote, then the distribution of the alleles influencing intelligence (represented by the capital letters) would form an approximately normal distribution. This is certainly an over-simplification of the genetic mechanism, for no notice is taken of dominance, or assortive mating, or of linkage. Lewis, however, points out that Fisher has shown that such a general mechanism may be postulated and a normal, or near normal, distribution of the contributing factors still obtained. Fisher argues from the distribution of stature, and Burt uses a similar argument, since he defined intelligence as *innate ability*. But it does not follow that, because it is innate, intelligence is simply normally distributed. It is sometimes claimed that the normal distribution of intelligence has been established as the result of intelligence testing. But the fact is, that it is almost impossible to produce a sufficient number of test items which adequately distinguish between different levels of ability and yet *at the same time* do not form an artificially arranged distribution.

It has been claimed that the test items from the Binet Scale support the normal distribution theory. But this test depends upon the principles by which the items are selected and that in turn influences the distribution of the scores.

Burt[5] has suggested that the curve which corresponds most closely to the actual distribution of intelligence may be asymmetrical and either positively or negatively skewed.

His views have been based not on single tests given to one particular set of children, but on very wide surveys. For example, since 1917 the normality of the frequency distributions obtained from surveys in the former London County Council area were regularly checked by the χ^2 method and in every case the distribution was found to diverge significantly from the normal.

Another investigation entailed administering the Stanford Binet Test to 1835 children in an unselected sample of the general school population between the ages of six and eleven. The mean I.Q. of this sample was 103, the medium was 101 and the standard deviation was 14·9. On testing this distribution for goodness of fit, it was found to differ significantly from a normal distribution. Even if the cases of mental deficiency are omitted from these figures, the curve still differed significantly from a normal Gaussian curve. Numerous surveys, carried out by various investigators, nearly always yield a similar type of curve, although occasionally, the deviations from the curve of normal distribution are not significant.

Fraser Roberts administered the Advanced Otis Scale to 2553 children between the ages of nine and twelve years in the City of Bath. He found that the distribution did not differ significantly from the normal. There was, however, a *negative skewing* of the curve, i.e. a definite 'heaping up' at the lower end of the scale, which is typical of the results of intelligence testing.

The scores obtained from the Binet Scale do give a more or less normal distribution, but these results are themselves dependent upon item selection. Hence the bell-shaped distribution of the Binet quotients cannot be used to verify the distribution of intelligence as a whole. Burt[5] apparently thinks that a moderately asymmetrical curve provides the 'best fit' for the available evidence.

There is also a very practical test. The assumption of approximate normality has been adopted for a wide variety of administrative purposes over a long period of years. In organising classes, in planning the number of schools to be built, in devising, or standardising schemes of marking, or grading and in numerous other ways, the distributions suggested by the normal curve have proved their usefulness. It is hardly likely that the normal distribution curve would have been such a reliable guide in practice, unless it corresponded fairly closely to the actual distribution of innate ability in the general population.

Other general arguments in support of the normal distribution of intelligence are as follows:

(1) It agrees with common-sense notions: namely the number of

geniuses is relatively small, and the number of mental defectives is small. (2) Most persons are average, or about average, in ability. (3) These views would require only a 'hump' type curve, of which the normal distribution is one particular example. But as a specialist in test construction once remarked, 'It is convenient to have intelligence follow the normal curve; we know so much about it' (Lewis[17]).

Dimensions of the Mind

Babcock[3] long ago pointed out the relationship between time and intelligence. She also distinguished between the *level* of intelligence and the *efficiency* with which intelligence functions. She regarded the level of intelligence as a dimension of the mind. The first dimension she called *sensory discrimination*. Without this the mind could not acquire any data with which to operate. This view is in line with the dictum: 'nil est in intellectu quod non antea fuit in sensibus' (nothing is in the mind which was not previously in the senses). The second dimension of the mind is *memory*. This is the 'mnemic', or conserving, capacity by which data is retained. In this way the mind acquires a store of data which can be manipulated as a result of intelligent activity. If the mind can 'work on' its stored information, new *combinations* of data are possible and the mind is truly creative. For although the original data were acquired via the senses, the new patterns of data which emerge are the direct result of mental activity. The third dimension of the mind is equated with the *level of intelligence*. The level of intelligence tends to determine the use that is made of other mental abilities. It determines the kind of data that a person can comprehend and it increases the amount that can be remembered. By classifying, and by the formation of concepts, a large amount of data can be handled effectively, stored easily and retrieved when necessary. (This view does not deny the fact that personality traits may seriously interfere with the storage of information.) The *level of intelligence* controls the formulation of principles and the grasping of similarities between apparently disparate sets of data. This leads to the verbalisation of the results, and hence the mind is able to answer increasingly difficult questions.

The fourth dimension of the mind may be regarded as the *mental tempo*. The speed with which the mind operates affects the number of memories it can store and the amount of experience it can undergo. These facts in turn affect the size of the mind's apperceptive background and determine the amount of available data on which it can work.

Divergent and Convergent Thinking

When a problem has several, possible equally, correct answers, *divergent thinking* is required in order to solve it. Suppose **S** is asked to name as many uses as he can for a given object, e.g. a shovel. He might say that a shovel is for shovelling up dirt; moving a heap of soil; loading up coal; shovelling away snow; mixing concrete and so on. All these answers are correct but they are of the same type. They give only *one basic use* for a shovel. As answers to a conventional intelligence test they would receive full marks. But since the question asks for 'as many uses as possible' the following series of answers would also be correct. A shovel may be used: to dig with; to carry something; to shovel snow; to put in the ground to mark a position; as a toy; for a present; as a weapon; as a lever; as a crude hammer; to beat out a fire; to signal with; as a model for painting, or drawing. This second series of answers gives a number of *basically different* uses for a shovel. Such basically different answers to a problem are typical of *divergent thinking*. They are creative, or original answers, typical of the 'man with ideas'. By contrast, the first set of answers are typical of *convergent thinking*, which has usually been regarded as an important aspect of general intellectual ability. The difference between the two types of thinking has long been recognised, but during the last few years an increasing amount of attention has been paid to divergent thinking and several attempts have been made to construct tests by which it may be assessed (Hudson[16]). Whilst many of these tests show promising results, the investigation is still in its early stages. Almost certainly, however, it is one of the important lines along which tests of intellectual ability are going to be developed. But too great an emphasis should not be placed upon the differences between divergent and convergent thinking. Most probably these two types of thought are the polar opposites of a continuum of thinking ability. Some people have more ability in one type and some in another, whilst most have a fair share of both.

TABLE I

Factors in the Structure of Intellect (Guilford[12])

Operations	Products	Contents
1. Cognition	Units	Symbols
2. Memory	Classes	Figures
3. Convergent thinking	Relations	Words
4. Divergent thinking	Systems	Behaviour
5. Evaluation	Transformations	—
6. —	Implications	—

The constituent parts of each factor are shown in the respective columns. Any one element from a column may be combined with any one element from each of the other two columns.

A 'Three-dimensional' View of Intellect

Guilford[12] has suggested that the 'structure of intellect' may be regarded as due to the interaction of three sets of factors. These factors are termed: operations; products; and contents.

An *operation* is a specific activity of the mind. It may be the activity involved in memory, or cognising, or logical or creative thinking. The *product* is the result of this activity and may take the form of a class, a unit, a system, a relation, a transformation or an implication. The operations need material to work on and this material is termed *content*. The *content* may consist of figures, symbols, words or behaviour. The constituent items of operations, products and contents are listed in Table I. In theory, any intellectual activity can be broken down into a combination of: operation, product and content. Suppose **S** is asked: What are 7 nines? The answer is 63. In this example, the *operation* is memory (or strictly speaking 'recall'); the *product* is a transformation (7×9 has been transformed in 63); and the *content* is symbolic. The following examples may help to clarify the manner in which operations, products and contents interact:

Example: Rearrange the following letters to make a proper word: AMDER.

Operation—cognition
Product—a unit
Content—symbolic

Example: The following letters form the initial letters of words in a sentence. Write the sentence in full.

t   d   r   f

Operation—divergent thinking
Product—a system (i.e. a properly organised sentence)
Content—words

(*Note*. More than one sentence is possible. There are no restrictions on the number of letters in each word.)

Example: Fill in the missing word or letter in the series:

(*a*) pots, stop, bard, drab, rats, ——
(*b*) KORA KORE KORI KORO KOR, ——

Operation—convergent thinking
Product—relation
Content—words (*a*) symbols (*b*)

This process may theoretically be extended to all operations, products and contents.

Each of the five operations may be associated with each of the six products and each of these thirty combinations may be associated with each of the four different contents. There are therefore $5 \times 6 \times 4 = 120$ possible types of problems which can be constructed in this way. It should be possible to devise scorable items for each of these 120 types. If it is possible to do this, the complete description of any one person's intellectual ability would require 120 different scores. In practice, some of the abilities may be inter-correlated, in spite of their theoretical independence. If so, a satisfactory assessment might be obtained, by using a sample of these 120 possible items, with a corresponding reduction in the number of scores required. Much more work is required on this theory before a final assessment of its utility can be made. It does, however, indicate one approach to the complex problem of analysing and assessing intelligence. Some of the main advantages and disadvantages of this theory are listed in Table II.

TABLE II

Some Advantages and Disadvantages of Guilford's[12]
View of Intellectual Ability

I. ADVANTAGES

Logical. Systematic
It employs discrete categories
Testable units of ability
Easily related to the general body of psychological knowledge
Employs everyday terms
No new terminology required
Testable hypotheses may be deduced from it
Embraces a wide range of related concepts far beyond the usual
    range of intelligence factors

II. DISADVANTAGES

A very large number of tests and scores are required
Theoretically deduced abilities may not have practical meaning
Resulting factors are generally too narrow
Highly specific factors may have little predictive value

Social Intelligence

Just as a person cannot be known unless he interacts with his fellows, so intelligence cannot be known in the abstract, but only as a result of the operations that S performs. In the consulting room, intelligence is assessed by means of standardised tests. In the experimental laboratory, it is investigated by means of specially designed problems, whilst in everyday life a person's intelligence is judged largely by the extent to which he successfully solves the problems of daily living. This everyday method of assessing intelligence gives rise to the concept of *social intelligence*, which Guilford[12] has included in his theory of the structure of intellect.

The idea of *social intelligence* is not new. It appears in the sub-tests of 'General Comprehension', and 'Picture Arrangement' in the Wechsler Intelligence Scales (Wechsler[29]). The items in these sub-tests require a knowledge of what to do in certain social situations and an understanding of simple inter-personal relationships. A much more elaborate scale of a similar nature has been constructed by Doll.[8] It is described in *The measurement of social competence*[8] and has an age range extending from babyhood to the superior adult level. It consists of a graded series of activities which are typical of different levels of social development. A

D

social quotient, S.Q., is obtained. Other factors besides intelligence are involved in social competence, and there appears to be no simple, consistent relationship between the S.Q. and the I.Q.

One great merit of Guilford's[12] approach to the concept of social intelligence is that he attempts to analyse a complex but rather amorphous notion into a number of fairly well-defined, specific abilities. Reference to Table I shows that the item *behaviour* (in the column headed *contents*) may be combined with five operations and six products to give thirty elements of behaviour. The details of these thirty elements have not yet been worked out, but they indicate that social behaviour may in theory be broken down into manageable units which can be evaluated by means of standardised tests. If this proves to be practicable, it could have an important bearing on the selection processes for people whose work brings them into intimate contact with others. Conversely, it would be of immense importance in advising individuals whether or not to contemplate a career which would involve them in close personal contacts with clients.

A concept similar to *social intelligence* was outlined by Adler and called by an almost untranslatable German word—*Gemeinschaftsgefühl*. There has been much discussion about the precise meaning of this term, but according to Ansbacher[1] it may best be translated as *social interest*. This includes feeling, an evaluative attitude to life and intelligence. Adler distinguishes between *reason* and *intelligence*. The former has a general validity and is directed towards achieving the general welfare of the community. Intelligence, on the other hand, may be used solely in the interests of the individual himself. *Social interest* implies that the individual's intellectual abilities are used in the service of the community. The neurotic, the rationaliser and the criminal are all frequently quite intelligent, but their intelligence is unsocialised and used for purely ego-centred purposes.

Wertheimer[30] put forward a view similar to Adler's, when discussing the transformations and reorientations that are frequently needed to solve a purely intellectual problem. He says, 'The problem may remain insoluble so long as one focuses on one's own wish or need.' It may become soluble only when the person views his own desire as a part of the total situation, so that one thinks in terms of what the *situation* demands and not simply in terms of one's own wishes. It is but a short step from Wertheimer's *situational thinking* to Adler's *social interest* and Guilford's *social intelligence*. The three concepts are closely linked and may well be fruitful areas for further research.

A considerable and increasing amount of attention is now being paid to the properties of small groups. Individual psychiatric management tends to be replaced by Family Psychiatry (Howells[15]), and an increasing emphasis is being placed upon the psycho-social origin of neurotic disorders. It therefore seems highly likely that the concept of *social intelligence* will play an increasing part in the evaluation and treatment of behavioural disorders. *Social intelligence* involves an understanding of what is useful to, and desirable for, society as a whole. This in turn requires an appreciation of human motives and relations and an evaluation of human actions. Much of the data to be evaluated is non-verbal and consists of attitudes, needs, desires, wishes, moods, intentions and other personality traits. All these have to be assessed within the context of inter-personal relationships, and against the background of individual personalities. So far, the assessment of much human behaviour has been by 'hunches', 'intuition' and 'guess-work'. Guilford's[12] concept of *social intelligence* provides a theoretical basis for replacing the present hit-or-miss approach by a rational, scientific scheme for evaluating human behaviour. His view has the further important advantage that intellectual abilities are not assessed in isolation from other personality traits. The interaction between the intellect and other personality variables has long been known. Most approaches to the study of intellect tend to assess it in isolation, and the widespread use of intelligence tests has reinforced this viewpoint. However, even 'I.Q. tests' are now known to be affected by many non-intellective factors. Guilford's theory of intelligence provides a possible basis for this empirical finding, in so far as he weaves aspects of *behaviour* into the general concept of intelligence.

3

Issues in the Assessment of Intelligence

The Intelligence Quotient

The familiar letters I.Q. stand for the *intelligence quotient*, which was originally defined as the ratio between a child's Mental Age (M.A.) and its Chronological Age (C.A.). Hence I.Q. = M.A./C.A. × 100. Although this method of calculating an I.Q. is still in use, it is most unsatisfactory, especially when assessing the intelligence of adolescents.

The basic criticism of the intelligence quotient is that it depends upon the unsatisfactory concept of a *mental age*. As Wechsler[29] points out, the mental age is simply a score which is obtained when an individual completes part of an intelligence test. Strictly speaking, it is not an 'age' at all, but simply a number which indicates that certain test items have been correctly completed. A second criticism of the mental age is that above a given score, mental age equivalents are quite unrealistic. The limit of the mental age is reached for any given test, when the mean scores made on the test cease to increase with increasing chronological age. Thus on the Mannikin Test in the W.I.S.C. the mean score ceases to increase above the age of eight years. On the vocabulary test, the mean score does not increase after about the age of twenty-two. The point at which an increase in score does not keep pace with an increase in age, depends partly upon the difficulty of the test and partly upon the developmental level which S has reached.

The Mannikin Test is too easy for children over the age of eight, and for most people the vocabulary test shows no significant increase after the age of twenty-two. By that age they will probably have attained their maximum vocabulary and even ten or twenty years later they will not be able to gain a higher score on this test. This kind of evidence has led to the view that the *mental age* reaches a maximum at a *chronological age* of sixteen. Hence in calculating the intelligence quotient for a person of, say, thirty, one has to assume that his mental age is sixteen. This is very unsatisfactory, because, on some intelligence tests, people of thirty or forty can, and do, obtain higher scores than would be warranted if their mental age did not increase beyond that of sixteen. Some authorities place the maximum value of the mental age slightly less than sixteen and others place it slightly higher. All are agreed, however, that if the *mental age* is to be used in conjunction with an already established test, then sixteen or thereabouts must be its maximum value. In recent years due to the researches of Wechsler[29] and others, evidence has been found for the view that intellectual ability declines quite perceptibly after the age of thirty-five or forty. These researches have shown that the *growth curve* of intellectual ability is a logistic curve and that equal increments of intellectual ability do not correspond to equal increments in age. Intellectual growth cannot therefore be represented by a linear function, and the simple relationship which had been assumed to exist between the mental age and the chronological age is not valid. A third reason for regarding the intelligence quotient as unsatisfactory is that it does appear to vary with time for any given individual. So far as mental defectives are concerned, their I.Q.s actually show a systematic decline with age (Wechsler[29]). The variability of the I.Q. is also due to a statistical feature which was overlooked in earlier investigations. This arose from assuming that since the mean values of I.Q.s remained constant, then the extreme values would also remain constant over a corresponding range of values. This assumption is quite unjustified and could lead to serious errors in calculating the I.Q. of the mentally sub-normal, or of the very brilliant child, if the mental age is used.

Perhaps the most serious criticism of the use of the mental age is that it provides no adequate means of expressing the intellectual ability of the adult. The intellectual ability of adults depends upon experience as well as upon cultural factors. Some intelligence tests are heavily weighted in favour of educational achievement. So, if a person has had a very poor schooling, he would tend to make a poor showing on this kind of test. On the other hand, if he were given tests involving practical ability, the manipulation of material, or the formation of designs, he might gain a much higher score, as a result of his experience in adult life. His mental age would then depend just as much upon the test employed as upon his actual ability. The only satisfactory method of assessing adult ability is to use a wide variety of test material and to *rank* Ss of the *same age-group* in order of ability. These two conditions are fulfilled by the Wechsler Adult Intelligence Scale.

Psychological Measurement

The attempt to extend to psychology the precision of measurement used in the exact sciences must be scrutinised with care. Some maintain that Whitehead's dictum, 'To talk sense is to talk in terms of quantities,' does not apply to psychology. Others doubt whether the concept of measurement is applicable at all to psychological qualities, and Zangwill[32] has suggested that nothing psychological is truly measurable. But measurement in psychology need not be identified with measurement in physics. Psychological measurement need not presuppose a scale consisting of a zero point and units of constant size. Measurement is possible with an *interval scale*, like the Fahrenheit scale for temperatures, which has no zero and on which the comparison of degrees is not strictly possible, since 100 degrees Fahrenheit is not 'twice as hot' as 50 degrees.

If measurement in psychology is regarded as essentially measurement on an *ordinal scale*, much of the objection to the term measurement is met. For intelligence could then be measured in the same way as the hardness of minerals is measured. This would be quite adequate for applied psychology, since classification and rank order are used instead of absolute measures. Some psychologists claim that intelligence quotients should be interpreted as measurements on an interval scale, and Peel has attempted to construct such a scale with constant additive units. This scale, however, depends upon intelligence being 'normally distributed'.

Speed as Indicative of Intelligence

An unusual approach to the assessment of intelligence has been suggested by Furneaux.[9] He claims that most intelligence tests which claim to measure a general factor 'g' and related attributes, do in fact measure the *interaction* of three relatively independent attributes. He calls these Speed (SP); Accuracy (A) and Continuance (C).

The *speed* with which a set of problems is solved has usually been measured either in terms of the number of correct answers given within a set time or the *total time* required to complete a test, irrespective of whether the answers were correct or not. Both these measures of speed clearly include what Furneaux calls Accuracy. It has, however, been shown that *speed of working* is distinguishable from accuracy and that Ss of approximately equal mental ability do work at appreciably different speeds. Furneaux[9] proposes to measure speed of working (SP) by counting the number of *correct* answers given within a certain time (t). If a group of Ss is presented with a number of problems which are all of equal difficulty, then the various times (t) taken by individual Ss for the solution of the problems will vary considerably. If values of log t are plotted for each person, the distribution will approximate to that of a normal curve.

If, however, the values of log t are plotted against the degree of difficulty of the problems, then a straight line is the result.

If the difficulty of the problems is increased, the time required to solve them also increases. If the required time exceeds a certain critical value (which is different for each S), then S tends to abandon that problem and attempt another. The extent to which he is willing to persist until he has solved the problem is a measure of his *continuance* (C). In order to measure SP uncontaminated by other factors, three requirements are necessary. (1) A large preponderance of *correct* answers must be given. (2) The problems must all be of approximately equal difficulty. (3) The scores must be stated as the logarithm of the response-time; not as absolute time. (From requirement (1) it follows that the items must be relatively easy for any given group of Ss.)

Speed tests can be given under two conditions, *stressed* or *unstressed*. The former condition requires S to work as quickly as possible. The unstressed condition allows him to work at his own natural rate. For most Ss there is a high correlation between the scores obtained under the two conditions. If the scores gained under stress show appreciable divergence from the unstressed scores, then some degree of psychological disturbance may be suspected in the persons concerned.

Scores on speed tests discriminate between psychotics and neurotics. The Accuracy (A) score allows predictions to be made about S's performance. For if the proportion of correct answers given by S at any given level is known, then his success at any other level can be predicted.

Each of the components, SP, A, C, can be measured separately by the Nufferno Tests,[20] or a combination of these factors may be assessed. The tests may be administered individually or to groups. They are suitable for use with Ss of eleven years and upward, according to the factors being measured. Accuracy norms are also provided for the eighteen- to thirty-year age group.

All tests are of the series completion type and employ only letters of the alphabet.

If speed were as fundamental a characteristic of intelligence as Furneaux suggests, then it seems that, given enough time and enough continuance (C), anyone could solve any problem. But degree of difficulty would appear to be a limiting factor in intelligence, as well as speed and persistence. The importance of speed in intellectual assessment is specifically recognised by the Wechsler tests of intelligence, since a considerable number of extra points are awarded for correct, speedy solutions of several of the subtests.

Some further support for the view that speed is a characteristic of intelligence is provided by experience with teaching machines. The evidence is by no means conclusive, but some researchers have found that there is a correlation between speed of learning and intelligence. This finding runs contrary to the original expectations, for it was hoped that programmed instruction might make the process of learning independent of intelligence (Lewis and Gregson[18]).

Creativeness

One of the more recent developments in the assessment of intellectual ability has been the attempt to evaluate the child's creative thinking (also known as divergent, or lateral thinking). Traditionally, creativeness has not been associated with tests of intelligence, although some authorities maintain that, apart from genius, creative ability is accounted for by the *general factor* of intelligence, or *g*.

In popular thought, creativeness is associated more with artists than with scientists. Yet both artist and scientist depend upon 'inspiration', and each has to work hard to develop the ideas which come to him 'in a flash'. There appear to be four fairly well-defined stages through which original ideas develop. These are: preparation, incubation, illumination and verification. Creative ideas may occur to an individual at any time, but they appear only after the mind has been stored with relevant data. Most people would probably agree with Arieti[2] when he says that the creative process enlarges human freedom and enriches human experience. Creativity is not in conflict with reality, although it may frequently give an unusual view of the real world. Creativity helps to satisfy human curiosity and the need for new and more rewarding experiences. Viewed in this way, it seems unlikely that creative ability can be assessed by any sort of test. Perhaps, in the end, it cannot; but some success in evaluating it has been obtained, and is discussed by Butcher[6] in a chapter on 'Creativity and Intelligence'.

Getzels and Jackson[11] studied children in a private school, where the mean value of the children's I.Q. was 132. There were 292 boys and 241 girls in the sample studied. They assessed the creative ability of the children by using the following five types of tests:

TYPE I. *Word associations.* The children were asked to give as many definitions as possible for words with multiple meanings (e.g. post, bolt). The score allowed for the number of definitions given and also for the number of radically different meanings.

TYPE II. *Uses.* As many different uses as possible were required for common objects. Both frequency and quality of responses were included in the score.

TYPE III. *Hidden shapes.* The task was to find a geometrical figure which was 'hidden' within a more complex pattern.

TYPE IV. *Fables.* Three different endings were required for each of four fables. One ending was to be moral, one to be humorous and one to be sad.

TYPE V. *Problems.* Four paragraphs of numerical statements were given to the child. He was required to make up as many problems as possible using these statements. He was not required to solve the problems.

The answers to these problems and the results of the intelligence test formed the basis for dividing the children into two groups. One group consisted of those scoring high on the creativity tests and relatively low in the I.Q. test. The other group scored relatively low on creativity and high on the traditional I.Q. test. This research shows that intelligence measured in the conventional manner is not necessarily identical with a creative approach to problem-solving.

Several other studies of the relation between divergent thinking and intelligence have shown that a rather small, but positive correlation exists between them. (r varying from 0·2 to 0·4.) One or two results have given a value of r as high as 0·6 or 0·7. Dacey[7] and his colleagues, in a recent study, suggested that the correlations between intelligence and creative thinking might be due to the *methods* employed in the investigations, rather than to a genuine relationship between them. They suggested that, 'true relationship between intelligence and divergent thinking factors cannot be determined with complete confidence' without further research into the possible relationship between the 'trait and methods factors'. It is possible, however, that the trait of divergent thinking is unaffected by educational, or cultural factors (Dacey *et al.*[7]).

It would be a great advantage from a social and educational point of view if it were possible to discover the more 'creative' children relatively early in their school careers. They might be allowed more opportunities to develop their gifts, with consequent advantage both to society and to themselves. Progress is being made with this 'open-ended' type of test and also with the study of divergent thinking. Some of the differences between the conventional intelligence test and the type of test used in assessing creativity are shown in Table III.

TABLE III

Some of the Main Differences Between the Problems in Conventional Intelligence Tests and Those in Tests for Creativeness

Conventional I.Q. Test	Tests of creativeness
Only one answer needed	Several answers needed
Problem precisely defined	Problem loosely defined
Forced-choice answers	Open-ended answers
Large element of traditional learned material	Learned material must be marshalled in new ways
One-to-one relationship encouraged	One-to-many relationships needed
'Original' answers penalised (even if logically correct)	'Original' answers needed
Precise instructions	Informal instructions

Tests for Superior Levels of Intelligence

Specially designed tests are necessary to distinguish between those adolescents who are of 'superior' ability and those who are still more intellectually gifted. Such tests have been devised by Valentine, Heim and Raven, and in general they distinguish between the 'pass' and 'honours' levels of intellectual ability.

Valentine's *Reasoning tests for higher levels of intelligence* consist of a series of propositions whose truth or falsehood the S can discover by logical reasoning. If he considers that a proposition is not correct, then he must indicate the reason why it is fallacious. The mean scores for 'honours' and 'pass' graduates are significantly different at the 1 per cent level. The test is also suitable for sixth form pupils of sixteen years of age and over.

Heim's test is known as *A.H.5* and is a group test in two parts. The first part consists of verbal and numerical items and the second part is composed of 36 diagrammatic items. Norms are provided for university students, high-grade apprentices and grammar school children in the thirteen- to eighteen-year range. There is also the *A.H.4* version of the test suitable for children over ten years of age.

Raven has devised two sets of Advanced Progressive Matrices. Set I is a ten-minute test consisting of 12 matrices. Set II is a series of 36 matrices, which may be used as a test of either intellectual efficiency, with a time limit, or as a test of intellectual capacity with no time limit.

(*Note*. Both Heim's and Raven's tests may be obtained by suitably qualified users from the National Foundation for Educational Research, Slough, England. Valentine's test is published by Oliver and Boyd of Edinburgh.)

Primary Mental Abilities

As a result of factor analysis Thurstone[27] claimed to have isolated seven *primary mental abilities*. These are: spatial ability (S); perceptual speed (P); numerical ability (N); verbal meaning (V); memory (M); verbal fluency (W); inductive reasoning (R). On the basis of these findings, he devised a series of tests using five of these primary abilities, namely: V, S, R, N, W. One of the tests is suitable for adolescents aged eleven to seventeen years. Since the scores on the five abilities are relatively independent, the test is very useful in vocational counselling, as it tends to indicate the specific abilities or weaknesses of the individual. In diagnostic and counselling procedures the *pattern* of the scores must be considered, not simply the overall result.

The British Intelligence Test

A new intelligence test is now being developed under the auspices of the British Psychological Society. It will be standardised upon a sample of English children and will cover the age range two to eighteen years. The new test incorporates some of the principles discussed in this chapter and should be available by 1971.

Although the full details of the test are not yet known its main structure has been disclosed and it will probably follow the pattern summarised in Table IV. The test result will be given as a *profile* instead of an 'I.Q.'. Most of the test items will not be timed, and considerable importance has been placed upon 'creative thinking', analysis of relationships, and the concept of 'conservation'. The test makes use of the work of Piaget and other recent research and rests upon a wide theoretical and practical basis. It retains many important features found in the Wechsler tests; the Stanford–Binet, and Raven's Matrices. Well-established items like vocabulary, memory tests and calculations are included in the new scale; but the actual content is almost all new.

TABLE IV

Probable General Outline of the New British Intelligence Scale

(*Note.* The names of the sub-divisions are not necessarily those actually used in the Scale.)

Sub-divisions of the Scale	Type of Items within each sub-division
Reasoning	Matrices Analysis of relationships Identification of objects Assessing statements
Verbal	Vocabulary General knowledge Concept formation
Space perception	Pattern-making Understanding plans and diagrams
Number	Concept of conservation. Calculations
Memory	Production of patterns and relations Number sequences Content of literary passages
Ideas and Fluency	Unusual uses for objects Unusual consequences Extent and quality of ideas

4

The Interpretation and Use of Intelligence Ratings

(*Note.* The following discussion concerns results obtained from the W.I.S.C. and W.A.I.S., unless otherwise stated. This is not to deny the importance of the three forms of the Terman–Merrill Tests. But for *diagnostic* purposes the Wechsler Tests are to be preferred. The T–M tests are excellent for the assessment of educational and general academic ability.)

Reporting the I.Q.

The result of an intelligence test is usually expressed as a number. This number is 'the I.Q.' and it is an essential part of the assessment process. So far as psychological records are concerned the numerical value of 'the I.Q.' is only *one* number among several others, all of which must be taken into consideration when interpreting the significance of the person's 'I.Q.' as given by the test.

When, however, the psychologist is *reporting* the results of a test, he has to bear in mind two classes of people who may read his report. They are: (*i*) those who understand the full significance of the *pattern* of scores disclosed by the test; (*ii*) those who still think in terms of 'an I.Q.'. In reporting to the former group the full pattern of scores should be given. In reporting to the second group, *only a rating* should be given. An 'I.Q.' should *never* be reported as a single number, nor even as the three separate numbers obtained from the W.I.S.C. and W.A.I.S. tests. There are several reasons for recommending this procedure.

1. The number itself is only the climax of a very complex process, during which several personality variables have been sampled. The *process* of taking the test may be regarded as the 'ground' against which the *final result* appears as a 'figure', after the manner of a 'figure-ground' Gestalt. The final result acquires its meaning only against the background of the total test procedure. It may even be argued that the test result is seen in its true significance only against the background of S's personal history.

2. A number is a convenient label, and once a person has been labelled, the label tends to stick. This may result in unfavourable comparisons being made between one person and another with consequent injustice, or the arousal of ill-feeling between members of a family.

3. The numerical I.Q. is neither a fixed nor an absolute value. It may vary over time, and it is always subject to experimental variations, as Burt's[4] Four-Factor Theory makes clear. The numerical difference within a small range of I.Q. values is of no consequence; the difference between an I.Q. of 99 and an I.Q. of 102 is of no importance whatever. Yet an I.Q. of 102 sounds better than one of 99. Whilst one is statistically below average and the other is above it, yet both values indicate a person of 'about average' ability, and this phrase is a sufficient description of them.

4. Another reason for avoiding the reporting of I.Q.s as simple numbers is that different tests, applied to the same subject, may quite properly give different numerical results.

5. In addition, it should be remembered that no intelligence test is a test of 'pure intellect'. It always samples some personality features as well, although these are not represented as scores in the test. Some allowance can often be made in the report for the psychological state of the person at the time of testing. The scores in the test may also indicate a difference between the present level of functioning and S's potential ability. Such a difference may even require the *intelligence rating* to be qualified in the report, let alone a numerical I.Q.

Intelligence Ratings

If the full results of an intelligence test are not to be reported, then a *rating* of S's intelligence must be given. The *rating* places S within a fairly broad band of I.Q. values, as shown in Fig. 2. Of course, there may be some results which do not fit strictly within these ratings. It is then incumbent upon E to qualify his rating in such a manner that, without doing the patient an injustice, he gives a clear indication of S's ability.

TABLE V

The Same Numerical I.Q. May Represent Widely Differing Disorders
(Reproduced, with the author's permission, from Gathercole[10])

Full scale I.Q.	Verbal I.Q.	Performance I.Q.	Condition of the subject
65	65	65	Mentally defective
65	80	50	Brain damaged
65	50	80	Illiterate delinquent

The Pattern of Scores

An excellent example of the misleading nature of a simple numerical I.Q. is provided by Gathercole[10] and shown in Table V. The full scale I.Q. shown in the first column is identical for the three widely differing conditions shown in the fourth column. If only 'the I.Q.', i.e. the Full Scale

TABLE VI

Pattern of Scores Showing Educational Retardation in a Child of Average Ability

Name ....
          ....
Age   ....
Test used—Wechsler Intelligence Scale for Children

Verbal Scale		Performance Scale	
Information	6	Picture completion	9
Comprehension	8	Picture arrangement	10
Arithmetic	2	Block design	11
Similarities	11	Object assembly	13
Vocabulary	7	Coding	7
Digit span	6	Mazes	10
TOTAL	40	TOTAL	60

Verbal I.Q. = 79   Performance I.Q. = 100
Full Scale I.Q. = 91

Intelligence rating—Of about *average ability*, but probably educationally backward and may be having difficulty in concentrating and learning.

Wechsler I.Q. were mentioned in a report, it would, in this example, be quite misleading, since it would not indicate the conditions underlying it. When a marked discrepancy occurs between the Verbal and the Performance I.Q.s, it is usually an indication that the subject is suffering from a more or less serious disorder which is reflected in, but *not diagnosed* by, the scores. Some of the disorders reflected in intelligence test scores are discussed later in this chapter.

Another important pattern of scores is shown in Table VI. The discrepancy between the Verbal I.Q. of 79 and the Performance I.Q. of 100 is largely due to S's poor educational achievements. Educational backwardness is reflected in the scores for Information, Arithmetic and Vocabularly. Since the scores for Digit Span and Coding are also relatvely low, this S's backwardness may be linked to lack of concentration and inability to learn quickly. A pattern of scores like this *does not prove* that S is suffering from these disabilities, but it does indicate that further investigation is essential, and also indicates the lines along which it might be undertaken.

Deterioration

Serious deterioration of intellectual ability sometimes occurs during adolescence. Organic pathology and, occasionally, incipient schizophrenia are the conditions most likely to lead to a deterioration which would be reflected in the scores of an intelligence test. There are two methods of detecting the possibility of such deterioration as shown by the pattern of the test scores. Both depend upon the fact that intellectual deterioration has a *differential effect* upon the scores in the sub-tests of the W.I.S.C. and the W.A.I.S. Scores depending upon material which has been thoroughly learned, like a vocabulary, tend to be little affected. Scores depending upon immediate perception and the manipulation of material are often considerably affected by intellectual deterioration.

Method I. According to Wechsler,[29] the sub-tests *least affected* by deterioration are: Vocabulary, Information, Object Assembly and Picture Completion. These are called, 'Hold tests' denoted by H. Sub-tests which *are* appreciably affected by deterioration are called 'Don't Hold Tests', denoted by D.H. An assessment of the extent of deterioration may be obtained by using the formula, $\dfrac{H - D.H.}{H}$. It is important, when using this formula, to use the *age-corrected* scores from the special tables in the manual accompanying the test. Whilst this formula gives an indication of possible deterioration in intellectual functioning, it does not indicate its specific cause or causes. This formula would be of no value with a semi-illiterate S, since at least two of the 'Hold' scores would inevitably be quite low. Under these circumstances it is possible to obtain a 'negative deterioration' score. This rarely happens, but when it does occur, the most likely explanation is that S is of about average basic ability, but with hardly any educational achievement to his credit.

Method II. Intellectual deterioration may be suspected as a result of a simple inspection of the *pattern* of scores. If the results of one or more of the Digit Span, Block Design or Digit Symbol sub-tests are well below the level of the other scores, then a suspicion of deterioration is aroused. In particular, if the score on Block Design is very much lower than the others, then the possibility of parietal lobe damage may be suspected. The verbal responses may also give an indication of a deteriorated condition *provided that* S was known to be previously of at least average ability. 'Clang' associations, bizarre replies, the inability to form concepts and repetitive answers may also be signs of intellectual deterioration.

Under-achievement

One of the currently fashionable descriptions of some school children is that of *under-achiever*. When this term is applied to a pupil, it simply means that he is not making as much educational progress as he 'should do'—and the phrase 'should do' is the key to the understanding of the term. There are four basic reasons for saying that he 'should' do better. (1) He has dropped behind his classmates. Instead of being in the highest quarter of the class list he is within, say, the lowest quarter. (2) There is a discrepancy between his ability, as estimated by an intelligence test, and his actual performance. (3) His parents or his teachers think he is not working hard enough. (4) He gains good marks in some subjects, but poor marks in others.

TABLE VII

Some Causes of Under-achievement at School

Personal factors	Family factors
Illnesses and therefore absent from school	No encouragement or interest from parents
Excessive anxiety	Reaction against rejection
Loss of interest	Bereavement
Over-active	Family disrupted
Attention-seeking behaviour	Parental quarrels
Boredom	Frequent moving
	No facilities for homework
School factors	**Social factors**
Dislike of a teacher	Member of wrong 'gang'
Changes of school	Too many out-of-school interests
Changes of method	Eager to be at work
Inappropriate teaching methods	Dislike of being 'better' than peers
Too little stimulation	

The reasons for under-achievement are multitudinous. A sample of the possible causes is given in Table VII. Purely as a matter of convenience, the causes of under-achievement are classified under the headings: personal; family; school; social. However, it is most important to remember that these causes are not necessarily independent, nor are they mutually exclusive. Not only may more than one cause be operating at one time, but different causes may interact with each other; and indeed, one event, like a bereavement, may bring a whole series of detrimental reactions in its train.

An assessment of the pupil's intelligence may determine whether he really is 'under-achieving', or whether in fact his educational attainments are in keeping with his general ability.

Over-achievement

Analogous to the group of under-achievers are those who *over-achieve*. These children 'do better' educationally, than their intelligence quotients would suggest. Frequently, they obtain a verbal I.Q. which is appreciably higher than their performance I.Q. They may also be relatively less successful at the university or in an occupation than they were at school.

TABLE VIII

Some Factors Conducive to Over-achievement in Schoolchildren

Personality	Family
Perseverance	Cultured background
Facility in learning	Ambitious parents
Need for compensating activity	Tradition
Desire to please parents	Emulation of sibling
Self-image	
Insecurity	
Social	**School**
Tends to be isolated	High standards
Lacking in social achievements	Strict discipline

Broadly speaking, their *over-achievement* is due to consistently careful work and to an indefatigable application to learning. They are the children who do their homework conscientiously, learn their vocabularies and know their 'bookwork'. They also spend much time in reading, or in pursuing some 'educational hobby'. In these several ways they are always learning and encountering ideas and information which most children would meet at a later developmental stage, if at all. To the casual observer they are 'model children' and give the impression of being intellectually bright. But when they are presented with a problem outside the range of what they have learned or read, these children tend to perform below expectation. The failure may be due partly to personality factors, but also because they lack basic intellectual ability, as distinct from the ability to learn. Their painstaking industry masks the fact that they are 'slow learners', and that itself is an indication of relatively low intellectual ability. Within the sheltered environment of school, their industry pays dividends. If they are of the introverted type they may compensate for lack of friends and social achievement by being good scholars. Once school is left behind, they are less successful and their lack of drive frequently prevents them from making the best use of the abilities they possess.

On the other hand, those who worked hard simply to please their parents, or because they were made to, will probably revolt as soon as they leave school, if not before!

If the child feels insecure, he may try to overcome this by building up an exaggerated image of his own abilities and then try to live up to his own expectations. A feeling of insecurity may also drive the child to work hard in order to gain the affection of his parents. The main reasons which lead to over-achievement are listed in Table VIII.

Over-achievement in itself is not necessarily harmful. It may be mildly beneficial, if it acts as a compensation for unavoidable deficits in development. It may, however, retard the child's social development and could be a source of disappointment after leaving school. It is sometimes one factor in neurotic breakdown, and may be a contributory cause of excessive anxiety.

A test of *creative ability* would probably distinguish between the over-achievers and the under-achievers, the latter scoring higher than the former.

Special Schooling

Sometimes it is advisable for a younger adolescent to have a change of school on psychological grounds. Such a change may be desirable because of unfavourable home relationships, delinquent, or potentially delinquent behaviour, or some specific personal defect. If the child is to be entered at a special school for maladjusted children, it is usual for an assessment of the child's intellectual ability to accompany the request for admission to the school. When a request for transfer to a special school is considered, it sometimes means that the child is an 'under-achiever'. Transfers may be made, however, when the child is working up to the level of his ability but is also showing signs of stress and strain.

Vocational Guidance

Occupation and intelligence. The assessment of intellectual ability plays an important part in any vocational guidance that may be offered. An intelligence rating *by itself* is not sufficient data on which to determine the advisability of a particular career. Interests, aptitudes, values, personality traits, educational achievements and family background must all be taken into account when advising the client about undertaking a particular occupation. An estimate of intellectual ability indicates whether further education should be attempted, and if so, what academic level is likely to be reached. It will also indicate the range of occupations which are within the compass of the individual's abilities. Super[23] gives the range of intelligence required for an extensive list of occupational groups, based upon tests given to about 90 000 members of the U.S. Armed Forces in 1944. The tables on pages 96–97 of his book give a broad idea of the level of ability required for a wide range of occupations. There is, however, a very large overlap between the levels of intelligence required for different occupations, as shown by Woodworth and Marquis.[31] Intellectual ability is only one factor, but a very important factor in determining an occupation.

Predicting Vocational Success

Future success in any occupation is probably more highly correlated with intellectual ability than with any other single factor. At least this seems to be a reasonable deduction from the massive longitudinal study of careers carried out by Terman[25] and his associates. Terman[25] began the research in 1921, and the latest publication in the series (Terman and Oden[25]) gives findings obtained thirty-five years later. About 1500 children were originally tested and in this latest follow-up study, 95 per cent of them actively participated in the program. Terman's studies are not strictly speaking studies of *genius*. No great creative artist or scientist emerged from the sample he studied. The group did, however, contain a large number of talented individuals. It also showed that, whereas various psychological and behavioural disorders occurred within the group, there was no correlation between these disorders and intellectual ability. The more intelligent individuals were not 'weak' or 'defective' in any way. Intelligence was in nowise a compensatory factor for other deficiencies. On the other hand, a few of the highly intelligent were doing semi-skilled jobs in middle-life. But *in general* intelligence ratings proved reliable guides to occupational success.

Forensic Value

Intelligence ratings may be valuable as evidence submitted to a Court of Law. There are three main areas where evidence of the patient's intellectual ability could be of considerable importance in legal proceedings.

TABLE IX

*Scores Obtained in Successive Tests on the W.A.I.S.,
by a seventeen-year-old Boy, Who had Sustained Severe
Damage to His Brain*

Date of test	Interval between tests	W.A.I.S. scores		
		Verbal I.Q.	Performance I.Q.	Full Scale I.Q.
Dec. 1961	—	untestable		
Feb. 1962	3m	86	60	73
June 1962	4m	91	75	83
Dec. 1962	6m	101	86	94
July 1963	7m	95	79	88
Jan. 1965	6m	93	88	90

1. The diagnosis of *mental subnormality* cannot (at least in England) be made solely on the basis of an intelligence test. It is defined as 'a state of arrested or incomplete development . . . which requires or is susceptible to medical treatment or other special care or training of the patient'. (Mental

Health Act, 1959, 4, 3.) However, the psychologist could certainly contribute an opinion regarding the 'other special care or treatment'.

2. Juvenile Courts frequently ask for psychiatric reports upon the adolescents who are brought before them. When such a report also requires an assessment of the offender's intellectual ability, it is submitted directly to the Clerk of the Court.

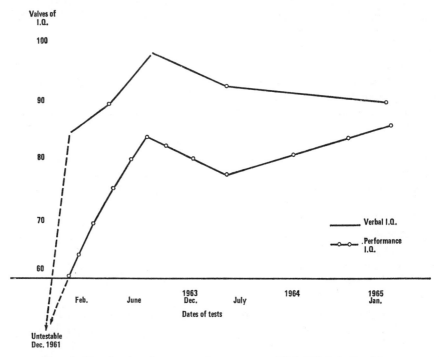

FIG. 3. Graphs showing successive scores on W.A.I.S. (obtained by a brain-damaged patient).

3. *Action for damages* may involve a claim based upon loss of ability or employment, due to temporary or permanent impairment of intellectual functioning. In these circumstances, the psychologist may be asked to assess the client's present intellectual state and to express his opinion, as an *expert witness* (McKellar[19]), about the possible consequences of the condition. It is essential that such a report should be made *direct* to the legal representative who requests it. It must not be incorporated in a report made by anyone else, or, as Haward[13] points out, it will be subject to the rule of *hearsay* and therefore not admissible as evidence.

A good example of the kind of evidence that might be called for is indicated by the data shown in Table IX. This data was submitted on behalf of a seventeen-year-old boy in support of a claim for damages as the result of a car accident. He was injured in June and remained unconscious for about eighty-five days. In December of the same year he was quite untestable, as he could not even place the blocks in a Gesell Formboard; a task easily accomplished by a three-year-old. Three months later, he had considerably recovered and showed a steady improvement for about a year (Fig. 3). Two subsequent tests indicated a slight deterioration in ability, although there was still a tendency for the Performance I.Q. to improve. No further test was carried out after January 1965, so that it is not known whether the curve reached a steady maximum value, or showed a subsequent decline. The graph in Fig. 3 makes it quite clear that this boy was functioning below his potential ability for a period of over three years. The differential recovery rates in the verbal and performance scales are also quite clearly shown.

Therapeutic Uses

A brief mention should be made of the contribution that intelligence ratings can make to various therapeutic procedures. Traditionally, only the more intelligent patients have been regarded as suitable for psychotherapy. Recent research, however, suggests that in psychotherapy the ability to learn is more important than sheer intellectual ability (Porter[21]). However, there appears to be a fairly high positive correlation between intelligence and speed of learning. Moreover, a patient's appearance, or even his social status may mask his real ability. An assessment of the patient's intelligence should help the therapist to decide whether the patient is likely to benefit from individual treatment, or whether some form of Vector Therapy (Howells[15]) may be more appropriate. Whilst some of the sub-tests in the Wechsler Scales may be used to assess the ability to learn simple processes, it is doubtful if they are reliable guides to the complex processes involved in re-educative and therapeutic work. Tests involving problem-solving and divergent thinking may be more useful in assessing the possibility of success in psychotherapy.

Another important function of an intelligence rating is its possible use as a means of *reassuring* the patient about his own ability. Sometimes, as a result of a series of failures or misfortunes, an adolescent may not only become depressed but also feel that he is lacking in ability and that he will never make a success of anything. An intelligence test will certainly show what potential ability he possesses, and its result may be used in several ways. 1. If the patient really has but very little ability, it will be necessary to help him to accept his limitations and to direct him into an occupation where he will be likely to succeed. 2. If he is an 'under-achiever', a suitably graded program of work should be devised to enable him to gain confidence and prove to himself that he really can succeed. 3. On the other hand, the psychologist may have to initiate a therapeutic program for the parents as well as for their child. Such a program is necessary if the parents are over-ambitious and therefore expect from their son or daughter achievements of which he or she is quite incapable. Parents are often reluctant to accept the fact that their child is not as 'brilliant' as they thought he was. In these circumstances, it may be necessary to give them a fairly detailed explanation of the significance of intelligence ratings, as well as a course of family therapy. Whichever procedure is adopted, the intelligence rating provides a reliable basis for a counselling, or a remedial, program. When the patient's future career may be at stake, it is advisable to base the rating upon the results of two or more tests (e.g. Wechsler, Raven and Thurstone). The results should corroborate each other, yet at the same time, they sample somewhat different areas of intellectual ability and thereby increase the confidence with which the recommendations are made.

Rehabilitation

It is usually necessary to carry out an intellectual assessment of a candidate for a rehabilitation program. The test results help to decide the level of work he should attempt—unskilled, semi-skilled or highly skilled. The pattern of the test results may also indicate specific weaknesses which might affect the training he receives.

Acknowledgments

I am grateful to Mr Christopher Gathercole of Rainhill Hospital for permission to quote the data in Table IV from his book *Assessment in Clinical Psychology*. I also must thank my colleague Mr Clive Sims for his very welcome suggestions and for reading the manuscript.

REFERENCES

1. ANSBACHER, H. L. and ANSBACHER, R. R. 1958. *The Individual Psychology of Alfred Adler*. London: Allen & Unwin.
2. ARIETI, S. 1966. *Creativity and its cultivation*. In *American handbook of psychiatry*, Ed. S. Arieti, vol. 3. New York: Basic Books.
3. BABCOCK, H. 1941. *Time and the mind*. Cambridge, Massachusetts: Harvard University Press.
4. BURT, SIR CYRIL. 1940. *The factors of the mind*. London: University of London Press.
5. BURT, SIR CYRIL. 1957. The distribution of intelligence. *Brit. J. Psychol.*, **48**, pt. 3.
6. BUTCHER, H. J. 1968. *Human intelligence: its nature and assessment*. London: Methuen.
7. DACEY, J., MADAUS, G. and ALLEN, A. 1969. The relationship of creativity and intelligence in Irish adolescents. *Brit. J. educ. Psychol.*, 39, 261.
8. DOLL, E. A. 1953. *The measurement of social competence*. Educational Test Bureau. Chicago: Educational Publishers.
9. FURNEAUX, W. D. 1960. Intellectual abilities and problem-solving behaviour. In *Handbook of abnormal psychology* (chap. 5), Ed. H. J. Eysenck. London: Pitman Medical.

10. GATHERCOLE, C. E. 1968. *Assessment in clinical psychology*. Harmondsworth: Penguin Books.
11. GETZELS, J. W. and JACKSON, P. W. 1962. *Creativity and intelligence*. New York: Wiley.
12. GUILFORD, J. P. 1959. Three faces of intellect. *Amer. Psychologist*, **14**, 469.
13. HAWARD, L. R. C. 1965. Hearsay and psychological reports. *Bull. Brit. Psychol. Soc.*, **18**, 21.
14. HEBB, D. O. 1949. *The organisation of behaviour*. New York: Wiley.
15. HOWELLS, J. G. 1968. *Theory and practice of family psychiatry*. Edinburgh: Oliver & Boyd.
16. HUDSON, L. 1966. *Contrary imaginations*. London: Methuen.
17. LEWIS, D. G. 1957. The normal distribution of intelligence: a critique. *Brit. J. Psychol.*, **48**, 98.
18. LEWIS, D. G. and GREGSON, A. 1965. The effects of frame size and intelligence on learning from a linear programme. *Programmed Learning*, **1**, 170.
19. McKELLAR, P. 1968. *Experience and behaviour*. Harmondsworth: Penguin Books.
20. *Nufferno Tests*, 1950 by FURNEAUX, W. D. London: University of London Press.
21. PORTER, R. (Ed.). 1968. *The role of learning in psychotherapy*. London: Churchill.
22. SPEARMAN, C. 1932. *The abilities of man*. London: University of London Press.
23. SUPER, D. E. 1949. *Appraising vocational fitness*. New York: Harper & Brothers.
24. TANNER, J. M. 1962. *Growth at adolescence* (2nd edition). Oxford: Blackwell's Scientific Publications.
25. TERMAN, L. M. and ODEN, M. H. 1959. *The gifted group at mid-life. Genetic studies of genius, V*. Stanford, California: Stanford University Press.
26. THOMSON, G. H. 1951. *The factorial analysis of human ability* (5th edition). London: University of London Press.
27. THURSTONE, L. L. and THURSTONE, T. G. 1963. *Manual for the primary mental abilities* (3rd edition). Chicago: Science Research Association.
28. VERNON, P. E. 1969. *Intelligence and cultural environment*. London: Methuen.
29. WECHSLER, D. 1958. *The measurement and appraisal of adult intelligence* (4th edition). Baltimore: Williams and Wilkins.
30. WERTHEIMER, M. 1961. *Productive thinking*. London: Tavistock.
31. WOODWORTH, R. S. and MARQUIS, D. G. 1963. *Psychology: a study of mental life*. London: Methuen.
32. ZANGWILL, O. 1950. *An introduction to modern psychology*. London: Methuen.

V

THE NEEDS OF ADOLESCENTS FOR EMOTIONAL HEALTH

S. A. Szurek

M.D.

Professor, Department of Psychiatry
University of California School of Medicine
San Francisco, California
Director, Children's Service
Langley Porter Neuropsychiatric Institute
San Francisco, California
U.S.A.

Our youth now love luxury; they have bad manners, contempt for authority; they show disrespect for elders and love chatter in place of exercise. Children are now tyrants, not the servants of their households. They no longer rise when elders enter the room. They contradict their parents, chatter before company, gobble up their food and tyrannize their teachers. Attributed to Socrates, Fifth Century, B.C.

1

Introduction

The lament of the ancients about the traits of their youth seems startlingly familiar and modern. It brings a sudden, deeper realization that every generation of parents and other adults has probably experienced in some degree similar difficulties with their adolescent children and vice versa.

Adolescence may come so suddenly that, like a storm, it may take both parent and child by surprise. Or it may come gradually over weeks, months, or several years. In either instance the change is often, if not generally, disconcertingly profound and needs to be met by a new philosophic understanding.[14]

Adolescence has been characterized in many ways. Erikson[1] speaks of it as 'that no man's land between childhood and adulthood more or less derisively called adolescence'. A headmaster of a great English school[15] described the ages between twelve or thirteen and fifteen or sixteen years as the 'tunnel'. He said that boys go in with a certain character and are then obscured from sight so that 'you never know what is going to come out at the other end'. Wicksteed[15] speaks of it as—'characteristically, if not invariably, a time of disillusionment for parents, often for teachers, and sometimes for the boys or girls themselves'. He notes 'a certain irresponsiveness to former appeals' which is very disheartening. It has also been called a 'half-way house'.[13]

The stress between the adults and the adolescents seems almost inevitable, since each is making a different demand. That of the adolescent is to shake off the semi-make-believe of childhood and to enter the world where his activities will have real and 'not merely imaginative consequences'.[15] More or less unconsciously for the parent and child, a change in their feelings appears. The charm of dependent smiles and tears of the early years begins 'to wane and the more deadly charm of the rival (to the parent and child of the same sex) is beginning to wax'.[16] This period is one of war over the body of the individual between man and nature—man for society and nature for posterity. It is a war of the generations in which both contenders must win in some measure and not be one of a fight to the finish for the race to continue and progress.

In this struggle the adolescent of both sexes becomes resistant to almost any extraneous demands and very characteristically secretive. The grown-up impositions of childhood, the restrictions and requirements of home and school sicken them and become absurd and unreal. 'To put it rather unkindly, the early adolescent boy growls and the girl giggles at the absurd and officious demands of maturity.'[16] They are striking root into a deeper level, need time to cut their psychic teeth and listen to nature rather than to their parents.

Thus Wicksteed[17] (italics the present writer's) speaks further of the situation between the parent and the young adolescent: 'We are riding on life's journey with a small boy walking by our side and holding on to the stirrup-strap for help. While we temper our speed to his weakness we look round—to see him suddenly seated upon a full-grown horse. But the boy, finding himself thus mounted, is entirely absorbed in his new, strange, and exciting adjustment to this mettlesome and unbroken mount he finds himself astride of. *We must not expect that because he is suddenly horsed, he will suddenly become a horseman, and it will be long before he can ride by our side in equality and renewed companionship.* To adapt the metaphor somewhat: we are all centaurs, but the horse in us abruptly matures, while the man is still half-grown.'

Adolescence, then, psychologically is a necessary loss by both parent and child of each other, while the adolescent's physical dependence is unchanged, or strengthened. To win a friend in the end in the place of a charge, the parent needs to endure the distressing loss of authority without losing responsibility.

Speaking of adolescence as the last and concluding stage of childhood, Erikson[2] also calls attention to the fact that the young individual needs, and societies offer, during this period of his life a more or less sanctioned *psychosocial moratorium.* He contrasts this with the psychosexual moratorium of the latency period before puberty. During adolescence the young person, sexually matured, is still more or less retarded in his psychosexual capacity for intimacy and his psychosocial readiness for parenthood. His task is formidable. In the process during this moratorium he seeks through subordination of childhood identifications to a new identification in his absorbing sociability and competitive apprenticeship with and among age mates. In the latter, the playfulness and zest of youth decrease. There is dire urgency to choices, decisions leading to self-definition and commitments for life. In all this, in fortunate circumstances, a lasting pattern of inner identity is formed as a sense of inner continuity and social sameness between what he was as a child and what he is about to become. This formation then reconciles his conception of himself and the community's recognition of him. During the moratorium he is free to experiment with roles in his search for a niche in 'some section of his society, a niche which is firmly defined and yet seems to be uniquely made for him'.

Others, like Wicksteed,[18] express a similar notion when they speak of our determination 'to graft on a new period of infancy to our human stock'. During this period when the adolescent is in the aforementioned 'tunnel', he is like a moulted crustacean—'having shuffled off his protecting armour he lurks in the shadows till his new coat of mail is grown'.

2

Early Adolescence

The needs of the adolescent center, then, around the problems of his status and his sexual impulses.[13] Neither problem is entirely new, but both acquire aspects of increased urgency from two general sources. As previously indicated, one of these arises as the consequence of the surge of biological maturation with pubescence. This brings not merely increase in body size, strength and appearance of secondary sexual characteristics but of a still greater impulse towards the autonomy of adulthood. The other source of this urgency, of course, is the increased expectation in regard to his learning, work and behavior from parents and other adults of his community. This external expectation has its reflection in his own inner greater self-expectation.

Conflicts and Strains for Adolescent and Adults

The poignancy of the inner conflict and strain in this phase of development, then, is almost inevitable in most present-day societies not only for the adolescent himself but also for his parents and often for many other adults of the community around him. The factors contributing to the conflict and strain likewise originate from elements both internal to the adolescent himself and in the external world of the adults around him. For some years his bodily and mental maturation and experiential resources will be incomplete. No longer appearing nor feeling like the prepubescent child, he still is not the adult in skills, in knowledge, in relatively greater assurance and poise. His parents, teachers and other adults, although expecting of him more responsible self-direction, still do not grant him, nor is he prepared in these years for, full independence of adult citizenship nor the opportunity for satisfaction of procreative urges which may be biologically matured. Unlike the adolescent of preliterate, non-industrialized cultures who is inducted much earlier in his life, often with appropriate rituals, into fuller participation in the life of the adult community, the adolescent of most technologically advanced cultures of the modern world waits for such admission till after the second decade of his life. Furthermore in the case of an increasing number of vocations, and of most professions, the entrance into the full-fledged status is delayed even for years beyond the point of legal citizenship.

Individual Variations in Degree of Strain

All these well-known internal and external factors operate generally, that is for all adolescents of both sexes to some degree. There are, of course, individual variations as to just when after eleven or twelve years of age the spurt of growth in body size or pubescence occurs. If there is some delay as to their occurrence in comparison with friends of his own age group, an individual teenaged boy or girl may experience some feelings of inferiority —or an intensification of any pre-existing sense of inadequacy for other reasons. On the other hand, any degree of precocity in appearance of pubertal changes—perhaps more frequently in the case of the girl—may likewise pose emotional problems for some in the direction of shame or embarrassment particularly if earlier attitudes towards sexuality have been seriously conflicted.

In some instances of delay in growth and pubescence in boys, the adolescent's own troubled feelings in contrasting himself to his friends may be further complicated and intensified by the neurotic anxieties of one or both of his parents about the matter. In one such instance the misery of the boy was greatly increased by his mother's severe worry about it, which drove her to many physicians intent upon some hormonal remedy. Some years later, after the son's physical growth spurt occurred and his social adaptation improved, the mother became similarly disturbed by the mild tendency to obesity and acne of her younger daughter. The daughter in this context suffered difficulty in concentration in schoolwork, rather strong feelings of inferiority to age mates, and depressive periods related to a sense of physical unattractiveness. Not unusually, the mother who had with great difficulty moderately reduced her own severe obesity was also tormented by strong feelings of hateful jealousy towards her own sister and of deprecation of her own husband. The husband in this period required therapeutic help for an episode of moderately severe anxious depression with suicidal impulses.

Individual Problems in Relation to Parents

The problems indicated that are common to all adolescents are naturally individually variously experienced in degree, depending upon the adolescent's relations with his parents not only during these teenage years but also those before puberty. If his experience with them throughout his life has been on the whole integrative, as is probably the case in most families, then his adolescent development may be less stormy and troubled. Although he may experience the need to repress any intensification of some perhaps unresolved oedipal strivings and conflicts with the pubertal surge of sexual drives, he usually gradually solves them by turning his interests toward girls in his group or younger. Although he may show greater reluctance about close affectionate gestures toward his mother, and may oscillate in some measure between dependent and independent tendencies towards her, he generally achieves finally some balanced attitude toward her usually with her wise and firm help. Although his relation with his father may manifest a still greater evidence than in earlier years of ambivalence, of fear and of oscillations between submission and rebelliousness, again with the father's firm, just, generally approving help for his actual achievements, the fortunate adolescent consolidates his identification with him.

This identification may or may not include eventually his choosing freely and realistically, in terms of his own abilities, interests and actual opportunities, his father's vocation or profession, or one admired or wished and hoped for him by his father. This identification with father (as well as with mother) is not in such instances limited to the issue of vocation. It often, of course, may include identifying with their attitudes towards sex, towards peers, towards social and economic problems, politics, religion, people in authority and the law.

Integrative Family Solutions

Such a course of development naturally presupposes a generally loving mutuality between the parents who are able to discuss openly and fully any differences they may have about their adolescent boy or their hopes for him, and to arrive at some agreements about them that are not too disparate from his actual potentialities and manifest ability. Such a relation between them gives support to each of them in the boy's need to feel their firm opposition to any exaggerated self-assertive defiance about some wish or behavior of his. In such an atmosphere between such parents the young adolescent's characteristic resistiveness is not generally hardened into a more or less completely secretive and serious estrangement from them. Their firm opposition to some wish of his that they judge potentially destructive to his own other interests is balanced by a sincere search *with him* for a safer, more constructive, alternative mode of satisfaction for his core desire. This means a search for a mode of its satisfaction which is feasible for them economically and with their attitudes and total situation, and yet congruent with his growing impulse for initiative and independence. If this proves impossible, such parents clearly express their considered reasoning (and *all* the reasons including their *anxieties* about his welfare) about their prohibition as well as their regret.

Such parents, of course, generally in such crises, or after some rebellious, and rather destructive, or potentially destructive, act of the adolescent, do not subsequently condemn him out of hand in some total way. They are able to acknowledge, together with their regretful disapproval and disagreement of his act, their satisfaction, pleasure and even joy about his actual achievements and positive attributes. They express their surprise that his basic wish and impulse seemed to the adolescent something too frightening to discuss with them beforehand. They emphasize then and on every other suitable occasion their equal interest in *his* wishes as well as in their own.

Thus his mistrust of the adult's capacity to entertain the adolescent's satisfaction of wishes no longer of great interest to them may be reduced. Mutual trust based on genuine consideration for the differences between generations may be strengthened. And perhaps most important of all, the adolescent's own self-consideration regarding his own needs and wishes may develop with a steadier tendency to subject them to evaluation as to the effect of their satisfaction upon *other* wishes of his *own* and to concentrate upon the realistic possibilities for attaining them. Under the influences of such processes his self-regard may develop more solidly and flexibly.

One is tempted to say also that when such solid self-regard begins to be integrated into the young personality, then his attitudes towards others are also more likely to be considerate, compassionate and empathetic. These attitudes towards the needs of others will then be as unambivalent as they are towards his own needs. Even his youthful enthusiasm for joining others will be tempered with a sturdier consideration for possible disadvantage to himself. There will be less need for heedlessness, for submission to destructive leadership, or on the other hand, for subjugation or dominating exploitation of others' needs, weaknesses or follies.

Similar development occurs under similar circumstances of the family in the case of the adolescent girl, with the exceptions that the defiant self-assertiveness may be somewhat less than that in the boy and that the rivalry and ambivalence during the period is often more prominent in her relations with her mother. This latter problem is usually gradually and eventually solved by the girl in a more thorough identification with her, particularly if there is no severe reactive, neurotically conflictful, repressive, response of the mother to the ambivalent behavior of her daughter. Important to such an outcome, naturally, is the father's firmness in response to the possible divisive tactics of the daughter to win him to her side in conflicts with her mother. As in the case of the boy, the adolescent daughter too, eventually solves, with both of her parents' unconflicted and unanxious help, her sexual interests in turning to boys during these years, generally those boys who are somewhat older than herself. The latter tendency to be interested in adolescent males older than herself reflects the earlier maturation among girls than among boys.

Such a rapid and sketchy characterization primarily of the usual outcomes of the adolescent phase of development leaves out much that is important and unique to this period of life.

Attitudes Towards Peers

As previously suggested, separated from childhood by the changes in his body and feelings on the one hand and excluded from, and in many ways unprepared for, the world of adults on the other hand, the adolescent turns to that of his age mates. His or her chum and other friends become the objects of intense and incessant interest and absorption. The desire either to be together or talk again together on the telephone, even a short time after separation, seems to be an all-consuming urge. This is often not easy for parents to understand or even to tolerate. The need to validate his own reactions, feelings, thoughts with another undergoing similar experiences appears insatiable. The world expands; the self expands and is discovered and rediscovered in such intimate exchanges. The adolescent's anxieties about the strange and unfamiliar, new inner changes decrease.

The adults seem sometimes not to understand fully the strength and even violence of the new impulses, the enthusiasm and the overwhelming importance of each event and activity, nor the intensely acute disappointments, rages or fears bordering on despair. The intensity and rapid oscillations of mood reflect the burgeoning growth of new energies and the great uncertainties and dangers about their fulfillment.

Characteristic Conflicts

These dangers about fulfillment are numerous and often obscure. They may be obscure not only to parents or other adults but not altogether clear to the adolescent himself. They may be obscure to the adults because of the adolescent's shame about feeling or showing his fear to others. A strong tendency to hide or deny the fear may stem not only from the fact of the extremely disagreeable nature of anxiety itself and the almost automatic effort to suppress it, to avoid the situations in which it is aroused and to develop a variety of compensatory defensive maneuvers to reduce it. It may also stem from (or be very greatly reinforced by) experiences in earlier childhood with adults who unthinkingly, unempathetically (or who suffer similar difficulties) may have contributed to the child's shame about feeling afraid. All these factors may be powerfully reinforced by the adolescent's need to live up to his own enormous wish, and those of his age mates, to appear assured, poised and 'strong'.

The dangers themselves may be unique to a given adolescent in combination or number arising from his own particular past experience and endowment. In general, however, the dangers are about his falling short of his own (often extremely heightened) standards or desires about his appearance and attractiveness, about his competence in and out of school, about his capacity to know things and to be familiar with all matters of the world. Such anxieties and shame about them make for the adolescent's shakiness in his pride, for his extreme sensitivities to any real or fancied criticism or disregard, as well as for his frequent, secret, sullen hurts, his tendencies to appear indifferent or openly rebellious. His difficulties in concentration in school or remembering his chores then are more understandable. Similarly understandable are the periods of lonely brooding and the dreamy preoccupations with phantasies of great achievement and marked daring.

In the early years of puberty, in many if not all adolescents, the sexual urges are not only keener than ever experienced before but also shrouded with considerable anxiety and often quite inhibited as to direct, open expression in respect to any actual age mate of the opposite sex. Instead, particularly among girls there appear 'crushes' upon an admired older teacher of the same or opposite sex. Perhaps a little later wildly exaggerated enthusiasms may appear for an actor, singer or some other particularly sexually attractive male, publicly known performer. This may be shared not merely with a single friend but often with large masses of other girls some of whom react with hysterical screaming or even fainting. Parental disapproval of such devotion at a distance often seems to add zest to the interest.

Boys of the post-pubertal years may also experience similar 'crushes' upon teachers, of the same or opposite sex, upon athletic heroes as well as upon public performers of the opposite sex. Their expression, especially in the last-mentioned instance, is less apt to be the open, more obvious, mass adoration of the girls. They may each experience some special attraction towards such actresses, singers and the like more secretly in their daydreams, as if they were more consciously aware of the sexual nature of their feelings than the girls seem to be. The boys seem to have a greater need to control their more active impulses learned earlier than is true of the girls; and their sensed need to be more active also perhaps contributes to their greater restraint of more overt expression of such feelings. In other words, for the male, sex is more a matter in which his initiative and activity —rather than a passive response—are important aspects of his feeling intensely involved. Hence he may feel less moved by a performance in which he plays no active part, despite his being stimulated by it.

Schisis between Sex and Tenderness

Thus the sexual impulses of adolescence, inhibited to varying degrees by fear, guilt, shame and embarrassment acquired in pre-pubertal years, are apt to be experienced as equally distressful and exciting. Felt as 'bad', the early sexual impulses after puberty may not be fused with tender, respectful, friendly or 'good' feelings. Hence in adolescents of both sexes, such sexual impulses may be split apart and he or she may experience them separately; that is, the sexual response may be felt only towards the 'bad' girl or boy, while the 'good' feelings towards other individuals with whom sex may not be possible to associate consciously. Both the adolescent boy and the girl only through a succession of such feelings towards members of the opposite sex may, as they become more accustomed to their own subjective experience, gradually be able to fuse all these feelings into a capacity for romantic attachment. In the early years such attraction may be entirely a matter of daydreams with no overt sign of them towards the actual person involved. There may be considerable torment experienced about one's own attractiveness during the early period when one's rapidly growing body is still not gracefully carried, when one is plagued by skin disorders and by doubts of one's actual capacity to converse suavely, and to carry off social situations with poise.

The Herd Phenomenon

The sense of exclusion from the world of adults and from their own pre-pubertal behavior of childhood, and the need of each adolescent to find himself in friends, give rise to the increased phenomena of the herd among them—phenomena already evident to some extent in the pre-adolescent child. All sorts of fashions and manners appear in each generation of adolescents, as if to emphasize in every way possible their unique identity as a group. Again special ways of wearing the hair—sometimes rapidly changing—appear. Particular styles of clothing, changes in uses of words, phrases, almost a new vocabulary springs up among them. Such hectic efforts to assert a rather defiant difference in their group and world include the adolescents' own waves of enthusiasms and interests in sports, recreation, music, dance and pranks.

Conflicts about Freedom and Authority

At home the adolescent often presses for more freedom and new privileges from his parents with a new intensity and openness. Denials of some even unreasonable demands evoke strong reactions of open or sullen resentments alternating with tearful hurt moods (especially among girls) or rather wild accusations of parents' unfairness, excessive sternness and old-fashioned rigidity of attitudes. Such episodes may inject some confusion, some doubting self-searching as well as hurt, anger and anxiety into the reactions of parents. It is not always easy for parents to recall the storms of their own adolescent years. It is not easy for them always to perceive beneath their children's exaggerated, rebellious self-assertions the inner tormenting uncertainties, self-doubts and anxieties about their attractiveness, their poise, their abilities—in short how shaky is their self-regard and self-assurance.

Need for Positive Balance of Satisfactions over Discontents

The need of the adolescent in this context is the same as the need of persons at any stage of the human life cycle, namely a positive balance of satisfactions over the discontents. It may be that the stresses of his particular period of life may increase his need for this positive balance.

Health

Basic to all the other needs is good health. The essential problem is not only of endowment but also the acquisition of all those habits, and the seeking of opportunities for their expression, of adequate self-care. Such self-care, of course, includes cleanliness, a balanced nutrition, attention to dental and skin hygiene and, not least in importance, vigorous muscular activity and systematic exercise. It does not seem to this writer that this need for vigorous muscular activity must be satisfied only in highly competitive, or potentially exhausting or injurious sports. There are many games and sports which can be enjoyed together—or even alone—which fulfill this bodily and emotional need.

Given good health and the maintenance of strength, stamina and physical fitness contribute much to the adolescent's greater ease of obtaining the satisfaction of his other needs. A healthy vigor is an essential element of attractive vitality in both sexes, even though marked physical beauty especially of facial features may not be part of the adolescent's endowment. It adds greatly to the adolescent's quiet, solid pride, self-contentment and therefore to his self-assurance and poise.

Such health expresses itself in greater eagerness to seek and find opportunities for other intellectually and emotionally satisfying activities which are constructively creative. Adults, parents, teachers and others who are ready to do so, respond to the adolescent's eagerness even more readily with opportunities and guidance for him to feel useful and creative in work or play, at home, at school or elsewhere in the community. It needs no emphasis that such activities themselves are the sources of the adolescent's deepest satisfaction. It is nevertheless also true that prompt reward in the form of recognition of the achievement, added monetary reward and balanced praise or the wholehearted pleasure of the adults concerned powerfully increases the adolescent's satisfaction.

Adolescents' Projections onto Parents

As emphasized previously, the adolescent typically is ashamed and very embarrassed by his own inner fearfulness and often can hardly acknowledge it to himself much less to his parents. Occasionally to a trusted teacher, school counselor, physician or other adult may he or she be able to speak of such self-derogated worries. But even in such conversations the parents may still be pictured as repressively restricting ogres who are then clearly recipients of the projected, internal, self-prohibiting anxieties against which he also rages often with tormenting impotence. The need of the adolescent in such storms for wise judicious firmness about clear rules for many aspects of living from his parents is often quite evident.

The Need for Firmness

This need for firmness presents many parents with a perplexing problem. The adolescent repeatedly forgets, or otherwise fails, to carry out some aspect of self-care, of orderliness, thoroughness or punctuality about his room, his possessions, appointments or assigned tasks and household chores, or his money. It is difficult for the parent not to react to such repetitious deficiencies, delays or failures with irritation, discouragement or some sense of personal failure. If such feelings get even partial expression in the parent's tone of voice or manner of speaking, the 'nagging' quality is translated by the adolescent as a sense of blaming and derogation of himself. In addition to his inner response of guilt, his reactive hurt and resentment immediately compounds his problem. It interferes with his ability to learn from the exchange and contributes to his emotional estrangement not only from his family but also from his own positive self-regard. It may give him some basis for seeing his parents as unjust or impatient to a degree greater than the occasion calls for. Hopefully, the parent from such experiences learns to check the adolescent's performance, remind him before or after the time with considerate courtesy and unremitting vigilance which may seem to the parent endless and unrewarding.

In reaction to such firmness the adolescent then experiences not only considerable relief but also support against his own often self-destructive, impulsiveness (again often not admitted), and gains in growth of self-direction and steadiness—until the next episode. For obvious reasons on the other hand, the adolescent experiences an increase in his anxious, rebellious self-assertiveness, when parents uneasily waver in their reaction to his pressures either while in the process of making their decision, or if they take too long to arrive at a clear definitive choice about what they permit and agree to or deny of his specific wishes. The turmoil of the whole family is easily imaginable and understandable if the demand of the adolescent succeeds in intensifying some unresolved difference between his parents about one or more particular issues.

The Need for Discriminate Reaction by Parents to Each Situation

Despite what may seem as innumerable and insurmountable problems of this sort, the need of the adolescent (and of his parents) is clearly to experience (and for the parents to deal with) each deficiency, failure or rebelliousness as a discrete, immediate situation. Even though there probably have been many previous similar instances, there is the possibility, if not a great probability, that consideration of the recurrences as evidences of some obscure characterological defect may become a self-fulfilling prophecy. Feelings of human beings tend to have a global quality. This quality often gains expression in recall of similar experiences and behavior (one's own or that of others) in the past. It is then generally felt as a fear of similar troubles in the future. Discrimination of the current issue or episode from the *affective* spread into the past and the future is both difficult and essential.

The Need for Restitution

An aspect of this necessary discrimination—which may reduce the anxiety of all concerned and check the tendency toward panic—is the need of the adolescent to have an opportunity to make adequate restitution. It needs to be a restitution which is actually possible for him and satisfying to both his parents and himself. If one is found which actually *restores* the situation completely, or as much as possible, to what it was before, and is agreed to by all those concerned, then the perpetuating destructiveness of prolonged guilt (and the rebellion against it) may be reduced or altogether avoided. It may be important to note that such guilt, which has no real resolution in restitutive action, affects not only the adolescent but also his parents. It certainly colors strongly all other aspects of their living together, often with extremely negative and destructive feelings.

The Need for Balanced Attitude from Parents

Part of all this atmosphere in the family which the adolescent requires in the face of his problems is a balanced attitude from his parents. If corrections when needed are made *with an effort to help him learn or acquire a needed skill or satisfaction*, they naturally are more integrative not only for him but for the entire family. If these corrections are offered with full acknowledgment for the adolescent's actual achievements and integrative qualities, the hurt to his self-regard will more likely be less. Such corrections, expressed more with the parents' regret and concern for his total welfare than with angry condemnation, tend to ease the adolescent's own painful and destructive sense of guilt. They then may reduce the adolescent's fear about being truthful with his parents about any future errors, failures or misdemeanors.

Such attitudes are more likely to maintain the adolescent's sense of *belonging* to his family. At the same time they increase his positive sense of self-respect. With this, such experiences tend to reduce any tendency to more prolonged depressive disability in function in other aspects of his living. Such disabilities generally lead to another and secondary by-product: that of a further increase in the negative balance in his satisfactions and discontents. This often results in substitutive symptomatic behavior. Not

E

the least important of this latter process is the not infrequent search for companions who are negativistically arrayed in a hostile if not destructive manner against adult mores. Such companionship may be originally primarily for consolation. It may however consolidate the negative, the hostile attitudes even more.

3

Later Adolescence

The later years of the second decade of life may in many adolescents be somewhat less turbulent than the early phase described above, but they are concerned with a major problem that becomes for many an increasingly pressing one as adulthood approaches. This is the search for and the acquisition of—in Erik Erikson's phrase—identity.

If the early years of adolescence have on the whole been lived through integratively with adequate parental help, the later adolescent is more accustomed and more familiar with both his own bodily changes and subjective feelings. He is progressively mastering what he learns in school, his new social role and the new freedoms and the responsibilities that are inextricably a part of them. The degree and steadiness of his mastery of these skills of self-direction may vary not only from that of others of his age mates but also in his own life from time to time of external pressure and in internal need. He or she dates the opposite sex with less anxious tension; he gets his household chores done more or less passably well along with school work; he may show fewer episodes of defiance with parents; and his earlier herd-like enthusiasms may become somewhat less intense.

The Need for Integrated Sense of Self

However, he not only becomes more and more preoccupied as to what he will be, but in this preoccupation he may still in any uncertainty of eventual vocational or professional goal, frequently experience struggle and disturbing feelings: 'Who am I?' 'Is this I?' and 'What is that?' The answer to such questions comes in these and later years of adolescence with still more experience of self-discovery. As Erikson[2] puts it, the task of adolescence may be fruitfully discussed in ego-psychological and psychosocial terms. He states, 'Man, to take his place in society, must acquire a "conflict-free" habitual use of a dominant *faculty*, to be elaborated in an *occupation*; a limitless *resource*, a feedback, as it were, from the immediate exercise of this occupation, from the *companionship* it provides, and its *tradition*; and finally, an intelligible *theory* of the processes of life.' This theory he prefers to call an *ideology*. All this he subsumes, as indicated previously, in the process he names as identity formation.

Erikson considers the process of identity formation in considerable detail from its beginnings in earlier childhood and its continuation into early adulthood. He considers it always as a process of intimate interaction between those events inside the individual and those which occur in relation to other persons. Among these other persons, of course, are included not only the parents and adults in and outside the immediate family but also younger and older children and youth as well as his peers and age mates, all of both sexes. This interaction permits him continuous opportunities for role experimentation in the variety of relations he will meet throughout life.

He speaks of the process as one of *mutuality* between these others and the emerging person who is progressively identified and recognized by society which also feels 'recognized' by him. These others of society feel this recognition by the individual who cares to ask for recognition. By the same token, these others can feel deeply vengeful and rejected by the individual who does not care for recognition.

Adolescence as Normative Crisis

Erikson emphasizes that, in spite of the similarity of adolescent 'symptoms' and episodes to those of neurosis and psychosis, 'adolescence is not an affliction but a *normative crisis*'. It is a phase of increased conflict but one characterized by a high potential for growth. Although such a normative crisis may arouse dormant anxiety, it is yet a phase that is 'relatively more reversible, or, better, traversable' by reason of the available abundance of energy to support new ego functions in searching and playful entrance into new associations and opportunities. This is in contrast to the waste of energy in the self-defeating circular conflicts of neurosis. Thus, unless scrutinized without prejudice, the aggravated crisis—which may appear to be a neurotic illness—may be self-liquidating and even contributive to identity formation.

The Process of Identity Formation

In this process of identity formation some aspects of the childhood identifications are assimilated and integrated, and others repudiated and rejected into a new *Gestalt* or configuration. As Erikson puts it, 'identity formation begins where the usefulness of identification ends'. The process of integrating psychosexual and psychosocial aspects is a continuous one. Not only is this integration occurring at each level of development, but new elements of identity need assimilation. Earlier crystalizations of identity are subject to renewed conflict. This occurs when changes occur in the quantity and quality of drive, in mental equipment, in new and often conflicting social demands. Such changes make previous adaptive integrations insufficient. Further, the growth process supplies new energy, as others in society offer new opportunities.

Erikson[3] then summarizes this process from the genetic point of view thus: '—identity formation emerges as an *evolving configuration*—a configuration which is gradually established by successive ego syntheses and resyntheses throughout childhood; it is a configuration gradually integrating *constitutional givens, idiosyncratic libidinal needs, favored capacities, significant identifications, effective defenses, successful sublimation* and *consistent roles.*' Whether or not all this occurs, or whether the adolescent regresses to more infantile conflict depends on at least two factors. It depends upon the opportunities and rewards which he may find in his clique of peers. It also depends upon those formal ways in which the society invites him to work experimentation from social play and to final commitments from rituals of transit. All of this, says Erikson,[4] needs to be based upon a mutual contract which is implicit between society and the individual.

4

Pathological Deviations of Adolescence

It is in the circumstances of family turmoil, particularly when it is prolonged or long-standing, or frequently recurrent in the whole of the child's life before adolescence, that clinicians see the various more severe maldevelopments of personality during the post-pubertal years. Since the emphasis here is upon the needs of the child for his emotional health, the more pathological deviations will be barely mentioned.

Specific Contributing Stresses

From what has been previously indicated, the stresses of adolescence, internal and external, contribute their own quota of determinants to the more serious episodes or periods of disorder in behavior and psychological functioning. Any tragically unfortunate events in the family in the sense that they are in no way connected with the problems of adolescence, however, are additional factors. Deaths in the family, particularly of one of the parents, economic difficulties, especially if they are not outgrowths of parental financial mismanagement, political and social disorders, as well as acute interparental turmoil with or without divorce and their accompanying difficulties, are some of the examples of categories of family difficulties that may in a given instance be contributing stresses.

Of course, depending upon all the circumstances and the personality resources of the persons of the family as well as that of the adolescent himself from previous experience, such stresses may be challenges to further integrating development of everyone involved. Nonetheless, if such stresses are either overwhelmingly difficult to surmount, or occur as another in a long history of previous family turmoils, the problems of adolescence may in this sense become critical.

General Malintegrative Influences

Before proceeding to the consideration of more specific clinical syndromes it may be well to review some general observations upon phenomena among youth in recent years.

Josselyn[8] makes the point that, since in a democratic society cultural change occurs by evolution rather than by revolution, it is often the adolescent or young adults who are generally the carriers, or the effectors, of such change. If some aspect of the previously more or less established ethos is not only opposed by the youth itself but is given sufficient support or even leadership from older members of the society, the stage is set for possible modification.

This change may naturally center about any one or about a closely related set of society's mores. It may involve attitudes toward sexual practices, toward relations between the sexes, toward some special policy of the government and of the dominant older majority in regard to society's internal economics or its external international relations. It often focuses on some inequity, injustice or social problem which has long been unsolved, or one which may have for various reasons become more acute. It may fuse in itself not only a general social condition but also one which personally may contribute to one or another frustration of the youth himself.

One general example, especially in the United States, has been the opposition by a significant and vocal minority to this country's involvement in the Viet Nam war. This has led to the appearance among a proportion of the youth not only of a similar opposition to military service but to individual acts of burning of draft cards. Josselyn emphasizes that the aspect of a general 'Cause' and the possibility of heroic martyrdom for such a cause may arouse the youth's fervor in seeking admiration from the dissenting minority. The participation in social action, this writer observes, probably generally also indicates some failure of the youth's family and other adults of the community to provide an alternative type of leadership which would have made the burning of the draft card impossible for the individual youth.

It is not altogether clear to the present writer to what to attribute the recent prominence of certain youth movements—or subcultures of youth—such as the beatnik[10] or the hippie. One can only speculate about the role of several possibilities. In the United States there are estimates that at present about 40 per cent of the population is composed of youth. Hence, what may appear like a greater number of youth tending to live in ways implied in the name beatnik and hippie may be no greater proportion of youth than in earlier generations also seeking modes of existence divergent from that of the majority. Another possibility is that it is commercially advantageous to provide youth with its particular whimsical tastes in clothing, hair dress, music and news coverage in an age of accelerated and expanded means of communication. Whether the appearance or rediscovery of psychedelic drugs and their spread by some members of the older generation is a factor, or only a partial factor, also needs mention.

In this context Josselyn mentions clinical experience and suggests a possibly greater number of present-day youth than in earlier decades imbued with a philosophy which is termed 'crassly egocentric'. A basic tenet of this philosophy is that one of the rights of the individual is license rather than freedom. Citing Philip Rieff,[11] this author states that this present philosophy considers boredom as the worse possible sin and individual gratifications of the moment as the highest goal. One hears quite often from many of the young how many activities and experiences are 'a drag', and of the incessant search 'for kicks' and failing this, the impulse 'to turn on' and 'drop out'.

Josselyn also points to the frequency of parents' complaints about their adolescents' poor school performance largely in terms of it being an obstacle to future material success in not earning admission to schools of higher education and eventually a poorer earning power in the labor market. In her experience, it is a rare parent who expresses this concern about his son's or daughter's loss of deeper and wider subjective satisfactions in living—satisfactions which can only result from experiencing the pleasure and joy of learning and of mastery. The two aims—economic success and subjective emotional richness which derive from education—are of course not mutually exclusive. It is perhaps a matter of emphasis, or a lack of emphasis, by the parents upon their own experienced satisfaction in the exercise of his vocation or profession. Josselyn surmises that the experience of the great economic depression in the youth of the present generation of parents may have contributed to their anxiety about economic success and security and to this relative silence or shyness on their part with their children—the current youthful generation. From this source may arise the beatnik's or hippie's hostility to the materialism of their elders and their own insistence on love, pleasure and tolerance of the other man's 'thing'.

Factors Diminishing Pleasure in Learning and Mastery

Work then, especially in school, may become a 'drag' particularly if in earlier years of adolescence and preadolescence learning was insufficiently associated with mutual pleasure on the part of both children and their parents. Clinical experience with those parents complaining about their ten- or twelve-year-olds' disorderliness or lack of sustained interest and performance in matters of self-care, in their household chores and in their use of time suggests some of the contributing factors. The point has already been made about the contribution to this problem by the characteristics of the adolescent physical and mental growth period and the child's self-absorption in these inner changes. However, troubles of the parent often contribute markedly towards intensifying the adolescent's difficulty. We need not consider the grosser forms of parental neglect, lack of interest or even some special indifference, or even covert hostility, to a given child. What one may be more impressed with in such clinical situations is lack of sufficient participation with the child by one or both parents during the early periods of the child's learning a chore, a manual or a mental skill.

The mother who in her own childhood did not acquire sufficient help in learning how to make a bed, how to cook, sew, mend, to take care of clothing or younger children, and much less in orderly management of household economics is often in desperate straits with her own children in similar matters. She may be struggling to learn such things herself under the most trying circumstances of her responsibilities. She cannot then feel much satisfaction in her own skills. She is often harried by her own lack, by being constantly uncertain about her ability, anxious about the pressing tasks not performed in a timely, efficient manner, by striving to keep up with a schedule of duties inadequately done and yet often late. Her capacity to achieve satisfaction in her daily life is thus greatly decreased by such tensions.

In such moods which sometimes seem either very frequent or almost continuous she has little patient interest or eagerness to help her own child to learn similar skills through repetitively doing them with him. She may be utterly disabled, too, in feeling or expressing any satisfaction in *his* acquiring the skill or in his regular performance of it until the child himself acquires the trait of its effective timely and self-satisfying performance.

Similar problems may interfere with a father's capacity to contribute to his son's—or daughter's—integrating not only particular skills but also the pleasure or quiet satisfaction in their performance. It may be even a more malintegrative experience for a child and the later adolescent if there appears, or has always existed, a deep difference of attitude between his mother and father towards learning of all skills, their orderly performance and the quality of achievement. The tension between them undermines or makes difficult or impossible in his experiencing much satisfaction in such performance. The dichotomy grows between *recreation* and creative work as far as a satisfying subjective experience is concerned.

Work is then a 'drag'. Work undone, poorly or hurriedly done, still hangs as a heavy albatross around his neck. His guilty tension is more or less successfully transformed into overt indifference, with secret hate and envy of the better-integrated age mate. Under these circumstances the irritable reminders of parents arouse a guilty rebelliousness tainted by self-contempt. To the extent the irritability of the parental efforts with him are also guilt-ridden from some murky subjective awareness of their own failure to live more effectively, with self-satisfaction and with some measure of tranquility, they cannot be firm. The adolescent often senses this only too clearly. He is not helped to internalize sufficiently solidly within his own subjective feelings the ideals or values by which his parents presumably are trying to live as members of their culture.

Additional General Malintegrative Influences

It is tempting to speculate that perhaps other factors have been more generally operative in the past two or three decades in Western societies in addition to the experience of the Great Depression during the earlier life of the present generation of parents. These are the factors of rapidly changing international relations in the world with their more threatening tensions in view of the rapidly increasing world population and the technological advances in respect to nuclear energy, to more rapid transportation and communication, as well as perhaps the related inflationary monetary processes. All these factors, to the extent they contribute to undermining the economic security of persons who experienced the anxieties during the Great Depression, also contribute to a continuing sense of helplessness and anxiety about not only survival but also the maintenance of subsistence necessities.

If a nation's currency is devalued or eroded in its buying power, the effect not only upon the father as breadwinner but also upon his whole family seems inevitable, even if these causes may not always be perceived clearly by those so affected. If the salary or wages earned, despite their apparently higher sums, seem not ever to be quite sufficient not only for subsistence but also for some modicum of the commodities produced by technological advance, the pressure upon the parents—especially the father —for increasing effort in taking an additional job, or working longer hours, or failing this a negative effect upon his or their self-regard seems also inevitable. Such tensions generally also decrease any person's capacity for enjoyment of all aspects of living outside of employment. The mother reacting to the father's tension and fatigue and vice versa further decreases their capacity for the satisfactions of mutuality and intimacy not only with each other but also with their children. The vicious circles involve their productivity and hence satisfaction both at work, at school and at home. They involve also the effects of one generation upon the other mutually.

Erikson's Concept of Identity Diffusion

It is in the contexts outlined above that the concept of identity diffusion and negative identity offered by Erikson[5] would, for the present writer, apply. Erikson seeks 'to concentrate on certain common features representative of the common life crises shared by' a whole group of adolescent, and young adult, patients. He specifically mentions young borderline cases, customarily diagnosed 'as preschizophrenias, or severe character disorders with paranoid, depressive, psychopathic or other trends'. He does not question 'such well-established diagnostic signposts'. The features he calls attention to are 'a result of a (temporary or final) inability of their egos to establish an identity: for they all suffer from *acute identity diffusion*'. He also makes the point that the individual patients known to him, from which he formulated this general conception, came from both extremes of socio-economic status in the United States. He speculates that the families of these patients, 'because of their extreme locations on the scale of class mobility and Americanization, may have conveyed to these particular children a certain hopelessness regarding their chances of participating in (or of successfully defying) the dominant American manners and symbols of success'.

Erikson's characterization of his composite sketch, of the features of this life crisis, is subdivided under five general aspects: (1) the time of breakdown; (2) the problem of intimacy; (3) diffusion of time perspective; (4) diffusion of industry; and (5) the choice of the negative identity.

The time of breakdown, or a state of an acute identity diffusion, occurs when the young individual meets several more or less simultaneous demands upon him. These demands are for commitment to *physical intimacy* which are 'not by any means always overtly sexual', to decisive *occupational choice*, to *energetic competition* and to *psychosocial self-definition*. When exposed to a group of age mates from radically different backgrounds from his own—as in college—a young person needs to choose from among them friends, or intimates of both sexes and to repudiate others. Otherwise, particularly in the presence of serious inner conflicts, he is driven to an avoidance of choices which leads to outer isolation and an inner vacuum. The problem is often made the more acute by the fact that some of the age mates who are 'different' may comfortably display manners, values and symbols about which the youth may be driven in opposite directions at once. Involvement, or even success, with any group of such age mates may seem both to be irreversible and to narrow down other tentative, explorative involvements. The disturbance under such circumstances may be a transitory adolescent regression to older involvements and behavior in an attempt to postpone or to avoid, as Erikson puts it, a psychosocial foreclosure. Such a state of paralysis may ensue which can be understood as an effort to 'maintain minimal actual choice and commitment with a maximum inner conviction of still being the chooser'.

Concerning the problem of intimacy, Erikson makes as his central point the known fact that it is a sturdy integration of the self which makes possible a true engagement with others. Conversely it follows that an attempt to engage in any intimacy, whether in friendship, in competition or in sexual intimacy, brings into the open any latent lack of such integration, or as he prefers to call it a 'weakness of identity'.

Thus, the youth who is divided in himself by conflict experiences 'a peculiar strain' in any of his efforts to find tentative forms of playful intimacy with age mates of both sexes. When such a state is severe in degree, he may experience even in tentative engagements of this sort a feeling of a great danger of a loss of sense of self. Erikson calls it 'an interpersonal fusion amounting to a loss of identity'. Such anxieties lead to a variety of efforts to circumvent the disaster. A tense inner reservation with a caution about commitment may characterize his attitudes towards others. He may isolate himself or enter only formalized or stereotyped relations with others. Or, on the other hand, he may in frenzied repetitions experience frequent failures in involvements 'with the most improbable partners'.

Whether in friendly social intercourse or in lovemaking, the youth with such an uncertain self-regard is threatened with a loss of clear subjective discrimination of his own sensations, affects, decisions or purposes in the engagement. He becomes unclear whether what he does or does not do, whether what he experiences or does not experience is for himself or for the other. His own wishes become blurred or buried in a storm of anxiety about pleasing or hurting the other, about whether he or his partner experienced satisfaction or disappointment and at the behest of which of them. He loses the capacity flexibly to abandon himself in sex tenderly, for it implies a fusion in which one is lost to another whose response guarantees his own sense of self-continuity. In Erikson's words, 'fusion with another becomes identity loss'. A collapse of capacity for mutuality is suddenly threatened, with an intense desire to start all over again and with a bewildered rage more characteristic of early childhood.

Such difficulties in choosing intimates is often associated with a difficulty or inability to repudiate or reject a different set of available age mates. An insufficiently clear, internal sense of one's own values, preferences or tastes makes discrimination of others' characteristics difficult and fuzzy. Hence Erikson points to both 'a weakness or excess in repudiation' as an intrinsic aspect of the inability to attain a comfortable sense of intimacy. He also emphasizes that such youth often pathetically feel that only merging with a 'leader' can save them—an adult who can offer them himself as an experimental and safe object to whom to surrender and use as a guide towards relearning the steps towards mutual intimacy and legitimate repudiation.

If the last-mentioned relationship fails—as its intensity and absoluteness often determines—the youth recoils to a period of intense self-testing, introspection and isolation. During this he may experience, if his state and the circumstances are severe, a loss of sense of self-continuity and sameness, a painful sense of separation from others, a great sense of shame, a difficulty in deriving any satisfaction from any activity. He may even feel that life is happening to him rather than being lived by his initiative. A basic mistrust pervades him. It is up to others to demonstrate that he 'does exist in a psychosocial sense, i.e. can count on an invitation to become himself'.

In regard to the third characteristic of identity diffusion, that of diffusion of time perspective, Erikson calls attention to the exacerbation of the psychopathology of everyday adolescence, namely to the disturbance in the experience of time. This is simultaneously a subjective sense of great urgency and an apparent loss of consideration of time in his actual living. The youth may feel both extremely young and very old.

In its more malignant form there is both a deep disbelief that change may come with time and an intense anxiety that it might. Such an adolescent has difficulty in getting started, moving through even simple tasks of self-care, or in stopping in transition to another activity. Both going to bed and arising are equally hard to face. Hours are spent by some in endless head-rocking, listening to music or other self-absorbed and stimulating activities. To decide beforehand as to the time when one will be at a given place, how long one will remain there, or just what one will do in what order are extremely difficult.

Such phrases as, 'I give up,' 'I quit,' 'I don't know,' frequently indicate not only some degree of depression but also of a despair in which death of the ego or self is a welcome surcease to the current torment. This is not an actual suicidal wish in many, except when in a relatively few instances the 'wish to be a suicide' becomes, as Erikson puts it, 'an inescapable identity choice in itself'. It is an aspect of a hope that a new beginning can be made. In therapy some of these youths seem to require the feeling that the therapist is not committing them to a continuation of life if the experience should fail to prove it worthwhile; otherwise, in the absence of a conviction on that no such commitment exists, 'the moratorium would not be a real one'.

The present writer has some clinical experience in which it seemed that such marked disturbances in respect to the experience of time in the adolescent and young adult were related to his exposure over many years to intense conflicts of each of his parents and inevitably between them. The father, given to a great orderliness in almost every aspect of his life and to the thorough performance of even the minutiae of each task, was often so exhausted at the end of the day or the week that he required quiet and almost complete isolation from family for rest. The mother, more interested in a less planful and more 'spontaneous' existence, found this extremely disagreeable, distressing and frequently unbearable. Intense conflicts about many aspects of common living led to intense hurts, resentments, periods of emotional estrangement between them and episodes of depression, especially in the father. Numerous violent disagreements between them also centered about many aspects of the rearing of their children. Their younger child particularly manifested difficulty in learning at school, numerous conflicting, relatively short-lived, interests and an erratic achievement in both. In later adolescence he suffered from intense difficulties about intimacy, particularly with the opposite sex, about occupational choice, but especially about his use of time. Constantly extremely anxious about being on time, he was very resentfully reluctant definitely to commit himself to any schedule of activities. At home he often manifested the behavior in the routine activities which Erikson so aptly phrases, 'as if he were moving in molasses'. His movement in therapy was similar.

Erikson's next feature of this syndrome, that of diffusion of industry, has been touched on in the previous discussion of problems of earlier adolescence. He calls it an acute upset in the sense of workmanship. It manifests itself either in an inability to concentrate, to perform regularly or thoroughly required or suggested tasks. On the other hand, it may be evidenced by an absorbing but self-destructive pre-occupation with one-sided activities such as reading, listening to music, or endless rating of musical recordings as 'hits'.

The point is made that work goals are not only useful in supporting suppression of infantile instinctual aims but also in enhancing integration of the personality. This is particularly true, since the exposure to, the practice, and final mastery, of many skills occurs outside the home away from parents, especially away from the mother, with age mates (e.g. at the fishing hole) or with other adults such as teachers at school, workshop or coaches on the physical education or recreational fields. Thus such activities promote acquiring satisfactions with actual tools and material in a communal experience that find opportunities in the external world of social reality.

Erikson points to the immediate oedipal antecedents of the beginnings of a work identity. For this reason those adolescents suffering from identity diffusion find their gears reversed towards oedipal competitiveness and sibling rivalry. Thus he explains that in such youth there is both the inability to concentrate and an excessive sensitivity and abhorrence of competitiveness. Despite their frequently good intelligence, ability in school, work or sports, they lose their capacity for work, exercise and sociability which as vehicles for social play are also important alternatives to vague, anxious and formless fantasy. Although the disturbance may be a revived oedipal struggle, with enhanced dangerous energy from increased 'aggressive power' and matured sexual equipment, it is not, according to Erikson, to be interpreted in exclusively or even primarily sexual terms. He prefers to emphasize the turning toward the earliest origins of the diffused early introjects as an effort to resolve this diffusion and 'to rebuild shaky childhood identifications'. As such return and attempt at resolution of earlier conflicts, he sees the disturbance as a wish to be born again and learn even the very first steps toward reality, mutuality, and regain the 'functions of contact, activity and competition'.

Perhaps the most severe form of the disturbance being discussed is the *loss* of a sense of identity with a choice of a negative identity. This takes the form of a hostile, snobbish and contemptuous rejection of any role offered by his family or immediate social community as both desirable and 'proper'. Erikson states that any part aspect or all parts of a given role may be the focus of the youth's 'acid disdain'. It may involve rejection of his ethnic origin, social class, nationality or sexual role. It may occur in families with oldest established traditions or in those newest in the social order. It is often expressed as a general dislike for everything characteristic of the young person's origins and the expected role and as an overestimation, quite obviously irrational, of everything foreign or opposite. In Erikson's phrase,[6] 'Life and strength seem to exist where one is not, while decay and danger threaten wherever one happens to be.'

Such patients sometimes suffer from a pervasive, generalized subjective sense of depreciation, or a sense of insincerity or 'phoniness' about almost every thought, act, possession or characteristic of their own. It may lead them only rarely to a complete denial of personal identity, although some seek refuge in an angry insistence on having a new label in the form of a nickname or new name. Occasionally Erikson met with 'confabulatory reconstructions of one's origin', in the form of elaborating a totally different ethnic or national background (based in one instance on an early integrative attachment to a neighbor) and a complete denial of any biologic relationship to one's own parents. More commonly the negative identity is expressed more subtly on a perverse acceptance of aspects of behavior presented by parents as bad or dangerous. This is particularly true if such behavior is itself conflictfully experienced by the parents. The youth, as Erikson and others[7] have found, perceives the unexpressed wishes and weaknesses of the parents with remarkably self-destructive accuracy.

The vindictiveness of such choices of negative identity, however, do not obscure for the clinician closely scrutinizing the past and present plight of the youth and his current subjective turmoil the fact that it is often the only possible solution to these factors. It is often clear that it is a desperate attempt at regaining some mastery in an otherwise psychodynamically impossible situation. When the inner capacities are so deadlocked by conflict that to attain that which one is supposed to be is unattainable, then the adolescent seeks to 'derive a sense of identity out of a *total* identification with that which one is *least* supposed to be'. When a sense of wholeness seems impossible, the youth may find relief in a 'totalistic' reorientation by free choice in being either a '*nobody, or somebody bad*, or indeed, *dead* . . .'. Many young people have groped, and are groping, to find such relief in cliques or gangs collectively, whether in the use of drugs, social cynicism, homosexuality or in efforts to construct a new philosophy which underlies more total ways of living different from that of their elders. Whether the epithet 'blacksheep' is applicable in all such instances requires even more and more continuous study than has thus far been accorded not only those who become 'patients' but also those who remain in communities more or less their own.

Specific Types of Disorder

The major types of disorder in the adolescent years are well known.[12,13] The relative frequency of these types, as far as this writer is concerned, has not been determined and perhaps varies from region to region and from one period of time to another in the same geographical area. For the sake of brevity, it might be said that there are three major types with mixtures of symptomatology in some individual instances. These types, of course, are: (*1*) aggressively hostile disorders of behavior, the so-called 'delinquent', or dissocial or asocial personality disorders; (*2*) the psychoneurotic, or internal disturbances of personality functioning; and (*3*) the psychotic disorders of schizophrenic or affective varieties. It is assumed here that the characteristics of these severe deviations of personality development will be discussed more thoroughly elsewhere in this volume and that they are probably in some measure known to the reader. A series of clinical studies has recently appeared on various aspects of such adolescent disorders which the reader may find useful.[9]

It is for these reasons sufficient here only to indicate that in the writer's clinical experience none of the instances of such pathological deviation in the adolescent years, that have come to his attention in which sufficient information has been available, appeared to have had their etiological factors limited to the period of life in which they occurred. In short, exacerbations of psychoneurotic turmoil, of psychotic degrees of schizophrenic illness, of severe suicidal depressive reactions, or of overt, hostile destructive behavior against the social or legal rules of the community (in males) or against the sexual mores (in females), have few of them appeared to have their beginnings in the post-pubertal years. Likewise, the prognostic indications have in such experience been intimately related to the duration of disorder in the preadolescent years and the integrative potential of the family in the same period of time.

Finally it might be added that most of the large types of disorder mentioned, or of mixtures of symptomatology from these types, have their counterparts during phases of preadolescent development. There are, of course, differences in detail of symptomatology related to individual differences in developmental or experiential factors. However, the dynamic expressions of conflict whether primarily directed against the self internally, or primarily against others, or oscillations between the two, are all seen. This is true, even if such symptoms as clearly suicidal acts are much less frequent, or all the details of schizophrenic turmoil of adolescent years may be different in the prepubescent period.

Such experience gives some basis for a long-standing hope that adequate preventive measures—if they can ever be sufficiently effective—in the earlier years of life of the child might at least reduce either the severity, the duration, or the frequency of the severe eruptions of deviation in the later years of adolescence.

REFERENCES

1. ERIKSON, E. H. 1959. *Identity and the life cycle.* Psychological Issues, Vol. 1, No. 1, Monograph 1. New York: International Universities Press.
2. *Ibid.,* pp. 110–111.
3. *Ibid.,* p. 116.
4. *Ibid.,* p. 118.
5. *Ibid.,* p. 122.
6. *Ibid.,* p. 219.
7. JOHNSON, A. M. and SZUREK, S. A. 1952. The genesis of antisocial acting out in children and adults. *Psychoanal. Quart.,* 21, No. 3.
8. JOSSELYN, I. M. 1966. *The adolescent today.* Unpublished paper presented at Alumni Meeting of Smith College of Social Work, San Francisco, California, November 18, 1966.

9. MASSERMAN, J. 1966. Adolescence, dreams and training. *Science and psycho-analysis*, **9**, 111–159. New York: Grune & Stratton.

10. MASSERMAN, J. 1967, The beatnik: up-, down-, and off-, *Arch. gen. Psychiat.*, **16**, 262–267.

11. RIEFF, P. 1965. *Triumph of the therapeutic: uses of faith after Freud.* New York: Harper.

12. SPOCK, B. 1964. *Dr. Spock talks with mothers—growth and guidance.* Greenwich, Connecticut: Fawcett Publications.

13. SZUREK, S. A. 1949. An attitude towards (child) psychiatry. *Quarterly Journal of Child Behavior*, **1**, 22, 375, 401, and in *Training in therapeutic work with children*, Eds S. A. Szurek and I. N. Berlin, Vol. II of The Langley Porter Child Psychiatry Series. Palo Alto, California: Science and Behavior Books, 1967.

14. WICKSTEED, J. H. 1936. *The challenge of childhood: an essay on nature and education.* London: Chapman and Hall.

15. *Ibid.*, p. 238.

16. *Ibid.*, p. 242.

17. *Ibid.*, p. 243.

18. *Ibid.*, p. 246.

VI

THE ADOLESCENT AS A SOCIAL BEING

JOHN BARRON MAYS
M.A., PH.D.

*Professor of Social Science in the University of Liverpool
England*

1

Introduction

There are two separate aspects of the relationship between adolescents and society. First, there is the degree to which the society meets or fails to meet the individual's basic needs and legitimate psycho-social requirements. Second, there is the broader, more sociological question of the need that the community has for the services and energies of adolescents in prosecuting and promoting society's ends and objectives. These two aspects overlap and interweave but are analytically distinctive. We ought to keep them both in view whenever we think about adolescents in modern society, whether we are asking what their appropriate role embodies or whether we are thinking more in terms of the social and psychological problems that a minority of adolescents present to the rest of the community. Sometimes, for example, it may be that tensions and difficulties arise because the social role being allocated to young people is adjudged by them to be unworthy of their capabilities and talents, with the result that they experience, individually and as members of a defined age group, a kind of insult. Yet again, tensions and difficulties may arise because the pressures which adolescents are being subjected to are denuding their personalities and depriving them of necessary satisfactions. An illustration of the first would be the rebellious younger university student, frustrated by non-participation in the organisation of his own academic affairs. An example of the second might be the overworked, examination-ridden pupil deprived of social activities and recreation by the exigencies of the curriculum. (As one commentator, Professor Frank Musgrove, put it in a trenchant essay, 'There is little joy in the Upper Sixth!'[17])

Hence it is that any consideration of youth's needs must be seen in relation to the needs of the community, and it is pre-eminently the task of the sociologist to attempt a descriptive analysis of the dynamic inter-relationship between these different, and at times distinctive, needs. Only if such an analysis is successful can we hope to put forward realistic policies and programmes which will, so to say, meet the needs of youth, or, in other terms, resolve the problems of youth.

One of the principal points that I want to make in this chapter is simply this: that young people can never be considered or understood in any depth as though they existed in social isolation or as if they comprised an age group located in a kind of sociological vacuum. This means rather more than saying that people are in a constant state of inter-relationship. It implies further that the *pattern* and *tone* of their inter-relationships are subject to external pressures and influences which emanate from the structure of society itself. Such sociological influences are both national and local in scale, long-term and immediate in their impact. Although their nature is impersonal and their origin social, their results and implications are, in the last analysis, experienced personally and, at times, quite profoundly by individuals as attitudes and motivations which seem to be entirely their own.

Youth, I am going on to argue, is most especially subject to social pressures and group influences, because it is a stage of development which is in some respects extremely free and in other respects extremely regimented. It is a period, moreover, which is especially vulnerable to stress, strain and breakdown on account of this very freedom which at times can prove to be an unnerving experience.

The freedom that is extended to youth is, however, a relative freedom. Autonomy is in the main confined within the sphere of youth itself and is tolerated so long as it does not spill over into or make egalitarian demands on what is considered to be the adult sector of society. The regimental aspect of youth is most obvious in educational institutions, in exigencies of examination systems preparatory to admittance to various professions, in apprenticeship schemes and, in some countries, the claims of military service.

The obvious loneliness and isolation of more highly educated sections of youth is partly the result of this age-segregation process. Being left to his own devices, the young person may sometimes feel abandoned and without adequate guidance. This is especially the case with students living away from home, living perhaps in not entirely congenial lodgings, and, at the same time subjected to strong external pressures in the way of academic demands. Suicide rates amongst such adolescents show a tendency to rise in spite of apparent environmental improvements. University students, especially those at colleges which are residential and also cut off from the main stream of normal social life, like Oxford and Cambridge, seem to show this stressful reaction to social pressures and loneliness most clearly.

Our concern for the physiological changes that uniquely distinguish adolescence, and for the psychological consequences that depend upon these physical changes and developments, must not be allowed to blind us to the vital social correlates that accompany this same developmental stage. But the manifestations of adolescence are often so florid that the less conspicuous social reality is obscured, at least temporarily, by the physical and psychic changes. One result of this is that we are apt, for example, to see intransigence amongst teenagers as resulting from their own unresolved inner personality problems, or perhaps, at a rather more sophisticated level, as arising as a result of inter-generational jealousy rather than from the irreconcilability of social roles and status with biological and psychological maturity. We may also fail to see how the social role and function of youth can pull against natural needs and impulses, with, at times, catastrophic consequences. The clinician's concern with individual psychic states may lead him to miss the significance of the tensions produced by structural elements in the social setting in which his patient is immersed. Or, worse still, he may dismiss such considerations as irrelevant to his task which he is defining solely in terms of enabling the patient to function more success-fully in the *status quo*. But this is to risk the danger of merely treating symptoms instead of causes, and is open to objection also on the grounds that the therapist is uncritically promoting social adjustment for its own sake (e.g. the 'I am a doctor not a social reformer' plea), when it may possibly be the case that the situation to which the adjustment is being attempted is not only disturbing but positively unjust and ethically unacceptable.

2

Social Adolescence

Social Crises

Earlier I suggested that there is a phase of life which may not improperly be termed 'social adolescence'. Its extent varies for different social classes and occupations. For some young people it comprises an apprenticeship stage; for others it involves a protracted period of academic training which may not cease until the student is in his mid-twenties. But for all young people this phase commences in school, when the first steps are made towards finding a job, preparing for a career and tentatively preparing to play a future economic role in the life of society. This is a period when young people experience some degree of doubt and tension which seems to arise to some extent from the fact that the individual is aware that one very well-understood period of his existence is almost over and another more challenging and hazardous phase is about to begin. That this is so may perhaps be deduced from the observed fact that amongst working-class children in England the peak age for delinquency is located in the final year of formal education, i.e. during their fourteenth year. Earlier, when the school-leaving age was a year younger, the peak age was also younger and was located in the thirteenth year. In fact the peak year for juvenile delinquency moved up by twelve months shortly after the statutory school leaving age was raised, almost as though there was a causal connection between the two phenomena. It will be a matter of considerable scientific interest if, in the early nineteen-seventies when the school-leaving age is to be sixteen, we discover that the peak age for delinquency also shifts to the fifteen-year-old age group. Should this occur, it would be additional support for the idea that the transitional period between leaving school and finding work is a source of stress and strain which some young people try to resolve by delinquent or by other kinds of troublesome behaviour.

At this time it may be hypothesised that the individual and the group as a whole undergo something like a crisis of social identity; when they feel they are no longer school children and are not yet young workers with a real job to do in the workaday world; when the future is experienced as to some degree threatening, however keen the desire may be to leave childish things behind. Here the loyalties and associations of peer groups and contemporaries during this interim stage are clearly sources of considerable emotional support for the disoriented individual. Some adolescents perhaps find the peer group at such a time their sole source of help and reassurance.

There is, I believe, a second crisis of social identity, which occurs a few years later after the individual has left school, has found a job and become gainfully employed. This time the crisis may be brought about by a realisation that youth itself is coming to an end; that the pleasant associations of the peer group are soon to be broken up and that full adult responsibility will shortly be attained. The older teenager sees that many others of his acquaintance and family circle seem to be obliged to settle down in their early twenties and to accept their role as mature, autonomous citizens as husbands and fathers as wholly inevitable if not entirely desirable. The day when they too will give hostages to fortune is not far off and can be seen looming large on their horizons. Meanwhile they turn with renewed fervour to teenage pursuits and seem to emphasise their freedom and irresponsibility by outbursts of pleasure-seeking, drunkenness, rowdiness, vandalism and other kinds of law-breaking. Thus it is that we find a secondary delinquent peak at the age of seventeen plus in the criminal statistics for England and Wales which begins to decline until by the mid-twenties there are unmistakable signs of a general settling down process. This secondary delinquent peak, moreover, is characterised by physically aggressive offences, drunkenness and similar kinds of tension-releasing forms of misdemeanour.

Peer Groups

The existence of peer groups, or, as they are sometimes also called, age-homogeneous groups, during the adolescent developmental period has been widely noted and commented upon. It is in fact one of the most distinctive social features of young people in contemporary society that they seem to be very much aware of themselves as members of a loosely knit status group. Membership of such groups, however fleeting, performs a number of important social functions in addition to providing the kind of emotional support and solidarity already mentioned. They offer opportunities, away from too close adult scrutiny or parental control, for various explorations in the field of personal relationships and for experimentation in social situations that normally structured, age-heterogeneous groups cannot possibly do. This is as true for friendship clusters and similar spontaneous groupings as it is for more formal adolescent organisations and youth service associations. Not only do they derive much of their *raison d'être* from the mutuality they foster, but they are also invaluable in giving young people the chance to experience some of the privileges and problems of relatively autonomous living, which is so necessary for future democratic citizenship. By doing things together, by making their own decisions and seeing the consequences of these decisions upon their own affairs, the members of such groups learn much about the interdependence of the members of a larger society and gain insight into the meaning of social responsibility at first hand.

Delinquent groups or gangs are, of course, of a somewhat different nature.

It is important to distinguish between the gang proper, the 'near-group' and the friendship cluster when we come to consider criminal and anti-social behaviour. There are also important social class differences which are more marked in some countries than in others. These class differences influence both the structure of the group in question and the nature of its activities. Generally speaking, criminal gangs are lower class in origin and, as far as the literature goes, they are more frequently found in the slum areas of the great cities, especially those of the U.S.A., than elsewhere. It is very doubtful, for instance, if there are any organised gangs in Britain which function in the way described by Thrasher in Chicago in the nineteen-twenties, or more recently in New York by Lewis Yablonsky.[26]

Delinquent juvenile gangs, in which the illegal behaviour is not sporadic but part of their actual ethos, have been analysed by Cohen[5] and other American sociologists at some length. The gangs they delineate seem to be social mechanisms for the release of social hate and resentment against frustrations and long-standing inequalities in a society which, in its civic philosophy at least, extols the virtues of brotherhood yet seems to rely upon competitiveness and coercion in most of its affairs and to offer widely differential rewards and opportunities to various sections of the population. They represent the revolt of the underprivileged, and hence are to some extent explicable in Marxist terms. Such gangs often seem to resort to violence against property and against the person, indulging in street clashes with other gangs and with the police in a kind of triangular tournament. Although membership of such violent gangs may provide psychological support for their members, they can also exert a pathologically coercive influence by forcing the individual to participate in criminal activities in order to 'prove' his group-worthiness and to demonstrate that he is not 'chicken'. They also provide psychologically disturbed youngsters with opportunities to vent their aggressiveness, to exert power over junior and fringe members and to enjoy the perverse satisfaction of inciting punitive and repressive reactions from the authorities.

There is disagreement between the experts regarding the extent to which criminal gangs are highly organised and closely structured. The conventional pattern of a leader supported by a group of obedient lieutenants has been challenged by Yablonsky in particular, who has put forward the idea of a gang as a 'near-group' composed of a core of sociopathic individuals and a much less committed number of associates who occupy marginal positions.[26]

Other kinds of gangs, composed of what have been termed socialised delinquents, have earlier been identified in both America and Britain. These groups of coevals tend to associate together in their leisure time and to take part in delinquent acts more or less incidentally as an expression of their group way of life which is tolerant of a limited amount of deviance. Following Whyte's[24] classic description of the youths in his Boston slum, they are usually referred to as 'corner boys'. Their delinquency is usually phasic in character and tends to die away at the end of adolescence. It is normally non-violent and consists of fairly minor offences against property, petty stealing and, in America, association with adult-sponsored betting and similar rackets. They probably resemble the friendship clusters of an earlier pre-adolescent stage and so contain a regressive element. The energies of the members can often be safely canalised off into more acceptable institutions such as youth clubs and supporters' groups following particular football teams. They certainly do not present the kind of challenge to the community that the violent juvenile gang or near-group does, mainly, one suspects, because the members of such groups are, from the psychological point of view, basically normal.

Middle-class groups are more likely to be associated with specific schools and colleges. Their activities are both supportive and experimental and seem in the U.S.A. to be closely associated with the youth culture and with the stress on masculinity. Their delinquencies seem to involve activities of a proving type, such as joy-riding and the search for 'kicks' in terms of sexual experimentation and drug-taking, which suggest a greedy anticipation of the adult role. Their protest hence is not against society so much as against immaturity status.

Thus we can see that peer groups amongst adolescents can have either benign or malign significance. For the vast majority of youngsters the existence of these groups is both personally and socially beneficial. There are also, however, associated disadvantages such as making too clear-cut a distinction between youth and the adult society and in permitting, if not fostering, certain dubious features of teenage culture such as the 'drug scene'. The group *qua* group, moreover, is most especially vulnerable to mass hysteria and to exploitation by cultural merchandisers and the mass media. The rock-'n-roll movement which swept across the world some years ago, even permeating the iron curtain of communist countries, is a good example of the way in which group fashions and addictions amongst contemporary youth tend to become world-wide movements. So, too, with other musical idioms, dance forms and clothes styles, and, more recently, with youthful political unrest.

Major Developmental Tasks

The two adolescent social crises discussed above need to be considered also in relation to the significant physiological and psychological changes which have been operating during the same period and which in their own right produce some degree of disturbance both in personality and in behaviour. If we think of youth as pre-eminently the period in which the individual is in search of an abiding identity and sustaining self-image, it is clear that what Havighurst and others have called the major developmental tasks are particularly involved during this fourteen to twenty-one age range. The youth needs not only to find and secure for himself a place in the social and economic life of his community; he needs also to come to terms with his own physical being, with his sexuality and with his aggression. Finally, there is also the philosophical task to be worked through, and this involves coming to terms with life and with reality as a whole and finding for himself some set of values and a code of ethics to live by.[10]

Sociologically these three major developmental tasks imply both individuation and group solidarity. At the psychological level they are manifested in a search for freedom and autonomy and a yearning for fellowship. So it is that the teenage period is experienced as profoundly peer-conscious and group-based and yet at the same time deeply lonely and uniquely personal. Moreover, the stresses and contradictions of the period are exaggerated and reinforced by certain other purely social forces which often seem almost accidentally to be working in the opposite direction to a young person's natural developmental progress. These contrary forces which, incidentally, constitute a considerable part of what we have called 'social adolescence', are injurious in so far as they tend to prolong the period of indeterminacy and dependence upon others which a protracted initiatory and further educational phase imposes. In a highly evolved industrial society such as ours, which demands from its successful citizens longer and longer periods of training in order that the appropriate technical, scientific, managerial and similar vital skills will be made available to supply the economy and the administration with the requisite variety of competent manpower, there is a danger that fully mature people will be treated as pupils merely because they are still engaged in a learning process and are financially dependent upon others. The results of this protraction of dependency can be seen in certain aspects of student and undergraduate unrest, in which the demand to be taken seriously and to be treated as adult responsible members of the community are clearly discernible. The report of the Latey Committee on The Age of Majority (Cmnd. 3342[19]) represents a genuine desire on the part of those in authority to come to terms with such youthful aspirations and their broad recommendation that majority age should be reduced from twenty-one to eighteen is a bold step which the British government has recently implemented by legislation. Furthermore, the government has also conferred political franchise at the same age, thus bringing the right to vote into line with other legal rights, including, of course, the right to marry without parental consent. These changes clearly go a considerable way in the direction of satisfying the frustrations of youth and in taking some of the steam out of the adolescent revolt. They also pose problems at the top end of secondary schools, many of which have sixthformers in their nineteenth year. Some of these pupils will almost certainly be married, some may even become parents during their school life. Teachers will be called upon to behave with considerable tact and skill in the light of such changes which clearly must revolutionise the traditional relations between teachers and taught.

Whatever the truth may be regarding the alleged earlier onset of puberty and physical maturity which the present generation in most western countries are said to be experiencing, there can be little doubt about the fact that today's teenagers think of themselves as being more mature than their predecessors were allowed to be. Psychologically, young people are now ready at an earlier age to look after themselves and take responsibility for the organisation of their own lives. One clear indication of this is the lower age at which many of them are marrying nowadays compared with their own parents and grandparents. Economic factors obviously reinforce psychological readiness here, and nowadays it is much more possible for young couples to set up home together. All this, of course, does not mean that they will not make mistakes; marry the wrong partner, for example, or make unwise vocational and financial decisions.

It has been shown that the earlier marriages are contracted the more likely they are to be broken up by subsequent divorce. What one deduces from such statistics depends to a considerable degree upon whether or not one regards divorce as a bad thing in itself and also as an index of irresponsibility. All we are in a position to say, I think, is that young people today want to marry younger, desire autonomy in vital aspects of their lives earlier and chafe against restrictions and inhibitions with a growing irritability. This may not indicate greater maturity at an earlier age; on the other hand it may do. Criteria of sociological maturity are in any event hard to establish.

Sexual Experience

It is widely accepted that there has been a very great change in recent years in the field of sexual behaviour. This is most especially noticeable in the increased permissiveness of the teenage group which seems to have been brought about by a new attitude to sexual experience on the part of the girls as the final act, perhaps, in the long cycle of feminine emancipation. Girls nowadays are not only more willing to accede to sexual advances from boys, they are prepared at times to initiate them. They no longer merely co-operate but positively enjoy sexual relations. All this has undoubtedly been brought about by vastly improved contraceptive techniques, in their wider availability and in an associated pleasure ethic which denies the virtue of chastity and is prepared to accept premarital sexual experience as the norm. In this, as in so many other respects, at the moment it is the girls, for a change, who appear to be the pace-setters of modern youth culture.

Evidence on sexual behaviour is notoriously difficult to obtain and the data derived from research is accordingly hard to evaluate. Perhaps the most reliable enquiry is that carried out by Michael Schofield[20,21] and his colleagues on a cross-section of English youth which suggests that, on the basis of the evidence obtained, the majority of young people in England were not sexually active during the middle or even late teens, and a more limited study of Scottish youth gives the same impression. However, social attitudes change rapidly and there does seem to be a growing trend in the direction of greater and greater sexual experience in adolescence and outside marriage. Furthermore, personal impressions suggest that, as far as the university student population is concerned, the traditional inhibitions have been breaking down fairly rapidly in the last five years and that the permissive trend is likely to become accelerated. Additional evidence, which tends to corroborate the claim that the new attitude towards sexual conduct is a definite change of code rather than a temporary falling away from conventional standards, is to be found in the increase in pregnancies outside marriage by younger unmarried girls and a rise in the incidence of venereal disease amongst teenagers.

All this adds up to a change in social patterns of behaviour of a radical nature and which cannot be ignored. Sexuality is clearly highly and openly prized by modern young people. The general approach to sex is franker than it used to be and young people's attitudes are more relaxed and less censorious of one another. This latter point is one of considerable significance. Concern for the quality rather than for the form of interpersonal relationships is now elevated to the level of a moral imperative. Sexuality can be diffuse, with the old-fashioned distinctions between appropriate male and female dress and behaviour much less clearly defined. Pop group members, for example, are clearly sexually attractive but not so obviously masculine in their appeal. So homosexuality like other deviations is not condemned nor is it so feared as in the past, provided it can be shown that it does not hurt other people. Tolerance of each other's behaviour, unwillingness to condemn or even to adjudge other people's conduct or to insist on a rigid normative order is characteristic of the younger generation, and this attitude is consistent with a growing concern for people as people. The current ethical view which, for instance, emerges from the Eppels'[8] study is founded upon a moral pragmatism which stresses the importance of good human relationships in all walks of life and in all social situations regardless of any systematic and abstract ideas of what is good or right.

For such a generation the claims of organised religion rank low. How people treat one another is seen as being more important than what they claim to believe. The trend is clearly in the direction of increasing tolerance based on humanistic understanding and sympathy. The leaders of the younger generation hence see themselves as being identified with the pains of all oppressed communities and obliged to stand out publicly against racial discrimination, against militarism everywhere and against any attempt by a superior power to intervene in the internal affairs of any other country either on ideological or strategic grounds. Youth, or at least the militant minority, is everywhere on the move and eager to get on with the task of helping to shape its own destiny.

Social Alienation

As the need for longer training and more skill demands a protracted educational experience for more and more young people we ought, at the same time, to take note of a very curious anomaly which is currently afflicting an advanced industrial society such as the United States. There, as far as we can see, the problem of youthful unemployment is very much on the increase. 'Across the nation, during the school months of 1962,' say two American commentators, 'from 600,000 to 800,000 young people between sixteen and twenty-one were out of school and looking for jobs; among teenage Negro youth unemployment is double that of white youth; the outlook for the future is even more disturbing, for we face an unprecedented growth in the number of young people and a substantial reduction in the number of jobs traditionally open to youth.'[14] Peter Marris and Martin Rein writing somewhat later paint a similarly disturbing picture of the excessively high unemployment rates among Negroes and teenagers, especially those who have had less than eight years schooling. Negro teenage boys growing up in urban slums are epitomised by these authors as 'a whole generation of misfits driven from the poverty of the South to the more humiliating frustration of an urban ghetto'.[13]

Supportive findings have been reported for a specific area by Robert Havighurst and his colleagues in their longitudinal study of an age group of boys and girls in a mid-western community.[11] They show how, in a society which offers less and less jobs for juveniles, young people are tending to become divisible into two main groups: the successful and the unsuccessful, the conformists and the drop-outs. Differential home back-grounds coupled with differential educational experiences result in a structure of differential opportunity for each main group. The unsuccessful children are involved in a steadily deteriorating process of alienation from society, which commences with early failure at school and ends in delin-quency and similar kinds of adolescent maladjustment. The authors concluded that the drifters comprised some 14 per cent of the age group while the pathologically alienated consisted of another 13 per cent—thus totalling well over a quarter of the rising generation in the city whose social lives are likely to be characterised by disaffection, under-achieve-ment and general failure and exposed to rejection by the successful and well-adjusted majority. We may conclude from this kind of evidence that American society is both reliant upon and embarrassed by its adolescents. They are its long-term investment and also its long-term problem group. Moreover, even the ultimately acceptable, well-adjusted group are to be held at arm's length until there is a place available for them in the adult economy. So college careers and extended further education are to some extent utilised in order to keep the adolescent fixated in the transitional adolescent phase until the social telegraph indicator calls for the full steam ahead of mature citizenship.

Conclusion

These, then, are some of the outstanding social facts of life and we are obliged to try to come to terms with them in one way or another. At the present time it looks as though in England, at any rate, there is a willing-ness on the part of the older generation to give in to the demands of youth and to allow them earlier majority and greater freedom from constraint than they themselves experienced. It is one effort to come to terms with the admitted problem presented on the one hand by earlier desire for autonomy and the need, for social and economic reasons, to keep young people in school, college and university to a greater extent than we have ever done in the past. It is one way to reduce the dangerously lengthening gap between childhood and adult status which is obviously one of the sociological explanations of growing unrest amongst contemporary youth in western society generally. However, even a bold and far-reaching step such as this may, in the event, turn out to be a failure unless, at the same time, we can engender an appropriate sense of responsibility in age groups which have been brought up by their parents to be predominantly self-regarding and self-justifying. Students, for instance, and later even sixth-formers, may well receive wages instead of grants related to parental resources. It is more than doubtful, however, if they will be equally willing to shake down to stricter work disciplines than they have been accustomed to in a past which was characterised by the liberalism and paternalism that so many of them seem to be reacting against at the moment. Institutions of higher education may get more like factories and workshops than many young people would find comfortable. All this, of course, is highly speculative, but we may note the trends and tendencies as part of the rapidly changing pattern and shifting background against which the activists of the present generation are already working out some aspects of their future destiny. One can also note a further point which Professor Musgrove[18] has recently drawn attention to: that in the nineteenth century the young attained adult status earlier than they do now because of their obvious economic value as earners and workers—a fact that underlines the unreality of the position of many young people who occupy positions of total dependency today.

3

Teenage Culture

So it is that the teenage culture is fostered by commercial interests which are primarily interested in the financial exploitation of youth growing up in an affluent society, and the society itself acquiesces in this exploitation because it offers young people something to do, a short-run hedonistic way of life, while they are waiting for maturity to be ceded to them. It is rather like finding work for idle hands to do, except that in this case most of the elements in teenage culture are clearly non-work. More insultingly it is as though the parental generation said to their able and aspirant children, 'Not yet a while. Mummy and Daddy are busy. Go away and play now and we'll call you later.' Indeed, peer group activities have been caustically referred to by some commentators as a 'playpen culture', aimlessly distracting young people's minds and energies during this social latency period. To some extent, therefore, we can think of it as part of a social process tending to arrest both social and psychological development, and it may well be that a certain amount of psychic damage is sustained during this period by a fixation of juvenile attitudes into later life with fairly obvious adverse consequences. Edgar Friedenberg[9] has been one of the most outspoken critics of conventional teenage culture, seeing it as the enemy of what he calls 'true' adolescence. By the latter term he means that positive, idealistic, assertive element in youth ('facing the world', as he says, 'with love and defiance') which is nowadays being superseded by this teenage pseudo-youth-culture during the interim years between childhood and full maturity.

Some social commentators have seen youth as in some ways a prototype of all citizens of the future in so far as they exhibit a feature which, as a result of increasing mechanisation and decrease in working hours, will affect more and more sections of the community—the investment of much of the individual's emotional life in leisure time activities. Leisure is in fact becoming increasingly industrialised as more and more people become occupationally involved in meeting such needs. The pleasure ethic fostered by this industrialised leisure is in close sympathy with teenage culture in general and quite clearly the one serves to underline and reinforce the other. Youth is thus seen in this as in other respects as the exemplar of future trends, evidencing tendencies which are likely to become generally more pronounced and more acceptable as the generations succeed one another, and the twenty-first century comes nearer.

For lower-class youth, however, and for the drop-outs and misfits particularly, teenage pop culture is more than an in-between-times-meal, it is much more like a staple social diet. True, they share it for a while with their more successful middle-class coevals and this gives a gloss of class-lessness to many aspects of teenage culture. They tend to listen to and to produce the same kinds of music, to wear similar clothes and favour distinctively youthful hair-styles. Nowadays, moreover, there is a much less clear-cut difference between the appearance of artisan apprentices and students. The ubiquitous jeans, for instance, are favoured by all socio-economic groups, as is the cult of casualness and the touch of informality.

But lower-class youth's adherence to 'pop' culture is much more thorough-going than that of the aspirant middle classes. It has been shown, for instance, that teenage culture is more or less antithetical to the values propounded in formal education and that it is closely associated with academic failure. As Sugarman[22] indicates, in a study of London school-boys, the greater the individual's commitment to the role of teenager the less is his commitment to the learning role. Teenage culture is hence basically anti-educational. It glamourises leisure rather than work. It seeks pleasure rather than achievement. It promotes self-display, self-expression and spontaneity in specifically teenage ways which are often, if not always, hostile to the norms and values of 'respectable' adult society. Some of the traditional elements of lower-class youth culture are positively linked to this new and more affluent 'pop' superculture. Walter Miller's focal concerns of lower-class youth centred around what he calls 'areas', such as 'trouble', 'toughness', 'smartness' (i.e. outwitting opponents), 'excitement', 'fate' (i.e. luck) and 'autonomy' (freedom from external constraint) are all discernible in many typical forms of contemporary teenage conduct.[15] There is, therefore, a continuity between lower-class youth culture in pre-affluent and post-affluent generations. Middle-class youth, on the other hand, are much more influenced by idealism and bohemianism in a self-conscious rejection of bourgeois society and their own familial background. Although, superficially, the two groups seem to have much in common, there are also important differences which make it extremely unlikely that the two will ever unite to challenge authority together.

Financial Exploitation of Youth

Teenage culture in every aspect is obviously supported by a massive market-orientated commercial substructure. It is also quite clearly of peculiar interest to the mass media programme organisers and writers. The advent of television has made the teenager a much more visible and easily identified figure than otherwise would have been the case. The mass media have, in their own way, tended, like the pop music market, tin-pan alley, the makers of transistor radios, couturiers, the rag trade and hair-stylists, to exploit an easily exploitable situation by making young people every-where more and more aware of the symbols of their identity and then proceeding to persuade them to part with their money in order to possess these same symbolic trappings. Yet it would be misleading to suggest that there is no more to the teenage cult than that. One of the things that is immediately apparent is that teenage culture is an international phenome-non, that it permeates cultural barriers and political iron curtains most successfully.

Youth as a Reference Group

Youth is much more visible that it used to be, much more conspicuous, partly because of the new stylised appearance but also perhaps, following the post-war bulge in the birthrate, there are in fact generally more young people about. Moreover, there is a network of communication especially devoted to that age group and clothes, songs, the possession of motorbikes, guitars, records and portable transistor radios keeps them in constant cultural touch with one another. But it would be an exaggeration to say that youth now comprises its own distinct society, since most of the elements which make for a true sociological community are absent. They are more like a class—a cultural collectivity—aware of each other's existence and sensitive to the same swings of fashion and interest.

At the personal level the existence of an age group of peers is emotionally reassuring. The age group becomes a vital reference group to which one turns for reassurance and it provides some kind of group-based identity during the transitional stage. So the role of the teenage 'success' becomes highly significant. The film star who becomes famous overnight, or the beat group that breaks into the hit parades, or the footballer who soars to international fame before the age of twenty, are perceived as vicariously fulfilling their own, often frustrated, hopes and dreams, and at the same time acting as a snub to the more academic youngsters who have climbed the ladder of social success via the long slog of examinations and who, the less successful and unacademic majority feel, regard them as failures and 'dim ones'. Bryan Wilson describes the role of teenager entertainment idol as 'the scapegoat in reverse . . . the totem of the tribe, the emblem who expresses vicariously the pleasures of quick and easy success, with money, kicks and sex as the prizes . . .', and the 'less cultivated he is, the more unschooled he is, the more effectively he represents the rejection by the young of the over-institutionalised society . . .'.[25]

Inter-generational Tensions

So we can see that the inner meaning of dress is related to the adolescent self-image which is in part a definition of personal and peer group identity and in part a rejection of paternal values and the established social order. Clashes over clothing and arguments over hair-styles thus become symbolic of the inter-generational misunderstanding and failure of sympathy which distinguishes the modern generation from almost every generation that has gone before it. When the headmaster tells a boy he won't let him come into *his* school wearing jeans, or when he insists on boys having their hair cut short, and when the headmistress lays down regulations about dress lengths or bans lipstick, these are but the manifestations of a more deep-seated problem. Young people now from almost every social class and in almost every country are demanding that their claim for autonomy be recognised. They are self-consciously making gestures of rebellion and flying their own flags of freedom. They are becoming deliberate deviants. Children of post-war comparative affluence, brought up on a rich diet of pleasures and leisure time pursuits, attuned to the consumer society, they see no reason to submit tamely to middle-aged ideas and the limitations of 'respectable' middle-class values. There are many contributing factors to this youthful insistence on their own right of self-expression and loyalty to their own scale of ethical standards.

Adolescent Disenchantments

Without wishing to place these in any particular order of importance, I would say that the first is an especially strong disenchantment with the professed values and actual behaviour of the older generation and with all those adults who have tended to preach one philosophy while practising another. We are apt to forget and overlook the basic deceitfulness of traditional socialisation processes and formal educational institutions. One often notices, however, amongst more thoughtful pupils and under-graduates, a sense of emptiness and dismay which seems to spring from the realisation, which comes in mid-adolescence, that parents and teachers never really believed whole-heartedly in the values they were verbally upholding, that the whole apparatus of religious observance and the daily assemblies and religious instruction periods on the timetable were often nothing more than elaborate rituals or even downright bluff. A child of eleven may accept morning prayers conducted by a half-hearted conformer: the lively, intelligent young sixth-former is much more likely to be disgusted and to bring some of this disgust with him into the university as an undergraduate. He remembers, for instance, that he was never forgiven seven times, let alone seventy times seven, for his breaches of the school's disciplinary code; and he may, with justice, seek to dismiss as sheer hypocrisy adult ambivalence when faced in everyday life by moral issues and ethical dilemmas in business affairs or in the political life of his country. (The supply of arms to Nigeria in the late nineteen-sixties, for example, may be regarded by some young people as an economic decision calculated to reduce the balance of payments gap rather than an act of mature statesmanship.) So it is that disenchantment with half-hearted and often merely formal and superficial socialisation in moral values leads the teenager to despair at the postures of his own parents, the pretentiousness of teachers and the manifest failure of organised religion.

All this, of course, contributes to the spirit of the age which contains both the elements of despair and more benign ingredients of scepticism. But there are, luckily, other countervailing influences which are much more in keeping with youth's traditionally more positive and creative role as the shaper rather than the perpetuator of the established culture. Perhaps the first bizarre glimmerings of these other influences emerged in the early post-war world when the beatniks of San Francisco and elsewhere first rejected the naked materialism of American society and dramatically withdrew into a twilight kingdom of romantic poverty, drug-addiction and squalor. What they were rebelling against was the 'American dream' (recently reaffirmed by President Richard Nixon) with its excessive concern for worldly success, money, gadgets, possessions and status symbols. Like all such gestures and repudiations of the established social system, the cult of the Beats was comparatively short-lived and only partly effectual. But its echoes are still to be heard amongst the 'Happy Hippies' of the mid-nineteen-sixties in California with their ethic of self-indulgent pleasure-seeking, their adherence to drugs and uninhibited sexuality, and the reverse of almost all the conduct norms of traditional middle-class culture. Hedonism and the pleasure motif has more recently materialised in such movements as 'The Beautiful People' and 'The Flower People'—all of which are bred of affluence and a repudiation of much of what affluence has brought and all of which have been commercially exploited by the merchandisers and the admassmen of the free enterprise capitalistic economic order from which they have emerged like efflorescent epiphenomena.

There are obvious parasitical undertones here too. Typical perhaps of the small group of young people who seem to succeed in doing practically nothing for twelve months in every year is the remark attributed in a press interview to 'Woodbine' Chris Donne, eighteen-year-old ex-public school-boy: 'You ask how we live in the winter, man. I tell you: we don't know. We just do. We ponce on others, we live from day to day, that's what.'[4]

Similarly, recourse to amphetamines and the smoking of cannabis owe some of their social appeal to the fact that they are forbidden; hence to be a member of a group which defies authority in this rather romantic way is also an assertion of independence from the convention-directed 'establishment'. In a sense, it is a demonstration of Friedenberg's 'defiance' untempered by what he implied by his use of the juxtaposed word, 'love'. Much of the social protest is now overpowered by the delight in being different and in publicly shocking the remnants of older generations. But the banner of reform has passed from these outlandish cultural manifestations into the hands of student activists who, while still cultivating informality and a general permissiveness in dress and behaviour, espouse a much more serious purpose and have a much more aggressive attitude towards authority.

Student Rebelliousness

Student unrest, which has rolled like a tidal wave across the world, affecting almost all societies and influencing young people almost everywhere, is itself a highly complex phenomenon compounded of many convergent influences and kindred movements. There is, of course, the conventional rejection of paternal values, that 'growing away from father and mother' element which is inevitable if young people are to establish their own identities and attain to their own beliefs and ethical standards successfully. This normal reaction at the present time seems to be abetted by a lack of decision in upbringing and by a failure of belief and loss of nerve on the part of many parents themselves who deliberately withdraw from giving advice and guidance at critical stages, thus frequently leaving their offspring in a kind of philosophical vacuum. Furthermore, the reaction of more activist student groups suggests something much deeper than the 'normal' rejection of parental attitudes. It has overtones of what Karl Bednarik,[2] in his very perceptive study of post-war disillusionment amongst the youth of defeated Austria, called 'socialised father-hate'—a projection of some of the feelings of anger and frustration experienced in the parent–child relationship on to a society which already seemed to epitomise the moral emptiness of the older generation. Later political developments, especially in China where the youthful Red Guards have been exploited by Chairman Mao to maintain his new cultural revolution at a high pitch of reformist zeal, seem to have permeated the West. Maoist and neo-Marxist or merely, as Professor Tom Burns puts it, 'Marxist-by-hearsay' influences appear to be operating amongst students in France, U.S.A., Germany, Britain, Spain and several other countries. Although so far they may be few in numbers there is little doubt that the influence of these militant students is considerable even at colleges and on campuses where living conditions are far from being unpleasant and where staff–student relations are anything but distant and authoritarian. These young revolutionaries have abandoned the idea of gradual social progress towards a more just social order and, in a mood of despair, are seeking a far more radical and immediate solution to the problems which they allege are troubling them. But in colleges and universities where overcrowding and inadequate facilities exist, or where the authorities are reactionary in their attitude to students' claims for greater participation in the organisation of collegiate affairs, the fuel of discontent is the more easily ignited by calls to participate in sit-ins and more violent demonstrations of discontent. The use of police and the employment of riot-dispersal tactics against student demonstrations *in political democracies* indicates that the authorities are seriously worried about such intransigent behaviour—more especially, it may be added, because in many cases this is a revolt of the privileged against the very system which has marked them out for adoption into a selective cohort being prepared for an elitist future social role. It is here that we can discern how the traditional idealism and romanticism of youth are acting as potent reinforcers of rebelliousness. Yet another factor operating in the situation arises from the comparative freedom of the young from other responsibilities which make them able to risk social victimisation by taking militant action which for older people would jeopardise the well-being of their dependents.

Social Problems

One cannot help being struck by the change in the focus of adult concern that has come over society in the post-war years. Until recently our worries were almost entirely concentrated on lower-class youth, on the delinquent gangs and the threat to social stability coming from economically alienated sections of the population. Fears about the Teddy Boys of the nineteen-fifties gave way to anxiety about Mods and Rockers in the nineteen-sixties. Lower-class youths in the big cities of the Western world were flexing their muscles in 'rumbles', clashing violently with one another and with the police, and taking part in acts of vandalism, in Professor Cohen's terms,[5] for the sheer hell of it, or as they themselves might explain it, for the kicks. Now the limelight has shifted to the dissident student and to the middle-class drug-taker. Delinquency is seen as an old-fashioned form of social deviance. It is something we had learned more or less to live with and to contain within the geographical limits of the city slums. Gang warfare was not a challenge to the community to fashion a new social order; it was a reaction of deprived people against social frustration and an expression of hatred against those who frustrated them; many offences against property were attempts to get the good things that others enjoyed and which were denied to the under-privileged. There was no serious political threat involved in this kind of 'anti-social' behaviour.

But with the students' revolt there is a political threat, a real challenge to the establishment. And with the establishment is included the whole apparatus of conventional political life and all its stale philosophies and values—that same 'botched civilisation' which long ago Ezra Pound summed up in *Hugh Selwyn Mauberley* as 'an old bitch gone in the teeth'.

The theme of adolescent protest is more romantically underlined in the activities of the Dutch Provos. The name itself implies deliberate provocation of all those in authority by sit-downs in public places and street demonstrations calculated to disturb the class-conscious, bourgeoisified consumer society and to challenge the stolid conservatism of Dutch politics. But the Provos are not solely reactionary. They positively favour certain styles, attitudes and fashions. They like riding bicycles and mopeds but not cars. They stress creativity and are pacifist. White is said to be their favourite colour.

Reverberations of protest and reforming zeal amongst older groups have expectedly filtered down into the High Schools and led to similar claims on the part of pupils for participant democracy. French lycées during the

F

mid-summer trouble in France in 1968 came out in solidarity with the students of the Sorbonne. In England the movement for school councils grows apace and attempts are being made to modify existing examination and disciplinary systems. This movement has the active support of some teachers and, as in the colleges and universities, once again the influence of left-wing members of staff is probably of critical importance both in framing demands and suggesting methods of protest.

Conformist Youth

So far in this chapter we have perhaps been over-concerned with the more pathological and the more conspicuous aspects of modern teenage culture. We have given the limelight to various problems associated with the adolescent developmental phase which seem to arise from youthful intransigence of various kinds, from negativistic attitudes, and even from malicious reactions against the imposition of any sort of inhibitions by any authority whatsoever. It is dangerously misleading, however, to think of modern youth wholly in terms of student rebels, artistic bohemians, juvenile delinquents, teenage drug-takers, academic drop-outs and social misfits. The great majority of youngsters from all social strata are none of these, or, if they do manifest such tendencies, it is only for a short while and in a mild and acceptable form.

The problem of getting a job, of finding a satisfactory economic role for the future and establishing the foundation for a viable career weighs much more heavily on the minds of the majority. As we have already indicated earlier in this chapter, the prospect of unemployment faces a small proportion of school leavers, most especially in the United States, but in all countries the problem remains of how to get not just a job but the right job. This is one of the crucial aspects of adolescence, for it is during this stage that vital decisions are taken. Later in life it is exceedingly difficult to change jobs and to enter employment for which the individual did not receive the basic training.

A great deal of parental concern and interest is aroused at the time when future work roles are being decided and discussed. Many parents, indeed, pay much more attention to giving their children vocational guidance than they do to giving them any kind of moral experience or religious training. Employment, because of its strong connection with salaries and wages and future security generally, has an obvious material importance which does not need to be argued. The business of choosing the kind of job to be aimed for and the actual process of application is still largely family-based and family-influenced. Parents, relatives, family friends are approached to use their good offices and to proffer advice to the young worker. The official vocational guidance and job-placement institutions, such as the Youth Employment Service in Britain, play only a secondary role as a kind of stand-by for those unlucky ones who have no other resource to which they they can turn at this critical time.

Differential Sexual Roles

It has been pointed out by various social scientists that boys and girls, since they occupy different social and vocational roles in society, acquire during their earlier socialisation differential self-images. Boys tend to think more of the future in terms of work than girls do. The idea of the 'good' job occupies their thoughts more than dreams of eminence, while the girls focus on making a success of marriage and preparing for family life. The nature of the roles to be played mean that boys are likely to be more aggressive in outlook than their sisters. They have to learn to be competitive and independent and this in turn demands a more marked challenging of parental control than is necessary for girls. So boys and girls during adolescence make differential use of the peer-group relationship: the girls are less group-minded and gregarious in their behaviour than their brothers and are apt to involve themselves more deeply in the sphere of personal relations rather than in the search for social autonomy. Their different self-images, based upon their different social roles, lead young people at this stage along distinctive yet complementary lines. On the whole young people do not seem to fight against their social–sexual typing and they come to be at peace with their own self-image which is frequently one based on a rational assessment of their own abilities and a sensible adjustment of their personal aspirations.

This movement towards the mean, a trimming of one's sails to the winds of fact rather than fantasy, is achieved by a socialisation process in which educational experience is critically important. Schools with their detailed apparatus of examinations, streaming, prizes and disincentives operate as a gigantic selective machine which progressively elimates large sections of the child population in terms of criteria which are generally legitimated. It is a process of preparing round pegs for the round holes of the future and in the creation of an academic and occupational élite who will perform the key managerial, administrative and professional roles which are needed to keep the society going and economically viable. Most families do not encourage their children to challenge the system: the great majority accept the system and try to get the best out of it for themselves. They do this by conforming to the consensus view that social differentials must exist, while, at the same time, sharpening their own competitive tools in ways which are not only permissible but widely encouraged. Thus, if parental aspirations for their children are kept within realistic proportions, a high level of general stability is maintained and the amount of frustration retained within manageable bounds. But the revolt of the privileged, as we termed it earlier in this chapter, the rebellion of the group destined for élite status, itself involves a totally novel element in a situation which profoundly challenges the *status quo* and may well—if it goes on indefinitely—have genuine revolutionary results.

Further Political Aspects

In spite of the growth of political activism in recent years amongst students and intellectuals, there are also indications that something very much like political apathy is, relatively speaking, a much more common attitude amongst young people generally. Various studies suggest that the mental timidity and conformity of what is still almost certainly the great majority of youth tend to produce conservative reactions and a desire for economic security above everything. Politics is not seen so much as a way of reshaping society but as a means to preserve material prosperity. Abrams and Little,[1] who made a study of British teenagers in 1964, claimed to have found a generation with little positive interest in political affairs. Most of them thought that politics was a bore and a great many believed that it did not really matter which party was in power. Their voting behaviour, perhaps predictably, was likely to follow the parental pattern. Douvan and Adelson's very detailed research into the attitudes and aspirations of 3000 American youths between the ages of fourteen and sixteen led them to a similar conclusion. 'Our interviews,' they wrote, 'confirm a mounting impression from other studies, that American adolescents are on the whole not deeply involved in ideology, nor are they prepared to do much individual thinking on value issues of any generality.'[6] So, too, a few years earlier, James Coleman[6] describes the members of what he calls 'the adolescent society', made up for the most part of college youngsters, as characteristically focused upon teenage interests and activities far, far removed from adult responsibilities. Professor Bernard summed all this up when she said: 'Interest in politics is not an integral part of teenage culture.'[3]

Such attitudes may well derive from a realistic appraisal of the situation. Such an appraisal indicates their own personal humility and a mild scepticism with regard to formal political systems. Just as most youngsters have sensible and realistic job aspirations, the majority are also modest about their own political significance. In the bland social climate of the affluent society, they have been conditioned to accept parental values almost without question. Even those who do question and evidence strong ideological commitment of one sort or another tend to do so *outside* the field of formal politics. For the most part, their truly political and moral activities are nowadays staged without reference to the enclaves of the parties. They prefer the open streets and market places for their protests and demonstrations. Here their immediate impact may be more noticeable but their long-term effect less thoroughgoing than they may wish. Youth's lack of interest and trust in formal political institutions suggests that traditional parliamentary democracy is seriously failing to meet their basic needs for emotional involvement and personal participation.

4

Some Practical Aspects

Faced with disturbed and maladjusted youngsters, the clinical psychiatrist must often long for the help of the sociologist to change the social environment so that his patients may be relieved to some degree of the strains and tensions contributing to their problems. The major contribution that the sociologist can make, however, is to suggest to clinicians ways in which environmental influences and existing neighbourhood institutions could become involved with the ameliorative process. Unfortunately—or perhaps fortunately!—the sociologist has no direct control over the social system, or even much say regarding what organisations should be provided to serve the 'healthy' community. At the training level he can, however, suggest what is lacking in the environment and seek the support of psychiatrists in a long-term propaganda campaign to rouse the public conscience.

Almost every locality is served by a variety of voluntary and statutory organisations, all of which, at some level, could become involved in what may be broadly termed 'environmental treatment'. Some neighbourhoods are richer in institutions than others; fortunately, some of the older and poorer districts have been quite well served in this way and have a long tradition of voluntary social welfare services still in being. New housing estates are, on the whole, the most sparsely served at this institutional level.

The clinical psychiatrist should, therefore, make it an essential part of his professional work to gain a working knowledge of the locality of the town or city from which his patients come. He should make every effort to establish good relationships with social workers, teachers, youth leaders, church officials and similar key people. As far as young people are concerned, the youth leaders, the teachers, settlement and community centre wardens, will be most important. In some places these workers can be contacted at local luncheon clubs or at councils of social service. But, however difficult and time-consuming it may be for the clinician to establish liaison with these other youth service workers, a sustained effort must be made in this direction. He must mix with social workers, know them personally so that he may be able to guide patients to them as and when necessary. It might even be worth while becoming a member of a local community centre or helping for the odd hour or so in the neighbouring youth club in order to achieve the mutual trust upon which alone such reciprocity can be founded. Time spent in this way, getting into the area and meeting key workers and officials, will almost certainly prove rewarding in the long run and significantly promote treatment objectives. A lonely adolescent, for example, may benefit enormously by membership of a relaxed and friendly youth club; but he may, initially, require a little help in crossing the threshold. Similarly, the boy deprived of a paternal model may find a surrogate in club leader, scoutmaster or adventure course instructor. What is required is that the psychiatrist should be aware of what services are available either for further education or merely for recreation and physical well-being, and further that he should know how these ancillary services can be contacted and exploited on behalf of his patients. He should, also, whenever he has an opportunity press for a wider provision of recreational and welfare facilities for the adolescents of his area, including, it goes without saying, experimental work with those unattached to the more traditional type of groups. Furthermore, the establishment of the Young People's Consultation Centre[27] on the model pioneered, for example in London, where young people can voluntarily attend for help and guidance with almost every kind of personal and social problem, is something to which a psychiatrist could surely give unqualified support. One could justifiably hope that his support would be more than merely moral and that he might also become one of the counsellors voluntarily attending such a clinic.

5

Conclusion

Sociologically speaking, adolescence is an important phase both for the social maturation of the individual and for the economic and industrial future of the community. During the teenage period the individual learns in the company of peers how to behave democratically and autonomously. He asserts his independence of the pastoral supervision of parents and teachers and begins to make decisions for himself. At the same time the boy in particular is preparing to take his place in the near future as worker and producer and is obliged to some extent to submit to the discipline imposed by the unavoidable transitional role of learner, student or apprentice. The differential feminine role which is culturally prescribed tends to make the girl less occupation conscious and more family-oriented with consequently less likelihood of strain. Both are nevertheless actively preparing themselves to play their socially invaluable future roles. Thus we can see that, even if adolescence as a clearly defined stage in human growth and psychic development did not exist, it would be necessary for purely social and economic reasons to invent it.

During this transitional phase the adolescent experiences doubts and anxieties about his social role and its associated status and for this reason is especially exposed to psychological stress. He is aware at times of being pulled in opposite directions. He is expected to behave with the responsibility of the mature adult, while being denied full autonomy. He is to be forward-looking and creative in outlook and yet submissive to superiors and deferential towards those in authority. In such circumstances it is inevitable that various problems will arise both for individuals as they pass through the phase of social adolescence and for the community as a whole which has a continuing interest in the outcome of the process. Apart from the incidence of delinquency and vandalism, which shows two peaks approximately at the ages of fourteen and seventeen, there are two other general responses which contain problematical elements today. Juvenile crime, however disturbing, is a long established feature of modern industrial societies and, in the main, has been regarded as a lower social class phenomenon.

The other reactions, however, seem to straddle the class lines and to be observable to some degree throughout all social strata. We might term them respectively the problems of over-conformity and non-conformity, or of excessive traditionalism and rebelliousness. One leads to a tame acceptance and adjustment to the *status quo*, the other to an angry rejection of all conventions, institutions and established values. One produces a politically quiescent meritocracy, the other unrealistic anarchy. These are, of course, the polar extremes. In between them lie the vast majority of adolescents who seem to make a sensible go of their lives. They are neither revolutionary innovators nor contented cabbages. All, however, have to face some kinds of adjustment problems and, since their goals are more or less identical, they tend to be extremely conscious of their membership of a specific age group and to be aware of loyalties and mutual sympathies *vis-à-vis* their immediate contemporaries. In such circumstances youth tends to become its own reference group for almost every norm and value, and, when these are manifested with unusual stridency and bizarreness, misunderstandings between the generations can arise which, if unwisely handled, can easily lead into active hostilities.

The fact that adolescence continues to be a period of potential difficulty is made evident in the comparatively high incidence of suicide and attempted suicide, in a growing experimentation in drug-taking and similar deviant behaviour amongst a certain section of teenagers. At a much less dramatic, but by no means unimportant, level this is also to be seen in the numbers of young people who are clearly out of touch with their own parents, unattached to any organised youth groups (perhaps because they resent the old-fashioned authoritarianism of the leaders) and who are adrift from any kind of stabilising pattern of values on which to base their lives. The researches of Dr Hemming,[12] Mary Morse[16] and several other investigators have revealed the degree to which many young people are lonely, isolated and without guidance in the modern world, the extent to which their lives seem to be being wasted and dissipated in apathy and under-achievement. Too many lack guidance, discipline and love. Failed by their parents and out of touch with the adult world generally, they are obliged, if at all, to seek help in the correspondence columns of the weekly press or in visits to the all too few advisory clinics and centres which the voluntary social services have successfully pioneered in one or two places.

Summarising, then, it may be said that adolescence today simultaneously presents aspects of both continuity and change. The same major developmental tasks of finding one's self, of gaining a secure place in society and of achieving a set of moral values to live by, remain for this as for all preceding generations the fundamental challenges which have to be met and mastered. Failure at each of these tasks can result in social and psychological maladjustments of a serious order. It is here that adult help is required, both in the form of parental concern and sympathetic guidance and, in extreme cases of social misfits and educational 'drop-outs' at the level of preventive community action. Moreover, it is probably truer today than it ever was to say that the future, and the near future at that, belongs in a special sense to youth. So the traditional aspect of the adolescent role as the shaper of culture is seen to have increased urgency in a world which is moving ever more rapidly into an epoch to be dominated by cybernetics and automation and challenged by space travel while human problems of poverty and starvation yet remain unsolved.

At the same time there have been obvious and sometimes drastic changes of outlook and behaviour on the part of the rising generation. It is not merely a matter of new clothes fashions and behaviour styles, but of a generally more open and more tolerant attitude towards one another, coupled with a firm rejection of paternalism and authoritarianism, wherever they may be met. Dissatisfaction with traditional political systems, an increasing desire for full and equal participation in decision-making and a willingness on the part of a minority to demonstrate forcibly for equality and justice, suggest that there are many hopeful factors at work which may well result in an enrichment of the general way of life and by the reduction of anxiety and competitiveness give a new impetus to democratic institutions.

REFERENCES

1. ABRAMS, P. and LITTLE, A. 1965. The young voter in British politics. *Brit. J. Sociol.*, **16**, 95.
2. BEDNARIK, K., 1953. *The young worker of today: a new type.* London: Faber.
3. BERNARD, JESSIE, 1961. Teenage culture: an overview. *The Annals of the American Academy of Political and Social Science*, **338**, I. Philadelphia.
4. CLARK, E. 1964. Beatnik casebook. *The Observer*, 4th December, London.
5. COHEN, A. 1956. *Delinquent boys: the culture of the gang.* London: Routledge and Kegan Paul.
6. COLEMAN, J. 1961. *The adolescent society.* New York: The Free Press of Glencoe.
7. DOUVAN, E. and ADELSON, J. 1966. *The adolescent experience.* New York: Wiley.
8. EPPEL, E. M. and M. 1966. *Adolescents and morality.* London: Routledge and Kegan Paul.
9. FRIEDENBERG, E. 1962. *The vanishing adolescent.* New York: Dell, Laurel Books.
10. HAVIGHURST, R. J. 1953. *Human development and education,* London: Longmans.
11. HAVIGHURST, R. J. *et al.* 1962. *Growing up in river city.* New York: Wiley.
12. HEMMING, J. 1960. *Problems of adolescent girls.* London: Heinemann.

13. MARRIS, P. and REIN, M. 1967. *Dilemmas of social reform*. London: Routledge and Kegan Paul.
14. MARTIN, J. and FITZPATRICK, J. 1964. *Delinquent behaviour: a redefinition of the problem*. New York: Random House.
15. MILLER, W. B. 1958. Lower-class culture as a generating milieu of gang delinquency. *J. soc. Issues*, **14**, 15.
16. MORSE, M. 1965. *The unattached*. Harmondsworth: Penguin Books.
17. MUSGROVE, F. 1966. *The family, education and society*. London: Routledge and Kegan Paul.
18. MUSGROVE, F. 1964. *Youth and the social order*. London: Routledge and Kegan Paul.
19. *Report of the Committee on the Age of Majority*. 1967. (Cmnd. 3342) London: H.M.S.O.
20. SCHOFIELD, M. 1965. *The sexual behaviour of young people*. London: Longmans.
21. SCHOFIELD, M. 1970. Normal sexuality in adolescence. In *Modern perspectives in adolescent psychiatry*, Ed. J. G Howells. Edinburgh: Oliver and Boyd. (Chapter III in this volume.)
22. SUGARMAN, B. 1967. Involvement in youth culture, academic achievement and conformity in school: an empirical study of London schoolboys. *Brit. J. Sociol.*, **18**, 2.
23. THRASHER, F. 1963. *The gang* (abridged edition). University of Chicago Press.
24. WHYTE, W. F. 1943. *Street corner society*. University of Chicago Press.
25. WILSON, B. 1965. *The social context of the youth problem*. 13th Charles Russel Memorial Lecture. London: N.A.B.C.
26. YABLONSKY, L. 1962. *The violent gang*. New York: Macmillan.
27. Youth Studies and Research Foundation, Second Report. 1965. *A description of the young people's consultation centre*. London.

VII

ADOLESCENCE IN CROSS-CULTURAL PERSPECTIVE

MARVIN K. OPLER
PH.D.

Professor of Social Psychiatry, School of Medicine
Professor of Anthropology and Sociology
the Graduate School, State University of New
York at Buffalo
U.S.A.

1

Introduction

Although psychiatrists view child psychiatry as a special field, they have been slower in according the same status to adolescence. Puberty and youth are not simply periods of transition between childhood and the adult stages. As an important stage of life in its own right, the adolescent and youth periods of growth and development represent a kind of biological revolution. While infancy and early childhood stages reveal a faster growth process in height and weight, adolescence is a close second in the total life process. What is more, it is a period second to none in sexual differentiation. The changes in skeletal structure, weight distribution, voice, hair and other secondary sexual characteristics show greater specialization is occurring. Certainly, on a sheer biological basis, adolescence is a distinctive stage of evolution in a lifetime within our species.

In comparisons with infancy and early childhood adolescence is likewise a major period of psychological transformation. In fact such leading theorists as Freud,[10] with his general stage of psychic accompaniments for genital maturity, and Erikson,[5] with his adolescent phase of identity integration or diffusion, both utilize the biological spurts as having chiefly psychological consequences. In our paradigm for this evolutionary stage of development, we prefer to view this important physical and physiological revolution as having, in a more central sense, immediate social relationships. The psychological potential derives less from the constant of a universal physiological change than from the cultural helps or hindrances which enable or prevent the adolescent from growing into the texture of society. Thus, rather than assuming that physical events give rise to characterological ones, we say instead that cultural settings generate the entire process of what adolescents are to become, including their characterological assets or liabilities.[27]

We require a more comprehensive psychology of the vicissitudes of human nature than either the Freudianism of the past or the ego identity schools of the present. Neither of these movements, which were important in founding a science of personality, can answer certain questions. Their causal chain goes from the biological level to the psychological and by so doing it eliminates from consideration the historical and cross-cultural transformations and differences in the adolescent experience.[28] Our question is: granted the physical revolution which is everywhere much the same in the species, how can one account for the remarkable social and individual differences (the well or the disturbed, for example) without recourse to social and cultural relativity? While not quarreling with the physically generated transformation in adolescence to which Freud called eloquent attention, we are reminded that it resurrects an overly simple medical model of organic causation, while we know at the same time adolescent behavior is always modified or ameliorated by a fundamentally different procedure. While Erikson moves farther away from simple biological determinism, like Freud he tends to retain certain universal psychic consequences in the response to physical growth and transformation. Yet the variability about the nature of adolescence around the world does not reveal one single healthy or one single form of disturbed reaction to the relatively fixed and simple set of physiological changes.

Cultural Evolution

Instead of the usual start with a biological or a psychological transformation, the author's theory of adolescence begins with the facts of cultural evolution. What has occurred in the technologically advanced countries and in their metropolitan centers is that the roles of young people have changed from work involvements in smaller economic spheres, such as family, farm or local in-group economic ventures, to a greater dependency upon 'careers' in the wider community. Educational demands have extended both in time and durational impact upon youth, while at the same time the explosion of knowledge and technique has confronted them with the seemingly limitless extension of academic hurdles and subject-matters. The general complexities of power bloc wars and internal conflicts in society have dismayed them, since they fall heir to the wars and erupting power struggles based on social and economic inequalities. Further, youth in modern societies sense that they are constantly demeaned by lock-step mass educational techniques, competitive and categorizing examinations which threaten their quest for individual identity, conditions of increasingly meaningless mass employment, and of course deferment of social sanctions for sexual and other gratifications which adults say must be postponed until the educational and employment labyrinths are conquered.

The answer of youth has been clear and direct for each of these barriers to maturity. Individualized experience, recently called 'mind-expanding', has been sought in drugs, much as the previous college generation sought it in occasional alcoholic escape. Students have rebelled against curricula historically designed inside the educational establishment with the counter claim that these lack relevance, meaning and even importance in our troubled world. The sexual moratorium has simply not been accepted, and in place of it youth has even symbolized its distance from the adult world by championing sexual freedom and experimentation, or by modifications in dress and hair-style which simultaneously symbolize an 'inter-sex' similarity which at the same time is intended to differentiate themselves from older persons. Attempts have also been made to construct a youth ethic, youth slang and new forms of youth music and dance—all of which have far more symbolic significance and durability than passing fads and fashions.

The author has alluded elsewhere to the kinds of factors which must be included beyond ego or self-identification (Erikson's theoretical posture) or sexual identification process so ably discovered by Freud earlier. We have labeled this important and concomitant identification process in all individuals 'social identification', the occasion being a theoretical analysis of what we called *Anthropological and cross-cultural aspects of homosexuality*.[27] For the general reader, less interested in the full scientific catalogue of the various types of self, sexual and social identification processes around the world, let me quickly call to mind some very obvious events in the current and daily news. With technological changes in communication, the metropolitan youth culture has sprung up on every continent. Their styles of youth attire, including hair-styles, their movements in music and art, or their concern with activity-programs within schools and universities whether in Tokyo, Prague, Moscow, Mexico City, San Francisco or New York—all this and much more should remind us that our modern urban and world conditions, based on new technology and communication media, make a profound impact on young people. To confront such generalized trends with canards about 'conspiracies' is to forget all we know about other social statistics such as rising rates of illegitimacy, younger marriages and more frequent divorces, fads for drug use or for exotic musical and philosophical imports from ancient Asian sources, and even the shocking fact of rising suicide rates among the youthful and adolescent population.

If we summarize our approach to this point, we begin by pointing out that the position of adolescents in society has changed because the culture has changed. In place of family, farm and small social group connections, young people see themselves as being part of a larger sphere of social events. Instead of the kind of education which has a clear and easily seen goal in the immediate social surroundings, both in subject-matter and in scope, young people are confronted with a larger world of technique, professionalism, specialization and a high degree of heterogeneity. At the same time, they are handled in the mass, with mass instruction, mass testing and evaluation and with seemingly remote and often meaningless modes of control. Beyond their adherence to youth groups as a category of persons facing the same problems, they are subjected to the further results of wars, the social structuring of inequalities and the apparently never fully confronted social problems of our times. We have already noted above certain of the typical responses in behavior, dress and social fashions to these challenges.

The 'Generation Gap'

It remains to comment upon the so-called 'generation gap', since adolescents live partly with their age group, but also part of the time function with parents or older relatives, with teachers or with employers or other representatives of the 'establishment'. In cultural evolution it must be recognized that the faster the tempo of social and economic change, the more obvious the distance between generations will become. If each successive generation is influenced by economic and social conditions impinging upon its members, then it follows that the transformations in these conditions of existence will all the more affect each generation differently.[27] While the older generation can glimpse this from its own experience with what it once regarded as 'old-fashioned' *versus* its own notions of modernity, it is difficult for them to understand the kinds of social transformations which loosen adult controls and family bonds more fundamentally. We all know that the family has been transformed from an extended complex of relatives, often living together over the generations and functioning more as a productive social unit with its own economic home industry, to one which is fragmented in every aspect we have just mentioned. An adolescent in a metropolis today has little real sense of family economics or productivity, and of course still less awareness of their place in such a scheme over time. Instead, since there are no clear markings of progress towards a joint enterprise such as were once defined by apprenticeship, family farm or business enterprise and the like, many adolescents construe such interest or allusions on the part of parents as being the unreal references of people who simply do not see things as they are. In sexual mores, as a parallel trend, the concerns of older people are seen as intrusions, as pruriency, and as 'overconcern' about essentially private matters. In regard to drugs, the claim is often that the older generation's tobacco and alcoholic beverages are both known to be notoriously damaging to health, whereas young people live in an allegedly more scientific environment in which even the television advertisements or newspaper advertisements proclaim any number of instant remedies and gratifications for anything, ranging from the simple headache to the 'energizer', 'tranquilizer', or the items for cleansing or apparel that 'fix' skin, teeth, odour and sexual desirability.

Economic Development and Ethnic Groups

While there is some point in considering general trends in cultural evolution as these affect youth, it must be recognized that the tempo of evolution itself in particular instances varies with the degree of economic development (as among nations) and also in its characteristics among different classes and ethnic groups. For this reason, a general psychological approach to adolescence is doomed to failure. For example Erik Erikson discusses youth in terms of fidelity and diversity, or elsewhere deals with the adolescent phase as either the induction of a firmer sense of ego identity, or else its destruction in ego-diffusion. Fidelity as he describes it is the strength of disciplined devotion, meaning in part the achievement of controls over drives and conscience as a style of human adaptation.[6] What makes this vague, of course, is that the social conditions surrounding adolescence divide into such general factors and trends as we have described above but they bifurcate in other instances into adolescent conflicts and struggles under differing social conditions. Black Americans in the U.S., for example, currently symbolize differences in dress and hair style which, they think, demarcate their special problems.[13] There are fashions in pseudo-African Muslim styles with distinctive hats and shirts for men and dresses for women. While African dress and hair styles in reality cover a wide range, an Afro-American haircut for males is often one which could not be found very frequently on that continent. Yet the intention or meaning is clear that the 'Afro cut' directly symbolizes the special problems which arise when an entire ethnic population has been segregated and subjected to both exploitation and discrimination for a long time. While adolescents as a whole lay claim to some sense of distance and grievance, Negro youth regard themselves as being doubly rejected, first as youth in opposition to the older establishment, and secondly as inadequately trained, educated or employed in the society.[13] One social consequence of this process, since White youth also react to educational lacks and barriers to involvement in the larger society is that both, for once, often make common cause of their partly mutual problems, and other evidences occur of solidarity through increasing inter-ethnic marriages, college programs of reform and common causes against such controlling forces in society as police, courts, draft boards or the recent national Party conventions in the U.S.

On the other hand, because of differing tempos of evolution in such places as developing countries, one can still see as a prevalent pattern shops run on the apprenticeship pattern, or families functioning with clear older generation control in such cities as Accra in Ghana or in Lagos, Nigeria.[27]

What we have described to this point as an evolutionary trend is a general process in which the transition to adult status depends less upon the calling forth of psychological 'forces' or biologic potentialities than it does upon the specific handling of the adolescent age group under particular cultural conditions. The applications of this new hypothesis seem limitless. For example, Karen Horney in her book, *The neurotic personality of our time*,[17] pointed out that the modern urban individual feels helpless and alienated because he is constantly confronted with ideal images of accomplishment and competition through the educational mass media, through advertising, through the cinema, the press, and we might add since the time of Horney's book, through television. These projected ego ideals are cast upon a larger screen against which the individual's minor successes and struggles with competition seem all the more weak and ineffectual. Consequently, Horney said, the rising rate of neurotic behavior in modern society is a price we pay for a highly competitive social structure.

Similarly, A. B. Wheelis in his book called *The quest for identity*[35] has taken the further step of pointing out that the older classical forms of neurosis, such as hysterias, anxiety neuroses and the like have shifted over to rising rates of character disorders and sociopathy, to paranoid schizophrenias, and to internalized psychosomatic ailments. In the author's writings on this epidemiological shift it is suggested that hysterias, catatonias and catathymic outburst states, simple confusional dissociative states and certain forms of anxiety attacks are all more directly expressive of the underlying conflicts in interpersonal relations. On the other hand, the character disorder, sociopathy, paranoid schizophrenias and psychosomatic illnesses are more the diseases of isolated and alienated man and have therefore been marked by greater distortions and more deeply disguised maneuvers in one's relationship to others.[27] Our question is: Are these changes in psychological defenses in some fashion related to changes in the structure and functioning of society?

The evolutionary answer is, of course, affirmative. But how to account for it in detail? Psychologically oriented anthropologists like Clyde Kluckhohn or the author, in writing about nonliterate tribal groups like the Navajo of Arizona or the Ute Indians of Colorado have noted that the wider extensions of extended family organization along with the general importance of all these relatives have surrounded both the child and the adolescent in these cultures with patterns of influence and authority wider than our own small nuclear family with its Oedipal components.[26] In a word, for them authority is more greatly diffused. Further, the problems in parents, in marital conflicts, or in failures to deal effectively with a growing child subject the latter in our culture to fewer alternatives or escapes. In the youth jargon of today, problems are called by the depressing term, 'hang-ups'. Further, modern suicide statistics indicate increasing rates among the very young.[30] As if that were not enough to indicate where the trouble lies, highly authoritarian family structures, like the German, the Hungarian, the Austrian and the Japanese point directly to the very nations noted for their higher suicide rates. Or, when the extended family structure breaks down on modern Indian reservations, the same high rates of suicide appear there among the younger generation.

Metropolitan Youth Culture

Just as the epidemiology of suicide rates points to isolating and differentiated problems of adolescents, so the political activism of young people from one culture to the next depends upon their segmentation from other groups in social structure. The experience with the Red Guard in mainland China proves perhaps better than the comparisons with Czech, Japanese, American and British youth that the phenomenon which we call metropolitan youth culture does exist. In the internal political struggles in China between the Maoists and moderates, the youthful Red Guard obviously got out of hand in their zeal for changing bureaucratic structure and were recently deflected from urban activities to a government-sponsored dispersal among the peasantry. What Erikson has called 'fidelity' as being 'disciplined devotion' is possibly exactly what the Maoist faction expected of the youthful Red Guard. But as we have pointed out above, both adolescents and youth in rebellion oversimplified problems, or they seek the kinds of simple and direct solutions which the older generation is usually reluctant to map out more carefully. Just as the urbanized Red Guard youth have been reported to chafe at the 'old-fashioned' values of the older peasant generation, so we in other countries have noticed our own youth forming their own phalanx of young people's organizations to provide the catalyst for solving modern social problems. We are not interested in making any moralistic judgments about who is right in these conflicts beyond the observation that young people have focused on crucial social problems and have provided the energy to propel society from old ruts. In the U.S., it was the Freedom Riders of Negro extraction and young in age who effectively started the entire so-called Civil Rights movement. On the problematic side, however, adolescents and youth are increasingly seen enmeshed in psychological disorders, sociopathy, and, as we have mentioned earlier, in rising suicide rates.

One final word, namely that metropolitan cultures have not devised attractive and meaningful structures for the adolescent. There are few schools which involve them with the larger society, and education for the most part turns away, as youth itself has discovered, from the relevant and the meaningful. One amusing instance in the U.S. occurred when Black students on campuses decided to call their organization by the term Black Students *Union*, not Association, with the word Union intended to blot out any connotation of the Boy Scouts of America! It is possible that schools, as such, could provide a large extension of activist functions in society if they had either the wit or the imagination. Instead they hew to their vocational and largely antiseptic persuasions and change more slowly than practically any other institution in our culture. Against this background of dead issues in our schools, in our economic structure and in our elitist social life, the brighter and more enterprising adolescents seek outlets in the more fluid conditions in the Arts, flee on assignment to underdeveloped countries, salve their individual consciences with activist politics, and declaim their defiance against the academic establishment throughout the world.

2

Psychiatric Problems of Adolescence

If adolescence is the period when some individuals strive to achieve more mature forms of social identification, then it is also the time when others fail to complete this process successfully. The first terminology for schizophrenia, as a matter of fact, labeled this breakdown 'dementia praecox', meaning an insidious disorder which appeared when one was still young in years. Another guidepost in terminology is the word 'delinquent', usually signifying a pattern of early sociopathy and suggesting an individual in adolescence or in the immediately following post-adolescent years. These two major hazards account for extremes of adolescent failures and the literature concerning them is far too elaborate and complex to be given in detail here. In a cross-cultural perspective, however, the need is less to produce a catalog of the disorders of this period in life history than it is to acquaint the reader with leading epidemiological differences from various kinds of social settings. It is not the nonliterate and simple societies that provide the instances of high rates either of the schizophrenias or of delinquent behavior. These extremes are a mark of our own affluent and class-differentiated economies and cultures.[33]

It is well to range these problems side by side with other specific maladjustments of those in adolescent and youth categories. There are school phobias and conduct disturbances such as truancy or destructiveness, stealing, cruelty, sexual offenses, and early excessive use of alcohol or drugs. All of these disturbances flag our attention to *social* misconduct or misbehavior and indicate a distance being set up between the child and modal cultural behavior. However, today, the difficulties with school, seen in school phobias, truancy, and drop-outs, the differences in ego identification achievement as seen in sexual offenses, in extremes of hostility or in the addictions, and the neurotic traits as seen in tics, stammering, hyperactivity or excessive shyness mark out the areas of impairments in adjustment to the school or to self and sexual identification processes. Even here one can discern subtle contrasts between the internalized personality disorders of the past and conduct problems which seem more in evidence today. The more introverted model used to be described as nervous, spoiled, irritable or irresponsible, as seclusive or daydreaming, as depressed or inefficient, or simply as queer. Today's young patient frequently has enough peer-group connections, if not enough other points of social identification, to have more obvious and on-the-surface conduct problems such as temper tantrums, fighting, swearing, violence, lying, truancy, stealing, addictions and sexual acting out. These contrasts in the style of problem illustrate what we meant above by the difference between earlier forms of neurotic behavior in children and what we now call character disorders. One suspects that in both historic instances there is the expectation of proper behavior, but that the earlier locus of the problem in the individual and in conflicts based often upon Oedipal patterns is now replaced by impairments in life functioning centering in school, peer-group relations and in a whole range of specifically *social* adjustments. Under the term social, we of course subsume such life goals as probable career, sexual adjustments, education and even political role. These are surrogate terms for jobs or individual role in the economy, the approach to sex and marriage,[28] the response to knowledge and technique, and the outlook on power relationships in the larger society. The normative acting-out behavior of normal youth in our culture is matched or paralleled by the large probability that some will encounter tremendous difficulties in the approach to such life functions as job, marriage, schooling and social response.

When we speak of the social gaps produced between parents and children by a speeded up tempo of cultural evolution, we can note by looking backwards at nonliterate societies that they frequently, through adolescence ceremonies and initiatory rites solidify the kinship and ethical-religious bonds or signalize heightened periods of courtship or sexual experimentation at precisely the points in time when we confront the adolescent with the remote rules and demands of vocation, sexual deferment, school and the social structuring of inequalities in the 'establishment'.

The Range of Cultural Influences on Personality

One of the inevitable consequences of rapid communication and technological development in modern times has been the apparent shrinking of world space. Youth and adolescents can be said to have experienced this smaller world outlook in the metropolitan centers. Young people are today, more than ever before, involved in world travel, or failing that, among less elite groups, their purview is extended by magazines, movies, television and the press. Through most of human history this present condition has hardly been the case. People were only dimly aware of the complex happenings in non-European and American cultures. When youth today insist on the inclusion in the U.S. of curricula dealing with African studies, or become incensed at the plight of starving Biafrans, they symbolize the point in education and politics that the world is, indeed, smaller and more interdependent in its regions.

At the same time, cultural anthropology on a scientific basis has become a part of world outlook among social and behavioral scientists. Only the most perfervid Freudian persists in allusions to instincts like 'innate aggression' or to a notion of uninfluenced sexual drive. Similarly, only poorly informed journalists write about 'animal territoriality' in crude attempts to define ecological adaptations in the human species. Meanwhile even the more current Freudians, like Hartmann[15] and Kris,[16] or Erikson,[7] utilize the concept of conflict-free areas of ego-adaptation to signify what we anthropologists would call cultural conditioning. Or, Erich Fromm as a neo-Freudian adds to the usual orthodox theory of dreams the further observation that some dream work may be problem-solving and that not all dream phenomena exemplify id and ego conflicts.

It is obvious that the above theoretical observations on original Freudianism do not go far enough in suggesting cultural influences on personality. Among anthropologists there has been greater emphasis upon modal personality differences from culture to culture and even within cultures. Thus, Ralph Linton describes for the Tanala of Madagascar[20] the way in which the eldest sons receive different treatment from birth on in such a way as to develop feelings of initiative and responsibility in them. Other siblings were curbed, disciplined and by implication repressed from achieving these traits. While the Tanala might look, at first glance, like a remote and isolated instance from the nonliterate world, it is well to remember that in another rice-growing (but also manufacturing) culture of the modern world, namely in the populous and powerful nation of Japan, roughly the same factors of personality development are exercised to stimulate the eldest son to the same achievements. Further, in the Japanese instance, the social role of eldest son is not predetermined by infancy disciplines at the start of the life cycle, but emerges as a difference particularly in adolescence. Both the Tanala and the Japanese examples are instructive, since they tell us immediately that a cultural system does not produce a single uniform level of behavior called 'adult personality', nor is this influence restricted to effects of infancy handling.

Social and Cultural Conflicts

In contrast with the infancy period and earlier childhood phases, adolescence is a period of development in which, as Erikson has put it, greater autonomy or emancipation is sought. Not only are there the obvious developmental changes in growth and sexuality, but the emotional life also shows clear signs of movement towards new balances. That this is not easy or without turmoil is indicated by the show of spurts of emotionality in various directions. Even the normal child evidences greater sensitivity, with consequent conflicts and upheavals. As we have noted above the high school years in the United States are a prime period for the eruption of acute schizophrenic behavior in some adolescents who are poorly prepared for advances to maturity. Between the normal and the pathological extremes, one finds an incidence of neurotic trends, or of characterological acting out such as we have noted above. For example, delinquency may mark a less stable integration of attempts to cope with the barriers we have listed as existing in family, school, intersexual contacts and role-development in the larger society. Again one can note even for normal development, more introspective attention to one's self and his relationships with meaningful others. Or one can note pronounced awkwardness and clumsiness. Some parents are surprised by the mood swings of their adolescents. When young people resolve such problems by withdrawals or by distortions of their status and role in reality, we may be sure that feelings of uncertainty, of inferiority or of compensatory attempts to feel superior are at work. Hence the awkwardness of adolescents signals insecurities as do narcissistic poses, or shyness, or today, the more dramatic rebellious reactions. Nonliterate cultures maximize the social and ethico-religious inputs at this time through the folk wisdom of initiation rites or the ceremonies concerned with age-grades.[36] But in modern metropolitan society the target of the adolescent rebellion is usually directed against the immediate family, and in particular against parental figures.

The Freudians have noted for the Oedipal family that the role behavior of the parent of same sex is the prime object for attack. Our schools have few methods for relieving this impact—for example through the kinds of clubs and associations where older youth might train the young. The styles of rebellion may range from those which are directly antagonistic to those which ignore parental authority. The parent, in turn, may react with stirrings of his own latent difficulties. Or, the child may set out for social contacts with peer group or gangs almost exclusively without any particular insight or guidance as to what this behavior really signifies, or in other words without stabilizing insights from either parents or peers. A. Aichhorn, in his work called *Delinquency and child guidance*,[1] furnishes accounts of how this emotional isolation develops and also what the tactics are for redeveloping contact with such youth in order to re-establish the mood for promoting insight and the interest in older stabilizing forces. A concomitant problem for adolescents, promoted in our culture, is the difficulty in handling guilt, since our chief social models are competitiveness, achievement and reward for performance. With our young separated by custom and social structure from economic and educative independence, the combinations of guilt and dependency provide further barriers to emancipation.

It is clear from our analysis to this point that the range of cultural influences on personality achieves paramount importance in adolescence. In societies which practice a more individualistic or shamanistic form of religion, the adolescent period is the prime occasion for religious conversions.[26,36] Even in our less religiously oriented metropolitan cultures, youth is, as we have seen, the time for various kinds of ideals to flourish. For these reasons, dramatic solutions are sought today in regard to educational conservatism on campuses, or in respect to racial inequalities, to middle-class hypocrisies about sex or to shocking inequities in the social and economic arrangements for the rich or the poor. Because the nonliterate cultures of the world tend to solve the problems of economics, of training and enculturation, of sexual expression and of ethical or religious rapport much more directly than we 'moderns', the youth of such societies are never accused of becoming a lost generation or even a rebellious one. By contrast, our youth are required to solve complex problems in regard to vocational choice, educational preparation, the approach to sexuality or the choices involved in politics. When we state that a sense of guilt and struggles with problems of dependency are the natural consequences of these perplexing dilemmas, we mean simply that the conditions for their development as problems are a consequence of the way in which adolescence is handled in metropolitan youth culture.

A more strictly linear view of development going from infancy stages through latency and on to puberty would hold that each stage, in order, is determinative of success or failure during the one which follows. Infancy determinism is, of course, an old point in Freudian doctrine.[9] But it also is a part of the point of view of Erik Erikson in his theory of ego-adaptation.[5] Both the Freudian viewpoint and Erikson's cohere in one essential and that pertains not so much to the idea of linear development for an individual (which of course harbors an essential truth); but they agree in being essentially psychogenic theories of etiology or causation. Ruth Benedict, in one of her most interesting writings on continuity and discontinuity in the life cycle, put the matter differently.[2] For Benedict, it was important to learn whether a culture stimulated behavior in a certain direction and then, later, produced a contradiction by halting or penalizing such behavior and through suddenly instituting entirely different demands. While Freud or Erikson would both claim that individual conflicts have their locus in the individual, the Freudian ego and id conflicts are somewhat modified by Erikson when he pictures the individual struggling with successive kinds of ego-adaptation. Yet besides these conflicts played out in an individual lifetime, there are tremendously important social and cultural conflicts which may be seen more directly as continuities and discontinuities in the learning of culture.

We are obviously emphasizing two kinds of conflict in society: one which concerns intrinsic contradictions in its values and its structures while the other type may arise from the linear discontinuities demanded of people in playing social roles. At any rate, both are deep-seated cultural conflicts, the first arising where youth, often bitterly, note the disparity between ideal stated values of the culture and real behavior.[6] Youth who are today filled with a ferment to see honest solutions take place for real problems in society exemplify one reaction to the first kind of culture conflict. The second form of conflict is more internalized, and while we do not claim that it always produces pathogenic consequences in an individual, nevertheless it does provide difficult hurdles which must be overcome.

Culture and Mental Illness

It would be unfortunate, however, to leave the matter of range of cultural influences in this partly defined state. It is a part of growth and development to be able to make choices in the most conflicted of social settings. Thus, all cultures, no matter how strained in disparities between the actual enactment of real values and ideal values, nevertheless contain persons who strive, cope and struggle successfully within the problematic setting. The epidemiology of mental illnesses may be worse for the society as a whole (as it is in modern metropolitan cultures in Europe and America). But there are always well persons to be noted in practically any culture. Similarly, discontinuities in a given type of life cycle may produce more disorder, but again there may often be many individual victories. To cite one commonly given example in the United States, it is claimed that the relatively permissive childhood training of the decades from 1930 to the present, when followed by greater strictness in educational and job requirements later produced such problems as the youth rebelliousness we have mentioned above. While the general statistics are true, the real test depends on the family and social modes of handling natural resentments, problems in communication and the development of insight. In social psychiatry it is claimed that newer methods of social intervention are necessary on the youth level, or that family therapy, specially designed youth services, and community psychology applied more effectively in schools and in activity programs would be most beneficial. In many cases, some with and others without the full panoply of such agencies, remarkable personality gains are made later on in the period following a problem-ridden adolescence. In order to understand such successes, more careful studies are required of the assets and liabilities, along with modes of handling, of the adolescent problem case.

Role discontinuity may therefore involve the individual in psychological stresses or it may mobilize latent pathology in such periods as adolescence and youth. A study by Livson and Peskin[21] in 1967 found characteristics in the junior high school period to be more predictive than similar variables in earlier childhood or in the slightly later adolescent period of the ages 14 through 16. Livson and Peskin in finding that the young people of 12 and 13 years old in junior high showed the greatest predictions for later behavior concluded that the way in which the child responded to the transition from grade school to the junior high was the best indication of such gross differences as 'actively inviting or withdrawing' from new experiences. Earlier, the author and colleagues in the Midtown Manhattan study[33] pointed out that the rate of mental disorders was highest at points of role transition and loss, such as the change from an active maternal to a post-maternal role in later life. In *Mental health in the metropolis*, we suggested that the impact of role discontinuity would, of course, be hardest upon vulnerable personalities, the latter defined as partly due to the cultural failures in providing training for an individual moving into or toward new social roles. However, it is well to remember that the Midtown age-trend data may be supplemented by other types of adult follow-up studies, such as Jean Macfarlane's conclusions concerning 166 persons in the Guidance Study at the Institute of Human Development.[22] Macfarlane noted clearly that many individuals in this study were able in time to overcome earlier difficulties. She stated that many of the most outstandingly mature were those confronted with very difficult situations and were in fact often those whose childhood and adolescent reactions seemed to multiply their problems. In other words, the struggles of adolescence may furnish the individual with new strengths, especially where guidance procedures have helped to overcome the hurdles.

Personal Resources and Environment

Such puzzles are found frequently in the literature, probably because adolescence as a performance stage is open to regressions as well as to movements toward maturity. Our own point of view has emphasized that there is a transactional interplay between personal resources and environment. M. B. Smith in 1966 confirmed this in a study of persons with the Peace Corps who were serving as teachers in Ghana.[32] The 44 teachers were rated predictively by psychiatrists through two 50-minute appraisal interviews before departure from the United States. Smith found that the mental health ratings predicting competence in field performance were later found to be entirely uncorrelated with the actual functioning in overseas work. The overall correlation of $-.02$ between the ratings and later administrative evaluations of actual performance further varied as between $.54$ correlations for the city teachers, $-.02$ for volunteers in semi-rural settings, and $-.36$ for those located 'in the bush'. The trend in these results suggests that the ratings were really specifically designed for the functioning of teachers in an urban setting whereas, apparently, greater flexibility than the tests predicted was required in the settings where cultural shock and different environment would be most marked. R. Coles in comments upon Civil Rights workers[4] in the United States has remarked that often the quiet and even timid become transformed into the most vigorous teachers and forceful fighters or organizers under conditions where they are confronted by the police and the establishment apparatus of the deep South. As a matter of fact, the studies of disaster situations recorded in the *Symposium on preventive and social psychiatry* by J. S. Tyhurst and others[34] have for a long time emphasized that a species of natural and adaptive leaders often springs up most unexpectedly when whole communities are confronted with catastrophes.

Studies of differentials in youth adjustment, however, do not seem to provide us with a basic understanding of adolescence in different societies.

In the two decades 1920–1940, the chief attempt to point out variations in adolescence itself was made by Margaret Mead in her books, *Coming of age in Samoa*[24] and *Growing up in New Guinea*.[25] Her emphasis on cultural relativity, especially as concerns the effects of culture on female puberty, was perhaps the chief influence on Ruth Benedict's work, *Continuities and discontinuities in cultural conditioning*.[2] Mead's general view of the untrammeled and sexually experimental Samoan girl later came under a certain amount of criticism since such a development of gradual and natural sexuality in a continuous line is not fully in accord with other large ethnographic studies of the curbs placed upon the Samoan female adolescents which include, for example, stoning them to death in high-ranking lineages if they are found to be non-virgins at the time of marriage. But the larger contrast of Mead was between the emphasis in our society upon the sexless nature of the child, along with our prudery about sexual growth and development; whereas in contrast the Samoan child does indeed know more about the biological events of life including birth, death and puberty. Mead added to this that what we consider perversions, homosexuality and promiscuity, are probably viewed more simply or naturally in the Samoan setting.

To the same general period belongs B. Malinowski's *Sex and repression in savage society*,[23] a work which has been less open to ethnological criticisms and which stated that the natives of the Trobriand Islands lived in matrilineal or clan society where the specific 'nuclear family' complexes obviously did not accommodate the notion of a universal Oedipus complex with dominating father-authority patterns. In the Trobriands, except in the rarer chiefly lines of succession in richer districts, like Kiriwina, which did indeed recognize patrilineal succession if not true biological fatherhood, most Trobrianders regarded their fathers as friendly caretakers and companions even though they were 'strangers' in their own matrilineal villages.

In Samoa small girls and boys were involved in the adult work of each sex group and at six or seven the former would care for and even discipline younger siblings while the boys did simple reef fishing and canoeing, both increasing responsibilities gradually. In the Trobriands, likewise, the learning of work relationships under surveillance of a mother's brother is a normal accompaniment of puberty. Ethnographic accounts are also full of examples of the cultural attitudes toward first female menstruation, the Apache Indian girl's first menses being followed by the famous Girl's Adolescence Rite in which she is carried through four stages of life into old age and guaranteed vigor and capability in shamanistic ceremonies. The Ute Indians of Colorado also signalize this event culturally, though they organized her protection in a separate encampment and likewise imposed regular ritual observances for any girl's or women's benefit.[26]

One could contrast such culturally evolved protective devices with the unconcern and neglect accorded Black adolescent girls in White America. Two Negro psychiatrists in their book *Black rage*[13] have noted that both for Negro female and male adolescents' maturation period, the difficulties lie not so much in lack of sexual and biological information as in the socially reinforced lack of self-esteem. Negro girls, growing up at a time when the ordinary female narcissistic needs and emotional supports are greatest, are confronted with the many degrading racial distinctions fostered in the dominant White community. While the same is, of course, true for the adolescent boy, the hazards to his ego development will be in terms of non-masculine images fostered in the White culture, whereas for the girl the stereotyped conceptions are usually brutal and non-feminine. When we reflect, again, upon the female needs and growth periods that are highly discontinuous, like female puberty, this withholding of a special accent upon female dependency, narcissism and emotional response accounts for the high rates of pregnancy and illegitimacy among Negro adolescent girls. Such events and their institutional consequences further damage self-esteem. If, then, we reflect again upon the customs in nonliterate societies which support and accent the emerging of adult female roles, it is more probable that the emphasis on discontinuity and change for Blacks, or supporting compensations for primitives, are closer to the mark than Mead's theory of natural or gradual development. Our own modification would put greater stress upon the practices in many societies to support this changing role; and we could add that boys' adolescent ceremonies likewise have the same social functions.

Biological Theories of Development

If one surveys theories of adolescence, one finds that most approaches have tended to minimize the effects of culture. G. Stanley Hall, in his two-volume work called *Adolescence*[14] emphasized in 1916 a physiologically based theory in which his developmental stages were infancy and childhood followed by youth and adolescence. The latter was the period from puberty until adulthood. Hall did notice the emotional and volatile swings in adolescent behavior based no doubt upon observations in our society. As we have pointed out above, Freud and his immediate followers tended also to emphasize the biological and instinctual nature of man, apart from cultural differences, in such a way that little room was left for regarding this life stage as modifiable through social factors. The neo-Freudians like Fromm, Horney and Sullivan evolved some departures from this universalistic theory. For example, Erich Fromm in his least noticed work, *Studies on authority and the family*,[12] did in 1936 emphasize that father and son are not rivals in their psychosexual dynamics in many societies. It is worth adding that the Mead and Malinowski work had already appeared.

To continue with the development of theory chronologically, Anna Freud in 1936 published *The ego and the mechanism of defense*[8] in which she noted that what she called a second Oedipus complex occurred with vehemence at the beginning of puberty, producing more sharply defined castration fears in boys and penis envy in girls as in earlier Oedipal conflicts, but now played out on a level of fantasy in which the super-ego called forth further defenses such as repression, denial and displacement and turning these, sometimes, against the self. Thus the fears of adolescence, the anxieties about social acceptance, the aggressions of delinquency, pregenital perversities and other neurotic symptoms could be exhibited for a time. A girl could sometimes exhibit astounding feelings of rage and hatred as well as the opposites of dependent and clinging feelings toward the mother. Or a boy's delinquency might test male authority with great zest, while at the same time showing forceful undercurrents of feelings of inadequacy, fear and helpless uncertainty. Certainly, these pitfalls are particularly true of our society, and therefore clinical instances of such turmoil can be multiplied. But the theoretical model, while it is an exciting indicator of possible kinds of psychodynamic process, obviously pays less attention to the ways in which society might increase the strength of id impulse, or through character training and super-ego development in the latency period could strengthen the ego ability to cope with impulsivity in general. Since 1936, when Anna Freud made her formulations, there is increasing evidence that middle-class adolescents in the United States have been subjected to social changes which increase the problem of impulsivity, while the forces that would strengthen independence have received much less attention.

Cultural Anthropology and Psychoanalysis

The debate between cultural anthropology and Freudian points of view has continued with Geza Roheim's book, *Psychoanalysis and anthropology*,[31] published in 1950. Roheim, in his initial chapter on Central Australian cultures, stresses such things as the male initiation rites of circumcision as if these were reenactments during adolescence of the initial Oedipal conflicts of the infant to be separated or untied from the mother. Of course, in Australia, as Roheim knows, there are also ceremonies of clitoridectomy, or parallel female initiatory rites from the same regions. But what Roheim simply reads off as 'symbolic castration' of the male and almost infantile separation from the mother has also very important elements of inculcation in the adult lore of the tribes concerned; solidarity, now as a young man, is achieved with important relatives of his social group. Films of youth undergoing the painful subincision emphasize the coping with pain and even more importantly this attainment of a more adult status. The faces of the youth undergoing the pain show unmistakable pride. As for the notion of subincision being symbolically equivalent to castration (and hence by some mysterious transmutation and change of male organ to 'vagina'), the actual fact is that initiation officially begins a Central Australian's serious sex life on a more adult level.

There have been other attempts, as in Kurt Lewin's field theory,[19] to define adolescence as a more fluid state between childhood and adulthood. Some of Lewin's theoretical points are similar to those we have used. This is the period of life, *par excellence*, when an individual expects to be involved in an expansion of his 'psychological field', or as we would prefer to put it, of his life space. He may experience this with his peer group, or as happens in our culture, the peer group is somewhat isolated from the work and the other adult roles of the culture. Lewin sensed this when he described adolescence as a marginal state. The space of 'free movement' accessible to an individual in adolescence was his psychological construct by which the relationship of the individual to his culture could be explained. While Lewin's 'free movement' seems vague on first encounter, he further defined it as being 'what is forbidden to a person' or 'what is beyond his ability'. In most primitive cultures, adolescence is viewed as the time when the adult roles are opened up to young people, in work, in special roles, in relationship to adult functions and in intersexual behavior. It is interesting that Lewin also reflects the prohibitive conditions in our culture by mentioning, first of all, 'what is forbidden'. We do not mean that nonliterate societies do not have proscriptions and taboos, but we are rather calling attention to the larger scale upon which we are 'taboo-ridden' whereas the nonliterate culture has highly particularized and often more carefully delimited proscriptions and rules. This is made clear when we note that the adult work of our society is deferred, sexual behavior is clandestine rather than sanctioned, and education which is our usual prescription for the adolescent and youth years seems unreal, overly technical or generally divorced from real life.

We therefore constantly stress in our culture 'what is beyond his ability' for the adolescent, whereas in other cultures, as we have stated above, work and social involvement are not seen by youth to be a special and separate precinct beyond their reach. Thus, while Lewin's notion of an increased involvement in the adolescent's life span involving new developmental tasks sounds enticing, it is perhaps better organized in nonliterate cultures than in our own. At the same time, 'metropolitan youth culture' and increasing opinion on our college campuses argue directly for a rapid expansion of youth involvement in our current politics, in our educational establishment, in our arts, and in our degree of attention to the long standing problems of our shrinking world.

Specific Challenges and Pathologies

Our particular theory of adolescent problems in our culture should explain our specific epidemiology of disorders for this age group. Above, we have accounted for the shifting to character disorders. Most of the views of this pathology find that it is rooted in a lack of *meaningful* relationships between the self and others. Our cultural tendency both to isolate and also to protract the adolescent period certainly provides a reinforcement of any cases which earlier lack proper familial relationships.

A lack of meaningful relationships can be traced back within the family line, but a more likely method of explanation would include the way in which the whole society may minimize the best in human behavior and hence in interpersonal relations. According to this latter point of view, the process of decay in modern metropolitan culture would lead to widespread impairments in life functioning of the members of society. While some anthropologists, the functionalists in particular, usually stress the positive elements in social systems making for continuity and support of the culture, the present author has always felt that one must understand pathologies of people as being the result of social and psychological stresses produced by the society. Here we are speaking of the compulsions and contradictions in a social system which can breed psychological processes of decay. Modern urban societies therefore seem to disregard elementary needs of human beings and to promote the social factors which lead to individual breakdowns. In cultural evolution, one would trace the development of psychic disorders against the background of changes in society which lead to individual impairments in life functioning.[29]

Elsewhere we have pointed out that the modern urbanized cultures of western Europe and America are precisely the ones which show the greatest amount of such impairments. The rise of character disorders and paranoid schizophrenias in increasing numbers helps to document this fact. In addition, the author, as a principal investigator of the Midtown Manhattan Mental Health research study, can document the process of decay from eight years of research in New York City. Here the epidemiology of adult impairments between ages 20 and 59 disclosed that only 18·5 per cent of the sample could be classified as Well, i.e. free from significant symptoms. The Mild and Moderate levels of symptom formation accounted for 36·3 and 21·8 per cent of the sample respectively. The Marked, Severe, and Incapacitated were 13·2, 7·5 and 2·7 per cent respectively. Thus over four-fifths of the sample were found to be suffering from some identifiable form of mental disturbance, and nearly a quarter were 'in the impaired range of the mental health continuum'.[33]

In a somewhat more impressionistic approach than the epidemiological method, Edgar Z. Friedenberg's book, *The vanishing adolescent*,[11] claims that this stage in life is being compressed in time in the sense that traditional adolescence *is* disappearing through increasing precocity of youth of high school age into roles as consumers, sex experimenters, 'committee men', social 'operators', etc. Our own point, contrasting to his view of the adolescent in suburbia, is that modern adolescence is very much protracted in time when compared with the induction of youth in nonliterate societies. This we have stated above. But while we both agree that the adolescent is increasingly enmeshed in the intricate machinery of education and a wide range of social agencies, we probably do not see eye to eye on the fact that young people are differentially exposed to the pressures of the larger society. In their book, *Black rage*, William Grier and Price Cobbs point to the adolescent brutalization of young Negro females as well as to the demasculinization of the young male; and both processes, however opposite in direction, are results of exploitative techniques imposed upon the American Blacks. What Friedenberg and the author are agreeing to is a social and economic disinterest in the adolescent except where the White variety becomes a consumer or the Black a member of a sometimes ignored labor pool. In other words, we both can note kinds of obsolescence affecting this stage of life, but in my own view one's place in the social structure will largely determine the psychological stresses.

Object Relations in Adolescence

Anna Freud in *The ego and the mechanisms of defense* feels that the most remarkable aspect of the adolescent period is its connection with object relations. Writing as she did in 1936, with English translation published in 1946, it is interesting that she commented upon the giving up of incestuous fantasies of the prepubertal period with the young person tending to isolate himself. She did add that the ego alienates itself from superego connections as well. But the isolated adolescent is most uncharacteristic of our modern times. In contrast to this picture of self-isolation, the adolescent of today is thrown together with others of his peer group and this, more than isolation, accompanies his abandonment of the earlier parental object relationships. Further, our youth today grow up at a greater distance in 'cultural time' from their parents than ever before, simply because the tempo of cultural change increases as technology and knowledge unfold. What the author calls metropolitan youth culture intensifies this youth communication just as the communication media themselves make it possible.

Youth, therefore, are not so much isolated as active in the mass. Their tempo is faster and their demands are more immediate. In pathological terms, their struggles with impulsivity would be more desperate. It is interesting that Anna Freud, when commenting upon the increasing adaptability of youth, quotes the work of Helene Deutsch in 1934 on the borderline neurotics which she called 'as if' personalities, because in the object relations of this adult type they acted *as if* they were acting out views and opinions on life with genuine feelings, whereas their friendships and attachments are not only volatile, but swing from strong dislike to passionate loves rapidly and in a transient fashion. Youth today show the latter forms of object relationships: changing sexual liaisons and experimentation, strong rejection of parents and 'establishment', and fickleness in regard to fads, fashions and tastes. But while impulsivity is a definite youth characteristic of our times, they are also passionately concerned with the external world, with ideal and quick solutions to long-festering problems and with a more solid kind of social idealism derived from youth leaders. In our view the factors which might strengthen the superego and the forces of the outside world are essential to their progress and to the avoidance of empty narcissism. That some succumb to character disorders and others struggle with psychosomatic ailments, paranoid schizophrenias, or evidence higher rates of suicide in depressive states is merely a way of recording the prevalent epidemiology of our times. Meanwhile, if our educational and social organization could only make more use of the idealistic components in these total social trends, that alone would bring youth into greater involvement in the problems and progress of the larger society.

3

Toward a General Theory of Adolescence

Economic Systems and Social Values

When anthropologists characterize societies, they emphasize two elements of prime importance, one being the economic and technical system, and the other being the social organization and values including the family system. Those emphasizing material and economic forces in society are often called Marxian, while those emphasizing family systems and values are variously typified as being sociological or Freudian in emphasis. In our view in this chapter, the evolution of society has been such that the connections between technical and social change and the various designs for living which also evolve are closely connected in their relational or reciprocal interdependence. What is most needed today are controls over technical and economic forces which go beyond the usual modes of 'control over the total forces of production' in such a way that our equally growing store of information about the social and humanistic requirements of man also have application. It is interesting that both adolescents and youth also attack such questions vigorously, or that experimental programs in social planning such as those concerning the *kibbutzim* of Israel likewise develop plans or designs for living. For instance, in many of the *kibbutzim* as reported by Bruno Bettelheim in his book, *Children of the dream,*[3] the adolescent is discouraged from sexual experimentation through adolescence and into youth, while at the same time the social group and work orientations are stressed. For most adolescents and youth in what we have called the metropolitan youth culture, the idea of sexual experimentation has been stressed in the opposite mode, and here of course the discovery of contraceptive pills has furthered that direction.[28] Even where we have stressed the intersex styles of dress and hair among some youth today, it is only fair to follow their definition that these items in appearance do not define the differences between sexes today, since these fashions are merely superficial trappings of the older 'establishment'.

However, adolescents and youth fail to recognize in such idealistic accounts of their own behavior that they are much more the creatures of their times and their culture than they ever expected. For instance, underlying these intersex fads of long loose hair, sandals, trousers and loosely fitting upper garments is the general cultural condition for some that they are living out a response to changes in education, the job market, which becomes increasingly technical, and the other social requirements which place a moratorium on success. Experimental communes, recourse to drugs and new fads in music or visual arts become their products. The more staid youth continue with technical education, but share in the general moratorium on achieving closure in social, sexual and even economic participation in the establishment.

We make these summaries of some central tendencies among adolescents and youth merely to contrast them with the different style of living and of morality in nonliterate cultures or in those of more slowly developing nations. In the nonliterate culture, one's involvement with the economic and social scene begins earlier and more naturally. One works directly in the economic life through participation in gradually broadening aspects of the total economy—much of which *is* within reach. Through imitation and apprenticeship, much is learned. Because of technical simplicity, often, the adult need not always 'do things' for the adolescent, but rather at the time of adolescence rites he is expected to enter into the adult life more fully. The same type of early, but *social*, involvement in relationships and sexual life may occur, but the cultural fabrics are woven so tightly that there is little meaning to terms like 'alienated youth,' 'identity crises', and 'existential struggles' from such nonliterate settings. On the contrary, among the chief problems of adolescents and youth in our modern urban cultures are matters of 'involvement', by which is ordinarily meant meaningful participation in the total or adult world. On campuses throughout the world, this is the constant cry which rings out in applications to the conduct of higher education, of politics, or struggles toward world peace.

Adolescent Psychiatry

In this light, the chief continuing need in adolescent and youth psychiatry is to develop social and group forms of expression and functioning which will bring young people into realistic relationships with the world in which they live. The group psychotherapeutic technique, psychodrama, the use of expressive arts in therapy and also community forms of functioning in groups for worthwhile purposes are probably among the most useful techniques at our disposal. Because knowledge is more segmented and technical than ever before, means must be found to develop generalizations about our cultural evolution which place the youth effort in its proper context. Means must be sought to speed up and shorten the technical education of some, so that the moratorium on adulthood is not too long deferred. Vocational options must be developed so that those seeking careers have a range of possibilities which are viable rather than a single narrow and distant goal. Meanwhile, the establishment, as it has been called, must obviously become more flexible and willing to accommodate to adolescent and youth needs. In educational programs a better 'mix' of the professional, the graduate student, the undergraduate and even promising adolescents beneath these levels would be helpful. In the same context the rigid separations between the educational establishment and the 'outer world', whether in sciences or humanities must go if we are to achieve a greater sense of involvement.

The disturbed adolescent, like his normal counterpart, is acting out a way of life characteristic of a pattern of social development before he became ill. The chief goals of a successful adjustment are: the achievement of a clear sense of sexual identity, but at the same time a widening awareness of both self and social identification. F. Kluckhohn deals with the social value systems which are formative in shaping the family.[18] However, the values that underlie family styles in different class and ethnic backgrounds account for kinds of conflict which may develop in contact with any dominant form such as evolving metropolitan culture, or its American variety ordinarily called middle-class, or as youth have it today, 'the establishment'. For the adolescent there is always shaping his self-image and sense of social identification his struggles with the symbols of authority. Both Erikson and Horney in describing the adolescent search for identity and autonomy tend to ignore the specific class or subcultural context, both of which have profound effects upon the patterns of family style and the types of community problem which confront the adolescent.

A general theory of adolescence which is more culturally relativistic would insist upon these realistic contexts while not forgetting the general values, aspirations and fears of the adult world that influence all adolescents as a group. Thus, most descriptions of this period which emphasize the pornographic and sexual fantasies of boys in contrast to what are called the more private and guarded fantasies of girls or, which like Anna Freud, describe intellectualization and asceticism as the opposite ideals, seem to be highly abstract and not fully characteristic of specific groups. Similarly, Erikson's 'psychosocial moratorium' as a prolonging of adolescence into the youth period hardly conforms with today's realities of political awareness among young radicals or sexual experimentation in the high school and college aged groups. Further, the adolescent of today because of his greater numerical visibility in the population is forcing new values and attitudes upon both the family and the educational scene. In social life also the clear split between those who combine intellectualism and activism for political and social ends and those who emphasize more asocial behavior such as withdrawal from the 'establishment' or defiance, represents two polarities in metropolitan youth culture at the present time. Paul Goodman has suggested that some delinquents and nonconformist youth are responding imaginatively in their distance from the adult world to its failure to provide decent standards of education, employment and values to which they could respond. At any rate, the much larger incidence of delinquency, drug addiction and schizophrenia among the most disadvantaged youth points directly to their lack of adequate homes, jobs and families.

One of the advantages of group psychotherapy with adolescents and youth is that it encourages them to reach into chaotic feelings and to clarify for themselves their own responses. The therapist, in dealing with the individual can often help them discover their unconscious attitudes simply by telling them what they feel. It is curious that less education in psychology is done at this stage of life than almost any other, since it is then, particularly, that self discoveries would be highly important. It is also notably a time when such different techniques as support or direction *versus* limit-setting have possibly the greatest usefulness. The therapist also must establish competence against a background of the adolescent's natural tendency to test the adult or to solidify a sense of suspiciousness about him. In puberty also, because the needs for independence and privacy increase, the adolescent often responds positively to confidentiality and to the assurance that healthy reality orientation is the goal. They therefore require both an honest directness and flexibility, and because adults or parents are likewise often involved, any family session techniques must be supplemented with the reassurance of private sessions with the adolescent patient himself. In some institutions where adolescents are already aggregated in groups, it is found that they also benefit from adult contacts rather than age-group separation, while at the same time the therapy group is often best confined to their own number. What we have suggested above, in education about the desirability of a 'mix' going from professional to undergraduate, is likewise true of the therapeutic institution where it is all too easy to segregate and isolate adolescents from other ages. Like the nonliterate society, in which he is best off by assuming social and economic roles amid all age groups, the most realistic institutional milieu will also mirror as much of the total outside workaday world as possible.

The New Environment and Mental Illness

Perhaps the real question for the cultural evolutionist is whether he has pointed out the general contours of social change as these have affected the adolescent so that the political turbulence and war, the temporary relationships and mobility, and the technical jobs which seem unconnected with a more fulfilling reality, along with the protracted and demanding education, all come into clear focus. Obviously, the planning of change requires recognizing this new environment for what it is, so that we can learn to relate it to the energy, idealism and boundless desires of youth. It can be said that many adolescents feel an inchoate fear that their elders not only fail to understand them, but that they inhabit a different and long since dead world of their own. Cross-cultural perspectives at least allow us to place this now changed world in its proper context and they might, if we had the welfare of the adolescence period of life in mind, give us the tools for preparing more interesting and productive lives.

The language of the young is today a combination of impulsive activism and the electronic symbol ('turn on', 'blow—or—expand your mind', 'do your own thing', 'get high'). Even the current popular American movie,

G

The Graduate, will portray a young and confused, but sincere, hero who wins his bride away from the smooth and successful medical student cast in the role of a banal 'establishment' figure, probably the successor of the man in the grey flannel suit. We make these points because in our electronic age of rapid communication we need new interpreters much like Freud and Sullivan were for their day, who can be subtle and artistic perceivers of the current kinds of sensory awareness.

Similarly, the connections between today's cultural backgrounds and our present-day types of mental illnesses must be made clear. When we look at character disorders or full-fledged sociopathy, we can see how easily prone young people would be to possess desired objects immediately or else experience tremendous discomfort. The simple sociopath wants what he wants with no possibility of delayed gratification, and his is the action mode for satisfying irresistible impulses. More must be done to teach young people to want and expect tenderness and less superficial relationships with further techniques for approving the postponement of gratification without experiencing frustration. Our permissiveness in child-rearing has been overplayed without the counter-balances of demonstrating longer processes of goal achievement, better techniques for handling anxiety and guilt, and especially the ethical values of tenderness and unselfish motivations.

The schizophrenic with paranoid reaction is likewise strongly represented in youth today and here we see both the intrapsychic and interpersonal breakdown of someone who has been made to feel that the whole world is unacceptable. While most writers have emphasized the existential anxiety about the self, we would prefer to note, as with the character disorder, that social and ethical relationships are also underplayed in the world of the schizophrenic. One can add that sexual identifications are badly damaged and that many young people succumb to homosexual trends. In fact, a 'homosexual streak' is frequently found in the admixtures of pathology of the sociopath. However, classically the schizophrenic experiences a deeper sense of panic; and with his weakened and inadequate social and self image, the burdens of anxiety, hostility and magical detachment involve him in a more completely disintegrating personality breakdown. This more total defeat or entrance into a private and delusional world is marked by the compensations of grandiose fantasies and psychotic notions of persecution. It is interesting that this psychotic reconstruction of the external world provides the paranoid schizophrenic with a wholly new, if delusional, social setting in which his defeats and self accusations are countered by the excuses that others harm him or that his immense powers go unrecognized. At the same time, the more depressed patient's feelings of failure, or the suicidal attempts of those who want help in their suffering are again eloquent commentaries on the failures of the social environment to provide the kind of emotional supplies needed by human beings.

Education and the Adolescent

Perhaps the greatest contribution of young people in the metropolitan youth culture has been their attack on hypocrisy and insincerity among the generation that went before them. Again a phrase of theirs, 'tell it as it is', points to this preponderant concern. Adolescents and youth recognize that the world they live in, its wars, unemployment, educational banalities and hypocritical mouthing of values, provide the conditions of existence that will shape their own lives in every important respect. The general mass response has been to seek more involvement and also more control over these forces of destiny. Their sensitivity to hypocritical 'cheating' is something like the youngster's who hysterically cannot learn to read because he feels his environment is dominated by some pervasive sense of insincerity or feigned concern which overwhelms him. This is best seen in the combinations of rage and hopelessness among Negro youth in White society, where the segregated schools, the de-emphasis on subtle and higher modes of education and the generally negative symbols for Blacks destroy their self-esteem and lead to ghetto youth dropping out of schools entirely. In the United States, the feeling among all educated youth is growing into a belief that this is just another betrayal of their age group; and consequently, they demand more Black teachers and professors, more Black students in every type of school, and more responses in the curriculum to subjects concerning Africa and Afro-Americans such as dignify the Negro cultural contribution. We already know that the Negro adolescent may be adversely influenced by White domination in schools or in tests, so that even his psychological test responses are affected by the color of the person doing the testing.[13]

In fact all learning disabilities are not so much affected as infected by the social environment. Yet it would be the most empty kind of pretense to suppose that the minority group adolescent, or adolescents in general can establish the necessary transformations in society acting as a single age group. Today, in the United States and elsewhere throughout the world, young people are asking for the right to revamp the educational and political establishments, including the hiring and firing of teachers and officials, the backing of political candidates and movements, and so forth. The best move that can be made in education, in politics and in economics would be to meet them half-way in a conjoint effort at needed social transformations. The more we involve adolescents and youth in the serious work of the total society, the more we shall begin to resemble the efforts of nonliterate societies to accept the young as contributing members of the culture. To do so, we require more roles for youth, a greater mixture in work of the already trained and the energetic trainee, and a psychology of adolescence which is not merely judgmental from the established standards but which also makes room for a clear view of the culture of metropolitan youth and their problems. Once these goals are accomplished, the present writer would predict that the rising rates of character disorders, psychosomatic ailments, and even schizophrenias with paranoid reaction may diminish. The very reforms of realistic involvement suggest the direction of therapeutic organization for adolescents in the future.

REFERENCES

1. AICHHORN, A. 1964. *Delinquency and child guidance.* New York: International Universities Press.
2. BENEDICT, R. 1954. Continuities and discontinuities in cultural conditioning. In *Readings in child development,* Eds. W. Martin and C. Stendler. New York: Harcourt, Brace.
3. BETTELHEIM, B. 1969. *Children of the dream.* New York: Macmillan.
4. COLES, R. 1966. A psychiatrist joins the movement. *Trans-action,* **3,** 21.
5. ERIKSON, E. H. 1959. *Identity and the life cycle: Selected Papers.* Psychological Issues, Monograph Series, No. 1. New York: International Universities Press.
6. ERIKSON, E. H. (Ed.) 1963. *Youth: change and challenge.* New York: Basic Books.
7. ERIKSON, E. 1968. *Identity: youth and crisis.* New York: W. W. Norton.
8. FREUD, A. 1936. *The ego and the mechanisms of defense.* New York: W. W. Morton.
9. FREUD, S. 1933. *New introductory lectures on psychoanalysis.* New York: W. W. Norton.
10. FREUD, S. 1949. *An outline of psychoanalysis.* New York: W. W. Norton.
11. FRIEDENBERG, E. Z. 1959. *The vanishing adolescent.* Boston: Beacon Press.
12. FROMM, E. 1936. *Studies on authority and the family.* Paris: Alcan.
13. GRIER, W. H. and COBBS, P. M. 1968. *Black rage.* New York: Basic Books.
14. HALL, G. S. 1916. *Adolescence.* New York: Appleton.
15. HARTMANN, H. 1958. *The ego and the problem of adaptation.* New York: International Universities Press.
16. HARTMANN, H., KRIS, E. and LOEWENSTEIN, R. M. 1946. Comments on the formation of psychic structure. In *The psychoanalytic study of the child,* **2.** New York: International Universities Press.
17. HORNEY, K. 1937. *The neurotic personality of our time.* New York: W. W. Norton.
18. KLUCKHOHN, F. and STRODTBECK, F. 1961. *Variations in value orientation.* New York: Harper-Row.
19. LEWIN, K. 1935. *A dynamic theory of personality.* New York: McGraw-Hill.
20. LINTON, R. 1939. The Tanala of Madagascar. In *The individual and his society,* Ed. A. Kardiner. New York: Columbia University Press.
21. LIVSON, N. and PESKIN, H. 1967. The prediction of adult psychological health in a longitudinal study. *J. abnorm. Psychol.,* **72,** 509.
22. MACFARLANE, J. W. 1964. Perspectives on personality consistency and change from the guidance study. *Vita Humana,* **7,** 115.
23. MALINOWSKI, B. 1927. *Sex and repression in savage society.* London: Routledge and Kegan Paul.
24. MEAD, M. 1928. *Coming of age in Samoa.* New York: Wm. Morrow.
25. MEAD, M. 1930. *Growing up in New Guinea.* New York: Wm. Morrow.
26. OPLER, MARVIN K. 1940. The Southern Ute Indians of Colorado. In *Acculturation in seven American Indian tribes,* Ed. R. Linton. New York: Appleton Century.
27. OPLER, M. K. 1967. *Culture and social psychiatry.* New York: Atherton Press.

28. OPLER, M. K. 1969. Cross-cultural aspects of kissing. *Human sexuality*, 3, No. 2, 11.
29. OPLER, M. K. 1969. Culture and child rearing. In *Modern perspectives in international child psychiatry*, Ed. J. G. Howells. Edinburgh: Oliver and Boyd.
30. OPLER, M. K. and SMALL, S. MOUCHLY. 1968. Cultural variables affecting somatic complaints and depression. *Psychosomatics*, 9, 261.
31. ROHEIM, G. 1950. *Psychoanalysis and anthropology*. New York: International Universities Press.
32. SMITH, M. B. 1966. Explorations in competence. *Amer. Psychologist*, 21, 555.
33. SROLE, L., OPLER, M. K., *et al.* 1962. *Mental health in the metropolis: the Midtown Manhattan study*. New York: McGraw-Hill.
34. TYHURST, J. S., OPLER, M. K., *et al.* 1957. *Symposium on preventive and social psychiatry*. Walter Reed Army Institute of Research, Washington.
35. WHEELIS, A. B. 1958. *The quest for identity*. New York: W. W. Norton.
36. YOUNG, F. W. 1965. *Initiation ceremonies*. Indianapolis: Bobbs-Merrill.

PART TWO

CLINICAL

VIII

EPIDEMIOLOGICAL ASPECTS OF ADOLESCENT PSYCHIATRY

A. S. HENDERSON

M.D., M.R.C.P., M.R.A.C.P., D.P.M.

Professor of Psychiatry
University of Tasmania, Australia

J. KRUPINSKI

M.D., DOCENT, F.A.C.M.A.

Epidemiologist, Mental Health Research Institute
Parkville, Victoria, Australia

A. STOLLER

M.R.C.S., F.A.N.Z.C.P., F.A.C.M.A., D.P.M.

Chairman, Mental Health Authority
Victoria, Australia

1

Introduction

The study of mental illness among adolescents lends itself well to an epidemiological approach. The main value of epidemiology is in identifying the determinants of illness or deviant behaviour and in ensuring the effective deployment of services available for treatment and prevention. It also affords the clinician an overview of his task, helping him to retain an objectivity in clinical work which all too readily is lost under the pressures of routine service work.

The adolescents in a community are specially suitable for epidemiological investigation for a number of reasons: they form a discrete age group, although one must acknowledge the duration of adolescence is difficult to define with precision; they are an important section of the population both socially and medically; while they are at school or college, they are readily accessible for study; lastly, the period of adolescence is characterised by considerable physical, emotional and social changes for the individual, so that alteration in patterns of behaviour are condensed into a short time-span. Careful study of such changes may lead to a better understanding of the primary causes of abnormal behaviour or of mental illness itself.

The epidemiologist examines the prevalence or the incidence of illnesses and attempts to relate data on the amount of morbidity to personal, social, geographical or temporal factors. By the term 'prevalence' is meant the number of persons in a defined population who can be identified as being ill at any point or period of time. The problem is in the definition of illness: what constitutes a case? Different observers will perceive the same behavioural phenomena in different ways. One will elicit symptoms or notice signs which another will ignore, either through lack of training, a different type of training or orientation, or a higher threshold for the recognition of morbid states. It is difficulties such as these which have prevented meaningful comparison of morbidity rates in surveys conducted by different observers. For adults, such obstacles are being overcome to some degree through the development of a standardized interview schedule by Wing and his collaborators.[67]

It will be obvious that a true measure of prevalence must be sought outside the confines of a medical institution such as a hospital, a clinic or a general practice. The survey must be carried out in the setting in which people naturally exist. Those persons examined must be a representative sample of the population being studied: the sample must be chosen in such a way that it is highly unlikely to differ from the larger body from which it was derived. In the sample itself, after each person has been examined or screened for the presence or absence of the group of conditions in question, we can arrive at a figure of how many of the total are identifiable as being ill, disturbed or maladjusted. Where the threshold for identifying these states is high, the majority of the sample will be regarded as healthy: as the threshold is lowered, the 'healthy' proportion will progressively decrease in size.

2

The Prevalence of Psychiatric Disorders in Adolescents

(a) Statistics from General Psychiatric Services

These provide initial information concerning the occurrence of psychiatric disorders in adolescents. First admissions of adolescents to institutions and out-patient clinics at least indicate the degree to which adolescents turn for help to psychiatric facilities because of psychological disturbances. As these data are usually presented in quinquennial age groups, first admissions of patients aged 15–19 per 10 000 of population in this age group can be used as a measure of the incidence of treated psychiatric disturbances in adolescents. One has to be aware that these are only minimum figures which relate to the most serious disorders, and the rate also depends on the availability and utilisation of services.

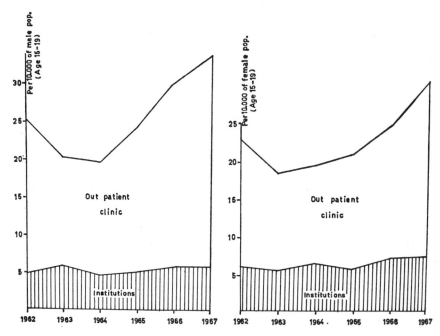

FIG. 1 First admissions of adolescents to institutions and out patient clinics in Victoria, Australia, 1962–1967, per 10 000 of male and female adolescents.

The historical study of hospital admissions in Victoria, Australia, from 1901 to 1947[31] showed variations in the admission rates of adolescents to psychiatric and mental hospitals in that there was an overall decreasing trend (from 3·9 in 1901 to 2·6 in 1947 per 10 000 males and from 3·0 to 1·5 per 10 000 females). The diagnostic breakdown of these figures was not, however, available, and it is even impossible to say whether these changes were due solely to variations in admission policies relating to mentally retarded persons.

More precise data are available for 1962–1967 in Victoria.[32] It has been shown that the increase of the overall incidence rate for both sexes depended solely on the increase of first admissions to out-patient clinics, whilst first admissions to hospitals remained relatively constant (Fig.1). When specific diagnostic categories were analysed, it became apparent that the incidence of schizophrenia had not shown any significant change during the period studied, whilst the incidence of transient situational disturbances had almost doubled (Fig. 2). This reflects the differences between patients admitted to institutions (Fig. 3) and out-patient clinics (Fig. 4).

Departmental statistics in Victoria provide information about the period-prevalence of psychiatric disorders in adolescents in terms of the number of persons under the care of the Department in a given year (Fig. 5). Again, the rates for schizophrenia showed only slight variations during this period, whilst there was an increase in the prevalence of almost all

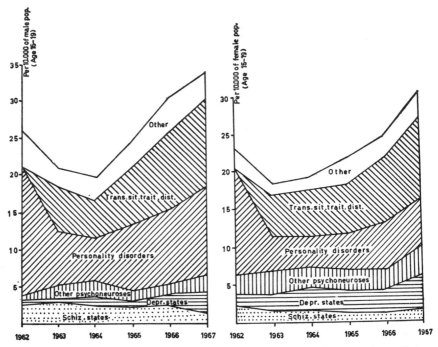

Fig. 2. First admissions of adolescents to institutions and out-patient clinics in Victoria, Australia, 1962–1967, in terms of specific diagnoses, per 10 000 of male and female adolescents.

other diagnostic categories. Thus, the overall prevalence of departmentally treated psychiatric disorders increased from 53·2 to 75·7 per 10 000 male, and from 43·5 to 59·6 per 10 000 female adolescents. On the other hand, resident rates in institutions declined (Fig. 6), indicating a change from custodial to community treatment of adolescent patients.

The comparison of first admission rates in different countries (Table I) shows a similar incidence of major mental illness in adolescents in England and Wales, Canada and New Zealand, whilst the rates for Victoria and Czechoslovakia are significantly lower. No explanation can be offered for this phenomenon, especially as the total incidence of schizophrenia, for all ages, is similar in all these four countries. The differences in the first

TABLE I

First Admissions of Adolescents (15–19 years old) per 10 000 Population in this Age Group

	Victoria, 1967. All first admissions		Victoria, 1967. Institutions only		New Zealand, 1967. Institutions only		Canada, 1965. Institutions only		England and Wales, 1966. Mental Hospitals		Czechoslovakia, 1966. Mental Hospitals	
	M	F	M	F	M	F	M	F	M	F	M	F
Schizophrenic states	1·8	1·6	1·2	0·9	3·4	4·0	3·5	2·9	3·1	2·3	1·6	1·5
Depressive psychoses	0·2	0·9	—	0·2	1·0	1·5	0·4	0·6	2·0	3·5	0·6	0·8
Other functional psychoses	0·1	0·2	0·1	0·1	0·4	0·6	0·4	0·5	0·2	0·5	—	0·1
Alcoholism	0·2	0·1	—	—	0·1	—	0·2	—	0·6	0·2	1·7	0·7
Other organic brain disorders	0·6	0·9	0·3	0·3	0·4	0·2	0·8	0·4	0·4	0·4	0·8	0·7
Depressive psychoneuroses	2·2	3·7	0·6	0·9	1·7	3·5	1·2	3·1	} 1·5	} 3·4	} 6·9	} 12·7
Other psychoneuroses	2·3	3·8	0·3	0·5	1·0	2·0	1·2	2·6	2·5	2·3	3·7	4·1
Personality disorders	11·7	6·4	1·5	2·1	6·6	6·5	4·8	4·7	2·5	2·3	3·7	4·1
Trans. situational trait disorders	11·8	10·9	1·4	1·9	0·6	1·5	0·4	0·3	—	—	0·5	0·6
No diagnosis	2·6	2·0	0·5	0·4	4·0	2·3	0·4	0·2	0·4	0·4	0·7	1·2
TOTAL	33·5	30·5	5·9	7·3	19·2	22·1	13·3	15·3	10·7*	13·2*	16·5	21·7

* There were additionally admitted 164 males and 284 females to teaching and general hospitals.

admission rates for non-psychotic disorders depend solely on facilities available and departmental policy in regard to admissions. This supposition can be supported by the increase of first admission rates in all countries for which appropriate data are available.

It is therefore necessary to supplement data obtained from psychiatric service statistics with information from other sources.

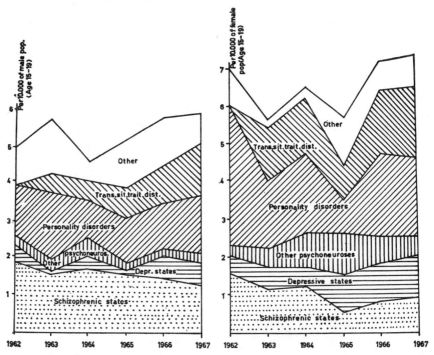

FIG. 3. First admissions of adolescents to institutions in Victoria, Australia, 1962–1967, in terms of specific diagnoses, per 10 000 of male and female adolescents.

(b) University and School Students' Surveys

Remarkably, there has been no comprehensive survey of the mental health of adolescents at school, so far as we are aware. In the United Kingdom, the School Health Service has for several decades concerned itself with the *physical* health of schoolchildren. It is exceptional, even now, to have an equivalent interest in the *mental* health of adolescents at school. For both prevention and research purposes we can look forward to the development of activity in this area. There are no other occasions in our society when nearly all members of an age group are so readily accessible for health assessment. There will, of course, be difficulties in putting such a system into operation; parents and teenagers are less likely to participate than they would in an inspection of physical health. An enquiry into the emotional adjustment of these young people might be seen as an unwarranted invasion of privacy. The experience of workers such as Masterson[41] and Offer,[45]* however, suggests that co-operation can be obtained by carefully conducted approaches to parents, teachers and teenagers themselves.

Unfortunately, insufficient work has been done to assess the psychiatric morbidity among adolescent school students. Some pilot studies indicate that approximately 9 per cent of school students have psychological disturbances, mainly labelled as adjustment reactions of childhood.

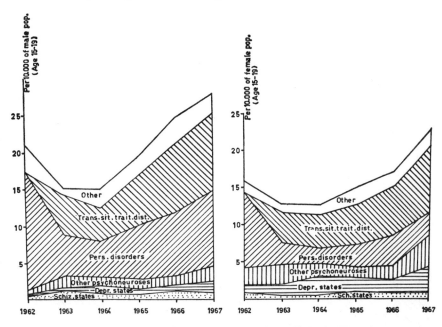

FIG. 4. First admissions of adolescents to out-patient clinics in Victoria, Australia, 1962–1967, in terms of specific diagnoses, per 10 000 of male and female adolescents.

More has been done in the way of a study of the mental health of college and university students. Survey of psychiatric morbidity among the students of both Belfast and Edinburgh Universities (Caldbeck-Meenan;[4] Kidd;[27] Kidd and Caldbeck-Meenan[28]) have shown similar rates of psychological disturbances in both centres: 9·1 per cent and 9·0 per cent of males and 13·5 per cent and 14·6 per cent of females respectively. Major psychiatric illnesses were extremely rare: there were only ten cases of psychosis among the 2530 students included in the investigation. The majority of detected cases (62·1 per cent) comprised students with psychological complaints of abnormal behaviour which did not warrant a formal psychiatric diagnosis. The prevalence of psychiatric disorders among Belfast and Edinburgh University students is comparable with the data of Davies et al.,[9] and of Ironside[24] concerning Australian and New Zealand

* See also chapter by Offer and Offer in this volume.

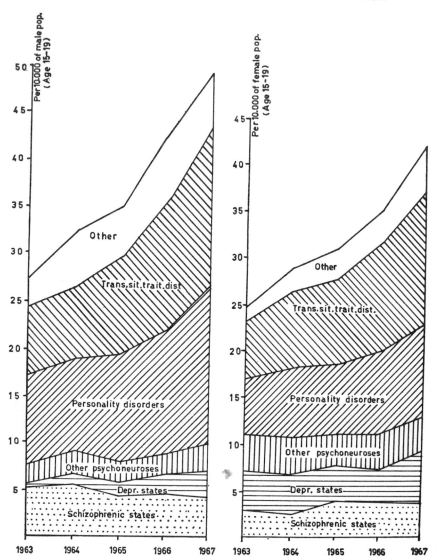

FIG. 5. Number of adolescents treated by the Mental Hygiene Department of Victoria, Australia, 1963–1967, in terms of specific diagnoses, per 10 000 of male and female adolescents.

medical students. The first survey showed that 11·4 per cent of male and 23·8 per cent of female Australian medical students passed the critical score of the Cornell Medical Index (more than 30 'yes' responses to the C.M.I. or more than 10 'yes' responses to the M-R sections), and could be regarded therefore as having significant psychiatric symptoms; the second indicated that 13·4 per cent of Otago medical students were in need of some psychiatric help.

Reifler[47] analysed the referrals of students to mental health services of the University of North Carolina and found that the proportion of students who were patients in these services had increased from 1·8 per cent in 1956 to 4·4 per cent in 1965. The author quotes in his paper other similar studies in U.S.A. and Canada, showing that referral rates varied between 1·5 per cent in British Columbia (Schwartz[53]) and 9·9 per cent in Yale (Arnstein[2]); referrals of psychotic patients showed much less variation;

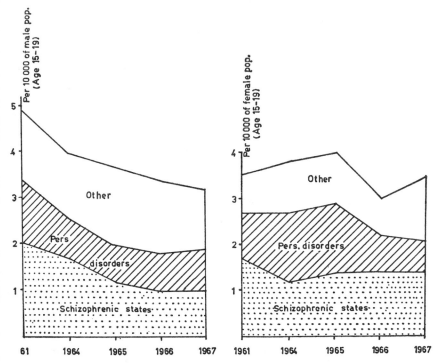

FIG. 6. Number of adolescents resident in Victorian institutions, in terms of specific diagnoses, per 10 000 of male and female adolescents.

0·1–0·4 per cent. All the above data, derived from psychiatric services for students, have to be contrasted with data obtained from a survey in Eastmet College (Smith et al.[57]) where the proportion of 'clinically disturbed' students was found to be 22·7 per cent for freshmen and 16·3 per cent for the same students in a one-year follow-up. This diminution in the proportion of 'clinically disturbed' persons among older students contrasts with the previously mentioned findings of Davies et al.,[9] who noted an increase of psychiatric disturbances between the first- and second-year students in both medical and law schools.

Psychiatric disorders contributed significantly to the drop-out of Harvard students (Nicholi[44]), where 38·3 per cent of drop-outs consulted the psychiatrist before leaving college, as compared with 8–10 per cent of the total undergraduate population. This is again in contrast with the findings of Davies *et al.*,[9] who showed that students who scored higher on the Eysenck Personality Inventory for neuroticism performed better academically. Even in Harvard, almost half of the psychiatric drop-outs graduated eventually, a figure identical to that of the non-psychiatric drop-outs.

(c) Community Health Surveys

These should provide the most comprehensive data regarding mental health and ill-health of adolescents. However, there are special difficulties in the psychiatric screening of adolescents.

TABLE II

Psychiatric Disturbances in Adolescents in the Victorian Surveys
(in percentages)

| | Heyfield | | Melbourne Metropolitan area | |
	M	F	M	F
No psychiatric diagnosis or neurotic symptoms	37·7	20·2	56·9	34·8
Isolated neurotic symptoms (no psychiatric illness)	45·9	60·5	28·3	51·4
Psychoneurotic and behavioural disorders	14·8	16·8	13·6	13·2
Organic brain disorders, functional psychoses, mental retardation	1·6	2·5	1·2	0·6
	100·0	100·0	100·0	100·0

Two prominent workers have drawn attention to the difficulty of recognising true disturbance in an age group where emotional discomfort or turmoil is held to be normal or even a necessary accompaniment of development. Erikson[13] writes that 'we look at adolescence not as an affliction but as a normative process, a normal phase of increased conflict, characterised by seeming fluctuations in the ego-strength and also by a high growth potential. What under prejudiced scrutiny may appear to be the onset of neurosis often is but an aggravated crisis which might prove to be self-liquidating and in fact contributive to the process of identity formation.' According to Anna Freud,[16] 'adolescence is by its nature an interruption of peaceful growth, and the upholding of a steady equilibrium during this process is in itself abnormal . . . The adolescent manifestations of growth come close to the symptom formations of the neurotic, psychotic or dissocial order and merge almost imperceptibly into borderline states, initial, frustrated or fully fledged forms of almost all the illnesses. Consequently, the differential diagnosis between these adolescent upsets and true pathology becomes a difficult task.' Clearly, therefore, a survey of morbidity in this age group requires to be carefully conducted with strict criteria for the presence of disturbance. Both the interviewers and the instruments used have to be sensitive, capable of eliciting information or signs or morbidity peculiar to this period. Ideally, the criteria used should allow comparison between different adolescent populations and different age groups. For the present, we have to acknowledge that such techniques are not available. A standardised interview schedule has not yet been devised for adolescents. Those used by Masterson[41] and by Offer[45] are applicable only to selected groups of the U.S. adolescent population.

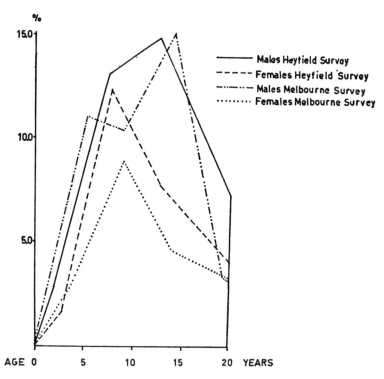

FIG. 7. Behaviour disorders in children and adolescents as established by two community health surveys conducted in Victoria.

For the comparison of morbidity rates between age groups, one difficulty is that criteria of disturbance change from childhood through adolescence to adulthood. A second is that most of the major epidemiological surveys, such as those by Srole et al.,[58] Leighton et al.,[37] Hagnell[21] and Taylor and Chave,[60] do not provide age-specific morbidity rates for the teenage years, but tend to use larger age groups, often spanning late adolescence and early adulthood. Since there are so many biological and psycho-social changes during adolescence, it is necessary to study the occurrence of mental illness using finer age groupings.

The two community health surveys, performed in Victoria in the rural town of Heyfield (Krupinski *et al.*[29,33]) and in the Melbourne Metropolitan area (Krupinski *et al.*[30]) separated adolescents from the rest of the population. The psychiatric morbidity of the adolescent population in both these surveys is presented in Table II.

Both surveys showed that behavioural disorders which are very frequent in children, tend to disappear in adolescents, and do so in girls at an earlier age than in boys (Fig. 7). In the Melbourne survey behavioural disorders in children occurred in 8·8 per cent of all interviewed children, whilst only 2·5 per cent of male, and 1·8 per cent of female adolescents were seen to have adjustment problems of adolescence.

Another 2·5 per cent of male and 1·8 per cent of female adolescents, however, were thought to have personality disorders of a more persistent character, diagnosed mainly as immature of inadequate personality. There were only two cases of sociopathic personality. Whilst male adolescents did not rate highly on the neurotic scale introduced into the Melbourne survey (Fig. 8), female adolescents showed a higher rate of neuroticism than the female adult population.

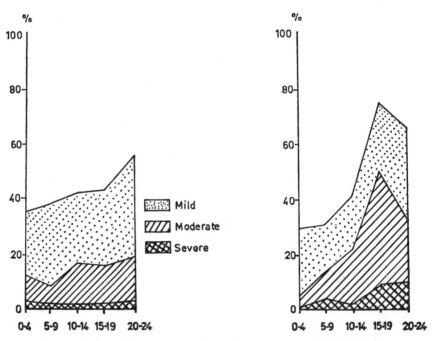

Fig. 8. Neuroticism in male and female adolescents in Melbourne as established from a community health survey (*Left:* males; *right:* females).

It is interesting to note that alcoholism, which had been noted in Heyfield only in male adults and with the peak prevalence in the mid-forties, seemed to start in the Melbourne area at a younger age, the rate in male adolescents being equal to that in male adults.

3

Juvenile Delinquency

Juvenile delinquency is regarded by many authors (Clinard;[5] Cloward;[6] Cloward and Ohlin;[7] Cohen;[8] Gelder;[17] Gibbens;[18] Guzman;[20] Johnson;[26] Kvaraceus;[35] Lee;[36] McCord and McCord;[38] Scott[54, 55]) as a measure of social maladjustment and psychological disturbance in children and adolescents. This attitude was also adopted by the first United Nations Congress on the Prevention of Crime and the Treatment of Offenders,[62] when the term 'pre-delinquent' was coined to describe those neglected, deprived, maladjusted and disturbed youngsters who can turn into delinquents in the legal meaning of the word. However, the Second United Nations Congress[63] defined juvenile delinquency for practical reasons as that kind of behaviour which, if committed by an adult, would be regarded as criminal. This operational definition of juvenile delinquency is unsatisfactory from the epidemiological point of view, as this same behaviour can be regarded in some countries as delinquent, and not in others, depending on the existing legal codes and the moral norms of the particular society. Gibbens and Ahrenfeldt[19] reviewed the situation in different countries and showed how difficult it is to compare criminal statistics internationally, even if in all cases police statistics could be used as the basic source material. Even in the same country, differences between racial and national groups could be attributed to different attitudes of the police to particular groups of offenders (Moses[42]).

Even data concerning delinquency rates in one country during a certain period of time have to be assessed with caution. Available statistics indicate an increase of juvenile delinquency in several countries. In Japan, there was noted an increase of juvenile delinquency between 1951 and 1961 from 10·2 to 14·2 offenders per 1000 persons aged 16–18 years, and from 6·7 to 11·7 per 1000 persons, aged 14–16 years (United Nations,[64]). In Israel, Markham[40] reported an increase of juvenile delinquents from 6·8 per 1000 in 1949 to 19·6 per 1000 in 1963, this being mainly due to the influx of African and Asian juveniles with the highest rates of delinquency. A similar trend was reported from other countries (United Nations, 1965 [64]). It was also noted in Victoria where the rate of offenders per 1000 persons, aged 7–16 years, has increased from 3·5 in 1947 to 5·1 in 1954, 8·0 in 1961 and 9·7 in 1967. In Victoria, where this increase could be analysed in terms of the type of offence, it depended mainly on the increase of minor offences and of the illegal use of motor-cars, which has recently become very common. Whereas the latter phenomenon can be related to the increase of the number of cars and their popularity amongst juveniles, it is difficult to say whether the apparent increase of offences against property, mainly minor thefts, was due to a better discovery rate or to greater opportunities for such offences in the big self-service stores.

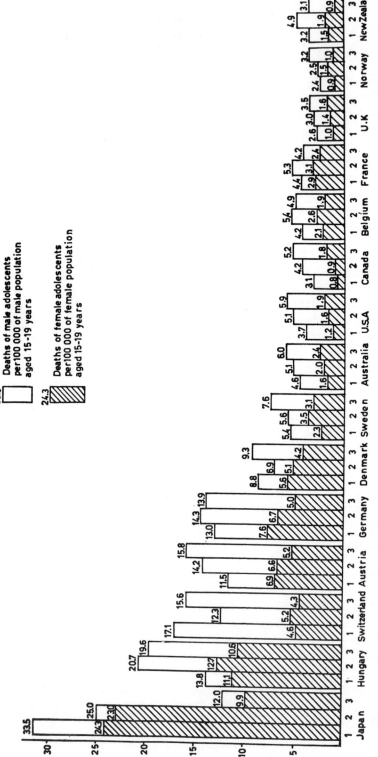

FIG. 9. Suicide rates per 10 000 adolescents in selected countries, in the period 1954–1964: 1—1954–57; 2—1958–1961; 3—1961–1964.

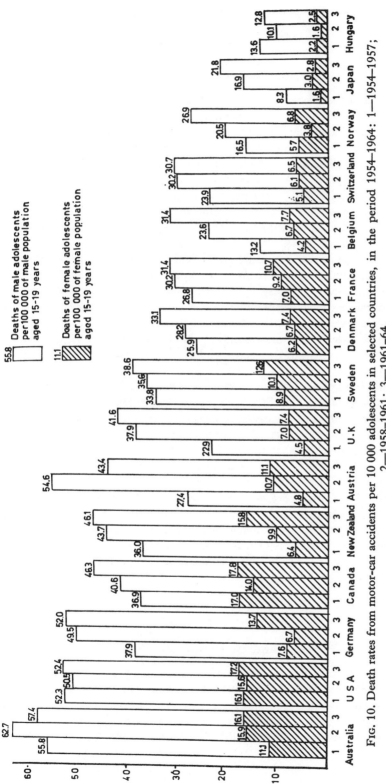

Fig. 10. Death rates from motor-car accidents per 10 000 adolescents in selected countries, in the period 1954-1964: 1—1954–1957; 2—1958–1961; 3—1961–64.

4

Suicides and Motor-car Accidents

Suicides and motor-car accidents can be regarded as a measure of psychological disturbances in adolescents. Teicher and Jacobs[61] and Jacobs and Teicher[25] analysed attempted suicides amongst adolescents in terms of certain causative factors. However, the statistics of attempted suicides are not comprehensive, and although attempted rather than completed suicides are typical for adolescents (Krupinski et al.[34]), only data on completed suicides per 100 000 of population in the 15–19 year age group are comparable for a specific period of time at an international level.

W.H.O. statistics provide relevant information only for the years 1954–1964. In all countries the suicides rates for males were higher than for females. There are striking differences between the particular countries as regards the number of adolescent suicides per 100 000 of the corresponding population. However, these rates have remained stable in each country through those eleven years. The two exceptions are Japan, where this rate has shown a significant decrease for both sexes, and Hungary, where an increase in males was noted since 1956. No explanation can be offered for these differences without a deep sociological study of Durkheim's[12] type (Fig. 9).

Involvement of adolescents in motor-car accidents could also be related to their psychological problems. However, the differences in death rates caused by motor-car accidents, between sexes and between countries, emphasise the dependence of these accidents on the availability of cars and on their predominant usage by adolescent boys. Affluent countries, such as Australia, U.S.A., Canada, West Germany and to a lesser degree England and Wales and the Scandinavian countries, are at the top of the list ranked for death rates from this cause. Since 1954, the increase of these rates in some countries is rather an indicator of rising affluence than a sign of a growing psychological maladjustment of adolescents. The fact that Australia has topped the list since 1954 and that the rate in that country has remained steady for eleven years, is of great concern for all interested in this field (Fig. 10).

5

Social and Environmental Factors

We would caution that current psychiatric thinking tends to place undue emphasis on the external environment of an individual, to the neglect of constitutional factors. Freeman,[14,15] a social anthropologist, has argued with great clarity and conviction that adaptation to the environment is likely to be determined by hereditary factors far more than behavioural science currently implies. Considered in phylogenetic perspective, human behaviour of the neurotic or personality disorder type is unlikely to be determined exclusively by experiential and social factors. An interactional approach seems specially relevant to adolescence.

Social variables which have been examined for their relationship to adolescent psychiatric illness include population density, social class, housing conditions, family size, nationality or race, delinquency and indices of social disorganisation. It is striking that, with the exception of delinquency, such studies were aimed at adult psychiatric populations in most cases; the picture for adolescent psychiatric illness has usually to be extracted from the overall findings.

The most comprehensive study of social and family factors in the adjustment of children is that by Douglas[10, 11] and his co-workers, Mulligan et al.[43] A cohort of 5362 children, born in England and Wales in one week of 1946, were followed until they were aged 20. It was confirmed that lower-class children have more delinquency and achieve less. There was no social class difference in the incidence of neurotic symptoms. When a comparison was made of the families of delinquent and non-delinquent lower-class children, a most interesting finding was that the non-delinquents' families were more personally stable and effective in life. In contrast, the delinquents' families were less educated, had more often quarrelled and separated and made much less use of the health services.

A recent study in Victoria showed that adolescents admitted to the Psychiatric Hospital at Royal Park live significantly more often in a non-family setting than 'normal' adolescents in Melbourne. A higher proportion of their parents were semi-skilled and unskilled workers, with a history of unemployment and occupational instability, than was the case for the 'normal' adolescents. Other factors such as bereavement, prolonged absence of one or both parents, family conflict and family disruption seemed to occur more frequently, but these data have not yet been compared with corresponding information from a control group of adolescents.

Robins[48] in a useful review of the determinants of abnormal behaviour in young persons, has described how it has been demonstrated (Wilner et al.[66]) that the provision of improved living standard does not lead to an improvement in behaviour. Apparently, in moving up in social class, or rather in the standard of living, the delinquent does not leave his delinquent behaviour behind. Another question is whether ineffective or behaviourally inadequate families produce an excess of delinquency, irrespective of social class. Robins and Lewis[49] found that having antisocial parents considerably increased the chances of educational failure or delinquency. This relationship held in both white-collar and blue-collar families. Furthermore, the effect was greater on the son the more antisocial relatives he had.

Parental deprivation has recently received much attention in adult psychiatry, being postulated as an adverse experience for later mental health. It is now fairly certain that childhood bereavement is to be found in excess in hospital cases of depression and, in some series, self-poisoning. As far as mental health in childhood and adolescence is concerned, it is now realised that there are so many contaminating factors: the sex of the child and of the parent who dies or goes away; the age at which this takes place; the previous relationship between the parents and between the child and the lost parent. Bowlby *et al*.[3] examined the children of mothers who had had to enter a sanatorium for tuberculosis. Such a cause for separation would be unrelated to the previous behaviour or personality of either the child or the mother. He found small differences only between such children and controls from the same school class. Such separation, however, was neither prolonged nor permanent, as is the case in separation, divorce or death. There is certainly room for caution in interpreting the significance of results in most studies of deprivation and it is well to keep in mind the multiplicity of interacting effects.

6

Paths to Treatment

The disturbed adolescent who decides to seek help is in a different position from the adult with personally unmanageable symptoms: the adolescent has to go to a member of the age group towards whom he is likely to entertain negative feelings. For this reason, consultation rates may be depressed whether the consultation be with a doctor, a teacher, youth leader or clergyman.

We do not have much understanding as yet about the perception of symptoms by adolescents and by their parents. One might anticipate that the concordance of views on the presence or absence of symptoms in the adolescent might be a most rewarding enquiry. Certainly we know that for children, individuals recognised by parents to be disturbed are often seen to be normally behaved at school; conversely, individuals identified by teachers as disturbed are not always seen to be so by parents. For children, mothers and teachers fail to agree on the presence of sadness, withdrawal, solitariness, obsessionality, overactivity, disobedience and bullying. They do agree, however, on the presence of more obvious symptoms such as stammering, nail-biting, school refusal, stealing and lying (Wolff;[68] Rutter and Graham[52]). These findings, of course, referred to children under the age of 12. Wolff has pointed out that such findings would suggest either different sensitivities on the part of parents or teachers, or truly different behaviour of children at home and at school. For adolescents, we need to have a similar investigation, comparing the parents' or teachers' perception of symptoms with those of the adolescents themselves.

So far we have discussed the awareness of symptoms by the adolescent and by others. Much importance should be attached to the subsequent action taken by either the adolescent or his parents or teacher. There is reason to suspect that lower social class adolescents tend to reach psychiatric help after an impulsive act of self-poisoning, whereas adolescents from more affluent families are seen to be disturbed and are referred directly by their family doctor to a psychiatrist. At any rate, perception of symptoms during adolescence is likely to vary appreciably with culture and social class. At present, most psychotic teenagers are likely in most Western countries to be in treatment. For the neurotic and personality disordered groups there is a wide range of facilities. Such teenagers might keep their symptoms to themselves, disclose them to parents or other relatives, to peers, a teacher, a youth counsellor, a clergyman or a doctor; alternatively they may declare their disturbance in carrying out antisocial acts.

Until carefully conducted morbidity studies are done at the field level, we shall have no information on what proportion or type of illness is channelled through the above helping media. There may indeed be appreciable misplacement, in the sense that teenagers may not spontaneously be finding the most appropriate help source. Many adolescents with neurotic symptoms may be adequately supported through a difficult phase by supervised lay workers, such as youth leaders and counsellors. Conversely, it is certain that the teenage clients of youth workers provide appreciable difficulties in management: working with adolescents is likely to be associated with marked transference phenomena. For this reason, it is always desirable to have a trained psychiatrist available for consultation and for liaison work. Such a facility is too seldom available.

(a) Youth Counselling Agencies

The value of youth counselling agencies remains unassessed. In most centres nowadays, these are established or planned for the immediate future, usually by voluntary organisations working in liaison with the social and psychiatric services of the area. They probably go some way towards offering help to adolescents who otherwise would not be able to present their emotional difficulties to family doctors or psychiatrists. Close collaboration with the psychiatric services ensures that adolescents with true mental illness and not just transient distress, reach medical help.

(b) The Family Doctor

Shepherd et al.,[56] in their study of general practice in London, described patients' consulting rates by age for psychiatric symptoms. From these data it can be seen that adolescents consult their family doctor rather less frequently than adults. This again raises the question whether teenagers fail to present psychiatric symptoms to their doctor, or if they truly have less illness than older age groups. From the surveys which allow comparison of rates for morbidity in young, middle-aged and elderly people, occurring at the field level (e.g. Hagnell[21]), it is unlikely that adolescents are failing to present psychiatric symptoms to their doctors. It is notable that in the study by Shepherd, the young patient was more likely than his elders to be treated by advice, reassurance or psychotherapy. The use of psychotropic drugs played a much smaller part in the general practitioners' preferred treatment for young people compared with their elders.

In Australia, the National Morbidity Survey (1966), concerned with illness treated in general practice, did not provide data for adolescents since the age group 15–24 was treated as an entity.

Psychiatric care in the future is likely to be carried out in large part by the general practitioner and his team. There is at present insufficient availability of training in adolescent psychiatry to allow interested general practitioners to prepare for a clinical task which is particularly taxing.

(c) Psychiatric Services for Adolescents

It has come to be widely accepted that special services for adolescents are desirable. The staff require special training. In the United Kingdom it is usually held to be essential that an adolescent psychiatrist should have had considerable experience in child psychiatry: in the United States, the adolescent psychiatrist frequently comes to the area from adult psychiatry. The principles of treatment, particularly of an in-patient or day-patient basis are sufficiently different from child to adult practice to warrant separate facilities. Unfortunately, too few of these exist and training programmes are available only in a few centres.

The most comprehensive review of the use of psychiatric services by young people is that carried out by Rosen et al.[50, 51] Their data refer to the use of psychiatric facilities by children and adolescents in the United States. The data are presented mainly as the number of persons attending for out-patient treatment, by sex and age, in 788 clinics. Because of the short duration of treatment for most patients, the data are considered to be generally descriptive of first consultation rates. Over the age range 10–19 years, the highest rate was for the 14–15-year-olds of both sexes; the lowest was for 18–19-year-olds, again of both sexes. Boys had consistently higher rates up until the late teens, when the rates approximated. Thereafter, females carried the higher treated morbidity rates, as has been repeatedly demonstrated in adult studies. As Rosen et al.[50] suggest, this finding that 'the 14- to 15-year-olds have the highest clinic utilisation rates, may represent a higher true incidence of emotional disorders or may reflect increased anxiety on the part of significant adults at their inability to cope with the adolescent when he reaches this age, particularly in the case of boys. Adolescent boys express their inter- and intra-personal conflicts in sullen moods and acts of defiance, while the 14- or 15-year-old girls are often referred because they are listless, depressed and "not making it" socially, rather than because of acting out.'

The reversal of rates for the two sexes, which occurs in the late teens, is said to be due to the combined effects of pathogenic social pressures on the one hand and the ease with which help can be sought on the other (Rosen et al.[50]). This latter factor, of course, does not operate when one is considering age- and sex-specific rates for morbidity ascertained at the field survey level. From such studies (Hagnell[21], Taylor and Chave[60]), we know that late adolescent girls and young women do indeed have more neurotic symptoms, quite apart from any difference between the sexes in the rates at which help is sought.

It is striking that in the 788 clinics seen by Rosen and her associates, schools were the primary source of referrals. This is a situation which is likely to vary appreciably between countries. Rosen confirms our own view that 'the school has a unique advantage, in relating to virtually all adolescents and thus being able to identify existing or potential disturbances'. For both service and research purposes, attention to schools is an obvious avenue for advance.

The use of all adolescent psychiatric facilities within a defined population was examined in Edinburgh. A survey was made of the clinical and demographic characteristics of all persons aged 14–19 who were in psychiatric treatment in Edinburgh during a twelve-month period (McCulloch, Henderson and Philip,[39] Henderson[22]). An inverse relationship was demonstrated in the rates in Edinburgh's twenty-three city wards for psychiatric contact by direct referral and after an act of self-poisoning or self-injury: city wards with high rates for self-poisoning acts among adolescents had a low ratio for direct referral of teenagers to psychiatrists by family doctors. Furthermore, the high self-poisoning rates were associated with a number of indices of social disorganisation, such as rent-arrears, children taken into care and overcrowding.

Data on the annual referral rate to psychiatric services (rates for the inception of treatment) were separately reported (McCulloch, Henderson and Philip[39]). For the adolescent population at risk in Edinburgh, the annual referral rate was 5·6 per thousand. One-third of these adolescents, mainly those in their late-teens, reached psychiatric help only after a deliberate act of self-poisoning or self-injury. One-half of the year's referrals came directly from their family doctors. Findings such as these point to the need to have a better awareness of disturbance in parent, teacher, family doctor and the adolescent himself.

7

Maturational Aspects

Everyone appreciates that adolescence is a period characterised by rapid physiological, emotional and social changes. These changes are themselves closely inter-related: thus the physical changes at puberty call for intrapsychic adjustment towards the handling of sexual feelings; at the same time, the social expectations made of the adolescent alter considerably so that he is required to make changes in his self-perception and attitudes in order to meet these demands. Some authors have drawn attention to the possible psychological effects of the secular trend in physiological maturation (Peskin[46]; Henderson[23]): puberty is coming earlier, by as much as four months per decade. One wonders what effect this may have in progressively shrinking the latency period of psychoanalytic theory.

An enquiry into physiological maturity and adolescent psychiatric illness was conducted by Henderson[23] as a first step in exploring the possible pathogenic effects of maturational change in all three major areas, physical, psychological and social: physiological changes, particularly if over-rapid or over-slow, were postulated to prove stressful for vulnerable individuals. Physiological maturity was assessed by measuring the skeletal age of the hand and wrist, using the standard of Tanner, Whitehouse and Healy.[59] Age at menarche was also used in girls. The subjects were 151 adolescent psychiatric patients, 76 juvenile delinquents and 241 normal teenagers. In this study, physiological maturity was found to be totally unrelated to mental health: adolescent psychiatric patients are neither more nor less physiologically mature than their behaviourally normal peers.

8

Follow-up studies of Adolescent Psychiatric Illness

Since mental illness in adolescence takes place at a time when personality development is incomplete, it would be logical to pay special attention to the outcome of illness in this period of transition. Warren[65] followed up 157 patients six or more years after their admission to the Adolescent Unit of the Bethlem Royal Hospital. There is likely to have been an appreciable degree of selection in the patients accepted for admission. He found that one-third of patients with neurotic disorders or conduct disorders continued to have further disturbance. Girls had a rather better outcome than boys, particularly in the neurotic group. One-half of the conduct disorders did well, but only one-quarter of the psychotic group improved. It is noteworthy that the prognoses given by doctors for patients with neurotic illnesses were unduly pessimistic.

Masterson[41] has described in detail his follow-up of seventy-two patients over five years. The conclusion he reached was that adolescent turmoil only rarely brings on psychiatric illness; it is more likely to aggravate and to have a pathoplastic effect on previously existent psychopathology. Sixty-two per cent of his series had moderate to severe impairment five years later.

The whole subject of outcome has been most thoroughly reviewed by Robins.[48,49] She describes studies of the prevalence, treatment and outcome of behaviour disorders in children up to the age of 18. Robins concludes that the outcome for childhood psychoses and extreme antisocial behaviour (delinquency) is poor, whatever the treatment. Neurotic and other behaviour disorders usually improve with time, again whether treated or not. This is confirmed time and again in both cohort and follow-up studies. Looking only at adolescents disturbed enough to require hospital admission, Annesley[1] found the schizophrenics had the poorest outcome, the sociopathic group were next and the neurotics did best of all.

9

Conclusion

Epidemiological techniques have successfully thrown light on a small number of the problems of aetiology and treatment in adolescent psychiatry. Further progress is likely to come from carefully conducted cross-sectional studies of morbidity, which will allow comparisons to be made across time and between different geographical areas. The present authors believe that it will be profitable to evolve more precise psychological measures of personality and illness: there is great need to improve the reliability and validity of our instruments for measuring morbidity, particularly in this age group. The longitudinal study of adolescent populations, although most taxing to carry out, is likely to be specially rewarding in identifying personal and social determinants of mental illnesses and the efficacy of services available for their treatment.

REFERENCES

1. ANNESLEY, P. T. 1961. Psychiatric illness in adolescence. Presentation and prognosis. *J. ment. Sci.*, **107**, 268–278.
2. ARNSTEIN, R. L. 1967. Psychiatric hospitalization and continued college attendance. *J. Amer. Coll. Health Ass.*, **16**, 135–139.
3. BOWLBY, J., AINSWORTH, B. and ROSENBLUTH, A. 1956. The effects of mother–child separation: a follow-up study. *Brit. J. med. Psychol.*, **29**, 211–244.
4. CALDBECK-MEENAN, J. 1966. Screening University students with C.M.T. *J. psychosom. Res.*, **9**, 331–337.
5. CLINARD, M. B. 1962. Contributions of sociology to understanding deviant behaviour. *Brit. J. Crim.*, **3**, 110–129.
6. CLOWARD, R. A. 1959. Illegitimate means, anomie, and deviant behaviour. *Amer. sociol. Rev.*, **24**, 164–176.
7. CLOWARD, R. A., and OHLIN, L. E. 1961. *Delinquency and opportunity: a theory of delinquent gangs*. Glencoe, Illinois: Free Press.
8. COHEN, A. K. 1955. *Delinquent boys: the culture of the gang*. Glencoe, Illinois: Free Press. Cf. especially, pp. 24–32 (The content of the delinquent subculture). (Also published: London, 1956.)
9. DAVIES, B., MOWBRAY, R. M. and JENSEN, D. 1968. A questionnaire survey of psychiatric symptoms in Australian medical students. *Aust. N.Z. J. Psychiat.*, **2**, 46–53.
10. DOUGLAS, J. W. B. 1964. *The home and the school*. London: MacGibbon and Kee.

11. DOUGLAS, J. W. B. 1966. The school progress of nervous and troublesome children. *Brit. J. Psychiat.*, **112**, 1115–1116.
12. DURKHEIM, E. 1951. *Suicide*. Trans. from French by J. A. Spaulding and G. Simpson. Glencoe, Illinois: Free Press.
13. ERIKSON, E. H. 1956. The problem of ego identity. *J. Amer. psychoanal. Ass.*, **4**, 56–121.
14. FREEMAN, D. 1966. Social anthropology and the scientific study of human behaviour. *Man*, **1**, (3), 330–340.
15. FREEMAN, D. 1969. Human nature and culture. In *Man and the new biology, The Australian National University Lectures, 1969*. A.N.U., Canberra.
16. FREUD, A. 1958. Adolescence. In *Psychoanalytic study of the child*, Vol. 13. New York: International Universities Press.
17. GELDER, M. G. 1965. Can behaviour therapy contribute to the treatment of delinquency? *Brit. J. Crim.*, **5**, 365–376. M. G. Gelder *et al.* 1964. Behaviour therapy and psychotherapy for phobic disorders (Paper presented at 6th Int. Congress of Psychotherapy, London).
18. GIBBENS, T. C. N. 1961. Trends in juvenile delinquency. World Health Org. *Public Health Papers, No. 5*, Geneva. 1963. Psychiatric studies of Borstal lads. (*Maudsley Monogr. No. 11*.) London.
19. GIBBENS, T. C. N. and AHRENFELDT, R. H. 1966. *Cultural factors in delinquency*. London: Tavistock Publications.
20. GUZMAN, S. 1962. Delincuencia y problemas medico-psicologicos del adolescente. *Rev. colomb. Pediat.*, **20**, 50–53. English abstract in *Excerpta criminol.*, 1963, **3**, 172.
21. HAGNELL, O. 1966. *A prospective study of the incidence of mental disorder*. Svenska Bokförlaget, Scandinavian University Books. Stockholm: Norstedts-Bonniers.
22. HENDERSON, A. S. 1968. Un examen epidemiologique de la maladie psychiatrique de l'adolescent. *La psychiatrie de l'enfant*, **11**, Fasc. 1, 269–296.
23. HENDERSON, A. S. 1969. The physiological maturity of adolescent psychiatric patients, juvenile delinquents and normal teenagers. *Brit. J. Psychiat.*, **115**, (525), 895–905.
24. IRONSIDE, W. 1966. Psychiatric morbidity in medical students of four successive fifth-year classes. *N.Z. med. J.*, **65**, 752.
25. JACOBS, J. and TEICHER, J. D. 1967. Broken homes and social isolation in attempted suicides of adolescents. *Int. J. soc. Psychiat.*, **13**, 139–149.
26. JOHNSON, A. 1959. Juvenile delinquency. In *American handbook of psychiatry*. Ed. S. Arieti, **1**, 840–856. New York: Basic Books.
27. KIDD, C. B. 1965. Psychiatric morbidity among students. *Brit. J. prev. soc. Med.*, **19**, 143.
28. KIDD, C. B. and CALDBECK-MEENAN, J. 1966. A comparative study of psychiatric morbidity among students at two different universities. *Brit. J. Psychiat.*, **112**, 57–64.
29. KRUPINSKI, J., BAIKIE, A. G., STOLLER, A., GRAVES, J., O'DAY, D. M. and POLKE, P. 1967. A community health survey of Heyfield, Victoria. Reprinted: *The Med. J. Aust.*, **1**, 1204 (June 17).
30. KRUPINSKI, J. and STOLLER, A. 1971. *The health of a metropolis*. Melbourne: Heinemann Educational.
31. KRUPINSKI, J. and STOLLER, A. 1962. Survey of institutional mental patients in Victoria, 1882–1959. *Med. J. Aust.*, **1**, 269, 314, 349.
32. KRUPINSKI, J. and STOLLER, A. 1962–1969. *Statistical Bulletins Numbers 1 to 8*. Mental Health Authority, Victoria, Melbourne.
33. KRUPINSKI, J., STOLLER, A., BAIKIE, A. G. and GRAVES, J. E. 1970. A community health survey of Heyfield, Victoria. Melbourne: *Mental Health Authority, Special Publications* No. 1.

34. KRUPINSKI, J., STOLLER, A. and POLKE, P. 1966. Attempted suicides admitted to the Mental Health Department, Victoria, Australia: a socio-epidemiological study. *Int. J. soc. Psychiat.*, **13**, No. 1, pp. 5–13.
35. KVARACEUS, W. C. 1964. *Juvenile delinquency: a problem for the modern world.* UNESCO, Paris.
36. LEE, R. H. 1952. Delinquent, neglected and dependent Chinese boys and girls of the San Francisco Bay region. *J. soc. Psychol.*, **36**, 15–34.
37. LEIGHTON, D. C., HARDING, J. S., MACKLIN, D. B., MacMILLAN, A. M. and LEIGHTON, A. 1963. *The character of danger.* New York: Basic Books.
38. McCORD, W. and McCORD, J. 1959. *Origins of crime: a new evaluation of the Cambridge–Somerville Youth Study,* New York.
39. McCULLOCH, J. W., HENDERSON, A. S. and PHILIP, A. E. 1966. Psychiatric illness in Edinburgh teenagers. *Scot. med. J.*, **11**, 277–281.
40. MARKMAN, R. A. 1966. Juvenile delinquency in Israel. *Amer. J. Psychiat.*, **123**, 4, Oct., pp. 463–468.
41. MASTERSON, JAMES F. 1967. *The psychiatric dilemma of adolescence.* Boston: Little, Brown & Company.
42. MOSES, E. R. 1947. Differentials in crime rates between negroes and whites based on comparisons of four socio-economically equated areas. *Amer. Sociol. Rev.*, **12**, 411–420.
43. MULLIGAN, G., DOUGLAS, J. W. B., HAMMOND, W. A. and TIZARD, J. 1963. Delinquency and symptoms of maladjustment: the findings of a longitudinal study. *Proc. roy. soc. Med.*, **56**, 1083–1086.
44. NICHOLI, A. M. 1967. Harvard dropouts: some psychiatric findings. *Amer. J. Psychiat.*, **124**, 651–658.
45. OFFER, D. 1969. *The psychological world of the teenager.* New York: Basic Books.
46. PESKIN, H. 1967. Pubertal onset and ego functioning. *J. abnorm. soc. Psychol.*, **72**, 1, 1–15.
47. REIFLER, C. B. 1967. Some psychiatric considerations in the care of college students. *Sth. med. J.*, **60**, 171–176.
48. ROBINS, LEE N. 1969. Follow-up studies of behaviour disorders in children. Paper presented to the W.P.A.–R.M.P.A. *Symposium on Psychiatric Epidemiology*, University of Aberdeen.
49. ROBINS, LEE N. and LEWIS, W. W. 1966. The role of the antisocial family in school completion and delinquency: a three-generation study. *Sociological Quarterly*, **7**, 500–514.
50. ROSEN, B. M., BAHN, A. K., SHELLOW, R. and BOWER, E. M. 1965. Adolescent patients served in outpatient psychiatric clinics. *Amer. J. publ. Hlth.*, **55**, (10), 1563–1577.
51. ROSEN, B. M., KRAMER, M., REDICK, R. W. and WILLNER, S. G. 1968. Utilization of psychiatric facilities by children: current status, trends, implications. National Institute of Mental Health. *Mental Health Statistics Series B*, No. 1.
52. RUTTER, M. and GRAHAM, P. 1966. Psychiatric disorder in 10- and 11-year-old children. *Proc. roy. Soc. Med.*, **59**, (4), 382–387.
53. SCHWARZ, C. J. 1964. A psychiatric service for university students. *Canad. Psychiat. Ass. J.*, **9**, 232–238.
54. SCOTT, P. D. 1960. Assessing the offender for the courts: the role of the psychiatrist. *Brit. J. Crim.*, **1**, 116–129.
55. SCOTT, P. D. 1960. The treatment of psychopaths. *Brit. med. J.*, **1**, 1641–1645.
56. SHEPHERD, M., COOPER, B., BROWN, A. C. and KALTON, G. W. 1966. *Psychiatric illness in general practice.* London: Oxford University Press.

H

57. SMITH, W. G., HANSELL, N. and ENGLISH, J. T. 1965, Values and mental health in a college population: a follow-up report. *J. nerv. ment. Dis.*, **140**, 92.

58. SROLE, L., LANGNER, T. S., MICHAEL, S. T., OPLER, M. K. and RENNIE, T. A. C. 1962. *Mental health in the metropolis: the mid-town Manhattan study.* London: McGraw Hill.

59. TANNER, J. M., WHITEHOUSE, R. H. and HEALY, M. J. R. 1962. *A new system for estimating skeletal maturity from the hand and wrists, with standards derived from a study of 2,600 healthy British children.* Parts I and II. Centre International de l'Enfance.

60. TAYLOR, Lord and CHAVE, S. 1964. *Mental health and environment.* London: Longmans.

61. TEICHER, J. D. and JACOBS, J. 1966. Adolescents who attempt suicide: preliminary finding. *Amer. J. Psychiat.*, **122**, 1248–1257.

62. UNITED NATIONS DEPT. OF ECONOMIC AND SOCIAL AFFAIRS. 1956. *First United Nations Congress on the prevention of crime and the treatment of offenders* (Geneva, 1955)—Report prepared by the Secretariat, New York.

63. UNITED NATIONS. 1960. *New forms of juvenile delinquency: their origin, prevention and treatment*—Report prepared by the Secretariat (2nd U.N. Congress on Prevention of Crime and Treatment of Offenders, London, 1960), New York (pp. 51—53 cited).

64. UNITED NATIONS DEPT. OF ECONOMIC AND SOCIAL AFFAIRS. 1965. *The young adult offender: a review of current practices and programmes in prevention and treatment.* New York.

65. WARREN, W. 1965. A study of adolescent psychiatric in-patients and the outcome of six or more years later. II. The follow-up study. *J. Child Psychol. Psychiat.*, **6**, 141–160.

66. WILNER, D. M., WALKLEY, T. C. P. and TAYBACK, M. 1962. *The housing environment and the family life.* Baltimore: The Johns Hopkins Press.

67. WING, J. K. 1970. A standard form of psychiatric present state examination. In *Psychiatric Epidemiology. Proceedings of an International Symposium.* Eds E. H. Hare and J. K. Wing. London: Oxford University Press.

68. WOLFF, S. 1967. Recognition of emotional disturbance among school children. *Public Health*, **82**, 11–22.

IX

CLASSIFICATION OF PSYCHIATRIC DISORDERS

Consideration of adolescence and all age groups

JOHN G. HOWELLS

Director, The Institute of Family Psychiatry
The Ipswich Hospital, Ipswich, England

1

Introduction

Developments in a field depend on a number of factors, but probably none so retards progess in psychiatry today as the confusions of its nosology and, linked with it, the lack of agreement on criteria for defining syndromes together with the imprecision of its nomenclature. Ignorance is a matter to be overcome by time and endeavour; the lack of order in known phenomena is something to be righted now. An aetiological classification is a paramount need because accurate delineation of dysfunction leads to logical investigation, and so to the meeting of the central obligation of medicine, viz. effective treatment.

From time to time, with each upsurge of knowledge clinicians have attempted reclassifications. Their history is too lengthy for review here. Starting with a *tabula rasa* and in the belief that any attempt at classification is worth while, a tentative new model is now put forward. This new model (*i*) is based on the aetiological modality, (*ii*) accepts the division of psychiatry into two main fields dependent respectively on psychic and organic pathology, (*iii*) caters for all age groups in one classification, and (*iv*) is served by terms bereft of the distorting influence of 'common usage'. This classification, like every communication on the subject, is limited by the absence of final truth in psychiatry.

As will become clear in this contribution, any classificatory system in psychiatry must be applicable to all age groups. Thus a contribution to a volume on adolescence is an appropriate vantage point from which to deliberate on a classification suitable not only for adolescence but also for childhood and adulthood.

2

General Considerations

The Value of Taxonomy

It is appropriate to ask here, why should one classify any phenomena?— a purposeless exercise unless it has value. The attributes of categorisation have through long practice proved to be: (1) the aid it gives to the understanding of phenomena by generalising from data; (2) the more effective control it gives over phenomena, which in turn can lead to improvement; (3) the assistance to more accurate prediction of the course of the phenomena. Phenomena can be assessed from many vantage points and classified by many modalities; the most appropriate is the one that most adequately serves a given purpose at a particular moment in time. The classifier must be knowledgeable about the material he intends to classify if he is to establish a worthwhile system and be able to test the practicability of his formulations. Taxonomy (tax, τάξις, order; nomy, νομός, law) then, the science of classification, has a value.

Why classify in medicine? Classification by the orderly assembly of data may reveal instances that have affinity and are meaningful as a group; light may be thrown on the nature and locus of dysfunction; therapy may come to have a logical and therefore useful basis; more precise evaluation of treatment becomes possible; research can be planned in a manner relevant to its purpose; research data are more easily comparable; areas of ignorance may be exposed. Thus classification is a tool for the essential purpose of medicine, to relieve suffering, and to produce harmonious functioning by treatment. Nosology (nosis, νόσος, disease; logy, λόγος, word), the classification of diseases and a branch of taxonomy, has value.

Data in medicine, as elsewhere, can be categorised by many modalities, e.g. the age of the patient; degree of physical disability; degree of social disability; body build; size of head; shape of hand; response to therapy; prognostic value; or even by a mathematical abstraction of easy digestion using a computer, etc. The overriding factor in the selection of a modality for classification is that it be the one most appropriate to the purpose in mind. Experience has amply demonstrated the special value of a nosology based on certain aetiology; such a classification has the virtue of leading to certain treatment, the end result of medical endeavour. The elucidation of the nature of cerebral syphilis as an infection, for instance, led to the utilisation of the appropriate powerful therapeutic agents and to measures to control and prevent this disorder.

The Present Position in Psychiatry

Classification of psychiatric disorders on a useful aetiological model calls for precision and agreement in three main areas, in all of which at present there are deficiencies.

The first area includes the identification of indicators of dysfunction (i.e. signs and symptoms), agreed criteria for evaluating these, and a systematic procedure for investigating the presence of such indicators. Freudenberg and Robertson[15] have reviewed attempts to identify meaningful signs and symptoms. Sandifer et al.[44] have demonstrated the disagreement on evaluation of symptoms between clinicians in the U.S.A. and the U.K.; the U.S. psychiatrists reported twice as many symptoms as the U.K. psychiatrists. Feinstein[12] has reported that the position is not completely satisfactory even in organic medicine. Wing et al.[58] have launched into important work on establishing more precise criteria for interviews and examinations.

The second area includes the correct grouping of states of dysfunction to produce meaningful syndromes. Kreitman,[28] Foulds,[14] Zubin[62] have reviewed the reliability of specific diagnoses. Boisen[4] in 1938 showed that the incidence of various types of schizophrenia varied widely between adjoining States in the U.S.A. and even between different hospitals in the same State. Amongst co-workers Beck et al.[1] obtained only 54 per cent agreement on specific diagnoses, although agreement was higher over individual symptoms. Vera Norris[35] showed that concordance of diagnosis between observation ward and hospital in London was less than 30 per cent. For the World Health Organisation Shepherd et al.[46] reported an interesting and valuable exercise to delineate basic issues in clinical diagnosis. This exercise particularly showed the need to establish agreement through clearly formulated diagnostic criteria. Rawnsley et al.[37] after an international diagnostic exercise concluded that at the level of sub-categories of diagnosis, international variations in usage are so great as completely to vitiate comparisons between countries. For instance, U.S. psychiatrists diagnosed schizophrenia much more frequently than U.K. psychiatrists, but the reverse was true of depression; and Kramer et al.[27] came to similar conclusions.

The third area includes agreement over the definitions of all the terms and categories employed in nomenclature. Stengel[48] emphasised the essential requirement of a glossary with agreed definition of clinical categories if any system of classification was to be useful. This plea was reiterated in the report of the W.H.O. study group, Shepherd et al.[46]

The supreme example of the monumental waste and frustration produced by inability to agree on diagnostic criteria is the research field of schizophrenia. Langfeldt,[30] a distinguished researcher and nosologist, wrote in this connection: 'However, in spite of the thousands of investigations, thus far no conclusion has been borne to the point of universal authority by further investigation. This circumstance is, in part, due to the fact that there is no agreement on the characteristics of the schizophrenic disorders.' Bleuler,[3] with his definition of 'schizophrenia', extended the term to include the vaguer concept of psychosis, and this in turn has come to embrace any major deviation of behaviour, regardless of aetiology. Only a handful of papers define their criteria so as to show beyond doubt that they deal with 'genuine' schizophrenia. The result is great doubt on the interpretation of findings. In the genetics of schizophrenia, for example, there has already been a sharp change of opinion—concordance rates in twin studies of schizophrenia are not what geneticists a few years ago claimed them to be. Perhaps the criteria are different. Who knows? Is it possible, for instance, that many of the patients included in the category of schizophrenia in the early studies were advanced neurotics? The strong correlations amongst family members would be understandable, as neurosis is eminently a familial disorder, but by communication rather than by inheritance. Howells[18] is forced to regard the research on the family psychopathology of schizophrenia as unproven, as in no instance was there an adequate criterion of schizophrenia; the data suggested that the researchers were studying atypical schizophrenia, probably severe neurosis.

The starting point in any consideration of the present classificatory scheme for mental disorder must be Stengel's[48] exhaustive review carried out for the World Health Organisation, together with his more recent critical summaries.[49, 50] Some of the issues in the nosology of mental disorders were explored at a conference held under the auspices of the American Psychopathological Association in 1959 (Zubin[61]). This led to a cross-national study (Kramer et al.[27]). The W.H.O. has also set up a working party for a ten-year period, and laudably this group has also based their work on the study of case material. Stengel[48] reviews fifty-eight different systems. The International Classification of Diseases (I.C.D.) is the most widely employed system, but it is regarded with general dissatisfaction. The latest revision (1965)[59] is still regarded as unsatisfactory, and no one is more aware of its limitations than its architects. The I.C.D. has a number of unsatisfactory features. It is based on concepts that are often outdated. It is a compromise between many conflicting movements and traditions. But its most serious limitation is that it is based on a large number of different modalities, which causes it to be an illogical, disorderly, confusing hotch-potch. This latter point can be demonstrated by listing some of the modalities employed. The numbers refer to the categories in the I.C.D.:

Age—with childbirth—294·4; behaviour disorders of childhood 308; involutional melancholia 296·0.

Agent—alcoholic psychosis 291; alcoholism 303; infection 292; trauma 293·5.

Organ—brain 292; skin 305·0.

Symptoms—schizophrenia 295; neurosis 300; sexual deviation 302.

Social Behaviour—exhibitionism 302; antisocial 301·7; transient situational 307.

Degree—mental retardation 310–315.

Temporal—acute paranoid reaction 298·3; episodic excessive drinking 303·0; acute schizophrenic episode 295·4.

Obstacles to Agreement

As stated above and by numerous other writers on the subject, the question of diagnosis is bedevilled by the inability to establish agreed criteria for the definition of clinical categories. Some of the inherent difficulties will be catalogued. Some of these are beyond our control. Others are capable of modification.

(1) When there is exact knowledge, definitions present less of a problem. Ignorance on many essential matters presents a real problem for psychiatry. Nevertheless, classification still lags behind the available knowledge.

(2) It is clearly shown in Rayner's study[38] that the use of the term 'psychosis', which in classifications stands for insanity, has been widened to cover highly abnormal or unusual behaviour. Highly abnormal behaviour, however, also occurs in neurosis; acute anxiety or anguish can precipitate a number of acute symptoms which are as bizarre and extreme as those in psychosis, e.g. the phobic anxiety-depersonalisation syndrome (Roth[40]). Neurotic behaviour may be just as disruptive and damaging as psychotic behaviour if not more so. Careful examination, however, reveals that the abnormal behaviour in neurosis is different from psychotic behaviour. In the absence of careful examination many severe conditions of neurosis are liable to be labelled 'psychotic'.

(3) There are misjudgements that spring from personal training and experience; individual psychiatrists see what they are trained to see. At one extreme, psychiatrists may have a background of training and experience in mental hospitals and are orientated towards psychosis; psychopathology may be ill-understood, if recognised at all. Thus, there is a tendency to label highly abnormal behaviour demanding hospital admission as 'psychotic', irrespective of the basic clinical picture. Thus psychosis is over-diagnosed. At the other extreme, psychiatrists may have a background in psychopathology and rarely see psychosis. Often they follow the fashion of regarding extreme states as psychotic—when acquaintance with psychotics would have exposed the qualitatively different clinical picture. Thus for both reasons psychosis tends to be over-diagnosed. This argues for a comprehensive training with experience in both fields.

(4) Every vocation has a heritage, and so has psychiatry. Misconceptions tend to go unchallenged and come to have the status of myths. Yet, practitioners in the past were even more ignorant than ourselves and therefore even less able to arrive at satisfactory criteria. For instance, Stierlin's[52] examination of Bleuler's[3] concept of schizophrenia exposed it as an attempt to integrate viewpoints from Kraepelin, Freud and Simon, and he left a

confusing heritage. Thus we must continually re-examine the assessments of the past.

(5) To base clinical requirements on hospital rather than on community practice can give a very wrong impression of clinical needs. Hospital practice may suggest the preponderance of psychotic material; community practice the reverse.

(6) Neurosis is more readily diagnosed if a direct link between the stress and the reaction can be established. Due to the exigencies of medical practice, time is limited. Thus, often either no attempt is made to explore psychopathology or no time is available. Therefore neurotic conditions may be overlooked. Particular examples are: conditions of paranoia with deep suspicion can be precipitated by anxiety and even by deafness; they are often interpretated to mean a psychotic state. Post-puerperal depression is an area that has recently come under the close scrutiny of psychopathologists, and what were previously thought to be endogenous psychotic depressions are now seen in the main to be reactive neurotic states.

(7) Symptoms can be shared by syndromes with a quite different aetiology. Dyspnoea may be due to anaemia or a pneumothorax. Equally, the depersonalisation of an agitated panic-stricken person may have a different basis from the bizarre depersonalisation of a schizophrenic.

(8) Hasty examination may cause the observer not to notice qualitative differences in common symptoms. The detachment of the lovelorn is qualitatively different from the detachment due to the stupor of catatonic schizophrenia or that of diabetic coma.

(9) Symptoms can be elevated into clinical syndromes. For example, 'enuresis' though a symptom, is often classed as a disease. 'Catatonia' is a symptom rather than a clinical category. 'Withdrawal' or 'autism' as a symptom may be due to preoccupation, depression, catatonic stupor or diabetic coma, but it is not itself a clinical syndrome. Slavish categorisation by the initial or presenting symptom will in particular lead to the above abuse. Thus investigation may stop short of an examination that would have revealed further signs of dysfunction, and an incomplete picture is obtained.

(10) A great disadvantage to psychiatry has been the break-up of its practice into age groups—infant, child, adolescent, adult and geriatric psychiatry. Thus, the flow of psychopathology from infancy to old age is not always comprehended. The temper tantrums of the infant become the awkwardness of the schoolboy, the delinquency of the adolescent, the criminal behaviour of the adult and the malevolent contrariness of the aged. As it is one process, the essential nomenclature should be the same. The late development of adolescent psychiatry has been particularly damaging as it sets up a gap between child and adult psychiatry. Terms associated with age periods, e.g. infantile psychosis, puerperal psychosis, climacteric psychosis, involutional melancholia, tend to establish discrete syndromes occurring at these periods and obscure the need to define the aetiological

picture. Sometimes the concepts of the practitioners of one age group are imposed upon those of another, when a total appreciation would have produced conclusions meaningful for all age groups and to the benefit of each.

(11) Terms may be misleading. Strömgren[54] has pointed out that 'amentia' in the United Kingdom is synonymous with mental retardation, whereas in continental Europe it is used for a specific form of delirium. Again, ideas may be shared by clinicians but the term employed for the idea may be different, e.g. 'psychogenic psychosis' in Denmark, 'constitutional psychosis' in Norway and 'reactive psychosis' elsewhere. Some words are borrowed from everyday language, e.g. 'confusion', and tend to be imprecise. A term, which by the concepts of one era sounds adequate, becomes inadequate with increasing knowledge; e.g. 'split mind' may have satisfied clinicians in Bleuler's day, and 'schizophrenia' was acceptable; but today the term hardly covers the central signs of this state of psychosis. Words coined to denote a particular category may be borrowed and used to cover related conditions; e.g. Korsakov's psychosis was first used to describe a state arising in alcoholic dementia but was later employed for similar states elsewhere in organic dementia.

3

Issues in Classification

The Medical Heritage

Medicine has a long history of grappling with classificatory systems for morbid phenomena and has arrived at a general plan which is satisfactory in its field of operation. Psychiatry should thus profit from Medicine's long experience. The definition of disease is as follows (dis-ease = without ease). 'A disease is the sum total of the reactions, physical and mental, made by a person to a noxious agent entering his body from without or arising within (such as micro-organism or a poison), and injury, a congenital or hereditary defect, a metabolic disorder, a food deficiency, or a degenerative process. These cause pathological changes in organs or tissues, which are revealed by characteristic signs and symptoms. Since a particular agent tends to produce a pathological and clinical picture peculiar to itself, although modified by individual variations in different patients, a mental concept of the average reactions or a composite picture can be formed which, for the convenience of description, is called a particular disease or clinical entity. But a disease has no separate existence apart from a patient, and the only entity is the patient' (*Butterworths Medical Dictionary*). Thus to delineate a clinical category there has to be an agent, a fabric which is disrupted by the agent and signs of the fabric's dysfunction. To identify the complete morbid process is to establish a clinical diagnosis. Feinstein's[12] recent re-examination of the procedures of clinical judgement does not quarrel with this system, but he calls for greater refinement and precision. Hereinafter the term 'signs' stands for 'symptoms' as well as 'signs'.

Before discussing in turn the agent, the fabric, the signs and the diagnosis some mention must be made of the phenomenology of psychiatry. Some would deny that there are meaningful signs of disturbances of psychic functioning. Krauple Taylor[56] has recently met the challenge of this attitude. There is no doubt that guilt at the murder of a mother is as much a phenomenological entity as a broken leg resulting from a fall. Dysfunction of the psyche manifests itself by anomalous behaviour which incapacitates, causes discomfort, pain and anguish, and makes the individual seek for relief, or makes the onlooker seek relief on his behalf. Hence the need for a psychiatrist (psyche, ψυχή, mind; iatros, ἰατρός, healer).

THE AGENT

As the result of long experience, five groups of harmful agents have been recognised in medicine. These are (1) infective, (2) neoplastic, (3) congenital and hereditary, (4) metabolic and degenerative, (5) traumatic.

Included in the last group should be emotional stress, which is overwhelmingly common, of great force of impact, capable of dire consequences and of influencing every component of the soma; yet emotional stress is comparatively neglected in Medicine. The terms *emotional, emotion, emotive* are difficult to define. They represent action of a non-organic kind arising from the non-organic part of the person. Emotional stress usually comes from an emotional source, i.e. another person. Where there is lack of precision due to ignorance, there is more advantage in a global term, such as *emotion*, than in an attempt to make a close definition which might result in a limitation of the term, or in pseudo-precision. The term 'love' comes into the same category; we are all aware of it and have a general idea of its quality; but few would dare to attempt a precise definition.

THE FABRIC

Harmful *organic* agents may disrupt any tissue in the body. The tissue of prime concern to the psychiatrist, or neuro-psychiatrist, is the encephalon (brain). Manifestations of the dysfunctioning of the encephalon are termed 'mental symptoms' and may come within the purview of the psychiatrist. In general the effects of organic agents on the encephalon are well documented. They may strike at the encephalon directly, or indirectly through the products of somatic dysfunction elsewhere.

Emotional agents may also strike at the fabric of the psyche and any part of the soma, including the encephalon.

Sometimes the two groups of reactions, organic and emotional, coexist, e.g. a physical blow may not only do direct physical damage, but may also arouse a psychic reaction by its threat value.

The 'process' precipitated in the organ by the harmful agent is of course different from the signs of pathology. The misfire of a motor-car is a useful sign of machine failure, but it is not an adequate description of the disturbed combustion in the engine. Pathological processes in the soma are now largely, but not completely, understood. Pathological processes in the psyche, as we shall soon discover, are a field of conflict, speculation and ignorance. The greater the ignorance, the more conflicting the views. Truth does not nourish speculation.

THE SIGNS

An increase in functioning *per se* is not a sign of dysfunction; for example, a rapid pulse rate in a runner is a sign of excellent functioning.

Signs may be shared by a number of different clinical categories; for example, dyspnoea can accompany carcinoma of the chest, anaemia or cardiac disease. A sign can be shared by emotional or physical disorders; dyspnoea can occur in anxiety and in physical disorders.

The signs of organic disorder are so well known that they do not need categorising here.

Emotional stress impinging on an individual releases three clusters[19] of signs of dysfunction: (1) Physical (termed psychosomatic). They may affect one organ alone, e.g. precipitating asthma, or a number of organs together, as in hypertension with colitis and migraine. The brain is not exempt and there may be dysfunctioning of the encephalon, e.g. migraine or epilepsy. (2) Mood changes. (3) Changes of behaviour. The signs of emotional stress are rarely, if ever, mono-symptomatic.

A number of signs appear in each group, and indeed it is rare for all three clusters not to be involved. But only careful and global examination will expose this fact. Too often examination stops at the presenting symptom.

THE DIAGNOSIS (διάγνωσις, discernment)

The isolation of the signs of disorder calls for a systematic investigation in a meaningful way, because, over time, careful endeavour in a field shows that particular signs are significant and these are incorporated in the plan of investigation. If the plan of investigation fails to examine for the significant signs, then it will fail to elicit these signs. In psychiatry there is disagreement over what is significant, and individual systems of examination are inadequate and incomplete. This is especially true in the emotional field.

Once elicited, the signs may be grouped together with the disrupted fabric and the responsible agent in a meaningful way and so be formed into a syndrome, a disease category. Hence the diagnosis is made. It is usually necessary to take account not only of the nature and degree of the signs but also of their historical development. It is relevant to point out that diagnoses are made by the presence of positive signs of disorder and not by the absence of signs. Frequently psychiatrists are encouraged by physicians to assume that the absence of physical signs must denote a psychiatric disorder. The latter can be diagnosed only by positive signs indicative of psychiatric disorder. The diagnosis implies a pathological process provoked by a known agent in a particular site or sites and leading to characteristic signs. Ideally, it leads to a logical plan of treatment.

Psychic and Somatic States

For centuries, with fluctuating clarity, attempts have been made to divide mental phenomena into those that result from dysfunction of psyche and those that spring from dysfunction of brain activity. In the sixteenth century Felix Platter[36] in Europe and Timothie Bright[5] in England and in the seventeenth century Richard Burton,[6] Willis[57] and Sydenham[55] all recognised emotional states. Hunter and Macalpine[21] recount that in 1600 there were in England practitioners licensed by the Bishops to practise on melancholy (neurosis) and on the mad (psychosis). Emotional disorder was well understood at this time (Howells and Osborn[20]). Harvey's[16] discovery of the circulation, in the early seventeenth century unleashed an era of intensive preoccupation with physiological activities; psychiatry survived only in as much as it dealt with insanity (psychosis), the demands of which could not be ignored. Psychiatrists became alienists largely divorced from the medical field. The end of the nineteenth century saw the reawakening of interest in psychic dysfunction. That trend continues apace today.

There is general acceptance that psychiatry has two areas of activity—emotional dysfunction and brain dysfunction. This is not accepted in all quarters where severe emotional disorder is believed to extend into psychosis. However, further discussion can be avoided here by reference to two authorities—a clinician Roth[41] and a clinical psychologist Eysenck[10] —who both from different viewpoints established a strong case for the dichotomy. It is noteworthy that a number of contemporary classifications reviewed by Stengel[48] also accept this dichotomy; for instance, it is implied in the classification of the American Psychiatric Association and again in the two classifications from the U.S.S.R.

One of the end results of lack of clarity over criteria is the tendency to confuse the signs of psychic dysfunction, for example anxiety, anguish, guilt, agitation, with signs of brain dysfunction, for example memory defects, confabulation, disorientation, hallucinations, perceptual anomalies, etc. The last group are known to spring from damage to areas of the brain, the first are not. On careful examination the two groups of symptoms are qualitatively different—but equally incapacitating to the individual.

A cause of bewilderment is that the clinical term employed to denote morbid disorder of mind, i.e. neurosis, suggests a disorder with an organic basis. Conversely, the term used to denote morbid disorder of the brain, psychosis, suggests a psychic basis. Can this be so? Remarkably, close study shows that this is so. Indeed the terms are virtually reversible.

The term neurosis is derived from the Greek νεῦρον, neuron (nerve), which with its suffix -osis (nosis—disorder) thus means a 'nerve disorder', i.e. a somatic condition. That this is so can be seen from the writings of the clinician who first used the term—Cullen, in 1776.[8] In his *Synopsis Nosologiae Methodical* he proposed to comprehend under the title of Neuroses 'all those preternatural affections of sense or motion which are without pyrexia as a part of the primary disease, and all those which depend not upon a topical affection of the organs but upon a more *general affection of the nervous system* . . . of such diseases I have established a class, under the title of Neuroses . . .'. (Author's italics.) Thus his class 'Neurosis' was intended to have a somatic basis. Further discussion will be found in Leigh.[32] But in time the term came to mean the reverse of Cullen's intention—it came to denote morbid states based on psychic dysfunction. An attempt at compensation was to add the prefix 'psycho' to neurosis, making psychoneurosis, which led to the absurdity 'psychic disorder of nerve'. Thus does haphazard 'common usage' bring inexactitude.

The term psychosis is also derived from the Greek ψυχή psyche, mind, which with its suffix -osis (nosis—disorder) thus means 'disorder of mind', i.e. psychic condition. Psyche is employed in the *Iliad* and meant 'breath'. It came to mean 'The breath of life' or the principle of life itself. Later it stood for mind, soul or spirit. Today it stands for mind. First employed by Von Feuchtersleben[13] in 1845, psychosis was not a widely used term in psychiatry before the early twentieth century, being preceded by 'insanity' and used interchangeably with it until about 1930. Thereafter 'psychosis' replaced 'insanity'. Thus again we find a central term in psychiatry coming by 'common usage' to mean its precise opposite.

Briefly, consideration must be given to terms used more or less synonymously with neurosis and psychosis. For the first there is 'mental disorder'. Mental comes from the Latin *mens* (the mind). Unfortunately, this term owing to incorrect 'common usage' embraces also symptomatology of brain dysfunction, for example memory loss. Thus its use is not advocated. 'Emotional disorder' has the disadvantage that there is no satisfactory definition of 'emotional', which probably forms only a part of psychic activity. For psychosis there is 'madness', 'insanity' and 'lunacy', all with evident disadvantages. For a number of centuries, 'madness' has lost all precise meaning and at worst is a term of abuse. 'Lunacy' is derived from 'moon sickness' thought to be associated with the moon in the mediaeval span of interest in astrology; it is too inexact for contemporary usage. 'Insanity' is derived from the Latin *insanus*, i.e. not sound (unsound in mind). Its direct meaning—unsoundness of mind—is thus the reverse of its commonly employed meaning and is no alternative to 'psychosis'. It seems that we are far from the era of astrology in time but not in nomenclature.

In seeking acceptable terms to cover conditions of psychic and somatic origin, the first possibility is to reverse the terms 'psychosis' and 'neurosis'. There would be the evident disadvantage of confusion, and in any event the term 'neurosis' describes a 'disorder of nerve' rather than a 'disorder of brain'. It would seem essential to go back to first principles. A common basis for both conditions in Greek or in Latin might seem desirable. From a Latin derivation 'brain' would force the term 'cerebrum' upon us; unhappily, it has ceased to mean brain, but stands for the cerebral hemispheres by 'common usage'. Greek is more helpful. We are offered 'encephalon' (encephalon, ἐγκέφαλος, marrow within the head, brain) which stands for 'brain'. Thus a morbid process of brain by adding the suffix -nosis (morbid process) to the above neatly becomes encephalonosis. A matching Greek term is now needed for the morbid psychic processes. Phrenosis is a possibility. 'Phrenic' is derived from the Greek term for diaphragm, which area was thought to be the seat of the emotions. Thus phren (phren, φρήν, mind) came to stand for mind. Frenzy, derived from it, at first covered emotional disturbance, but unfortunately the term soon became identified with mental disturbance, e.g. phrenitis stood for delirium. The term also has an unhappy link with phrenology. Another Greek term for mind is psyche, ψυχή. Psychosis is unthinkable because of the confusion it would cause. Psychopathology (psycho, ψυχή, mind; pathy, πάθος, morbid process; logo, λόγος, discourse) would fit, but regrettably it has a special meaning in contemporary forensic practice. Greek, however, is accommodating. The suffix -nosis (from νόσος disease) stands for a morbid process. Thus disorder of psyche becomes psychonosis.

So we have our preferred terms—encephalonosis (morbid process of brain) and psychonosis (morbid process of mind). These will now be employed in the remainder of this chapter with the old terms in brackets.

Areas for Delineation

Before attempting a finer sub-classification of psychonosis (neurosis) and encephalonosis (psychosis), some attention must be paid to some diagnostic categories which present difficulty in classification.

It will be noted that the issues in the first six categories below turn around differentiating extreme behaviour characteristic of psychonosis (neurosis) from psychosis. Instead of being labelled psychonosis (neurosis) they are all regarded as atypical schizophrenia and thus included under encephalonosis. Here it is relevant to mention that Robins and Guze,[39] after a study of these atypical schizophrenias, conclude that they are not true schizophrenias but quite different diseases. The high incidence of affective disorders in the relations of such patients would be in conformity with the view that the patients suffer from psychonosis (neurosis).

(1) *Pseudo-neurotic schizophrenia.* This condition was described by Hoch and Polatin[17] in 1949. It is a borderline state which causes problems in diagnosis. The characteristic features are a variety of psychic symptoms, chaotic sexuality, transient hallucinations and a good prognosis. The subject has been exhaustively discussed by Roth[41] and, like him, one is forced to come to the conclusion that these conditions are usually states of psychonosis (neurosis).

(2) *Schizo-affective psychoses.* These were described by Kasanin[26] in 1933. Their principal feature, according to Kasanin, was 'characterised by a very sudden onset in a setting of marked emotional turmoil with a distortion of the outside world . . . The psychosis lasts a few weeks to a few months and is followed by a recovery.' The similarity to pseudo-neurotic schizophrenia is evident. In time the condition came to stand for mixed affective and presumed schizophrenic states. In clinical practice it appears that, given time, it is possible to disentangle psychopathology in such patients and come to the conclusion that they are all essentially psychonotic (neurotic) states. Indeed, the very existence of affect is not indicative of a diagnosis of schizophrenia in that one of the characteristic features of this condition is the absence of affect in the patient.

(3) *Psychogenic psychosis.* A Danish psychiatrist Faergeman[11] has described this condition in some detail, and the term is widely used in Scandinavia. Sometimes the term 'reactive psychosis' or 'ambulatory psychosis' or 'constitutional psychosis' are used with the same meaning. The term psychogenic psychosis is useful in that it emphasises that extreme behaviour can occur as a result of emotional stimuli. But the term 'psychosis' is unfortunate in its present connotation. One is forced again to accept that these conditions are essentially psychonotic states (neurotic). They appear to present extreme, unusual, bizarre variants of neurosis. Some patients react in an unexpected way and this may be dependent upon their unusual childhood experiences. Reactive psychoses in the Russian classifications quoted by Stengel[48] are associated with psychonoses (neuroses).

(4) *Schizophreniform psychosis.* This condition was described by Langfeldt[29] in 1937. He distinguishes 'genuine schizophrenia' from an atypical form termed schizophreniform. Other terms applied to psychoses which are equivalent to 'genuine' are 'process', 'central' and 'nuclear'. The symptoms in Langfeldt's 'genuine' class are close to those regarded by Schneider[45] as of prime importance in the diagnosis of schizophrenia. The atypical schizophreniform psychosis like 'non-process' psychosis has a good prognosis; Stephens and Astrup[51] verified this for 'non-process' psychosis. It would appear that these conditions represent atypical, puzzling, or bewildering conditions of psychonosis (neurosis).

(5) *Paranoia.* Our increasing knowledge of psychopathology has shown that this condition can be set up in states of anxiety and can even reach an extreme degree, e.g. a bitter, disabled man up against, and thwarted by, authority. The suspicions and delusions are explicable in terms of real life situations. In the absence of other signs denoting schizophrenia, paranoia existing alone invariably indicates a psychonotic (neurotic) state.

(6) *Severe stress conditions.* It is reasonable to wonder whether severe stress can cause dysfunctioning of the brain and thus produce encephalonosis. Such an hypothesis is reasonable and must be considered in the genesis of schizophrenia, but it needs verification. It would seem that most

of the states described, e.g. phobic reaction, are reversible; and in this event it would seem better to regard the phenomenology as being indicative of a severe psychic reaction, i.e. severe psychonosis (neurosis).

Slight anxiety may cause anguish, an increased pulse rate, sweating of the skin, etc. Therefore very extreme anxiety would be expected to create an even more severe reaction. This reaction may be exaggerated by the fact that the somatic changes (e.g. thyroid, or adrenal secretion) may of themselves set up a toxic state. Thus the condition could be regarded as a psychosomatic disorder within psychonosis.

(7) *Paraphrenia*. This has come to mean schizophrenia occurring in the aged. It has the disadvantage of implying a separate aetiology from schizophrenia occurring at other age groups and is a term best deleted from clinical practice.

(8) *'Borderline' and 'latent' psychoses*. These terms have as little value as would the terms 'latent' or 'borderline' pneumonia. A condition either is or is not.

(9) *Psychopathy*. Strictly defined, this term means pathological states of mind or morbid conditions of mind. However, together with such terms as psychopathic states it has come to mean an anti-social or socio-pathic individual and it has a special meaning in forensic psychiatry. Such an individual if at variance with the society in which he lives is abnormal or sick. That is to say his dysfunction has been caused by emotional stress, and his behaviour is a part of his defensive reaction to it. Few would now accept Morel's[34] implication of constitutional moral degeneracy. As will be seen later in the discussion of psychonosis, this condition must properly form a part of psychonosis.

(10) *Character disorders*. Among these it is usual to include such conditions as homosexuality, sexual deviations and alcoholism. Clarification may come through a brief discussion of alcoholism. Habitual drinking of a social kind, although it may not be conducive to the well-being of the soma, cannot be regarded as a psychiatric disability. Indeed, should the habitual drinking take on a severe degree, it might still, strictly speaking, not be regarded as a psychiatric disability. However, for an individual to indulge in extreme habitual drinking threatening his own welfare is usually *per se* an indication of an emotional disorder. Experience shows that severe alcoholism indicates an emotional disorder and that the excessive drinking is part and parcel of his reaction to stressful events in his life experience.

Homosexuality is a developmental anomaly, and such an individual does not have psychiatric ill-health. In an environment prepared to tolerate his way of life he need not develop a psychonosis (neurosis). However, he may become ill in one or both of two situations: (1) if his disability or anomaly causes him to clash with his environment, (2) like anyone else, he may develop a psychonosis (neurosis) as a result of the usual stresses and strains of life. Again sexual deviations (e.g. fetishism), which are regarded as unusual in one society, may be regarded as perfectly normal in another and thus indicate health. Thus the deviation *per se* does not indicate morbidity. However if, as is usual, a deviation in our particular society is a defensive reaction to stressful events, then it usually forms part of a co-existing emotional disorder (psychonosis).

(*11*) *Multiple diagnoses.* These may arise in two circumstances: (*a*) a justifiable doubt about a diagnosis when two or more possibilities may be listed, (*b*) because there is a truly mixed condition, e.g. a neurosis (psychonosis) accompanied by amphetamine intoxication, i.e. psychonosis and encephalonosis together.

Elements of a Satisfactory Classification

From the discussion so far it is possible to identify the conditions for the satisfactory classification of syndromes in psychiatry.

(1) As far as possible, and certainly within its main divisions, the classification should be based on one modality.

(2) The most purposeful modality in medicine is that based on aetiology.

(3) The classification should be applicable to all age groups.

(4) There should be precise definition of all terminology. There is much advantage in using as far as possible, terms derived from classical Greek because of its universal usage, especially in medical terminology. Words should fit as closely as possible to the ideas they represent while appreciating that often a word can only approximate to the idea that it represents. Emotive words such as 'lunacy', 'idiocy', etc., should be kept to a minimum.

(5) Practicability in the clinical field is essential.

(6) The classification should be capable of existing alongside classifications based upon secondary modalities, e.g. degree of disorder, measures of social adjustment, measures of intellectual deficit.

(7) Multiple diagnoses should be possible.

(8) Miscellaneous terms should be kept to a minimum.

(9) The classification should be easily adjusted in the light of changing concepts of aetiology in psychiatry in the course of time.

4

Psychonosis

Definition

Psychonosis is defined as a morbid process of mind (psyche, ψυχή, mind; nosis, νόσος, disorder of).

The essential process in psychonosis is that the psyche suffers a stress with the result that there is disruption of its functioning, and evidence of dysfunctioning is seen in signs and symptoms. Psychic events are phenomena but we do not here need to get lost in a discussion of the form of the psyche.

Stress

The psychic stress may be of two varieties: (1) it may be a stress specific to an individual, a stress that has an especially destructive meaning for him, because of his sensitisation to the stress; (2) it may be a general stress to which most people are susceptible. The impact of the stress is greater if the personality is more vulnerable because of previous adverse stressful experiences.

Psychopathology

This consists of more than manifest signs and symptoms, in the same way that the symptoms of thyrotoxicosis do not give a complete picture of the process going on within the fabric of the thyroid gland. The process, psychopathology, is complex and diffuse and has been a matter for discussion between psychopathologists for many generations. The ways of describing psychopathology are legion, e.g. Freudian, Jungian, Behavioural, phenomenological, etc. There is no general agreement. Indeed there are so many elements, mechanisms and transactions at work that no agreed classification becomes possible. It may be that each case is unique to itself. In time, however, knowledge may reveal some general patterns that may allow a classificatory description of the psychopathological process. In the meantime, to seek agreement in this area can only bring frustration.

Signs

These can conveniently be divided into three clusters: (1) the psycho-somatic group, (2) the change of mood group, (3) the change of behaviour group.

The first, the psychosomatic group, includes all those signs of organ dysfunction. One or more systems of the body, including the central nervous system, may be implicated at any one time.

The second group includes all those signs of change of mood, e.g. anxiety, depression, apathy, obsessions, phobic states, etc.

The third group includes those defensive reactions such as timidity, withdrawal, and assertive changes of behaviour such as temper tantrums, awkwardness, antisocial behaviour, etc.

It is characteristic of psychonosis that it is never mono-symptomatic; indeed it is pathognomonic (characteristic) of psychonosis that it always manifests itself in a number of symptoms. Furthermore, it can be said that rarely does the symptomatology present in one of the above three groups alone. There is usually a total disturbance of the personality which embraces elements in all three groups, but which becomes apparent only on close and complete examination.

It might be asked why this truth is sometimes overlooked. This is because there has been a tendency to classify according to the presenting sign and not to proceed to a complete examination of the psyche. Hence such terms as anxiety, hysterical, obsessional, neurasthenic, depressive, states, are used. This is categorisation by the presenting sign and should be avoided. Indeed it would leave us at the era of the mediaeval practitioners who labelled such symptoms as 'fever' and 'melancholie' as clinical disorders.

The inability to agree about psychopathology has imperceptibly shifted attention to describing the process in terms of the signs; this is illusionary as the signs are a mere index and no more. Further knowledge may not allow categorisation of the psychopathological process. On the other hand, it may reveal that it is as clear-cut as the inflammatory process, is confined to one system, the psyche, and has variations in its expression which are dependent on the life situation, i.e. symptoms and signs may be governed by the demands and dictates of the life situation in the past and the present.

Diagnosis

The aim of classification is to produce order that leads to more useful treatment. It would seem that in the field of psychonosis (neurosis) any classification based upon the character of the stress, or the psychopathological process, or the symptomatology alone, limits rather than helps. As so many factors are involved when an individual in his life situation meets stress, a simple categorisation of the result is not possible and indeed limits the appreciation of this experience. Thus it is better to rely upon a descriptive account which outlines (1) the source and nature of the stresses, (2) the characteristics of the individual, and (3) the signs of dysfunction which are apparent.

In practice there may be virtue in using *secondary evaluations*. The *degree* of severity of the psychonosis may be considered, e.g. mild, moderate, and severe. The degree should be an index of the incapacity of the individual in his life situation at that time; some persons are so handicapped as to remain largely in the same degree of incapacity throughout their lives. The *speed of onset* may be another useful secondary evaluation, e.g. acute (sudden) or chronic (insidious).

A brief diagnosis could read: A married female aged forty under marital stress has a severely incapacitating and acute psychonosis in which she manifests lack of concentration, anxiety, depersonalisation, frequent haemorrhage and dermatitis, irritability and angry outbursts. This could be expanded by greater detail in each area or abbreviated to 'Psychonosis—acute and severe'.

Should the unit under consideration be the family rather than the individual, the same procedure is effective; for then the process in the group psyche of the family needs description.[19]

Three topics, psychopathy, personality disorders and child psychiatry, deserve brief special consideration before relating psychonosis to the International Classification of Diseases.

Psychopathy

It has already been stated that psychopathy and character disorders present special problems and that both conditions are best classified under psychonosis (neurosis). This is a feature of the Dutch classification noted by Stengel.[48]

The psychopath is an individual faced with an intolerable life situation which has provoked a psychonosis (neurosis), and by the nature of the life situation it has also provoked anti-social or asocial behaviour. Unfortunately the severity of his symptoms leads to concentration on his anti-social behaviour. But by proceeding to a full assessment of personality it is possible to see that there are manifestations of a total personality disturbance. Classification by the presenting symptom has in this area been a major limiting factor in the appreciation and management of this disability.

Personality Disorders

In this group are included terms to denote types of personality, e.g. paranoid, affective, hysterical, explosive, etc. Terms such as paranoid and hysterical have a clinical connotation and really describe mild degrees of psychopathology. There would be an advantage in reserving clinical terms for clinical states and classifying personality traits on a non-clinical schema such as one of a number devised by psychologists.

Child Psychiatry

Any useful final classification must embrace all age groups from infancy to old age. The child interacts with a situation, largely but not completely, within his family; the adult is involved in the same basic situation. Both child and adult manifest, flavoured by age, the same changes. Age must influence the expression of symptoms as development affects the equipment of expression, e.g. speech is susceptible during its formative period in early childhood; again an infant can have a temper tantrum but not rob a bank.

Child psychiatry has suffered a number of historical misfortunes from which it is rapidly emerging. Dependence on paediatrics led to focusing on the individual with a bias to neuropsychiatry that limited the evaluation of the child's interaction with parental and family psychopathology; indeed child psychiatrists often had no experience of adult psychopathology. The late development of adolescent psychiatry accentuated the isolation of child psychiatry; from this springs the tendency not to see the link between child and adult psychiatry and their common denominators, and hence a reluctance to use common terms. Furthermore it led to a tendency to regard childhood manifestations of psychonosis (neurosis) as being less dangerous than the adult forms, when in fact they are equally so. Psychonosis (neurosis) in the infant is not only widespread but also can be severe and even lead to sudden death, as for example in severe deprivatory psychic states. The dependence of the services on school authorities led to (1) limited experience with the under-fives, (2) an attenuated awareness of the furious and primary influence of family dynamics.

A number of contemporary authorities have written in this field, e.g. Cameron,[7] Mackay and Bigras,[33] Group for the Advancement of Psychiatry,[31] Jenkins, [23,24] Jenkins and Cole,[25] and Rutter.[42] The varying viewpoints found expression in the W.H.O. seminar.[43] Considerable progress was made there, and special mention must be made of the resolve that childhood and adult classification should be compatible, that neurosis should not be subdivided, and that reactive depression should be included under neurosis.

Comment on some terms employed in the children's field is necessary for clarification. It is noticed that terms such as 'normal variation' describe mild transient psychonosis, 'adaption reaction' and 'reactive disorder' describe moderate psychonosis, and 'personality disorder'—severe and persistent psychonosis. Thus terms denoting the degree of severity of the disorder (i.e. mild, moderate and severe) would be more suitable. 'Habit' or 'developmental' disorders because of their imprecision hardly deserve to be retained. To regard enuresis as a 'developmental disorder' as it commonly occurs in childhood is as useful as regarding gastic ulceration as a developmental disorder as it occurs in adulthood. There is of course no room for such terms as 'maladjusted' in the clinical field, as this term is a vague reference to social adaptability. The 'hyperkinetic syndrome' describes a child whose restlessness is produced by the coercion and restriction of his environment, and is usually seen only in a severe psychonosis.

Relationship of Psychonosis to the International Classification of Diseases (I.C.D.)

A number of categories listed in the Eighth Revision, 1965, would fall under psychonosis (Table I).

TABLE I

Neurosis	300
Reactive depressive psychosis	298·0
Reactive excitation	298·1
Reactive confusion	298·2
Acute paranoid reaction	298·3
Paranoia	297·0
Reactive psychosis unspecified	298·9
Sexual deviation	302
Alcoholism	303
Drug dependence	304
Physical disorders of presumably psychogenic origin	305
Transient situational disturbances	307
Behaviour disorders of childhood	308
Mental retardation (with psycho-social deprivation)	310–315·8

5

Encephalonosis

Definition

Encephalonosis is defined as a disorder or morbid process of brain (encephalon, ἐγκέφαλος, brain; nosis, νόσος, disease). The term includes all disorders of brain, but as it has not been employed in other directions it can be reserved for those conditions seen in psychiatric practice.

Encephalonosis is a disorder set in being by an organic agent acting on the organ brain resulting in a number of well-defined signs and symptoms.

Agents

Traditionally in clinical practice these are grouped into five types: (1) infective, (2) neoplastic, (3) congenital and hereditary, (4) metabolic and degenerative, (5) traumatic (including emotional stress). The agent involved influences the pathology and thus the ultimate signs.

Pathology

The influence of the agent on the organ may be either direct, i.e. primary, or indirect, i.e. secondary. In the secondary group the agent affects some organ in the body, which in turn sets up a toxic agent which influences brain functioning, e.g. adrenalin of the suprarenal gland may influence brain functioning. The pathology depends upon the area of brain damaged together with the nature of the agent and the duration of its action.

Signs

These include hallucinations, illusions, disorientation, emotional lability, perseveration, echolalia, amnesic symptoms, etc. Signs may be common to a number of syndromes. They are commonly covered by the term 'mental'. However, they are different from the symptoms of psychonosis (neurosis) in that (1) they are qualitatively distinct, (2) they are largely unaffected by changes in the psychic environment.

Diagnosis

As the organic agent plays a part in determining the organic process, there is merit, indeed it is usual, to classify these conditions according to the five groups of agents, viz. infective, neoplastic, genetic, degenerative and traumatic. Although the division is not complete, some states have an acute onset and tend to be reversible, and others take a slow or chronic course and tend to be irreversible. Thus classification can proceed by two main divisions—acute and chronic—and each may be subdivided into five categories according to the agent. In addition there are conditions of unknown aetiology—cryptogenic (crypto, κρυπτός, hidden; -genic, γένεσις, origin) encephalonosis. Incidentally, the term 'amentia' and the term 'dementia' are best avoided, as they imply disorders of mind (a = absence; de = out of; mens = mind).

Conditions can be further subdivided according to their *severity*, e.g. conditions of intellectual retardation could be subdivided into groups of severity such as mild, moderate and severe. Similarly, conditions can be graded according to the degree of social disability, for example employable, unemployable, etc.

Four topics, cryptogenic states, mental retardation, epilepsy and child psychiatry, now deserve special consideration before ending by relating encephalonosis to the International Classification of Diseases.

Cryptogenic (of unknown origin) States

There are two conditions in psychiatry sometimes covered by the term 'functional' which deserve special consideration; these are (1) schizophrenia and (2) manic-depressive disorder. It is noted that in one of the Russian classifications outlined by Stengel,[48] these conditions are included under the term 'of unknown aetiology'. The term *cryptogenic* is preferable to *functional*, in that it has an aetiological connotation.

The condition to be referred to later as encephalo-ataxia (schizophrenia) is a continuing challenge to psychiatrists. Its symptomatology by its nature, novelty and complexity lays claim to being the most fascinating syndrome in Medicine. Countless researchers have laid siege to it without its final resolution. Though it forms but a small percentage of psychiatric disorders, it is yet of major concern because of the severity and permanence of its disability. So that there be no confusion, it must be made clear that in this section the condition under discussion is 'nuclear', 'process', 'genuine', 'essential', schizophrenia.

As Rayner[38] recalls, the term schizophrenia was coined by Bleuler as a compromise to meet the organic-pathologists and psycho-pathologists, and stands for 'split mind'. This term might have some slight advantage in the early phases of schizophrenia, in as much as some aspects of reality are retained and thus the individual seems to be functioning at two levels. Recent work, however, has shown with little doubt that the central feature of schizophrenia is not the splitting of the mind, but the disorganisation of brain functioning. Thus a term should be employed to indicate disorganisation, disorder or confusion. Such a term would be encephalo-ataxia (encephalon, ἐγκέφαλος, brain; ataxia, ἀταξία, disorganisation).

It has become traditional to consider four sub-groups of encephalo-ataxia (schizophrenia)—simple, hebephrenic, catatonic and paranoid. These sub-categories are now outmoded by contemporary researchers. The Moscow group, led by Snezhnevsky,[47] studied over 5000 schizophrenics (encephalo-ataxics). In this report[47] the fluid, flexible, ever-changing polymorphic nature of the symptomatology is emphasised. There is an unfolding of stages in the disorder leading in some to a terminal stable stage. The progression of stages occurs at different speeds with three main courses of development, which however are not distinct as they appear to belong to one continuous process. It would be tempting to attach names to the varying patterns but this is unrewarding, as over 100 different states were observed. The same workers point to the links with acute encephalonosis on the one hand and with manic-depressive disorder on the other. Thus, whether or not there is one disorder involved or a number, in the present state of our knowledge it does not seem worthwhile to subcategorise this syndrome.

Manic-depressive psychosis is becoming a diminishing group due to the fact that many of the conditions once called cryptogenic are now seen to have a psychopathological basis and thus are included in the group psychonosis (neurosis). It may become even more diminished in the future by the realisation that those with the more bizarre behaviour belong to the group encephalo-ataxia. Until there is further elucidation it would seem desirable to maintain this category, but to give it a more rational descriptive title. Cyclothymiosis (cyclo, κύκλος, circle; thymos, θυμός, mind) indicates the cyclical nature of the mood changes of elation and depression. Encephalolampsia (encephalon, ἐγκέφαλος, brain; lampsia, λάμπω, to shine) indicates the state of elation, agitation and sensitivity. This was formerly termed 'mania'. Encephalobaria (encephalon, ἐγκέφαλος, brain; baria, βαρέω, to weigh down) indicates the state of depression.

The conditions considered cryptogenic are placed under encephalonosis because, all the evidence considered and in the present state of knowledge, it is a reasonable hypothesis to regard them as dependent upon organic pathology. Should time reveal otherwise, the conditions can without difficulty, in whole or in part, be moved to another section of the classification. Likewise, the nomenclature can be adjusted, e.g. assuming a psychopathology for the states, then encephalo-ataxia becomes psycho-ataxia, encephalolampsia becomes psycholampsia and encephalobaria becomes psychobaria.

Mental Retardation

Conditions giving rise to intellectual defect have always set problems in categorisation. They can be diagnosed on an aetiological basis emphasising the clinical aspect, or in terms of social disability—a social evaluation. Clearly the clinical classification must be adopted here. Intellectual retardation as such is not a clinical syndrome but a sign only of dysfunctioning of brain, and one sign amongst many. Intellectual defect occurs as the result of two conditions in general: (*a*) the primary condition due to multifactorial hereditary elements, i.e. those patients who lie at the lower end of the curve of distribution of intelligence; and (*b*) those patients whose defects are secondary to brain damage due to the five groups of agents mentioned above.

A classification based on aetiology bypasses the controversy over the term best employed to cover states of mental retardation. Terms advocated include 'mental handicap', 'mental subnormality' (with the defect that it suggests cultural subnormality), 'mental deficiency', and 'mental retardation' (but slowing up or retardation is present in many conditions). The essential situation is that the brain is damaged, at any age, and amongst those showing signs of brain dysfunction are to be found some subjects who show defect of intelligence. In fact, it is not the mind (mens, mental) that is handicapped, but the brain; those with intellectual defect may exhibit no disorder of mind.

There would seem to be no good reason for categorising conditions leading to intellectual loss in any way other than those mentioned above for all conditions of encephalonosis. This is the method followed in the classification of the American Psychiatric Association as reported by Stengel.[48] Indeed the failure to emphasise the clinical basis of mental retardation has been a weakness in this field. This has resulted in failure to appreciate the great contribution of the neurologist and the importance of cerebral studies.

Secondary evaluation in terms of loss of intellectual capacity is useful, and can include such grades as borderline, mild, severe, profound and very profound.

Brain damage occurring in childhood or infancy is no different from brain damage occurring in adolescence, adulthood or old age, and thus these conditions in all age groups should be considered together.

Organic states with mental retardation can co-exist with other syndromes, e.g. psychonosis (neurosis). This is particularly so in the higher grades of mental retardation. Furthermore, states of pseudo-retardation may occur as a result of gross emotional deprivation; such conditions of pseudo-amentia, however, should be considered under psychonosis (neurosis).

Epilepsy

This is not a disease category but a sign, composed of a sudden discharge of cerebral cells, due to organic pathology in the cells. The psychiatric connotations of epilepsy are as follows: (1) Emotional stress may precipitate or aggravate epilepsy. In such situations epilepsy is a psychosomatic symptom indicative of a psychonosis (neurosis). (2) An epileptic discharge focused in some areas of the brain gives rise to episodic 'mental' phenomena, such as dream states, etc.; these should be classed under encephalonosis (psychosis). (3) Following the positive discharge there is a negative phase, as originally described by Jackson,[22] in which the exhaustion of cells manifests itself in confused behaviour. Such a state is classified under encephalonosis (psychosis). (4) An epileptic may react to his disability by the development of a psychonosis (neurosis); clinical experience shows that frequently the psychonosis predates the epilepsy and has contributed to the incidence and degree of the attacks.

Child Psychiatry

Acute and chronic encephalonosis occurs in childhood, and its essential features are no different from those in any other age group. Cryptogenic encephalonosis may also occur—though cyclothymiosis is rarely noted in childhood. States akin to encephalo-ataxia (schizophrenia) do occur. Links with adulthood are suggested by the similarity of symptomatology; the known start of adult states in early childhood (Yudin[60] and Streltsova[53]), and the follow-up studies of childhood psychosis (made by some investigators, e.g. Bennett and Klein[2]) show a resultant state indistinguishable from adult encephalo-ataxia. Others claim a distinct condition in childhood, pointing to a separate peak of incidence in early childhood. The matter can be resolved to the satisfaction of all by calling these early conditions encephalo-ataxic-like states.

Much confusion is caused by the use of the term 'autism'. Dein[9] has traced its origins. At best it indicates 'withdrawal with phantasy'; sometimes it is a euphemism for childhood encephalo-ataxic-like states. Under its umbrella are gathered a heterogeneous group of conditions that can include severe psychonosis (neurosis) due to emotional deprivation, aphasic states, deafness, brain damage syndromes, as well as encephalo-ataxia. The sad payment for ignoring classification by aetiology is that all these children are treated alike.

Relationship of Encephalonosis to the International Classification of Diseases (I.C.D.)

A number of categories listed in the Eighth Revision, 1965, would fall under encephalonosis (Table II).

TABLE II

Psychoses	290–299
Schizophrenia	295
Affective psychoses	296
Involutional paraphrenia	297·1
Unspecified psychotic states	309
Mental retardation	310–315

6

Conclusion

It is suggested that psychiatric disorders be classified in two main aetiological groups: (1) *psychonosis*, dependent on psychopathology and (2) *encephalonosis*, dependent on organic pathology. The former, psychonosis, is subdivided into mild, moderate and severe forms. The latter, encephalonosis, is subdivided into acute, chronic and cryptogenic forms. The same classification is suggested for all age groups. Secondary evaluations are employed to a limited extent. Multiple diagnoses are possible. The figure on p. 233 shows the categories in diagrammatic form.

For those who would wish to leave open the question of the aetiology of the cryptogenic group, an alternative classification is possible. Psychiatric disorders can be subdivided into three groups: (1) psychonosis (neurosis)—mild, moderate and severe; (2) encephalonosis (psychosis)—acute and chronic; (3) cryptogenic states.

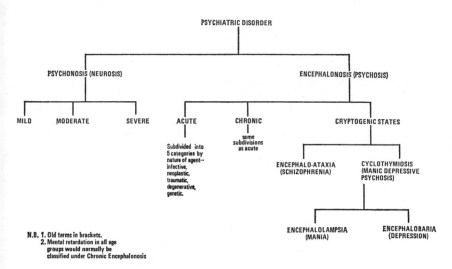

An essential requirement of a classification, it was suggested earlier, should be adaptability to new concepts of aetiology. To foretell the trends of the future is difficult. Clearly the conditions now grouped under 'cryptogenic' are those most likely to call for regrouping. Some argue for a metabolic aetiology for encephalo-ataxia, in which event it would be classified under chronic encephalonosis. Some conditions of encephalolampsia (mania) may well be thought to show the psychopathology of agitation and be reclassified under psychonosis (neurosis). Conditions of encephalobaria are often being reclassified as reactive disorders and would find themselves reclassified under psychonosis (neurosis). The conditions remaining under cyclothymiosis will then be regarded as essentially organic and endogenous.

Acknowledgments

I wish to acknowledge help from Mr J. R. Lickorish and Mrs M. L. Osborn; the former's Greek scholarship and the latter's pleasure at etymological exactitude have been of great benefit to me.
The following reference works were consulted with profit:

The Oxford Dictionary of English Etymology
The Shorter Oxford Dictionary on Historical Principles

The Oxford Classical Dictionary
The Origin of Medical Terms (Skinner, H. A.)
Butterworths Medical Dictionary (MacNalty, A. S.)
The American Illustrated Medical Dictionary (Dorland, W. A. N.)

REFERENCES

1. BECK, A. T., WARD, C. H., MENDELSON, M., MOCK, J. E. and ERBAUGH, J. K. 1962. Reliability of psychiatric diagnoses. 2. A study of consistency of clinical judgments and ratings. *Amer. J. Psychiat.*, **119**, 351–357.
2. BENNETT, S. and KLEIN, H. 1966. Childhood schizophrenia: thirty years later. *Amer. J. Psychiat.*, **122**, 1121.
3. BLEULER, E. 1911. *Dementia praecox oder Gruppe der Schizophrenien*. Leipzig and Vienna: F. Deuticke.
4. BOISEN, A. 1938. *Psychiatry*, **1**, 233.
5. BRIGHT, T. 1586. *A treatise of melancholie*. Facsimile edition in press. London: Pitman.
6. BURTON, R. 1628. *The anatomy of melancholy*. Everyman's Library, 1964. London: Dent.
7. CAMERON, K. 1955. Diagnostic categories in child psychiatry. *Brit. J. med. Psychol.*, **28**, 67–71.
8. CULLEN, W. 1776–1784. *First lines of the practice of physic* (4 vols). Edinburgh: C. Elliott.
9. DEIN, E. 1966. On the concept of autism. *Acta psychiat. scand., Suppl.* 191, **42**, 124–135.
10. EYSENCK, S. B. G. 1956. Neurosis and psychosis: an experimental analysis. *J. ment. Sci.*, **102**, 517.
11. FAERGEMAN, R. 1963. *Psychogenic psychoses*. London: Butterworth.
12. FEINSTEIN, A. R. 1967. *Clinical judgement*. Baltimore: Williams & Wilkins.
13. FEUCHTERSLEBEN, E. F. VON. 1845. *Lehrbuch der ärztlichen Seelenkunde*. Vienna: Carl Gerold.
14. FOULDS, G. A. 1955. The reliability of psychiatric, and the validity of psychological diagnoses. *J. ment. Sci.*, **101**, 851–862.
15. FREUDENBERG, R. K. and ROBERTSON, J. P. S. 1956. Symptoms in relation to psychiatric diagnosis and treatment. *Arch. Neurol. Psychiat.* (Chic.), **76**, 14–22.
16. HARVEY, W. 1628. De motu cordis. Transl. by Franklin, K. J., 1963, in *The circulation of the blood and other writings*. Everyman's Library. London: Dent.
17. HOCH, P. and POLATIN, P. 1949. Pseudoneurotic forms of schizophrenia. *Psychiat. Quart.*, **23**, 248.
18. HOWELLS, J. G. 1968. Family psychopathology and schizophrenia. In *Modern perspectives in world psychiatry*, Ed. J. G. Howells. Edinburgh: Oliver & Boyd.
19. HOWELLS, J. G. 1968. *Theory and practice of family psychiatry*. Edinburgh: Oliver & Boyd.
20. HOWELLS, J. G. and OSBORN, M. L. 1970. The incidence of emotional disorder in a 17th-century medical practice. *Medical History*, **14**, 192–198.
21. HUNTER, R. and MACALPINE, I. 1964. *Three hundred years of psychiatry*. London: Oxford University Press.

22. JACKSON, J. H. 1958. *Selected writings of John Hughlings Jackson*. New York: Basic Books.
23. JENKINS, R. L. 1964. Diagnoses, dynamics and treatment in child psychiatry. In Diagnostic classification in child psychiatry. Eds R. L. Jenkins and J. O. Cole. *Psychiat. Res. Rep.*, **18**, 91–120.
24. JENKINS, R. L. 1969. Classification of behavior problems of children. *Amer. J. Psychiat.*, **125**, 1032–1039.
25. JENKINS, R. L. and COLE, J. O. (Eds). 1964. Diagnostic classification in child psychiatry. *Psychiat. Res. Rep.*, **18**.
26. KASANIN, J. 1933. The acute schizoaffective psychosis. *Amer. J. Psychiat.*, **90**, 97–126.
27. KRAMER, M. *et al.* 1969. Cross-national study of diagnosis of the mental disorders. *Supplement, Amer. J. Psychiat.*, **125**.
28. KREITMAN, N., SAINSBURY, P., MORRISSEY, J., TOWERS, J. and SCRIVENER, J. 1961. The reliability of psychiatric assessment: an analysis. *J. ment. Sci.*, **107**, 887–908.
29. LANGFELDT, G. 1937. *The prognosis in schizophrenia and the factors influencing the course of the disease* (Monograph). London: Humphrey Melford.
30. LANGFELDT, G. 1969. Schizophrenia: diagnosis and prognosis. *Behavioral Science*, **14**, 173–182.
31. LANGFORD, W. S. 1964. Reflections on classification in child psychiatry as related to the activities of the Committee on Child Psychiatry of the Group for the Advancement of Psychiatry. In Diagnostic classification in child psychiatry, Eds R. L. Jenkins and J. O. Cole. *Psychiat. Res. Rep.*, **18**.
32. LEIGH, D. 1968. The form complete. The present state of psychosomatic medicine. *Proc. roy. Soc. Med.*, **61**, 375–384.
33. MACKAY, J. and BIGRAS, J. 1967. Classification des diagnostics pedo-psychiatriques. *Canad. psychiat. Ass. J.*, **12**, 305–315.
34. MOREL, B. A. 1860. *Traité des maladies mentales*. Paris: Masson.
35. NORRIS, V. 1959. *Mental illness in London*. Maudsley Monogr., **6**.
36. PLATTER, F. 1662. *A golden practice of physick*. London: Peter Cole.
37. RAWNSLEY, K. 1966. An international diagnostic exercise. Proc. IVth World Congress of Psychiatry. *Excerpta Medica Int. Congr.*, Series No. 117, p. 360.
38. RAYNER, E. W. 1966. The concept of psychosis. *Medical Proceedings*, **12**, 443–449.
39. ROBINS, E. and GUZE, S. B. 1970. Establishment of diagnostic validity in psychiatric illness. Its application to schizophrenia. *Amer. J. Psychiat.*, **126**, 983–987.
40. ROTH, M. 1960. The phobic anxiety-depersonalization syndrome and some general aetiological problems in psychiatry. *J. Neuropsychiat.*, **1**, 293.
41. ROTH, M. 1963. Neurosis, psychosis and the concept of disease in psychiatry. *Acta psychiat. scand.*, **39**, 128–145.
42. RUTTER, M. 1965. Classification and categorization in child psychiatry. *J. child Psychol. Psychiat.*, **6**, 71–83.
43. RUTTER, M., LEBOVICI, S., EISENBERG, L., SNEZNEVSKY, A. V., SADOUN, R., BROOKE, E. and LIN, T. 1969. A tri-axial classification of mental disorders in childhood. An international study. *J. child Psychol. Psychiat.*, **10**, 41–61.
44. SANDIFER, M. G., HORDERN, A., TIMBURY, G. C. and GREEN, L. M. 1969. Similarities and differences in patient evaluation by U.S. and U.K. psychiatrists. *Amer. J. Psychiat.*, **126**, 206–212.
45. SCHNEIDER, K. 1959. *Clinical psychopathology*. London/New York: Grune & Stratton.
46. SHEPHERD, M., BROOKE, E. M., COOPER, J. E. and LIN, T. 1968. An experimental approach to psychiatric diagnosis. An international study. *Acta psychiat. scand.*, **44**, Suppl. 201.

47. SNEZHNEVSKY, A. V. 1968. The symptomatology, clinical forms and nosology of schizophrenia. In *Modern perspectives in world psychiatry*, Ed J. G. Howells. Edinburgh: Oliver & Boyd.
48. STENGEL, E. 1959. Classification of mental disorders. *Bulletin of World Health Organization*, 21, 601–663.
49. STENGEL, E. 1960. A comparative study of psychiatric classifications. *Proc. roy. soc. Med.*, 53, 123–130.
50. STENGEL, E. 1967. Recent developments in classification. In *Recent developments in schizophrenia*, Eds A. Coppen and A. Walk. Ashford: Headley Brothers Ltd.
51. STEPHENS, J. H. and ASTRUP, C. 1963. Prognosis in 'process' and 'non-process' schizophrenia. *Amer. J. Psychiat.*, 119, 945.
52. STIERLIN, H. 1967. Bleuler's concept of schizophrenia: a confusing heritage. *Amer. J. Psychiat.*, 123, 996–1001.
53. STRELTSOVA, N. 1964. *The Korsakoff Journal of Neuropathology and Psychiatry*, 64, 1.
54. STRÖMGREN, E. 1969. Uses and abuses of concepts in psychiatry. *Amer. J. Psychiat.*, 126, 777–788.
55. SYDENHAM, T. 1682. Dissertatio epistolaris ad Gulielmum Cole, M.D. . . . de affectione hysterica. Quoted by R. Hunter and I. Macalpine, 1964, in *Three hundred years of psychiatry*. London: Oxford University Press.
56. TAYLOR, F. K. 1967. The role of phenomenology in psychiatry. *Brit. J. Psychiat.*, 113, 765–770.
57. WILLIS, T. 1672. De Anima Brutorum. Quoted by R. Hunter and I. Macalpine, 1964, in *Three hundred years of psychiatry*. London: Oxford University Press.
58. WING, J. K., BIRLEY, J. L. T., COOPER, J. E., GRAHAM, P. and ISAACS, A. D. 1967. Reliability of a procedure for measuring and classifying 'present psychiatric state'. *Brit. J. Psychiat.*, 113, 499–515.
59. WORLD HEALTH ORGANIZATION, 1967. *Manual of the International Statistical Classification of Diseases, Injuries, and Causes of Death*. 8th Revision, 1965, Vol. 1, Section V—Mental Disorders. Geneva, W.H.O.
60. YUDIN, M. 1941. Schizophrenia as a primary defect—psychosis. *Papers of the Central Psychiatric Institute*, 2.
61. ZUBIN, J. (Ed). 1961. *Field studies in the mental disorders*. New York/London: Grune & Stratton.
62. ZUBIN, J. 1967. Classification of the behavior disorders. *Ann. Rev. Psychol.*, 18, 373–401.

X

THE RANGE OF PSYCHOSOMATIC DISORDERS IN ADOLESCENCE

HERBERT I. HARRIS

B.S., M.D.

Adolescent Unit,
Children's Hospital Medical Center, Boston, Mass., U.S.A.

1

Introduction

The use of the term 'psychosomatic' implies that only disorders so named have an emotional disturbance that accompanies the physical disorder.[3] I believe that every disturbance that occurs in the body will be found to have an emotional component. The emotional ingredient may not be apparent to the sufferer but, however slight, it is somewhere registered in the central nervous system. For this reason, I consider it essential that every physician should be able to treat the emotional reverberations caused by any disorder in any part of the body.

In order to understand the range of psychosomatic disorders in adolescence it is well to describe the nature of adolescence and the phases of it in which different illnesses occur. The age of youth should not be regarded as a homogeneous block of years during which the process of maturing from childhood to adulthood takes place. So many maturational processes overlap, that it is with difficulty we can distinguish definite phases of adolescence. Rough divisions are possible, however, and are helpful in shaping treatment procedures.

Time-duration

We tend to lose sight of the fact that time-duration in adolescence is a different value from that found in childhood or adulthood. A Colles fracture at the age of six years is an entirely different emotional experience from that of the same fracture at age sixteen or at age twenty-six. There is a tendency to forget the tremendous evolutionary pace that obtains in childhood and only begins to slow down in adolescence. It is a relatively easy imaginative effort to conceive of the millions of years of evolution recapitulated by the human foetus during its nine months *in utero*. It is more difficult to grasp the gradual deceleration in the speed of evolutionary recapitulation in infancy, childhood and adolescence. The spinal cord, for example, is not fully myelinated until the eighteenth month post partum. What kind of diffuse stimuli are being recorded by the cerebrum during this period of neural development? So that the length of time a disability is experienced by an adolescent has an emotional impact that is quite different from that same time experience felt in childhood or adult life. Just as a chronic disease like diabetes has a profound emotional impact at any time of life, so a seemingly brief attack of chicken pox in adolescence may have profound traumatic effect, depending upon what period in adolescence it occurs.

Developmental Phases

The onset of adolescence at puberty is marked psychologically by difficulty in expressing thought and feeling. This period is one in which psychically there appears to be a change taking place in the way in which the person uses words. It seems as if in childhood and latency the emotional color of words is limited or, when rich, applies to a relatively small number of words; during childhood and latency, words are little used to express strong feeling. It is only with the onset of puberty that the person suppresses the various physical means to express strong feeling (hitting, crying, etc) and begins to try to express his emotions with words. Expressing emotion in words is no easy matter, as our greatest poets and writers will testify. It is not surprising, then, to find our adolescent encountering difficulties in expressing himself and so appearing to be extremely taciturn or monosyllabic in early adolescence. Psychotherapy during this phase is difficult, but if patience is exercised and the therapist tries to supply the groping speaker with suitable words to express his feelings, gratifying results can sometimes be obtained.

The first three years of adolescence (approximately) are likely to be averbal. This paucity of words is compensated for by joining a group or gang whose common vocabulary is sparse, shared by the group and may act as a sign of membership in the group. This is the time in adolescence when secret languages are devised, as much to draw the group together as to exclude adults. The great emotional task of the middle years of adolescence is the resolution of the remaining bonds to the parents. Most of the psychosomatic problems encountered in this phase of adolescence will be found to contain elements of this important conflict. The diminishing dependency on the parents carried over the latency years from infancy together with whatever remains of imitation of the parent of the opposite sex is sloughed off at this time, to be replaced by manners and attitudes copied from some more immediate hero or heroine of the same sex as the maturing adolescent. These changes prepare the youth or maiden for the final task of adolescence

—the capacity to love a contemporary of the opposite sex and accept and engage in heterosexual love. This task completed, there remains little more than the gradual assumption of the role of a mature and responsible adult.

The homosexual adolescent of either sex has failed to complete this final phase of oedipal conflict resolution and so remains incapable of loving any but those of his or her own sex. Because the full libidinal potential of the personality has not been mobilized by complete identification with his or her own sex, homosexual love at its most intensive never reaches the level of passion, devotion and self-abnegation of heterosexual love. A stable level of identification so steadies the emotional activity of late adolescence that the occurrence of psychic or somatic disorders is markedly diminished.

It is plain that a large number of our adolescents do not succeed in passing smoothly through these phases of adolescence. In fact, I incline to the view that most of the emotional problems of adults, with or without physical components, stem from failures to accomplish the tasks of adolescence and reach emotional maturity or adulthood.

The Emotional Component

The psychosomatic problems that bring adolescents to the physician usually have a significant burden of emotion. It is important to remember that the emotions involved in the doctor–patient relationship tend to seek earlier levels of emotional development no matter how slight the disability. The sufferer tends to seek, in his memories of an earlier, happier time, the comfort that his disability denies him in the present. The man of the house, for example, in bed with a bad cold, becomes fussy, petty and morose, and a trial to his mothering wife.

The same tendency to use emotionally immature ways of coping with illness is even more striking and unpredictable in adolescence. The emotional turbulence of the adolescent, because of the inner pressures it creates, is only too ready to attach itself to any somatic disorder, intensifying its symptomatology to such a degree that the clinician will often be surprised by the intensity of the symptoms with such minor physical changes.

Whatever the degree of physical disorder and the emotional discord accompanying it, the range of psychosomatic disorders in adolescence is wide and varied; and the familiar axiom that the 'gravity of the symptom parallels the gravity of the disease' is of uncertain value when applied to adolescent illness.

The emotional changes that occur in adolescence help to explain the incongruity of the symptoms that accompany psychosomatic disorders in this age group. For the adolescent youth or maiden is subject to a kind of recapitulation of the stages of emotional development which they passed through in infancy—the first five years of life.[6] Most clinicians are familiar with these stages, which were originally called by Freud[4] the oral, anal, urethro-phallic and genital in the order of their appearance, in the course of the infant's development. Coloring all the time of infancy, and indeed never

I

totally abandoning any of us, is the self-love and self-regard that seems to be at its most intense at birth [5] and which, as the objects in the infant's environment impinge upon him, becomes diluted and changed so that much of its original energy is probably transmuted into the capacity to love.

In adolescence, however, there is a resurgence of self-love or narcissism which, when physical or emotional illness occurs, can be further intensified to become the anxious self-regard of hypochondria. Few clinicians, perceptive and discerning as they may be, are aware of the severity of the hypochondria that may be found in adolescent illness. Adolescent males, for example, are encouraged to be able to 'take it' or to keep 'a stiff upper lip' when experiencing pain. Many adolescents are able to hold to this attitude only by dint of exerting great emotional tension, whose effects may extend far beyond the immediate traumatic experience. As with the adult, any interruption in health causes a degree of emotional regression in the adolescent and, because of greater instability, the adolescent may react far more regressively than the average adult. In such emotional regression, recourse to narcissistic attitudes may produce a much more severe hypochondria than a comparable illness would excite in an adult. It is well for the clinician to maintain a sensitive restraint in working with his adolescent patients and to exert every effort to discover and illuminate the emotional component that accompanies it.

Approaching the various systems of the body in the psychosomatic ills of adolescence the symbolic meanings of parts of the body are helpful in assessing how much emotion has been invested in a body part or system by the patient. It is remarkable, for example, how many children regard their bodies as a phallus and continue this attitude throughout adolescence. As a result of this usually unconscious attitude, symptomatology connected with the head carries with it a considerable amount of castration anxiety. While the headache may be nothing more than an expression of suppressed anger, it is well to treat it with the gravity that all complaints centered in this region deserve.

2

Range of Psychosomatic Disorders

With the continuing prevalence of electronic rock bands and the various psychedelic sound effects calculated to 'turn on' the adolescent, we must expect to find *hearing losses* of up to 45 per cent and the psychological concomitants of such loss in young people. The loss of hearing in a young or middle-aged adult is a severe psychic trauma. A sensory input that helped to maintain emotional and nervous homeostasis is lost. Complete sensory deprivation of sight, hearing, touch produces psychotic-like manifestations in the majority of persons so deprived.[9] The sudden or gradual loss of hearing is a major sensory loss, because sound input is continuous and unable to be shut off by the receiving organ. So that hearing loss is a more serious sensory loss than the loss of some of the other sensory modalities.

The commonest psychopathologic response to hearing loss is the development of suspiciousness that can progress to a measure of paranoia. The sufferer may see two people talking and smiling and, being unable to hear what they are saying, refers their actions to himself—he is being laughed at.

Loss of hearing by an adolescent can be even more emotionally disturbing. I have already referred to the constant preoccupation with themselves that is so widespread among this age group. Narcissistic self-regard is easily observed in the way in which hours are spent in front of the mirror by the average adolescent boy or girl. The resurgence of narcissism in adolescence provides fertile ground for paranoid behavior to develop, so that we may expect hearing loss to be extremely disturbing to the average adolescent. If we add to the self-love of the adolescent the reactivation of latent homosexuality that occurs in this age range, further pressure for the development of paranoid attitudes develops.

A disturbance in *vision* requires careful evaluation by the clinician in his effort to measure the emotional component accompanying it. Most eye problems are rather promptly referred to the ophthalmologist, so that the physician to adolescents does not have many opportunities to treat eye conditions and the psychopathy that goes with them. The eye has long been an organ invested with strong feeling and the many figures of speech in our language testify to the aggressive and phallic properties associated with the eye. 'His hot gaze pierced her through and through', 'He darted a glance . . .', 'She looked daggers at her rival', 'His eyes blazed with passion', 'Her barbed glances', and many others attest to the association with phallic penetration with which we regard the eye and the look. The paired disorders of voyeurism and exhibitionism further reveal how much healthy and unhealthy emotion is invested in vision. In the adolescent, damage to the eye may cause strong emotional reactions since, for some adolescents, the pervasive anxiety of castration may be centered in the eyes. The familiar psychotherapeutic manœuvres of ventilation and interpretation often work surprisingly rapidly when used in treating a psychosomatic eye condition.

The narcissistic preoccupation with one's personal appearance that besets most adolescents often chooses the nose as a focus of discontent. A vulnerable Kieselbach's area may produce annoying nose-bleeds which serve to invest the nose with even more emotion. The occasional girl who has nasal vascularity that oozes at the time of menstruation will also be found to have excessive investment of feeling about her nose. At this period of life, too, the whole question of plastic surgery to alter the appearance of the nose reaches a critical state. It is most important to have a careful psychological evaluation of the adolescent patient who wishes his nose altered, preferably continuing over several sessions with an understanding therapist.

The *mouth* is so highly charged with deep-seated feelings—witness the smoking addicts—that the psychosomatic ills that focus on it are numerous. Perhaps the most striking of these is the well-known anorexia nervosa.

'C.W.', 22 years old, Epsom, England, ballet dancer, hated food and died of malnutrition because her religious belief forbade her to ask medical help, a coroner's inquest was told. Miss W., a Christian Scientist, had been suffering from anorexia nervosa, a psychological disease in which victims—mostly young women—slowly starve themselves to death. She died last March weighing sixty pounds.

This brief paragraph is a vivid reminder of the gravity with which psycho-somatic disorders must be approached. In the cases of anorexia I have treated I have found a common psychological mechanism which comprises a nearly psychotic hatred of the mother, an equally exaggerated fear of 'putting on weight' and a peculiar kind of harsh punitive attitude toward the body—probably in part because it is a female one like the mother's. In the successful treatment of this condition the therapist's personality is of paramount importance. The therapist should be warm and active, en-couraging the development of a strong transference in the patient. The warmth of the patient's regard for her therapist displaces the primitive infantile rage for the mother and the patient eats and regains weight to win the praise, esteem and love of her therapist.

The opposite condition to anorexia nervosa, namely bulimia with obesity has, dynamically, a similar need in the patient. In these cases the leading force that moves them is the internalized rage (usually at the mother), with depression and recourse to food to ameliorate the depression. One objective of the excessive eating in these cases is to devour and reduce to waste matter the people in the patient's immediate experience who are the targets of her rage.

The *teeth* are an important site of emotional disturbance which can cause marked changes in the personality of the adolescent and mobilize such strong expressions of feeling that it is difficult to believe that small objects like teeth can produce such profound reactions. Again we have evidence from many recorded and analyzed dreams that the teeth, in some indi-viduals, are strongly erotized and represent phallic symbols. It can be seen that the extraction of teeth can awaken the old childhood fears of castration which reach a high pitch of intensity in adolescence because of the rising recapitulation of infantile stages of emotional development mentioned above.

The *throat* and neck in adolescence are often the seat of psychosomatic disorders. Two common colloquialisms indicate emotional bases for their occurrence. A person is described as 'choking with rage' and an obnoxious person is referred to as 'a pain in the neck'. Rage, and the anxiety that often accompanies it, may produce a variety of responses from a slight cough referred to as 'a catch in the throat' through hyperventilation to attacks of severe bronchial asthma. Again, the clinician cannot be too often reminded that all psychosomatic conditions occur in a spectrum of gradation from mild to severe depending upon at least three factors: (1) the amount of previous trauma the disordered site has received, at the time of symptom onset; (2) the length of time the noxious psychic and/or physical stimuli have been affecting the site; and (3) the nature of the ameliorating influences affecting the individual at the same time.

Intimately related to the throat and neck, the oesophagus and its appendage, the *gastro-intestinal tract*, is the seat of many psychosomatic disorders. The popular colloquialism, 'he can't stomach that', in which the noun is verbalized, embodies the typical psychosomatic state in which strong feeling activates an organ or region and produces a disorder of function. Heartburn or 'waterbrash' is commonly found in gastritis of any type and may occur in oesophagitis, too. It may at times be a larval form of vomiting and represent a wish to reject either a person or a situation that has acquired emotional overtones which the patient cannot tolerate.

In approaching the psychosomatic disorders of the splanchnic region one must constantly bear in mind the wide spectrum of ills that one will encounter from this area. Anyone who has had to make a public appearance has probably experienced symptoms caused by the acute stress he is under. Our language is full of idiomatic references to the symptoms caused by the influence of strong feelings on the splanchnic region. One of the commonest expressions is, 'butterflies in the stomach'. A 'lump in the stomach', like 'lump in the throat', expresses an intensity of emotion that may be accompanied by 'eyes filling up' (larval weeping) and tremors. The symptoms that arise from this region can be both acute and chronic. The acute and usually transitory symptoms illustrate more vividly the psychosomatic nature of many of these conditions. The elaborate sympathetic and parasympathetic innervation of the splanchnic region is the background against which the many psychosomatic disorders develop. This same elaborate innervation helps to explain why so many stomachic conditions are so chronic and resistant to treatment. I would assert categorically at this point that no abdominal disorder will heal effectively and permanently unless both organic and psychic treatment proceed hand in hand. Even the radical surgical procedures do not effect any appreciable change in the patient's basic emotional problem, with the exception of one condition farther along the gastro-intestinal tract—ulcerative colitis and colostomy.

There seems to be little cause to doubt the many observations by many different investigators that a large number of peptic ulcers are caused by the persistence in the patient of infantile attitudes never discarded despite the physical and psychic maturation of other aspects of the personality. These attitudes derive chiefly from the earliest or oral stage of infantile emotional development and represent an unrequited demand for love and attention that was not supplied in infancy. This finding is confirmed by studies of the mothers of peptic ulcer patients who were found to be in many respects similar to the mothers of schizophrenic patients.[1] They seem to be unable to provide their infants with the kind of warmth and attention that enables the infant personality to unfold and reach out to the world around it, obtaining ever greater supplies of warmth and attention as the people in the child's environment respond to its outward-reaching attitudes.

The *liver* appears to be singularly immune to emotional reverberations, although this may appear to be so because we have not yet developed sufficiently refined diagnostic skills to demonstrate a correlation between emotional disturbances and hepatic activity. True, we will find a degree of depression accompanying jaundice of almost any kind but we incline to consider this more of a somato-psychic response.

When we study disturbances of *pancreatic function*, especially diabetes, however, we encounter impressive emotional responses accompanying this disorder in adolescence. This large emotional factor occurs in part because of the reactivation of narcissistic activity in this age group. This self-regarding tendency, when accompanied by anxiety, can give rise to true hypochondria. In diabetes, the adolescent boy or girl, much concerned with self, finds himself beset with an illness from which he will never recover and which requires constant care and attention to diet and medication. Such repetitive demands are a reminder that one has a handicap unlike his fellows and, while it is not as obvious (on the surface) as a crippled limb, it does damage the adolescent's image of himself. This damage is so severe that at times the rage against fate which a handicap like diabetes arouses is turned inward by the adolescent producing suicidal thoughts and attempts. One sixteen-year-old diabetic boy I knew used to skip his insulin and then run as far and as fast as he could to bring on a hypoglycemic attack which represented a very close approach to death itself. A paper published some years ago described the cases of four diabetic adolescent girls, each of whom was depressed, had suicidal thoughts and made suicidal attempts.[7] The psychotherapy of cases of this kind is usually difficult and time-consuming. It is in psychosomatic disorders like this that the well-rounded clinician who can treat the disease and the emotional decompensation that accompanies it, is indeed the flower of our profession.

Mucous and ulcerative *colitis* have large emotional components which are shown most dramatically by the striking change in manner and even personality observed in sufferers from ulcerative colitis who have had a colostomy and wear a colostomy bag. These people are almost excessively cheerful and thoughtful of others, and become quite gregarious. The clubs that spring up in hospitals where a number of patients attend post-colostomy clinics are noteworthy for the cheerful helpfulness that prevails among them. I am not familiar with any continuing psychological studies in depth that have followed these patients before and after colostomy.

I viewed the psychodynamics surrounding the colostomy and the bag as one involving infantile and hence primitive, feeling and attitude. Expressions of primitive feeling and the development of profound (anaclitic) dependence on the therapist are commonly met with in the therapy of the colitides. Therefore, the internalized rage that causes the mucosa of the colon to 'blaze' with fury becomes symbolically externalized by the ritual of the colostomy operation and the visual evidence of the bag and its contents. The bag, like a totem, is taken by the primitive unconscious of the patient as witness to the removal of the bad part of his personality. Relieved of this burden, the patient's personality is freed to work with the positive elements it possesses, and the striking changes we witness in the post-colostomized patient take place. Psychotherapy with these patients brings out a most intense anaclitic relationship to the therapist who is besieged with insatiable demands from the patient.[10] Following colostomy, this intense dependency recedes, to be replaced, we must assume, by the gregariousness that characterizes so many of these patients.

Constipation would appear to be the obverse face of the coin of ulcerative colitis. It is a common symptom in the emotionally disturbed adolescent and, when the patient is deeply disturbed, may be accompanied by *encopresis*. While encopresis in the child may signal the development of a severe disorder (and this observation holds for most adolescents, too), there are times when the sign represents a relatively benign and easily treated condition.

A fifteen-year-old boy was presented by his mother with the complaint of encopresis of five years' duration. He had been difficult to toilet train as a child but was completely trained by age five. He was of low normal intelligence and showed no other physical or emotional defects. The encopresis had begun shortly after his parents had divorced and he had not seen his father since the divorce. Acting on the possibility that his symptom might represent a grieving for his father, the patient was encouraged to speak at length about his sire. Within a few sessions he began to express not only his grieving for his absent father but also his hidden rage toward his mother whom he considered responsible for 'sending his father away'. The ventilation of this matter was followed by a considerable change in the patient's manner and appearance. He began to groom himself and sometime about the fifth or sixth visit he reported that the encopresis had stopped. He was seen in follow-up six months later and reported no return of the symptom and no further difficulties at home or at school.

The genito-urinary system is the seat of many psychosomatic conditions although in adolescence they are on the whole less frequent than in adult life. One of the most commonly encountered is enuresis, usually persisting sporadically from childhood and becoming more troublesome when the young person gets into states of increased emotional tension. When all the possible physical causes for bed-wetting have been ruled out, a careful study of the emotional make-up of the patient should be made. Commonest of the psychic causes for persistent enuresis is repressed rage. The case of a sixteen-year-old girl illustrates this kind of enuresis. She was the only one in her family afflicted with this disorder and came to The Adolescents'

Unit in some desperation, because she had just been accepted by a nearby college for matriculation in the Fall. Fear that she would wet her bed in the girls' dormitory was intense. Various forms of treatment had failed and she and her family were discouraged about her future college career. By good fortune she reported, at the beginning of her second interview, a vivid dream in which her father was leading a parade down a street while she shot at and killed him from an upstairs window. It was not difficult with this hint to encourage the patient to bespeak her hidden fury towards her father. He was at times overbearing and at times affectionate and her feelings for him were confused but vengeful. After she had enlarged upon the rage which her father aroused in her, her relation to him moderated and her enuresis ceased. She reported two months later, just before entering college, symptom-free and in eager anticipation of the excitement of college life.

Another common psychosomatic disorder in adolescence is dysmenorrhea. I have found this condition in a number of girls who were having difficulty making an appropriate sexual identification. Many of these girls were tomboys and showed little concern for their appearance. It seemed as if their dysmenorrhea was body language which expressed the anger they felt because they were not boys. Some of these cases showed a prompt response to psychotherapy when the therapist was a young and attractive physician. Positive transference feelings for him promptly set in and the girls began to cast off the tomboy attire and 'fix themselves up' with lipstick and feminine decor. The added effect of this primping was that boys in school with them began to pay attention to them, their social activities increased and the dysmenorrhea disappeared.

Of the genito-urinary ills that beset the adolescent, pregnancy and venereal disease have impressive emotional concomites. The number of unmarried pregnant girls in Western society has never been higher. Fueled by the explosive population pressure, social forces have been released that are overwhelming age-old value systems related to pregnancy, abortion and marriage. The hippie movement has produced forms of compound marriage and, to avoid the draft, a large number of unregistered children. Former religious values are regarded by many young people to be a product of the Establishment and hence rejected. Much of the emotion surrounding pregnancy may be in the anxiety-driven urge to escape from the turmoil of adolescence into the hopefully less turbulent state of adulthood. As a consequence, teenage girls are in some cases eager to become mothers and leave the uncertainties about their adolescence behind them. Unfortunately, pregnancy and motherhood do not invariably solve the problems of emotional maturation, and we find young mothers who treat their infants like toys or, in some cases, like rival sibs with the hostility that such a relationship provokes. It is likely that some of the battered-infant cases are caused by emotionally immature adolescent parents treating their infants as a baby brother or sister.

The emotional responses to venereal disease range, as one might expect, from casual disregard of gonorrhea as 'a cold' to abject terror and syphilophobia. The art of treatment of these cases requires a nice balance between intensifying the concern and anxiety of the casual (and hence careless) adolescent and the reassurance and, if necessary, psychotherapy of the syphilophobe.

The disturbed emotional tone of the *epileptic* is comparable in some respects to that encountered with any chronic disease, like diabetes. The emotional disturbances generated by the repeated shocks of epilepsy are often severe and have, in some cases produced a personality profile considered consistent with an epileptic diathesis. The frequent history of migraine in the background of epileptic patients confirms the large emotional component one may expect to find in this disorder. Some patients suffering from migraine have been shown to be expressing violent rage with their attacks of hemicrania. The epileptic attack has been shown to be, on occasion, a defense mechanism used to neutralize attacks of violent fury toward some emotionally significant person in the patient's life. Epilepsy in adolescence is unusually burdensome because of its suddenness, its loss of consciousness and the postictal confusion. The adolescent beset with this disease may be expected to show poor schoolwork, confused thinking, sometimes a paranoid coloring to his personality, and depression. Again, the damage to the adolescent's ideal of himself is especially severe in this disorder because he is repeatedly rendered as helpless as he was in infancy by the recurrent attacks. Whether the condition is severe with Jacksonian characteristics and psycho-motor equivalents or mild with repeated brief blackouts, continuing support and psychotherapy as an adjunct to the medication can be of great value for the patient's present and future adjustment to his disease.

In like manner, *migraine*, a disease which usually has its onset late in adolescence will profit greatly by appropriate psychotherapeutic manoeuvers. Dr Jacob Finesinger, whose teaching of psychotherapy was much admired at The Massachusetts General Hospital, had a characteristic admonition that he used with his student, 'Go after her hostility!' If the student was successful in enabling his patient to ventilate her hostility, he was usually rewarded by a striking amelioration of the hemicrania.

Migraine and epilepsy are rarely associated with *hysteria* and the true hysterical personality in which conversion symptoms are encountered is something of a rarity in this age of debunking. Transitory attacks of hysteria may be encountered in adolescence but as a rule these are short-lived and respond promptly to psychotherapy. The case of a menarchial girl thirteen years of age who was having attacks of hallucinations is instructive. It has much of the quality of a tale from an earlier time in our history. The young young girl's hallucinations were that of a 'little man' who appeared to her usually at bed-time dancing on the end of her bed or on other articles of furniture in her bedroom. Her parents, the family priest and other interested adults had attempted to exorcize the apparition to no avail. A short talk with the patient convinced the author that the girl was hysteric and a suspicion of the nature and origin of the hallucination was confirmed when he asked the girl to draw him a picture of the 'little man'. With utter naivete the patient drew a strikingly accurate picture of an erect penis. By this time, in the first and only interview I had with her, excellent rapport had been established. Mustering all the gravity I could, I informed her that she would find that, having been able to put the 'little man' on paper—much like pinning down a voodoo wax model—she would find that she had rid herself of this troublesome apparition. One month later her mother reported over the phone with touching gratitude that her daughter was free of the hallucination and that, in fact, it never returned after the patient's one session. The remarkable suggestibility of the true hysteric was never more vividly portrayed to me.

I have not encountered any true conversion symptoms in adolescent patients. I have seen cases of adolescents who, having developed some form of muscle spasm, have rid themselves of it with difficulty because some secondary gain was derived from the symptom. The pain and spasm in a stiff neck is sometimes used to enable an adolescent to avoid unpleasant situations like school or required physical activities, but the number of malingerers, conscious or unconscious, is few.

The incidence of *arthritis* in adolescence is relatively low. It is almost axiomatic that, if a patient is found with rheumatoid arthritis in adolescence, it has been present since some time in childhood. This finding is not to be wondered at, since the emotional elements in rheumatoid arthritis are numerous. Much of the emotional tone that accompanies arthritis derives from the earliest levels of infantile development. In some cases which develop without any discoverable infection or traumatic insult there can be demonstrated intense repressed rage at persons close to the sufferer. It is as if the joints were immobilized by the arthritic process to prevent their owner from making violent physical attacks upon those close to him. Having been made a site of lowered resistance, the joint may then become prey to any traumatic or infective insult that attacks the host. Certainly the joint and muscle pains that attack one when beset with an influenzal virus suggest the likelihood of these organisms working greater damage on an arthritic joint than they would on a normal one.

While psychic influence upon the joints can be excessive and hence traumatic, the effects of the emotions on the *endocrine* organization can well-nigh approach the overwhelming. Consider the effects of prolonged fright and anxiety on the thyroid gland. Observing a typical adolescent patient with hyperthyroidism one cannot help remarking the patent signs of anxiety and fear that the endocrine influences produce in the sufferer. The onset of some cases of adolescent hyperthyroidism are so often related to some severe psychic or emotional trauma that sometimes we are tempted to seek this cause before examining the actual endocrine abnormalities that have taken place.

There is still so much excess emotion attached to the study of the activities of the gonads in adolescence that we would be remiss if we did not point to the blatant changes—physical, psychic and emotional—that take place in adolescence whenever the gonads undergo the maturational changes that occur at puberty. Here is a time when the art of the physician, i.e. his ability to do psychotherapy, is of profound importance. It is not widely known, and naturally less widely accepted, how important the proper handling of the pubertal adolescent can become. Years ago Mohr[8] reported the case of a girl whose pubescence was inhibited by a number of traumatic experiences. Ten years after puberty was supposed to have begun, the nature of the emotional factors preventing its fruition was brought to light. Within a few months after the emotional basis of this pubertal retardation was revealed to the patient, puberty was completed with appropriate breast development, menarche, increased thyroid gland size and the disappearance of hair from the chin.

The treatment of hypogonadism with various forms of testosterone and its equivalents shows dramatically how greatly endocrine changes can bring about psychic and character changes. The typical hypogonadal adolescent may have a high-pitched voice, be frail and therefore timorous and poorly coordinated. A few months treatment with the appropriate hormone may bring about striking changes in almost every facet of his physique and personality. As our diagnostic skills improve in this highly sensitive area and the refinements in treatment are enabled to follow, the psychosomatic range of adolescent endocrinology will be decisively extended.

Included in the range of psychosomatic disorders in adolescence are, of course, the *infectious diseases*. The adolescent patient's emotional response to any infective insult will depend upon the strength of his ego, i.e. how effectively he can keep repressed the powerful unconscious impulses which appear ordinarily only in delirium or in depressions as hallucinations and delusions. Furthermore, one may expect the adolescent to be more psychically vulnerable to infectious illnesses than the adult, because he is still in the process of personality formation and coping with the unsettling emotional tasks of adolescence.

Many cases of infectious disease may be expected to be complicated by tranquilizers and the effects of psychotomimetic drugs such as L.S.D. and peyote. I do not know of any instances, but it seems entirely reasonable to expect a severe febrile infection to excite a 'flashback' or recurrence of the L.S.D. 'trip' without recourse to additional Lysergic Acid. There are, in addition, many other modern drugs that have been found to produce psychiatric illness, and these may appear in conjunction with a systemic infection and perhaps be reinforced by it. Isoniazid, various tranquilizers, some antibiotics and corticosteroids have all been known to produce psychic disturbances.

The various viral illnesses which attack the brain produce the largest number of psychic disorders. Encephalitides almost invariably cause some mental disturbance in the course of the attack and some of the post-encephalitic syndromata produce serious mental decompensation.

Adolescents who are grieving may, if the grief has never been openly expressed, develop a remarkable *variety of symptoms* in the effort to relieve the inner pressure it creates. An adolescent college student who had turned in a remarkable scholastic performance for the first two years of his undergraduate career, slumped dramatically in his third year and developed vague somatic symptoms. Headache, indigestion and mild insomnia were unrelieved by symptomatic treatment. There was no obvious cause for this striking change in his working ability. In the course of the second interview he mentioned the heavy responsibilities his mother had had to assume since his father's death. It then came out that the previous summer his father had had a severe coronary attack while the family were around their swimming pool. The student had ridden in the ambulance to the hospital with his father who died in his arms on the way. The patient, the oldest child, had made all the funeral arrangements, supervised the reorganization of his father's business so that his mother could continue with it and then, when assured that everything was proceeding satisfactorily, returned to school. He had, throughout this entire period, no experience of grief or mourning but remembered suppressing some feelings of grief at various times. Encouraged to enlarge upon his memories of his father and his love for him, it came out that they had been very close and that the father's death had hurt him very deeply. Extensive ventilation of his hidden feeling worked a dramatic change in the patient and within a short time he was able to resume his college work with his former effectiveness and his somatic complaints vanished.

3

Treatment

The kinds of treatment used for psychosomatic disorders are as many and as varied as those used for the entire range of medical and emotional illness. This wide variety precludes any elucidation of treatment modalities in this limited space. Furthermore, new developments in therapy are appearing frequently, so that much of what is written here might be out of date by the time this is published. Some of the newer forms of treatment have not yet been tested over a sufficient length of time to insure the permanence or the safety of their effects.

The one form of treatment that is effective and has universal applicability is psychotherapy. I firmly believe that it could and should be used to a greater or less extent by every physician treating every patient in his entire clientele. True, many 'natural' psychotherapists do employ little gestures of reassurance and counsel that are part of the great body of psychotherapy. But the great need is that physicians everywhere and in every specialty be aware of the importance of the emotional factors in their patients' illness and be able to recognize signs of emotional distress related to illness, in order to take positive steps to relieve it. The relief of the emotional stress incident to an acute appendicitis is as much a part of the treatment of the syndrome as the incision at McBurney's point and the removal of the inflamed organ. I feel that we still have wide areas for improvement in the practice of medicine. If the recognition and treatment of the emotional tension which accompanies every illness that attacks mankind is included in the therapeutic program, the quality of medical praxis will be greatly improved.

The treatment technique is best learned by a kind of apprentice relationship with a practising psychiatrist. If several physicians band together to work with one psychiatrist, an ideal group arrangement can be worked out. Knowledge of group psychodynamics is readily accessible to most psychiatrists and can contribute importantly to the teaching program.

For the most important possession of the psychotherapist, be he specialist or general practitioner, is the capacity to accept, without outward signs of disapproval or rejection, anything the adolescent patient may say. This age group is inordinately sensitive to non-verbal cues and tends to react to any of the more subtle signs of disapproval by flight from treatment. The capacity to tolerate and accept the extreme attitudes voiced by modern youth is not easily acquired. Participation in a group of physicians led by a psychiatrist in which free and spontaneous exchange of thought and feeling takes place is probably the most effective way to acquire the tolerance and capacity to accept the adolescent patient. It is more than likely, too, that if the physician is emotionally and intellectually unable to accept the adolescent's views he will not be able to treat adolescent illness

When the adolescent college student of today clamors for 'relevance' in his studies, his teachers and his college, he is bespeaking the failure in communication that has developed between his and the older generation.[2] The same breakdown in communication will develop between the physician and his adolescent patient if the former is unable to tolerate and so understand the many emotional facets of the latter's personality. Rebellious anger, erotic sensuality, latent homosexual anxiety, and even eruptions of material that seems psychotic, are all present in the anxious or diffident patient that faces you. Such a patient will sense almost immediately whether or not the physician can accept him, and will respond accordingly. It is only through acceptance and its perception by physician and patient that successful psychotherapy can proceed. Once a physician has experienced group give and take, his acceptance of his adolescent patients increases remarkably and he will find that they are eager to talk with him. The catharsis that uninhibited expression provides is highly therapeutic and provides a flow of speech in the course of which clarification of feeling and often true insight occurs. If, in addition, the physician occasionally repeats some interesting or unusual statement by his patient, he may very well confront him with a view of himself he has not had. In this way, the amelioration of the emotional tension accompanying any and every illness can take place and the patient's recovery can thereby be hastened.

4

Conclusion

In conclusion, I should like to speak of the lamentable schism that has developed between the psychoanalytic therapists at one end of the spectrum and the organicists at the other end. This extreme dichotomy represents a kind of primitive or infantile form of thinking and feeling which tends to classify different schools of therapy into the 'good guys' and the 'bad guys'. Sargants' and Eysenck's vituperations about the psychoanalysts are no less infantile than some of the analytic condemnations of Sargant and Eysenck. The new 'schools' of therapy, viz. behavior, 'desensitizing' and 'flooding' techniques, have all been employed long ago and derive much of their value from the works of Mesmer, Pavlov and Jacobson.

What is lost sight of by all these 'out strouting cluster fists', as Doctor Rabelais called them, is the patient. My concern over the past twenty-five years has been for the patient and the doctor who treats him. I have therefore devoted much of my time to the teaching of physicians—general practitioners, pediatricians and internists—in the simple and human ways of listening to people in distress. This is called 'psychotherapy', a poly-syllable for a process that is as old as mankind. It is remarkable, too, that this process of listening constitutes the art of medicine, and no bureaucracy or assembly-line method of treating the ills of human kind will ever be able to take its place. The adolescent patient comes to the physician with mixed and turbulent feelings. We have but to listen in all honesty to hear the age-old saga of youth trying to become man. If we listen well and with compassion, we shall find that this seemingly simple process will fill the adolescent patient with life and love and enable him to reach out like Blake's 'Glad Day' to embrace maturity with the challenge, the passion and the glory it deserves.

REFERENCES

1. ALEXANDER, FRANZ. 1934. The influence of psychological factors upon gastro-intestinal disturbances. *Psychoanal. Quart.*, 3.
2. CROWSON, R. A. 1967. Science and phenomenology. *Nature, Lond.*, 223, 1318–1319.
3. DUNBAR, F. 1954. *Emotions and bodily changes* (4th edition). New York: Columbia University Press.
4. FREUD, S. 1938. *Infantile sexuality*. In *The basic writings of Sigmund Freud*. Trans. by A. A. Brill. New York: Random House.
5. FREUD, S. 1946. 'On narcissism'. *Collected Papers*, vol. 4. London: Hogarth.

6. JONES, E. 1950. *Papers on psychoanalysis* (5th edition). London: Baillière, Tindall & Cox.

7. MASON, P. 1954. *Psychoanal. Rev.*, **41**, 48.

8. MOHR, FRITZ. 1925. *Psychophysiche Behandslung Methoden.* Leipzig: Huizel.

9. SOLOMON, P., KUBZANSKY, P. E., LEIDERMAN, P. H., MENDELSON, J., TRUMBULL, R., and WEXLER, D. (Eds). 1961. *Sensory deprivation.* Cambridge, Mass.: Harvard University Press.

10. SPERLING, M. 1946. Psychoanalytic study of ulcerative colitis in children. *Psychoanal. Quart.*, **15**, 302.

XI

OBESITY IN ADOLESCENCE

HILDE BRUCH

M.D.

Professor of Psychiatry, Baylor College of Medicine
Houston, Texas
U.S.A.

1

Introduction

There has been in recent years growing awareness that obesity, the excessive accumulation of fat tissues, is a complex condition which presents challenging diagnostic and therapeutic problems. There is even a problem of definition, of at what stage weight and fat accumulation should be rated as excessive. There are adolescents who are desperately unhappy because their weight is slightly above the so-called average, or even about their normal curvatous development, and others who seem to be indifferent to even enormous weight excesses, or who appear helpless in their efforts to fight their ever-increasing weight. Some adolescents have been fat all their lives, since infancy or after entering school; in others the weight increase represents no more than a temporary imbalance during the active growth processes of puberty, or is an expression of their inability to face new tasks and problems from which they withdraw into the state of obesity.

There is also increasing awareness that obesity is a rather complex, far from uniform clinical condition, with disturbances in many areas. There is evidence of hereditary factors in some cases, of disordered regulatory mechanisms in others, of variations in the number of fat cells, of disturbances in deposition and release of fatty acids, and of other metabolic malfunctioning.[1,10] In spite of increasing knowledge, the degree of confusion does not seem to diminish, because the tendency persists to generalize from observations in one group of patients to all forms of obesity. In most instances the underlying constitutional factors are not well defined, nor accessible to specific treatment. For practical management recognition of social and psychological factors appears to be of greater importance.[2]

Obesity due to definite organic causes is quite rare in adolescence. In my wide experience I have seen no case of thus far unrecognized tumor at the base of the brain associated with obesity, and only two, probably three, young patients in whom severe obesity developed following encephalitis, characterized by many changes in behavior, including an uncontrollable desire for food. Such patients will eat whenever food is available, without relationship to any recognizable event or emotional stress. Similar patterns of continuous eating are observed in animals with hypothalamic lesions.

There are also vast differences in the psychological problems associated with obesity. Frequently, the very development of obesity is an expression of underlying emotional problems. Invariably there will be other manifestations of disturbed adjustment. Often such cases are characterized by rapid increases in weight during times of emotional stress, alternating with frantic efforts at reducing. In such patients the study of the weight curve may give clues to the underlying problems and conflicts. With stable weight, too, an evaluation of the total life situation is important for a long-range prognosis and effective treatment. Psychiatric symptoms of obese patients cover a wide range, from minor adjustment difficulties and neurotic disorders to borderline states of frank psychosis. They may be intrinsically related to the weight disturbance, or are only coincidental. There is no personality structure that would apply to all fat people, and the manifold symptoms are difficult to fit into the standard psychiatric classification. The condition is complicated by society's critical and condemning reaction to the obese state, which creates secondary psychological problems. Physicians frequently share this cultural attitude and thus may be handicapped in recognizing the underlying intrapsychic problems, and in maintaining an objective and supportive therapeutic attitude. A more tolerant cultural attitude is of greatest importance for the health profession to avoid reinforcing the damaging problems fat youngsters encounter.

2

Social Aspects

Western culture, on the whole, has been critical, even contemptuous of obesity. In the United States preoccupation with weight, with the demand to be slim, has reached such proportions that every fat person faces some problems in his social relations. Adolescents, in particular, are vulnerable to the social rejection and cultural condemnation which being obese implies. Even those without a weight problem are eternally concerned with their physique and appearance, the adequacy of their development and with how they look to others.

Though recognition of this condemning attitude is long-standing,[2] systematic studies are of recent origin. By comparing a group of obese girls in a reducing camp with girls in a typical summer camp, Monello and Mayer[11] could illustrate, through administration of a series of projective tests, the damaging effect of this cultural pressure, of being victims of intense prejudice, on obese adolescents. They showed heightened sensitivity to and obsessive preoccupation with the state of being fat, combined with a tendency to be passive and to withdraw in the face of group isolation. These obese girls shared 'acceptance of dominant values', and considered obesity, hence their own body, as undesirable and harmful.

In evaluating the 'body image' of obese people, the positive or negative attitude towards their own appearance, Stunkard and Mendelson[17] found that obese adults who had been normal during adolescence felt much less derogatory towards their appearance than those who had been exposed to social rejection and blame for being fat during childhood and adolescence.

There is also a marked variation with social class in the occurrence of and attitude towards obesity. A survey in midtown Manhattan revealed that obesity occurs seven times more often in lower-class women than in the upper class.[12] Conversely, a fat upper-class youngster will encounter more serious psychological and sociological problems than one of lower-class status growing up in surroundings more tolerant of obesity.

Cahnman[9] conducted a sociological study focused on the stigma of obesity and concluded that the obese teenager is discriminated against and made to understand that he deserves it and thus he comes to accept this treatment as just. As a result, he is unable to escape his condition and settles down to live with it. He becomes timidly withdrawn, eager to please and tolerant of abuse. He may escape into intellectual pursuits, assume the role of a funny character, resort to empty boasting or submit to spells of despondency. Whatever avenues of escape he chooses, he interprets himself in the way that is indicated to him, and responds to expectations by accepting dominant values.

The intensity of the rejection of the obese youngster in the American culture was illustrated by Richardson and his associates,[14] who showed drawings of six different types of children (depicting a normal child and five with various abnormalities and disfigurements, incuding an obese child) to 10- and 11-year-old children and asked them to rank the drawings in order of their preference. The majority selected the *obese child* as their *last choice* for a friend, though boys were equally wary of the amputated child.

The importance of these observations cannot be overlooked. The following case reports must be read against the background of this rejecting social attitude. Yet a clinician must also recognize that generalized conclusions may becloud the underlying issues in an individual patient.

Cahnman[9] feels that rejection on account of overweight outranks rejection on account of color, and gives as example the biographical account of a 20-year-old overweight colored girl who was an A-student in college and whose ability was not in question. Describing her social difficulties she felt that problems of racial prejudice became confused with problems of being overweight. 'The latter is a much more severe problem. For instance, I know that colored girls were employed in certain offices where I applied for a job—so my being rejected there could not be attributed to color. At one company, the interviewer said it won't look right for the company to have a lot of overweight people as checkers.' She added: 'The feeling of being discriminated against usually lapses into a feeling of guilt or depression.' Contrary to what she would have done if she had met with color prejudice, she was unable to sustain her protest.

In my experience, in spite of this widespread prejudice, individual obese youngsters will react according to their sense of competence and independence. Many obese adolescents have been obese children. Many, though by no means all, have serious emotional problems. Those with a fairly healthy mental attitude can face their social difficulties with a certain equanimity, or will take it as a challenge to begin a reducing regime, on their own decision. In a large group of obese children who were followed into adulthood, about one-third had outgrown the condition during adolescence.[3] In re-evaluating their early records, in particular the differences in parental attitude, it could be shown that they were the ones who had been accepted by their parents as being heavy, without being exposed to much pressure to reduce. Psychological tests showed them as fairly stable and well-integrated in the development of various mental functions, in contrast to the marked variations in performance of those who were emotionally disturbed.[4] In contrast, those obese youngsters who arrived at adolescence with a low self-esteem, with a sense of helplessness and of not being in control, had reacted with more guilt and depression to the critical cultural attitude. They are the disturbed fat youngsters who will come to the attention of psychiatrists.

As an alternative to Cahnman's example I should like to cite the case of a 24-year-old Negro woman who was outstanding in her intellectual and academic achievement and held the position of instructor at a university. She felt that her obesity had developed in response to her feeling not accepted socially, and that this antedated her obesity. She was the only daughter of parents who held secure semi-professional positions and lived in their own house in a comfortable neighborhood. She was slim as a child and attended a parochial school. Though this was a private school for colored children, she felt discriminated against because she was 'darker' than the others, wore glasses and felt at all times excluded, not part of the group, even the object of jokes. She felt she was always running after the others, never member of the group. When about 8 years old she started to become plump, 'the eating became sort of a compensation', and gained more rapidly after her menarche, at age 11. She weighed 150 pounds when 14 years old. Her parents tried to help her control her food intake by not having any sweets at home, and by restricting her spending money. She reacted with rebellion, tried to get money of her own and to eat as many sweets as possible. This 'craving sugar' persists and she still feels this is a protest against her mother's never having any sweets around. Weight increase was rapid, to 200 pounds at age 16 and over 300 at age 21. Her obesity had not interfered with her professional progress, but she still felt socially a loner, that she is pursuing people, and continuously withdraws in fear of rejection.

Having moved throughout her life within a group of educated Negroes, she felt the early rejection had come from her own group. Though the obesity was now handicapping, she was convinced that weight loss alone would not solve her problem of social inadequacy. She requested a psychiatric consultation when her physician had advised a radical reducing regime.

3

Clinical Case Histories

In view of the great diversity of psychiatric problems in adolescent obesity, a series of sketches will be presented as illustrations of the wide range of such involvement, ranging from normal adjustment, though overweight, to obsessive concern with weight, inability to form personal relations, withdrawal into a fantasy life, and, finally, to psychotic disorganization.

Not all forms of overweight during adolescence are abnormal; a certain weight excess is part of the rapid growth and development during puberty. The blossoming of adolescence has always been known and was admired as beauty, in other times and cultures, or, at least, it was accepted as part of the growing-up process, or as an individual's reaction to this event. In the United States, with the overemphasis on slimness, this leads to continuous preoccupation of adolescents with diets and reducing. Many healthy adolescents are successful in this effort and maintain the desired weight, with or without medical supervision. Others accept their plumpness as part of their makeup. A psychiatrist will see only those who encounter difficulties in living which may, or may not, be related to the obesity, though invariably the obesity will be blamed as the cause of all difficulties.

CASE 1

Normal adjustment

This is one of the rare instances where psychiatric consultation was requested for an essentially normal plump adolescent. Amy was 18 years old, 5 feet 1 inch tall and weighed 175 pounds. She looked attractive, was well-groomed and well-dressed in clothes that were designed to flatter her figure.

Her mother had arranged for this consultation while a two-year younger sister was in therapy. Though slim, this girl had serious problems in school, academically and socially. She blamed her difficulties on her mother who, she felt, had been overcontrolling and overdemanding throughout her life.

Amy agreed that mother was somewhat difficult but she knew how to handle her; in addition, she always had had a supportive friend in her grandmother. The consultation about her obesity was just one example of mother's trying to run everybody's life. She knew that her appearance was not fashionable but she was not too concerned about it. She felt she had inherited her grandmother's makeup, her quiet and considerate temperament and her short stocky figure. Grandmother was quite an outstanding person, not only on account of her husband's prominent social position but in her own right, having stimulated and organized a number of worthwhile social projects. Amy was aware of the change in taste, that being plump fifty years ago was not the same social handicap as it was now. Nevertheless, she had found out that she functioned better, was more interested in what was going on in the world, did better in her studies and, in particular, was socially more responsive, when she had what she felt was her natural weight. Under mother's pressure, she had repeatedly tried to reduce, and had even lost 10 or 20 pounds. However, she felt so tense and uneasy that she had come to the decision that to maintain her present weight was the wiser choice.

She was grateful for support of her view that her general functioning was more important than her appearance.[5] About a year later she came to tell me about her engagement to an attractive young man with whom she had many interests in common. When she had raised the question that her weight might be socially embarrassing to him, he had replied that he was marrying *a person*, not *a figure*. Their marriage turned out well. There were two children, without excess weight gain during or after the pregnancy. Ten years later her weight was exactly the same as it had been at age 18, too plump by contemporary fashionable standards but not interfering with an active and meaningful life.

CASE 2

Obsessive concern

Brenda's story may serve as contrast. When 18 years old she became acutely depressed during her senior year in High School. She felt she was destined to lead a lonely life because no man could love her because she was 'too fat'—and a brilliant student. She was tall, 5 feet 8 inches. Her weight had never been above 135 pounds, but since age 15 she had been obsessed with dieting. She had forced her weight down to 110 pounds but then was acutely unhappy because whe was embarrassed by remarks about her being too skiny. She tried also to be less conscientious about her school work in order to be 'like everybody else', but then was unhappy when her grades dropped. For a while she dated a young man and took part in social activities of her group. He seemed to be in love with her but she had no real feelings for him. She became alarmed when she gained some weight, to about 125 pounds, during this more relaxed period. Now she missed the remarks about how thin she looked. She became so depressed that she needed to interrupt her schooling.

Obsessive concern with her weight and figure was in this girl a camouflage for deep-seated self-doubt and confusion. Though more extreme than usual, her concern is akin to that of many modern adolescents who feel attractiveness is measured in pounds and inches, and will use any degree of plumpness as alibi to avoid the possibility of sexual contact.

CASE 3

Phobic concern

In Carla's case, aged 13, fear of fatness interfered with her puberal development. She had always been a tense child, closer to her father than to her mother. She was an only child until age 7, when twin sisters were born, and a brother a year later. She was an excellent student and had a small circle of friends; recently she had become concerned about not being 'popular'. During the past year she had clung to a diet because she had noted that during the preceding year she had gained 12 pounds, from 70 to 82 pounds. She was afraid that if this continued she would become 'too fat'. She rigidly watched every bite she ate so that her weight would not exceed 82 pounds. There had been beginning breast formation but no further progress of puberal development since she had started dieting. Her academic work continued at a high level, but she had withdrawn from her friends, felt they were ridiculing her, and she would stay away from school whenever her feelings were hurt. At home she was restless and unhappy, obsessively preoccupied with cleanliness and more critical of her mother than before.

In this girl the 'fear of fatness' was the first manifest symptom of serious emotional maladjustment. She was aware that her fear of fatness was not realistic, that it indicated her need to be 'different' from other girls who enjoyed their feminine development and had changed in their interests.

CASE 4

Family pressure

Albert was 13½ years old when he was seen in consultation. Both parents angrily complained about his being 'fat', that he had been gaining weight rapidly for five years and refused to do anything about it. They described him as very intelligent and a good student, but were concerned about his being 'different' from other boys. The father had tried to get his son interested in athletics since early childhood and more forcibly after his entering school. He expressed keen disappointment about his son not being interested in sports, not even as a spectator. This issue of athletics had become so acute that Albert had withdrawn from all activities and had become depressed.

This father, a successful businessman who had done better than anybody else in his family, was tall, slender, bronzed and athletic-looking, and spoke with great satisfaction about his own achievement, in the business world and in athletic competition. The mother appeared critical of her husband's overpowering interest in athletics. She had been affectionate and indulgent towards the boy, with some awareness that he was too old to be so demonstrative towards her. There was some concern about his jealousy towards a younger sister who was considered by both parents to be the 'perfect child'. Albert was tall and heavy-set, approximately 20 per cent overweight, not 'fat' as his father's description had indicated. Puberty development was well advanced. He was suspicious and resentful about the psychiatric consultation, but relaxed when he recognized that this was not another attempt to coerce him to go on a diet or to become an athlete. The therapeutic work was directed towards helping the father accept that he could not force his image of success and perfection on his son. He was able to relax his excessive expectations and to show approval and regard for what his son enjoyed and did best. As the pressure to be athletic diminished, the boy became again outgoing and made friends who shared his own literary interests. He acknowledged his clumsiness and took private dancing lessons before venturing into new social activities. During the last year in High School, he himself felt that his excess weight was a hindrance and asked for a diet, and followed through on it. When he graduated at age 17, he was tall, well developed, not too heavy, but not athletic-looking either. Leaving for college was an escape from an overdemanding home. He has done well in his chosen profession and scarcely remembers his so-called obesity.

The interesting aspect of this case is that it was the demand for athletic activity and competitive sport that was superimposed on a boy with different interests. The weight excess developed when he withdrew from this inappropriate pressure. He had grown up in a suburban home and was not truly 'inactive' as it is often observed in the lower-class patients whose anxious parents keep them from playing in the streets or public parks.

Case 5

Family possessiveness

Much more serious were the psychiatric problems and abnormal involvements in the case of Bruce, who was 16 years old when first seen, weighing nearly 200 pounds. This case also illustrates the therapeutic difficulties provoked by a possessive family. The immediate reason for the psychiatric consultation was his having suddenly declared that he did not want to finish High School. He had become so slack in his work that he was in danger of failing in spite of excellent intelligence. His attitude towards life in general was one of complete resignation. There was no sense in planning for the future, or in trying to achieve anything. His attitude towards treatment was just as lackadaisical: something his parents wanted him to go through, but there was no hope or future for him.

Bruce had a long history of chronic illness and had been quite skinny as a child. He had needed repeated hospitalization, and there was an endless stream of consultants to handle his medical problems, recurrent infections and untractable dermatitis. The mother was vituperous in her outbursts against the various physicians whom she had consulted, and of whom she spoke as 'just having messed up the case', or 'not knowing what it was all about'.

Every word and action of the mother indicated that she felt her son had survived only due to her devoted efforts, and that he was her showpiece and possession. That he had become fat during puberty was an insult to her, and his failing in school was the final rejection. She felt Bruce had been happy in spite of all the illnesses, and she denied any adverse psychological effects from his chronic ill-health. She, of course, had suffered from terrific fears; and if she had been overprotective, it was well justified but it had not adversely influenced his development. She admitted that maybe she had pushed food on him in an effort to keep him well; maybe she had over- done it. But she was also convinced that there must be other causes for her son's obesity than just overeating. She was particularly indignant about an endocrinologist who had called the obesity 'pure unadulterated fat'; and the dermatologist who had finally been of help with the skin condition and who made the crowning insulting remark by saying to Bruce: 'Your mother and I have put too much into you to let you go to pot now.' She reported the boy's rage—'He could have killed him'—with an intensity that made one feel that she could have done the same.

For the past two years she had been in search of a psychiatrist and had consulted a good many; not one of them had understood the boy's problems, she felt. Since I had a special interest in obese youngsters, she had decided to honor me with this consultation.

It seemed obvious that treatment would be futile unless there were regular conferences with the mother. It was also felt that Bruce should not be compelled to do something against his will, and the frequency of visits were left to him. The mother was indignant when these two points were made. She could not see why she should come, as she was as cooperative as anyone could wish her to be. As to her son, everybody had told her that he needed at least three sessions a week and I appeared to be indefinite about this. She did come for a few weeks; then she declared that she had gotten so much benefit that she saw no need to continue. Bruce responded well to the non-authoritarian attitude and soon established a once-a-week pattern and became interested in what he could learn about himself. Some time later he expressed the wish for more sessions. This time the parents were indignant about the increase and demanded a reduction in fee.

There was good therapeutic progress and, during vacation in a summer camp, Bruce felt that for the first time he had acted like an independent human being. Shortly thereafter he gave up his usual restraint and answered the question: 'What would be worthwhile?' with a passionate outburst: 'What is the sense of doing homework? If you can't get 90 or 100 in all subjects, why try to do anything! Just to be average, just to be good, just to do what everybody else does—there is no sense to living that way. And even if I go on studying, who will guarantee that my name will be remembered 500 years from now? Why should I work and exert myself just to be an average lawyer, doctor or businessman? I cannot see the sense to that.' This outburst of secret unrealistic ambitions in this extremely passive and pathetic boy was rather surprising, though such overambitious daydreams are not unusual in emotionally disturbed fat youngsters. He could learn to recognize how these unrealistic ambitions were related to the enormous sense of obligation he felt he owed his mother for having saved his life over and over again, and that it was impossible to live up to such dreams of glory. He recognized that his excessive eating was related to experiences of acute disappointment for not being as outstanding as he felt he had to be.

This type of eating to relieve tension and despair fulfills the primitive hope that eating in some way will make up for the defect. Yet, however much food is taken, eating never gives the satisfaction such a youngster craves; it does not accomplish the very special thing it is supposed to accomplish. The resulting increase in size fulfills on a primitive symbolic level the desire to be big, though in reality it leads to new difficulties. One day Bruce expressed it as 'I am just not big enough for what I am cut out to do,' then stopped at the word 'big' and added: 'I mean in my mind— just look at me—I certainly do *look big enough.*'

As he became more realistic about his goals in life he became interested again in his studies and finished High School with good grades, but not 'outstanding'. He was unable to lose weight as long as he lived at home where 'every bite was watched'. He decided to go to a Southern college where he felt the demands would not be as great as in one of the Eastern colleges. He knew that this was a disappointment to his parents' ambitions, but felt it was wiser for him to make decisions according to what he could do. He also wanted to put distance between himself and his home. Though he encountered some difficulties in college, he was able to finish his study and enter a career of his own choosing.

CASE 6

Family obligations

Dora had been a rather poor eater and skinny 'like a beanstalk' until she was 12 years old, when she went to summer camp for the first time and discovered that 'eating could be fun' and she indulged in all kinds of new foods. In her wealthy home, meals had been served with utmost frugality, though there was always more than enough food; but eating more than what was absolutely necessary was just not done. Emancipation from home became identical with the idea of 'abundance', namely, eating as much as one wanted of things that thus far had been doled out meagerly, such as cake and candy. There was a rapid gain in weight to nearly 200 pounds, when she was 14 years old.

The next years were a continuous struggle about her weight. She was away most of the time at boarding school, where there was continuous criticism of her eating habits. She might lose some weight but it would always rise as soon as she escaped the strictest supervision. She was a brilliant student with enormous capacity for work, a driving compulsion to master any subject, 'devouring' books and knowledge. Social relations, however, were poor and there were repeated fights about her attending the school dances, which she refused to do because she felt awkward and fat. There were periods of depression and great loneliness. She spent one summer vacation at one of the reducing salons. She accepted this in the spirit of defiance and resentment; she would show 'them' that she could do it, and she lost 30 pounds but considered this experience the most unhappy period of her life. She gained little or no satisfaction from losing weight and regained it in brief order.

When 17 years old she came for psychoanalytic treatment, which was characterized by extreme negativism, suspiciousness and aloofness. The mere mentioning of her eating habits, or of any other practical aspects of her living, would provoke deepest resentment and depression. Her concept of life, as it gradually evolved, was that everything and anything that she had ever done had been forced upon her. There were frequent hints that she was engaged in more rewarding and satisfying daydreams, without divulging the content of her fantasies. She might say as much as 'There are so many of us', or 'Oh, we know how to amuse ourselves'. At times the clinical picture resembled that of depersonalization, without awareness of her true identity, and with doubts about the reality of the people around her.

Progress in her concept of self-awareness and reality was slow. During the second year of treatment she enrolled in college and again mastered the academic subjects with great success, complaining at the same time that everything was forced upon her. The subject of her weight or dieting was strictly avoided, yet there seemed to be no further increase in weight, although she had gained continuously during the preceding years.

During the second year of treatment an episode occurred which shed light on the underlying problems. She had seen the play, *The Cocktail Party*, by Eliot, and was enraged that the psychiatrist in the play told people what to do, that he made 'choices' for them. In her own life there had been a continuous conflict between 'choice' and 'duty'. *Duty* was defined as something *one has to do* because it involves other people. *Choice* is what *one does for one's own sake alone.* Her continuous complaints about being forced to do things were revolts against this excessive sense of duty.

Returning from the theatre she saw a beggar in the street and felt guilty because she walked by. Then it occurred to her that she would have felt just as guilty had she given him some money because, in a way, nothing would have been changed. She realized that this continued sense of guilt, this overwhelming feeling of what she ought to do, was an expression of the image she had of herself, namely, that she had gigantic power. It was her duty, more than anybody else's, to correct the ills of the world because she had this gigantic power. Her passivity, her just sitting by, continuously led to a sense of frustration of not fulfilling her fate.

She related this sense of her enormous responsibility to her childhood experiences. Instead of not having been loved enough, as many of the popular theories on neurosis try to explain, she felt that she had been loved too much, that she had been the center of all of her parents' attention. This family lived on a large country estate, and she had grown up without companions who were her equals. Her parents did not have an active social life and they were centered on each other. She felt she received a tremendous amount of love and admiration. This aroused in her the expectation that she should make up to her parents their own frustrations and losses; to her mother that she had not been the beauty she had wanted to be as a young girl, and to her father the loss of his former high social position and vast possessions.

Her isolation and loneliness during childhood had deprived her of experiences that might have led to a correction of these unrealistic ideas of her tremendous responsibility. She had contempt for a possible life of middle-class contentment and so-called happiness which would mean a denial of her extraordinary tasks and duties and also of her gigantic power. She had tried, over and over, to find support for her efforts at doing good in religion, but was always disappointed.

Her reaction to this new insight was one of relief, of no longer being confronted with tasks which always had remained undone, which always had given her a sense of being too little and which had created this deep sense of inadequacy and frustration. She recognized the relationship between this inner disappointment and her eating habits and large size.

Shortly thereafter, during a brief interruption of treatment, she began reducing on her own decision. She lost more than 10 pounds during two weeks. She had made this decision, or as she called it, a *choice*, in order to demonstrate to herself that she was free now of this obsession of her special tasks and bigness. Although she had begun the diet 'on her own', it soon became apparent that it was only a 'part' decision. The other part of her self experienced it as a 'command' and rebelled. She felt as if there had been a vote and that the 'absent member' was now protesting.

By the time treatment was resumed she was in a state of extreme tension. She still followed her self-imposed diet and was worried about not being able to break it even if she wanted to. The diet interfered with her sleep because the thought of food kept her awake. She had an insane desire for all kinds of food, even those she ordinarily loathed. She felt tired and dizzy during the day-time, her knees felt weak and she felt she had to watch every step, in a physical sense as well as in regard to eating. 'There is a feeling of walking right off the edge of something—a feeling of no volition.' The gravest danger was that 'of drifting into eating something', particularly when she did not feel very hungry. Temptation, as 'an active thing', was around all the time. She consumed large quantities of tea, smoked constantly, tried escape by reading magazines and talked to herself in an indulgent voice. At the same time she would tell herself to stay on the diet—'a command is a command, no matter where it comes from'.

The result of this continuous struggle and tension was a complete deterioration of her daily activities. She was unable to do her work—and 'mastering' her studies had been another aspect of her special power. She withdrew from whatever friendships and social contacts she had gradually built up. She discontinued the efforts at dieting after three weeks with awareness that the real danger was the danger of losing her hold on reality.

After discounting the diet her weight quickly returned to the former level. The panic and tension subsided within a few days. As treatment progressed and her sense of reality was more firmly integrated, she gradually lost weight without specifically dieting. She was tall and large when she graduated from college. She subsequently married, had three children and gained satisfaction from having a family. About fifteen years later she faced some marital problem and consulted another psychiatrist who was somewhat puzzled that she had ever been in treatment for untractable obesity.

CASE 7

Megalomania compensation

Enid had succeeded in reducing her weight by regurgitation after every meal, from 170 down to 115 pounds, which she considered her ideal weight. When she came for treatment she was panicky with fear of growing fat again because her weight had risen to 125 pounds. Actually she was tall and slim, and her preoccupation with 'fatness' had a phobic character.

Although she had thus succeeded in creating a perfect figure, her adjustment to life had not only not improved but had deteriorated to a race between eating as much as she wanted and maintaining her perfect figure. In the course of treatment she expressed that this point was very important because it was proof of her power to defy Nature, that she was doing something nobody else could do and get away with it. Whenever she gained a pound she became depressed because 'her power was slipping'. Her whole approach to life was characterized by the need to be continuously reassured of 'complete perfection in every respect'.

She was the second of three children of a wealthy and socially prominent family, which gave the impression of compatible and stable relationships. The other two children had developed into competent, well-adjusted people. She had been a happy and pretty little girl, the favorite of her father.

When she was nearly 4 years old, a younger sister was born, at a time when she and her brother were sick with otitis and were hospitalized. She needed an operation and remained at the hospital for several weeks. When she came home, her mother was busy with the new baby and her care was left to a nurse. A great change of behavior occurred during this period. Instead of friendly and outgoing, she became shy and clinging and much more attached to her mother. However, she made a good adjustment to school and became a leader due to her intelligence and her great prowess in athletics.

When she was 13 years old the family moved to another city and she entered a High School as a 'new' student. She felt she had to work hard in every respect to be perfect and her diaries from this time abound with resolutions on how to make herself perfect. Her parents noticed the great enthusiasm with which she would enter into new activities, all kind of activities, only to give them up as soon as she was successful. During this time she became somewhat plump, which to her was the explanation why she could not be popular with boys.

The real difficulties began when she went to college, leaving home for the first time. Being prominent and popular became a compelling need and she worked hard, 'like a politician', so that she was chosen president of her dormitory. Once she had accomplished this, her interest in the other girls lagged. She became quite depressed because she was unable to maintain her high academic record, but tried to hide this from everybody. To relieve her tension she would eat and eat, and gained a considerable amount of weight. From now on fatness became the core problem which, she felt, stood in her way of outstanding accomplishment. At this time she was introduced to the method of regurgitation after big meals. This appealed to her as the ideal solution of her problem, and she practised it to such an extent that she lost weight rapidly. She felt reassured in her attractiveness when, during the next few years, she collected a long string of young men, who were attracted to her and spoke of marriage. She was ready to agree to an engagement, but then her interest in the relationship ceased. Within five years she accumulated approximately twenty broken engagements. Her only interest lay in attracting a man, in getting his declaration of love; then he had fulfilled his function. Her need to be reassured that she was more attractive than any other girl was appeased for a time.

Whenever reassurance about being superior and perfect was not forthcoming she would go on an eating spree. Such 'binges' would take several hours, during which she consumed gargantuan amounts of food, until her stomach would bulge. Then she would relieve herself by vomiting. The slightest disregard for her feelings, an unplanned evening, any disappointment or the fear of not living up to somebody's expectations, was sufficient to provoke such a binge. In periods of stress she would go on three or four binges a day. She was unable to finish college or to maintain a job, because she would run away for an eating binge when the slightest event undermined her feeling of superiority. She was preoccupied with world-saving ideas of doing good for all the oppressed people, or of saving and elevating individuals whom she met in the course of her many activities.

She succeeded for a while to hide her condition from her parents, but gradually the disturbed nature of her never finishing anything and her many meaningless activities was recognized. There were repeated attempts at psychiatric treatment, each of which was given up, for various external reasons, after four to six months. In the course of her treatment with me it became gradually clear that she had used her previous therapists as tools to help her accomplish this Godlike perfection which she described as the one and only goal of her life. Whenever she felt that a therapist was not helping her enough, she would find a good face-saving reason for breaking off treatment. It was only after this delusional goal of her therapeutic efforts had been clarified, that something like a valid treatment relationship could be established and that she could develop beyond this state of megalomanic compensation for her inner convictions of helplessness and worthlessness.

CASE 8

Psychosis

The demand for superiority and perfection led to psychotic disorganization in Flora's case when she was 16 years old. She came from a socially prominent and cultured home, and her mother had fought against her daughter being fat throughout her life. Now Flora had defied her and weighed more than 200 pounds. No longer able to differentiate between her fantasies and the realities of life, she was unable to attend school or to maintain even the slightest social façade, and would spend hours in what she called 'trances'. She was preoccupied with dreams of the prince who would come and release her from ugliness; or of spending her time on a beautiful mountainside covered with bushes which produced the most delicious food, of which she could eat as much as she wanted without becoming fat, and without having the compulsive hateful feeling that she had when she ate sweets and other foods forbidden to her. Gradually, she imagined a whole secret world of her own, with language, laws, religion and mores of her own creation.

The outer manifestations of her breakdown was her becoming extremely careless of her appearance and her eating inedible material. As far back as she could remember, her mother had been 'phobic' about her figure and had tried to supervise every bite she ate. She had some vague memories that when she was little she was permitted to eat such 'forbidden' things as chocolate pudding or cake. But she was sure that since age 6 or 7 these things had never been allowed, and her whole life had been a struggle to feast on them. When all food was locked away, with a lock even on the refrigerator, she commenced to eat the staples—unprepared jello or uncooked cereals or spaghetti. She also would chew pieces of string and eat concert tickets and programs. Her behavior became so disturbed that hospitalization became necessary.

She was sufficiently in contact to give a picture of her family life. She felt that her mother's slimness and smartness were the result of eternal denial of food, and that her anxiety over her daughter's figure was an effort to exercise complete control over her. Although the family had given her a great deal of cultural stimulation, she felt that they had not been really interested in her, only in her appearance and brilliance. The father had only two absorbing interests: his business, in which he was very successful, and a complete devotion to mother. His concern about his daughter's queer behavior was also, in her feeling, only an expression of his devotion to the mother and, of course, anger that his daughter, one of his possessions, was not as perfect as she was supposed to be.

The relationship to the mother had been very close, but entirely in terms of the mother's wishes and needs. They had a great common interest, music. The daughter received a good musical education, but there was an exhausting struggle to make her conform to traditional standards. Her ambition was to compose unconventional works. This meant to her that she was expressing her own individuality through her artistic development. She wanted and needed an accomplishment of her own, and despite the self-belittling terms in which she talked about herself, she was also convinced of her essential greatness. She wanted to achieve something quite extraordinary that would be recognized by everybody. She compared herself to great composers of the past who had achieved fame at an early age. She felt her life would be wasted unless she accomplished something that would be on the genius level. This demand for recognition on the superlative level is frequent in obese adolescents. Characteristically, it must be an innate gift and it must fulfill itself without effort on their own part. This very special talent must be so outstanding that the whole world will admire their genius, and thus serve as a compensation for the sense of essential worthlessness from which they suffer.

At this stage in her development, she no longer cared about being fat. To be sure, she still dreamt of having the fatness taken away by the magic prince, but actually it would not help. It would not change the fact that she was inwardly mean, filthy and dirty. When she dropped some ashes on her dress during the interview, she became panicky: 'That's me! I'm always filthy and I fill the chair and I flow over it. It's just my meanness coming out.'

It seemed that when she could hide no longer behind her fatness as a cause of dissatisfaction and failure and became convinced that even reducing could not change her problem, reality checks broke down. The deep problems of the schizophrenic became manifest: the desperate search for her own identity, physical and psychological, for effective means of orienting herself about her own behavior and interaction with other people and of facing the world with an adequate sense of mastery and self-respect.

CASE 9

Sexual adjustment

Weight excess is commonly blamed as an interfering factor in making a sexual adjustment. That it is not the weight excess itself, but the attitude towards it, is illustrated by the example of Gladys, a 17-year-old girl, the third among eight children, mostly girls, who had been markedly overweight since age 7. Gladys resembled her father, a huge man, outstanding in his career, who had tried unsuccessfully to control his weight. The family was socially prominent and there was much pressure that the daughter should reduce. When fifteen, she became rather depressed about her appearance and was sent to an out-of-town reducing service. Her weight dropped in six months from 250 pounds to 180 pounds. She was terribly disappointed when her family felt this was not slim enough and continued to put pressure on her to reduce more.

The pressure increased when she met a young man who fell in love with her and spoke of marriage or elopement. With increased tension she gave up all efforts at dieting and her weight rose rapidly. Exactly one year after discharge she came back to the same medical service, now weighing 280 pounds, reluctant to enter the reducing regimen but determined to marry her young man. She was seen by a psychiatrist and she came to recognize the rebellion and anger in her behavior. She also realized that her parents' concern about her desire to marry the first man who came along had some justification, since she had felt unattractive. There were also true feelings of love and loyalty towards her boy-friend. Finally her parents gave their consent to the marriage. By that time her weight was down to 230 pounds. She had no feeling of concern that her fatness would interfere with her sexual enjoyment; there was great desire and mutual attraction. A year later she reported a good marital adjustment and asked for advice about ambulatory reducing programs. This was the first time that she herself felt the need to bring her weight under control.

4

Psychopathology

These examples may suffice as illustrations of the manifold clinical pictures and problems underlying or associated with excess weight. In no case was there evidence of an organic or endocrine disorder. In addition to these obese adolescents with their varied difficulties in living, there are numerous obese youngsters who, though overweight, are essentially healthy in their adjustment. Since they are capable of handling their weight, by reducing or adjusting to it, they will not come to the attention of psychiatrists. Only one example of such a normal adjustment was given (Case 1), though these ordinary fat youngsters probably outnumber those with emotional problems. It would be erroneous to generalize from the psychiatric observations to all fat youngsters.

In the disturbed group with their great individual differences, certain common features can be recognized. In all cases the development of obesity is related to the fact that food and eating are used to appease non-nutritional needs and tensions which are erroneously interpreted as 'desire to eat'. In some instances the ordinary demands of adolescence are experienced as threatening and dangerous. More often, disturbed obese adolescents interpret these demands in an unrealistic way and withdraw from them. Not infrequently they approach new tasks and problems with exaggerated ambition, with concepts of achievement that are unrealistic and unfulfillable. Thus they are continuously confronted with disappointment and failure.

Such misconceptions about his importance and obligation appear to be related to early experiences in which a child feels that he is expected to compensate his parents for the frustrations and unfulfilled ambitions of their own lives.[6] Such parents, in particular mothers, are apt to superimpose their feelings and values on the developing child, expressing this in every detail of his physical and psychological care. Thus a child will arrive at adolescence lacking, with wide individual variations, in preparatory experiences essential for developing independence and his own identity. Specifically he may be deficient in the awareness of being a differentiated self-directed separate organism with the ability to identify and control bodily urges, and to define his needs and present them in a way that can lead to appropriate and satisfying response. If severe, such deficiencies may be experienced as a sense of not owning his own body, as not having a 'body identity'. Traditionally obese people have been accused of 'lacking in will power' when they are unable to adhere to a diet though bemoaning the obese state. This appears to be related to the falsified awareness of their bodily sensations and functions, specifically to the inability to correctly identify hunger and satiation.[7]

This deficit in perceptual and conceptual awareness of 'hunger' is a prerequisite for the misuse of the eating function in the service of various non-nutritional needs, with widely different symbolic meanings. Corroborative evidence for this clinical conclusion has come from direct observations. Stunkard[16] observed that fasting obese women, during contractions of their empty stomachs, failed to report awareness of hunger, wheras non-obese women would usually report such sensations. Through a series of ingenious experiments in which external factors were manipulated, Schachter[13] and Nisbett[15] could demonstrate that obese subjects, chiefly college students, are affected in their eating habits by external cues such as the sight of food, its states and availability, or apparent passage of time, whereas subjects of normal weight will eat according to enteroceptive determinants.

In the cases here presented it would be easy to extrapolate from the available information that there had been abnormal transactional patterns

K

between the fat child and his parents, with failure of appropriate, 'empathic', response to expressions of the child's needs.[8] The result is not only disturbed hunger awareness but also gross deficits in initiative and active self-experience. Such an adolescent child will be unprepared and helpless when confronted with new situations and intrapsychic or interpersonal problems. Helpless under the impact of his needs and urges, he will become involved in 'compulsive' eating when confronted with to him insoluble problems.

Though obesity in adolescence is a serious social and psychological handicap, weight loss alone is unable to solve the underlying problems of living of emotionally disturbed adolescents. Invariably obese adolescents before they come to a psychiatrist, had unsuccessfully attempted to reduce, or had become more disturbed while doing so. In the here presented series of cases, severe psychiatric difficulties were observed in those who rigidly adhered to reducing regimes (Cases 2, 3), or who had attempted dieting before emotional readiness (Case 6), or who had forced their weight down through bizarre eating arrangements (Case 7).

In order to control their weight successfully, such youngsters need to become aware of the conflicts and circumstances under which the excess eating takes place, and they need help in overcoming their basic sense of incompetence and helplessness. In the psychiatric treatment of such a patient there is need for explicit and consistent emphasis on his developing awareness of thoughts and impulses originating in himself. Through alert and consistent, confirming or correcting responses to any self-initiated behavior or thought he will become able to actively participate in the therapeutic process, and thus in the way he lives his life. It is only then that he can make a valid decision whether to follow a reducing regime, or whether to accept himself as an overweight person.

REFERENCES

1. BRUCH, H. 1968. Obesity. In *International encyclopedia of the social sciences.* New York: Macmillan, and The Free Press.
2. BRUCH, H. 1957. *The importance of overweight.* New York: W. W. Norton.
3. BRUCH, H. 1955. Fat children grown up. *Amer. J. Dis. Child.* 90, 201.
4. BRUCH, H. 1970. Juvenile obesity: its course and outcome. *Int. Psychiat. Clinics,* 7, 231–254.
5. BRUCH, H. 1957. The emotional significance of the preferred weight. *Amer. J. clin. Nutr.,* 5, 192–196.
6. BRUCH, H. 1940. Obesity in childhood: V. The family frame of obese children (together with G. Touraine). *Psychosom. Med.,* 2, 141–206.
7. BRUCH, H. 1961. Transformation of oral impulses in eating disorders: a conceptual approach. *Psychiat. Quart.,* 35, 458–481.
8. BRUCH, H. 1962. Falsification of bodily needs and body concept in schizophrenia. *Arch. gen. Psychiat.,* 6, 18–24.
9. CAHNMAN, W. J. 1968. The stigma of obesity. *The Sociological Quarterly,* Summer issue, 283–299.

10. MAYER, J. 1966. Some aspects of the problems of regulation of food intake and obesity. *New England J. Med.*, **274**, 610, 662, 722.

11. MONELLO, L. F. and MAYER, J. 1963. Obese adolescent girls: unrecognized minority group? *Amer. J. clin. Nutr.*, **13**, 35–38.

12. MOORE, M. E., STUNKARD, A. and SROLE, L. 1962. Obesity, social class and mental illness. *J. Amer. med. Ass.*, **181**, 962–965.

13. NISBETT, R. E. 1968. Determinants of food intake in obesity. *Science*, **159**, 1254–1255.

14. RICHARDSON, A., GOODMAN, N., HASTORF, A. H. and DORNBUSH, S. M. 1963. Variant reactions to physical disabilities. *Amer. Sociological Review*, **28**, 429–435.

15. SCHACHTER, S. 1968. Obesity and eating. *Science*, **161**, 751–756.

16. STUNKARD, A. 1959. Obesity and the denial of hunger. *Psychosom. Med.*, **21**, 281–290.

17. STUNKARD, A. J. and MENDELSON, M. 1961. Disturbances in body image of some obese persons. *J. Amer. diet. Ass.*, **38**, 328–332.

XII

ANOREXIA NERVOSA*

G. K. USHAKOV

Professor of Psychiatry
Department of Psychiatry, 2nd Moscow Medical Institute
Moscow, U.S.S.R.

1

Introduction

Clinical investigations have revealed a number of aetiological factors of anorexia (the refusal to eat) in patients suffering from a variety of psychiatric disorders. As a syndrome, anorexia can be found in a wide age range and presents a picture familiar to the psychiatrist; it may present in association with negativism, with hallucinations—particularly of a compulsive nature, with delusions—especially of being poisoned—or with depression, etc. In anorexia, together with each type of symptomatology, are usually found changes in the secretive and mechanical functions of the alimentary tract. These changes may precede the psychiatric disorder, or may be caused by complicated modifications of the brain activity, due to the brain being influenced by cortico-visceral mechanisms.

The clinical picture of anorexia nervosa in adolescence shows such constant and well-defined stages of development that it can be safely assumed that it is a distinct clinical entity; also it is highly significant that the clinical manifestations of anorexia nervosa have particular characteristics in adolescence.

Currently, there are two schools of thought about the clinical nature of anorexia nervosa. One school regards it as a separate nosological entity, as anorexia nervosa is notable for the uniformity of its clinical manifestations, its psychogenesis, its predictable course and resolution. The other school points to the apparent similarity of symptomatology in the many variants of anorexia and regards it as a cluster of symptoms typical of many

* Translated by Mrs Ushakova, Moscow, U.S.S.R., and Maria-Livia Osborn, Research Assistant, The Institute of Family Psychiatry, Ipswich, England.

diseases. This duality of thought on the evolution of the same phenomenon stems from the fact that not all investigators share the same definition as to what constitutes the anorexia syndrome. If we attribute all cases of refusal to eat in psychiatric patients to anorexia nervosa, then we would have to agree with those who consider it as a mere symptom; cases of food refusal are extremely common and have many clinical aspects and varied aetiology. However, as mentioned above, anorexia nervosa is a particular form of food rejection found in adolescents and has, as we shall endeavour to demonstrate, all the characteristics of an independent clinical entity.

2

Historical

The anorexia syndrome was first described in the second half of the seventeenth century by Morton,[14] whose interest was aroused by a progressive wasting, accompanied by loss of appetite and depression of the digestive functions, but without any signs of fever, cough or dyspnoea. When cachexia is extreme, those patients resemble 'a skeleton wrapped up in skin'. Morton called this disease 'nervous consumption'. In 1789 Nodow described a nervous disorder, whose main feature was an extraordinary aversion to food. He associated its manifestation with a peculiar 'hysterical affectedness'. The clinical picture of this disorder resembled that given by Morton.

However, the systematic study of anorexia nervosa began in the later part of the nineteenth century, in France with the work of Charles Lasègue[10] in 1873, and in England with William Gull's work[6] in 1874. The clinical descriptions of the disease given independently by these two workers, were strikingly similar. Gull called it *'anorexia nervosa'* and this term has been adopted and used ever since in English, German and Russian medical literature. In France, however, the term *'anorexie mentale'* is more commonly found. This was first used by Gushara and replaced Lasègue's term *'anorexie hystérique'*. Lasègue had noticed the gradual, almost imperceptible onset of the disorder, the increasing loss of interest in food by the patient and his vague complaints of unpleasant sensations around the stomach. Lasègue considered the following symptoms to be characteristic of the disease: partial or total rejection of food, constancy of symptomatology, difficulty in therapy, as the patient does not respond to either persuasion or threats, and increasing cachexia. In the early descriptions of the disease amenorrhoea was mentioned as a typical symptom, and it is obvious that subsequently the workers who first described and isolated it as a disease entity were aware of the well-known triad of symptoms—the so-called three 'As'—*'anorexie'*, *'amaigrissement'* (wasting) and *'amenorrhoea'*. Lasègue identified three stages in the course of the disease. In the first, or 'gastric' stage, the patient refuses to eat, pleading pain during meals; but Lasègue found no signs of dyspepsia; the patient's own explanation was that he could not eat because eating would cause him pain. In the second, or 'struggling' stage, the painful sensations disappear and the patient's emotional rationalization would be: 'I have abstained from eating, I starved—now I am better. One not only can, but must, famish. I don't feel hungry—hence I am in good health.' As Lasègue points out, by the time this stage is reached the patient's anorexia is a subject of great concern and discussion in the family and this situation further stimulates the hysterical tendencies of the patient. The third, or 'cachectic' stage is characterized by extreme emaciation: the skin loses its elasticity, the abdomen is drawn in, the patient is pale, amenorrhoea and constipation are present, and weakness confines the patient to bed. Clearly, since anorexia nervosa was first described, its symptomatology has not changed, but rather a different interpretation has been put on its various components. This is demonstrated by the first description of anorexia in Russia by A. A. Kissyel in 1894.[8]

Investigators of anorexia nervosa have noticed that the rejection of food usually begins in adolescence, between the ages of 12 and 15, and presents predominantly in girls. In his study of the premorbid period, Frölich[5] found the girls in his sample to be of slight physique, or of infantile body structure. Although tall, they usually have small bones and flaccid muscles, a slender figure with flat chest and rounded shoulders, often showing signs of kyphoscoliosis (curvature of the spine). Schizoid traits are typical of their personality. These children are usually quiet, reserved and solitary from early childhood. They are lonely without any close friends; their affective reactions are shallow and they tend to be obsessional and to over-value certain ideas. In the premorbid period they manifest hysterical traits.

Concomitant with the onset of fasting there is a general change of interests and a diminution of activity. Cases have been described where adolescent girls become almost stuporose, or were in a state very similar to stupor. As well as being inactive and showing little interest in anything, the girls tend to lose their natural coquetry, regress to infantile behaviour, and become more attached to their mothers.

Amenorrhoea, which often precedes or is concurrent with the anorexia and, especially, with the cachexia, is an early and frequent sign of the disease. This is perhaps one of the reasons why European investigators tend to regard anorexia nervosa as a psychosomatic disorder (Decourt[3]).

The findings of an investigation on a large number of patients suffering from anorexia nervosa mostly agree with the two-stage development of the disease put forward by Löffler.[12] The first stage he calls the *passive* stage, during which the patient renounces food and will not be nourished, i.e. shows symptoms of negativism. During the second, or *active* stage, the patient finds various ways to further slimming and rejection of food by inducing vomit, taking purgatives, doing strenuous exercise, etc. However, in systematizing the stages of development of anorexia nervosa, it is better not to limit them only to the two stages described by Löffler.[12]

3

Precipitating Factors and Premorbid Personality

Our investigation on sixty-five patients has shown that the commonest age of onset for anorexia nervosa is around 14 or 15 years. The rate of hospital admission for girls is approximately five times higher than that for boys. On average, boys show manifestations of the disease at the same age as girls, but an earlier onset (10–13 years) is more common in boys.

In the group investigated, three cases were found to have one parent who, during puberty, had gone through long periods of food rejection with the aim of slimming. These symptoms had gone untreated as, at that time, child psychiatry services were less sophisticated. However, these three cases demonstrate that anorexia nervosa can be regarded as a familial syndrome, communicated from one generation to another, here spanning two generations.

Most of the adolescents observed came from prosperous families, with a highly cultured background, good living conditions and a quiet family environment. They were usually the product of a first or second perfectly normal pregnancy, and there were no pathological features in their birth or early development. On the contrary, these children were forward in meaningful speech, so much so that the parents of more than half the sample reported that their children could already speak clearly by the age of 18 months. Their physical development was normal, they were strong children, who ate in moderation and with good appetite; although their medical histories revealed that they had some food fads.

The majority of patients in the sample showed the following premorbid features: excessive body weight in relation to their age and height, they were stout children, of high intelligence, self-controlled, reserved, purposeful, over-sensitive, persistent on any set task, very active and precise. Good educational attainments set them apart from their school mates—more than half of them had always had excellent marks only. They tended to be rigid and dogmatic in their attitudes, had a highly developed sense of responsibility and were very conscientious in their studies. These children made good progress at school and possessed a wide general knowledge; they steadily achieved their goals in matters in which they were interested, and were able to solve any problem which excited their affective curiosity. They were meticulous to the point where their punctilliousness became ludicrous; their high principles were excessive for their ages; they had an unequivocal honesty and an exaggerated sense of duty, expecting the same attitude towards life from everybody. They found it difficult to compromise and showed an authoritative attitude towards their equals, actively participating in all social activities, but always wanting to lead.

In addition to the traits mentioned above, these children were selective in their friendships, even in the pre-school period; they were also reserved,

unsociable, often played alone, and many had no close friends and preferred reading to games. Even when participating in games, they remained
apart, as one girl verbalized by saying that she regarded herself as a
'looker-on', rather than a participant in the lively games of other children.
Although always attached to their parents, these children remained restrained and cold, never taking the parents into their confidence; often they
were selfish, egocentric and extremely demanding. Their feelings for other
members of the family were sound and quite deep, but they avoided any
demonstration of affection.

The girls did not show any interest in the opposite sex. Many of the
parents reported that they had noticed how their children had lacked the
natural unsophistication of childhood, and were 'excessively conscientious'
and 'excessively respectable', which is unusual in children of pre-school
and school age.

4

Symptomatology

We have observed that the initial symptoms of the disease often occur
long before the actual syndrome of anorexia nervosa shows any of its
manifestations. One or two years before the true onset the adolescent
tends to become more irritable, is less self-controlled, is over-sensitive,
is direct to the point of tactlessness, and abrupt in his relationship with his
peers and his family, and often causes conflict. At the same time uncharacteristic mood-swings begin to appear, but as they are still rather mild they
cause little concern to the parents. If these changes of mood are traced over
a long period of time preceding the anorexia, it is found that they become
more frequent and pronounced as the period of overt anorexia approaches,
and that they usually appear without obvious reasons. In some children
mood-swings become especially noticeable when the child is separated
from his parents, or when he finds himself in situations that, although of no
particular significance, cause him some emotional trauma. With the onset
of manifestations of anorexia, personality changes become more obvious
and they increase in intensity during the course of the disease. A previously amenable child becomes tactless and rude, showing irritability if
pressed to eat; his resistance and negativism lead to bitterness in the
parents. Later on, the child's apathy and his indifference to mother's
anxiety and tears are a typical development.

In the sample studied the first manifestations of anorexia nervosa were
often precipitated by occasional teasing with such epithets as 'pudge',
'tubby', or 'fatso'. Early manifestations were a restricted food intake: at
first, the children took smaller portions at meal-times, or cut out certain
items; for instance, soup, bread, butter or meat. They became very
interested in the calorific value of food and in popularly recommended
rules of nutrition. To find out more about this, they read on their own

initiative relevant articles in magazines and newspapers, and, in their eagerness to have more information on the subject, they even wrote letters to the papers asking for more details. Soon even the amount of food with no-calorific value became progressively smaller, and by the time of admission to hospital even the daily rations of these selected items had been reduced to a minimum; e.g. half a bottle of lemonade and a lollipop, or one cucumber, one spoonful of sour cream, or 20–30 grammes of bread, or 4–5 sweets, or a few ice-creams. One patient had taken a meal only once in three days.

This sudden, unmotivated change of diet in the adolescents attracted the attention of the parents, who consequently paid more attention to the feeding habits of their children. Parental vigilance, however, had little effect, as the adolescents would hide their food, throw it away and persistently reject it, showing great ingenuity to achieve their ends. When forced to eat more, they would take refuge in the toilet, where by artificial means they would cause vomiting, or wash out the stomach. During this period of the disease, it was observed that patients constantly rejected food and become emaciated, with a pale, greyish complexion. Despite this, however, they did not lose their customary appetite and felt hungry by the usual meal-times. Some patients even cried with hunger, but still persisted in 'restraining' themselves, saying that they could eat much more, but did not want to. To suppress the feeling of hunger, they tried to chew food for a long time, or kept it in the mouth for as long as possible, swallowing it by bits over several hours. A patient who had chosen sour cream for her diet used to spread it over the sides of a glass and then scrape it up in small quantities to 'prolong the pleasure'! It was observed that in a few patients, the feeling of hunger was not lost throughout the course of the disease; but in the majority of them it diminished after three to five months, and they did not experience any natural inducement to eat.

It was also noticed that during the initial period and during the first stage of food rejection the patients were hyperactive in all they did, although their behaviour maintained an appearance of purposefulness. They moved about a great deal, ran, did housework with a persistence and energy previously unusual in them. They cleaned already clean floors; did physical exercises, frequently till exhausted; skipped with a rope; after meals they kept squatting and jumping up and down and often took their meals standing. During the course of the illness, naps were never taken, and patients who had previously enjoyed an after-dinner nap would seldom lie down or even sit. Many of them even did their homework standing or walking to and fro. Body weight had considerably decreased by the time of admission to hospital, one patient showing a loss of 30 kg of his normal weight.

It is of interest to note that many of the girls in the sample not only skimped on food in order to slim but took also further measures to look slender, graceful and slim. They tightened belts round their waists; bound their breasts; some of them began, without any need for it, to wear tight corsets; and most of them—'not to look fatter'—wore no underwear; their posture had become peculiarly constrained and affected; the abdomen constantly drawn in deeply, the shoulders exaggeratedly squared, the head held up rigidly or even tossed back. This posture had quickly become a habit. The hair-style of these girls was rather extraordinary too, aimed at giving the impression of an elongated face.

These adolescents showed overt hostility towards any stout people they met and were indignant at the good appetite of other members of the family. Yet many of them took an active part in preparing meals; they helped to cook willingly, laid the table, saw to it that the family ate well and pressed excessive quantities of food on their younger siblings, becoming extremely upset if the latter resisted. As mentioned above, in the pre-morbid state these patients had been most honest and trustworthy; but we observed that during the disease they easily resorted to fraud and stubbornly tried to convince other people that their actions were right and their behaviour justified.

Mild depressive conditions and a frequent feeling of tension and anxiety have been observed during the whole period in which the disease was manifest. At the beginning, symptoms of heightened irritability, tenseness and mild depression were a very noticeable reaction whenever the children were pressed or forced to eat. Later, these changes of mood were present irrespective of the meal ritual. Eventually the adolescents became cold and antagonistic in their relationships with other members of the family, showing increased irritability and intolerance in their presence. They became less sociable both towards the family and their friends, tending to sever contacts with other people and becoming quite self-centred. Their now limited interests were also introverted upon their own feelings, whilst delusions and suicidal thoughts accompanied their increasing depression.

Describing the onset of the disease, the adolescents pointed out how elated their mood had been during that period and how any target seemed easily achievable. It seemed to them that from the very first days of their slimming regime everybody looked at them and noticed their graceful and elegant figures. But this initial lighthearted period was followed by one of dejection, and they themselves described the depression and the anxiety that overcame them, irrespective of their attitude to food.

With an increased rejection of food, they became emaciated and depressed, more flabby, with loss of flesh, adynamic, apathetic, with narrow interests and loss of previous incentives. 'Relatives and friends irritate me,' they would say; 'I don't want to see them.' 'To read . . . but what for?'

But although strikingly asthenic and emaciated, the adolescents were extremely persistent in continuing to accomplish any set task, reacting violently to any opposition and tackling physical work beyond their strength. Despite increased weariness and difficulty in assimilating their lessons, they went on doing well at school, although it would take them longer and longer to do their homework.

When they were eventually admitted as inpatients they came very unwillingly, resisting all they could, crying and begging their parents not to leave them in the hospital, and threatening suicide. Once admitted, it was noticed that after the first few days their weakness gave way to activity. This is mainly expressed in resistance to their enforced stay in hospital and to the physician's prescriptions. Furthermore, they refused to keep to bed, jumping out of it and continually walking about in the ward or the garden; day after day they would try to help in the domestic work of the ward and try to persuade the staff to let them keep order in a group of children. They would eat very little, spreading the food all over the place and eating it slowly, in small morsels, with an expression of disgust and sufferance; they would become much irritated if they noticed that they were watched, and argued loudly over every mouthful of food they swallowed. To this was added their dexterity in hiding food, which would find its way into the bedside tables, into the mattresses, pillow-cases or paper-bags specially brought in for that purpose; they would stick butter under the plate to avoid eating it. By the end of the meal these adolescent patients were very irritable and would impatiently jump up from the table to go to the toilet, where often they would induce vomiting and do some strenuous physical exercises.

It is difficult to make contact with these patients whilst they are in hospital; they look gloomy, tense and hostile, and maintain an arrogant and dour attitude. Many of them cry like babies, calling for their mother. When talking to them the physician finds himself hampered by their constant questions about the date of discharge, the terms of their stay in hospital, and how much weight exactly they must gain in order to be discharged. They are insistent in wanting positive answers and they make it almost impossible to change the subject of the conversation. Furthermore, in letters to their parents they would often describe the 'horrors' of the hospital regime; the 'terrible tortures' of injections they suffer; or the imaginary beatings inflicted on them; they beg the parents to take them away for whatever reason they can think of. Some patients keep things brought by their parents with great care, saying 'This is from daddy' or 'mummy', but nevertheless when parents come to visit they are often rude, tactless, resentful and overdemanding. The fact that the parents bring them gifts and sweets seems to offend them and they regard it as a personal affront.

When cachexy is at its maximum, the physical state of these patients changes suddenly. Dystrophy reaches its first or second stage; the skin becomes dry and peels off, its colour is sallow with pigmentation round the waist; the extremities are cold; some cases suffer from hypertrichiasis; cardiac sounds are muffled, and bradycardia and hypotension are often present. Neurological examination shows some pathology, for instance deficiency of convergence, an asymmetric grin and irregular reflexes. Often, when dystrophy is very severe, Babinsky's and Romberg's signs have been observed.

Two or three months after admission to hospital, most patients become more amenable and approachable. They start by associating with their peers, while still remaining unapproachable to the doctor. Later, they soften even towards him, and they begin to talk to him about their illness, confessing to a desire to slim; but still keeping their feelings to themselves. Their wish to be discharged is still there, but they no longer press for it so insistently as before. They eat better, often to the point of over-eating, although some patients remain choosy about their food right to the end of their stay in hospital, refusing bread in particular. Many of the adolescents confessed that they had begun to eat in order to be discharged sooner, with the aim of again abstaining from food once they were home. In fact, despite their protestations, their appetite gradually improved, but the fear of gaining weight still persisted.

After convalescence, many patients reported that during the last period of their disease they had been desperately homesick, an unusual experience for them. This feeling had been so strong that the very walls of the hospital seemed nasty; the whole environment made them feel irritable and they could not explain to themselves why it all seemed so 'miserable and unpleasant'.

5

Course and Prognosis

Following recovery from an episode of anorexia nervosa, some patients were found to be cured and free from any symptoms; in fact a follow-up covering many years, confirmed that they were fully and permanently cured. But in the majority of cases remission, even of long duration, was usually followed by one or more relapses. These relapses usually proved to be less acute and of shorter duration; which led the observer to speak of 'waves' of anorexia nervosa, because of the way in which the disease seems to rise and fall and eventually spend itself out. The last of these so-called 'waves' seems to occur, usually with a milder and incomplete symptomatology, when the patient is 17–19 years old; the author and his co-workers have found no evidence of anorexia nervosa in older age groups.

The undulatory course of anorexia nervosa is well demonstrated by the following case history:

The patient came from a prosperous family and was the product of a full-term pregnancy; she had developed normally. She started to read at the age of four and could read perfectly by the time she was six years old: she went to a nursery school, was well behaved, but lacked that spontaneity and vivacity typical of children. She started regular school at the age of seven and did very well; she read a lot, wrote poems, enjoyed the admiration of her classmates and was always ready to help those who lagged behind. She was very attached to her mother, but did not always confide in her. Her relationship with her father was cold. At the age of ten, following the death of a friend of the family, she became afraid of the dark, this fear lasting for about a month. She started menstruating at thirteen, but her menses were irregular. During all her life she was a poor eater, finicky and of poor appetite. When thirteen years of age, she spent a summer holiday in the country; she felt well, was cheerful and was gaining weight. It was during this period that one of her girl friends remarked that she had grown fatter. This remark led to the patient's frequent scrutiny of her figure in front of a mirror and to the development of anxiety, fear, irritability and short temper. She began to diet. If forced to eat, she would cry, shout and become very irate. When these episodes were at their worse, she would grip her own throat and try to strangle herself with a towel. She ate very little, but did not reject food altogether. She became constipated.

At the beginning, afraid of putting on weight, she would suppress any feeling of hunger; later, she complained of lack of appetite. It became difficult for her to concentrate, and she suffered from frequent headaches; she was depressed and grew indifferent to her environment. She no longer showed any signs of affection towards her family; was quite unmoved by the illness of a close relative and did not show any sorrow when the latter died. She started to say that she considered herself 'ugly'; she kept rubbing her chin to reduce its 'fat'. She became abrupt with her family.

At the age of fourteen, because of her persistent rejection of food, she was admitted to the child psychiatry department for treatment. She found the surroundings unbearable, cried often, protesting that she could not stand life in hospital, and from the very first day she insisted in fixing the date of her discharge. She explained that she avoided food because she was afraid of growing fatter. By the time of her discharge she had gained weight and was eating normally.

On the very first day of her return home, her mother noticed that the girl was still worried about putting on weight; she ate with reluctance, touching the food with distaste. She would eat very little so that she would not 'get fatter' and jump up and down for long periods of time as a form of slimming exercise. At first it was possible to force her to eat, but later she almost completely refused to take food.

She was readmitted to hospital, where quite soon she began to eat; the anorexia disappeared and she gained weight once more. However, once discharged home, her behaviour changed for the worse. With the help of a table of calories she calculated the minimum amount of food that she needed and rapidly reduced her food intake. Her headaches became more severe, she started to miss school, where her performance deteriorated. Vomiting followed and she became progressively thinner. Her relationship with her elder brother was poor; she was on better terms with her younger brother, but she used him to express her resentment and would force him to eat until he vomited.

Once again she was admitted to hospital and again displayed the same behaviour. She was reserved, apathetic, friendly only to some of the other girls, avoided going for walks, disregarded after-dinner rest periods, tried to go to bed later than the other children, ate slowly and reluctantly. She was aloof with her peers and did not show any interest in the life of the ward. Much of her time was spent on school work and reading, although sometimes she would condescend to join in the games. She was bored by her stay, and from the very first day demanded that a date be fixed for discharge. She pressed her parents into visiting every day, but when they came she was rude, impertinent and tactless.

Rapport was easily made with this girl, but it was always superficial. Her replies were correct, to the point, brief and cold, and came in short, polite and restrained sentences. Her behaviour towards her parents was resentful and she would blame them for the lack of attention and of the respect that she felt was due to her 'as a person'. She was inclined to be over-sensitive in her own analysis of her emotional experiences and her illness. She correctly explained that the onset of her illness was due to her fear of growing fat, but it was not so much her growing fat, as what people would say about her, that worried her. It suited her to remain thin, pale and ill because in that way she would get more attention. For the same reason she did not want to recover.

After a third admission to hospital of a duration of six weeks, she was much improved; she gained 6 kg and her constipation disappeared. She herself stated that whereas she had been thinking all the time about food, how to slim and how not to put on weight, now she remembered food at meal-times only, felt at ease, and was more active, sociable and approachable.

As demonstrated above, in the majority of cases the prognosis of anorexia nervosa is favourable, despite the severe and complex metabolic impairments that characterize its course.

Laboratory investigations have shown that the basal metabolism of these patients is very low, falling on occasions to an index of 40 per cent. During observations on protein metabolism the investigators noticed delay in the process of deamination; this they associated with dystrophic changes and impairment of liver function. The measurement of blood sugar after glucose load, indicated that sugar content was not returning to the normal level after three or four hours. Predominant were also alkalosis with hypochloraemia and hypopotassaemia (Staehelin, Reber, Bühlmann[15]).

In one case the outcome was fatal: the patient, an adolescent girl, persuaded her parents to reject the doctor's recommendation to hospitalize her and she died of malnutrition.

Thus in the course of the disease the following stages can be determined:

1. An initial stage of neurotic and psychopathic-like symptoms, which precede by a year and a half to two years the manifestations of anorexia.

    A further degree of development of this stage presents with dismorphic and phobic disorders, which immediately precede the manifestations of the disease. ('I am fat', 'I am stout', 'I am hideously plump', etc.)

During the above period, according to the prevalence of corresponding symptoms, it is possible to discern three variations in the development of the disease: an hysterical, a psychoasthenic and an asthenic development.

2. During the second stage overt manifestations of the disease occur.

   (a) The first part of this period shows the onset of *anorexia* with a predominance of obsessions and a fanatical determination to slim. The feeling of hunger remains, but is overcome by the patient's pathological auto-suggestion.

   (b) A period of *cachexia* follows, characterized by a progressive loss of flesh and an abundance of somatic disorders. At this time the obsessional desire to slim is not so intense, hence the patient could be persuaded to eat; the feeling of hunger is more frequent, but now the patient finds it 'impossible' to take food. He would say that 'the stomach doesn't take anything'; 'it is overloaded; even after a little food I cannot breathe'; 'I would eat sometimes, but I cannot'; 'Before, I was very hungry but I would not eat; I used to overcome hunger tenaciously. Now I am never hungry, and eating is a painful and nasty procedure. It is much easier not to eat.'

During this period, when the clinical disorder was very severe, we were able to observe isolated psychosomatic disorders concurrent with neurotic symptoms, cachexia and continuing anorexia.

3. In the third stage the processes of the disease are reversed in one of the following ways:

   (a) A rapid reversing of symptomatology leading to full recovery and a return to a sense of proportion about food.

   (b) A slow reversing of symptomatology leading to a full recovery and a gradual return to a sense of proportion about food.

   (c) An oscillating, gradual reversing of symptomatology, with some relapses.

6

Treatment

Treatment, besides psychotherapy and discussion with the patient, includes hormonal therapy, using adrenocorticotrophins, de-oxycorticosterone; small doses of insulin to stimulate the appetite and, of course, an appropriate diet. Among the tranquillizers, librium, valium and galloperidol proved the most effective. Symptomatic relief was obtained, when indicated, by the use of sedatives, stimulants and cardiac and vascular analeptics.

7
Differential Diagnosis

A diagnosis of anorexia nervosa can be arrived at with a good degree of accuracy by taking into consideration the age of onset, the clinical picture presented by the manifestations, and the characteristic course of its development. However, criteria for a differential diagnosis are necessary, as there are other diseases which include amongst their symptoms a progressive loss of weight and anorexia.

In 1914 Simmonds described cachexia in women, accompanied by amenorrhoea and atrophy of the genital organs, due to the partial destruction of the anterior lobe of the pituitary gland. As cachexia and amenorrhoea are typical of both *Simmonds' disease* and anorexia nervosa, both diseases were later to draw the attention of endocrinologists.

The criteria for the clinical differential diagnosis of anorexia nervosa from Simmonds' disease (or hypophyseal insufficiency) have already been fully discussed by Van Balen;[1] McCullagh and Tupper;[13] Escamilla and Lisser;[4] and others. The criteria proposed by these authors are as follows:

(*a*) anorexia nervosa presents mostly in early adolescence;
(*b*) more frequent in girls than in boys;
(*c*) lack of pronounced changes of secondary sex characters;
(*d*) lack of signs of premature senility;
(*e*) loss of hair and teeth extremely rare;
(*f*) psychogenic reasons for food rejection, without loss of appetite;
(*g*) direct relation of loss of weight with food rejection, as against the progressive emaciation characteristic of Simmonds' disease;
(*h*) the patient is hypersensitive to any offer of help and is eager to slim; persistently resists any treatment, which is regarded as an obstacle to slimming—these characteristics do not apply to patients with Simmonds' disease.
(*i*) absence of weakness, even with a significant degree of emaciation, is typical of the initial and later stages of development of hypophyseal deficiency;
(*j*) in anorexia nervosa the patients remain active, very sensitive, and have morbid aspirations towards their goal; in contrast, patients with Simmonds' disease are passive, apathetic and disinterested.

Research on adolescents suffering from anorexia nervosa has shown that in about 5 per cent of them the syndrome coexists with symptoms consistent with the clinical picture of *schizophrenia*. In these patients the syndrome of anorexia is not a neurotic phenomenon which determines its clinical characteristics. We have found no anorexia nervosa in typical adolescent schizophrenics, whether their schizophrenia was 'nuclear' (hebephrenia, paranoid schizophrenia with hallucinations and delusions), 'periodical' (catatonic schizophrenia, circular schizophrenia or manic-depressive psychosis) or other forms of psychosis. We are, or course, not referring here to anorexia resulting from hallucinations and paranoia. However, overt anorexia has been observed in clinical variants of schizophrenia with a slow development which resemble a neurotic, psychopathic or mild paranoid disorder.

The following criteria for a differential diagnosis distinguish schizophrenic anorexia from anorexia nervosa:

(a) slow progressive changes towards a schizoid personality and gradual display of a symptomatology consistent with schizophrenia (increasing autism, infantilism, derangement, dissociation of thought processes, loss of mental activity, affective disorders and shallowness, neurotic and psychopathic disorders, or any other psychotic symptoms);

(b) co-existence of anorexia with the processes symptomatic of schizophrenia of slow development;

(c) lingering, mild but constant development of the anorexia syndrome itself, with the absence of discernible motivation for food rejection, which by contrast is typical in anorexia nervosa;

(d) undulating development of the anorexia syndrome and of resistance to therapy.

8

Causal Mechanisms of Anorexia Nervosa

Despite much research, the pathogenesis of anorexia nervosa still remains obscure, but clinical investigations so far undertaken have brought us nearer to understanding its mechanisms and its development. We now accept that the psychopathology of anorexia nervosa is complex, as it represents the expression of a supervalent thought.

From what has been said about anorexia nervosa in the preceding pages, it becomes obvious that the desire to slim is directly related to specific situations at the age of puberty, which is a period characterized by excessive value being given to certain thoughts. This is unlike paranoid thinking, which is devoid of logic in relation to actual situations. The thought of slimming becomes uppermost in the patient's mind; it becomes supervalent thought which is regarded by him as a personal intimate emotional experience. Despite this, the desire to slim can usually be corrected at various stages of the disease.

The theory that the wish to slim in these patients is based on a supervalent thought becomes even more valid if we compare the characteristics of their thinking with the typical traits of supervalent thoughts. A supervalent thought is a leading force, a controlling centre, which has a particular power to colour the affect, monopolizing it in favour of a single idea, that becomes the ruling element in the whole life and activity of an individual. This process always merges with the personality, which becomes identified with it, as if it was dissolved in it. The supervalent thought grows into an all-important nucleus, the very essence of the personality, which focuses a mighty power on a single point.

The thoughts of slimming in our patients has all these properties. Furthermore, we must stress the fact that during the period when the manifestations of anorexia nervosa were developing, patients often displayed dysmorphophobic phenomena, regarding themselves as 'fat', 'stout', 'ugly', 'plump', etc. This insane fear of becoming deformed was usually of short duration, but it spread, not only to the external features of the face but included the whole body; it was gradually replaced by more severe symptoms of anorexia. One of the characteristics of this syndrome is that the patient is anxious not so much about those features of his body which he already possesses, but rather about the possibility of future obesity. Despite this, the dysmorphophobia has no paranoid characteristics, but is also a supervalent thought. The frequent co-existence of dysmorphophobia and anorexia in the total picture of anorexia nervosa led M. V. Korkina[9] to regard the latter as 'secondary anorexia in dysmorphophobia'.

The dynamics of the development of anorexia nervosa show a transition from obsessional dysmorphophobia to supervalent thoughts about the shape of the body, and from obsessional anorexia to a period when food rejection is of overwhelming importance. Janet[7] included anorexia nervosa among disorders of an hysterical nature, as it presented 'in the guise of shame for the body', and named it 'phychoasthenic sitieirgia'.

In contrast to typical hysterical anorexia, in which the act of food intake is impossible (Loo[11]), in anorexia nervosa food intake is actively inhibited by the overwhelming desire to slim and to abstain from food.

Our investigations have confirmed that both dysmorphophobia and anorexia nervosa are syndromes typical to adolescents and young people. Moreover, as demonstrated above, these syndromes present mainly in adolescents 12–15 years old; that is to say in an age group which has just emerged from an important stage of personality development, marked by the evolution of abstract thinking, self-awareness, a transformation from individual being to social being, and a reorientation of affective relationships as new claims confront the adolescent. This complex moulding and reorientation of personality creates conditions which are especially favourable for the emergence of those character traits and, in the case of disease, of symptoms, which are not usually observed in an earlier age group.

These observations justify the conclusion that *one of the causal mechanisms of anorexia nervosa is a deficiency in a particular area in the process of personality development, i.e. a psychogenic mechanism.* The fact that anorexia nervosa has usually a favourable prognosis and is not found in adults suggests that this deficiency is transitory and is compensated as the adolescent grows older. Decourt[3] discusses the possible significance of reorientation of affects in a developing personality in relation to anorexia nervosa.

It is very important to determine the mechanism responsible for the pattern of dysmorphophobia and anorexia, as seen in our patients. The criteria for a differential diagnosis between Simmonds' disease and anorexia nervosa have already been mentioned above; however, in addition to those basic criteria, the medical history of many of the patients in the sample studied revealed past episodes of lack of interest in food, poor appetite, food fads, etc. These observations, the auto-suggestion and the psychogenic ability for total inhibition of the wish to eat, that we found in our patients, together with the endocrine and metabolic disorders noted by many workers, are findings that agree with those of Bergmann and Berlin[2] on the 'hypophyseal insufficiency' of these patients.

Thus a uniform pattern in the clinical course of anorexia nervosa suggests that the second causal mechanism in anorexia nervosa is a constitutional neuro-endocrine deficiency, with hypophyseal failure as its main feature. Hence two complex interlocking mechanisms, one psychogenic and the other somatogenic, co-exist in the pathogenesis of anorexia nervosa.

It is hoped that further investigations will help us towards a better understanding of the morbid process of anorexia nervosa, and produce effective therapeutic techniques for its prevention and treatment.

REFERENCES

1. BALEN VAN. 1939. Anorexia nervosa und hypophysare magerkeit. *Acta med. scand.*, **101**, 433.
2. BERGMANN, G. VON and BERLIN, I. N. 1934. Magerkeit und Magersucht. *Dtsch. med. Wschr.*, **4**, 129.
3. DECOURT, J. 1951. Nosologie de l'anorexie mentale. *Presse méd.*, **59**, 797.
4. ESCAMILLA, R. F. and LISSER, H. 1942. Simmonds' disease. *J. clin. Endocrin.*, **2**, 65.
5. FRÖLICH, M. S. 1953. Probleme der anorexia nervosa. *Schweiz. med. Wschr.*, **35**, 811–817; **36**, 837–841.
6. GULL, W. W. 1888. Anorexia nervosa. *Lancet*, i, 516.
7. JANET, P. 1911. *Neurosis.* Moscow: Cosmos.
8. KISSYEL, A. A. 1894. A case of a severe hysterical anorexia in a girl of 11. *Medicinskoie obozrenie*, **42**, 17.
9. KORKINA, M. V. 1961. On prognostic significance of 'dysmorphophobia' syndrome, *Problems of schizophrenia, neurosis, reactive conditions.* Moscow.
10. LASÈGUE, C. 1873. De l'anorexie hystérique. *Arch. gén. Méd.*, **1**, 385.
11. LOO, P. 1958. L'anorexie mentale. *Ann. méd.-psychol.*, **2**, 4.
12. LÜFFLER, W. 1955. Die anorexia mentalis. *Helv. med. Acta*, vols. 4–5.
13. McCULLAGH, E. P. and TUPPER, W. R. 1940. Anorexia nervosa. *Ann. intern. Med.*, **14**, 817.
14. MORTON, R. Quoted from E. L. Bliss and C. Branch, 1960. *Anorexia nervosa.* New York: Hoeber.
15. STAEHELIN, D. VON, REBER, K. and BÜHLMANN, A. 1955. Das Säure-Basen-Gleichgewicht bei anorexie mentalis and bei akuten Hungerzustand. *Helv. med. Acta*, vols. 4–5.

XIII

DRUG ABUSE AND ADDICTION IN ADOLESCENTS

PHILIP R. BOYD

M.B., B.S., M.R.C.S. L.R.C.P.

Lecturer in Adolescent Psychotherapy
The Middlesex Hospital Medical School, London
Clinical Assistant-in-charge
Simmons House, St Luke's-Woodside Hospital, London
England

1

Introduction

Many variables determine the advent of drug addiction in any particular individual but the seriously involved youthful addict seldom takes his tortuous and tortured path as an unfeeling degenerate remote from his own kind. Rather he is a frightened and unhappy youngster at odds with himself and the society into which he is emerging. In his search for assistance and in the context of a significant idiom of his own culture, he turns away from a world of seemingly hostile people and vainly tries to medicate himself and to seek solace in the society of like-minded rejects.

Such youngsters, of course, form only a very small section of the vast and normal teenage community, most of which will either avoid the web altogether or only temporarily indulge in the experimental challenge of drugs with an inherent caution that mercifully protects them. Nevertheless it can be argued that no person is really safe from infection and that all such drug-taking is essentially dangerous, placing any individual at risk to a malignant process for which, when it is entrenched, there is no certainty of cure. This indeed may be so, for there are no absolute boundaries in the spectrum of the human psyche between what is normal and abnormal.

Yet it is the addicted adolescent with whom we are primarily concerned here and not the relatively healthy youngster who can draw back from a hazardous experiment before he becomes himself the slave of his own experimental adventure. As Isbell[37] has pointed out, emotionally normal and mature individuals practically never become addicted. The same is true of the adolescent who is making sound progress in his development towards maturity.

2

Definitions

This is not the place for a detailed résumé on the whole subject of drug addiction. Nevertheless certain definitions and historical facts are necessary to get the picture of present-day drugs into perspective. We first require to be certain of the descriptive terms which are employed in this field, into which so many different professional and lay people have delved. The difficulty here has been that labels have been used by individual groups to bring succinctly together those qualities of addictive drugs which seem significant to their own special experience. Hence we hear the following terms which are confusing because they sound similar when in fact they are not. Drugs have been called 'dangerous' and 'safe', 'illicit' and 'licit', 'hard' and 'soft', drugs of 'addiction' and drugs of 'habituation' and finally, drugs of 'dependency'. In addition we talk about the 'misuse' of drugs and the 'abuse' of drugs. Even the very word 'drug' itself is beginning to have a pejorative meaning, as it is used incessantly in the newspapers, in the courts, and even in the clinics themselves, to mean a drug of addiction.

Almost any pharmaceutical drug can be dangerous if used for the wrong purpose, in excess or in the wrong way. Young drug-takers in particular demonstrate one important aspect of this fact when they crush down tablets of a relatively harmless medicament, suspend the material in tap-water and inject it intravenously into their arms. In this way a drug, which can be bought without hindrance of any kind, becomes an exceedingly dangerous substance. All the drugs of addiction which will be described can in some ways therefore be dangerous.

As for the term 'illicit' drug, this should only be used to describe a drug which is either prescribed illegally, dispensed illegally, or obtained and carried on the person illegally. The term should not be used as a synonym for any drug obtained for addictive use just because it is taken for a purpose for which it is not primarily intended, or against medical advice.

Similarly there is confusion between the terms 'drug misuse' and 'drug abuse'. The word 'abuse' rightly has the more severe connotation. The word 'misuse' might as well convey the idea of an unintentional mis-application of a drug as an intentional one. Yet one of the important Acts in the U.K. making the possession of certain drugs without prescription illegal, employs the term 'misuse'. The word 'abuse' indicates clearly the deliberate intention to use the drug for the wrong purpose, and is therefore more appropriate in the legal and drug addictive setting. The two words should not be used to describe different degrees of severity of addictive behaviour.

The terms 'hard' and 'soft' were first used by drug-takers themselves and then taken up by newspapers and lay persons to categorise drugs of addiction into two groups, making a mistaken assumption of equivalents of severity between the organic addictive features on the one hand and the dangerous effects of a particular drug on the other. This has tended to over-simplify and misrepresent the complex medical and social issues of drug-taking, and to mislead many people, adult and juvenile, about the hazards involved.

There has also been a problem among professional workers with the three technical words of 'addiction', 'habituation' and 'dependence'. The use of the word 'addiction' attached to the chronic use of and reliance on certain drugs goes back deeply into history, that of 'habituation' and 'dependence' are relative innovations. Until recent times 'addiction' had been used to describe a syndrome about which little was clearly defined. However, in 1950 the W.H.O.[70] offered a very good definition as follows: 'Drug addiction is a state of periodic or chronic intoxication detrimental to the individual and to society, produced by the repeated consumption of a drug (actual or synthetic). Its characteristics include: (1) an overpowering desire or need (compulsion) to continue taking the drug and to obtain it by any means; (2) a tendency to increase the dose; (3) a psychic (psychological) and, sometimes, a physical dependence on the effects of the drug.'

Later an attempt was made to deal with the separate concepts of the physical and psychological factors in addiction, and to relate these to the drugs concerned and their qualitative differences, both in terms of the individual's need for the drug and the effects produced by its withdrawal. Hence in 1956 the W.H.O.[71] introduced separate definitions for 'addiction' and 'habituation'. The latter was meant to be used for addictive drugs in which compulsion, tolerance and organic necessity were not essential qualities, and where it was thought that the effects were detrimental only to the addict himself. No doubt it was this division in terminology that eventually led to the lay terms of 'hard' and 'soft' drugs.

However, recent knowledge and clinical experience with the many drugs now being taken had shown that the term 'habituation' was really unsatisfactory. It is no simple matter to try and establish whether the taking of certain drugs does or does not cause some degree of physical need and tolerance; and the factor of compulsion is not at all a primary question of organic necessity. The problem of organic involvement is in fact a relatively minor one when it comes to the real issues of treatment of adolescents who are on relatively small doses of such drugs as heroin or methadone. Withdrawal symptoms are so variable, and so determined and coloured by emotional forces derived from the fear of the loss of a precious attachment, that the psychological aspects of addiction are clearly the paramount issue.

In 1964 the W.H.O.[72] suggested that both the words 'addiction' and 'habituation' should be replaced by the one word 'dependence', and that drug dependence should be described in terms of the specific pattern of the generic type of drug involved. This, however, really only offers a list of drugs according to their essential chemical composition.

An attempt to provide a more useful classification is made in Table I. One further point of definition, however, should be mentioned. The term 'narcotic drug' is often used. Strictly speaking this should describe any drug capable of causing narcosis, which is defined variously as a state of profound stupor, unconsciousness or sound sleep. Many different categories of drug will do this and the term is therefore unreliable in the general context of addiction. Its use stems from the original laws in the U.S.A. designed to deal with the problem of opiate and cocaine control and in that country it refers specifically to these two drugs. The latter, however, is clearly not a narcotic in any real sense of the word. Cannabis has also frequently been included under this term as it has been incorporated into the same legislation. In the U.K. these drugs come under what is called The Dangerous Drugs Act.

Bearing these issues in mind it would still seem that the word 'addiction' is the best one to use. The term 'dependence', although rightly stressing the dependent nature of the addict's personality, removes the essential connotation of a malignant and compulsive force at work and as we shall inevitably have to continue to describe the patient himself as an 'addict' (he can hardly be called a 'dependent'), the term 'addiction' should be retained for the persistent and compulsive taking of any drug when such a habit is entrenched in the personality and the behaviour of the individual succumbing to it, and when it places that individual or others in his environment at risk.

3

Classification

The drugs and substances with which we are concerned do not easily lend themselves to a simple classification. It is of course possible for an individual to use any substance or even an object or a person in an addictive way. Here, however, we are concerned with those substances, medical drugs, industrial chemicals and plant derivatives alike which youth employs in its search for a special experience, usually called a 'kick' or a 'buzz', and which apparently become an intensely vital and necessary source of gratification.

The classification shown in Table I is not entirely comprehensive but will serve to outline the major categories of addictive substances, their main central nervous effect and the usual degree of toxicity which they effect in the adolescent in general. It should be noted that these categories do not imply exclusive clinical effects. For example the amphetamines can cause hallucinations, and Lysergide ('L.S.D.') can provoke a psychosis.

TABLE I

Common Drugs of Abuse and Addiction (C.N.S. Intoxicants) Employed by Adolescents

Usual toxic effects	Physical and psychological addiction	Mainly psychological addiction	
	I C.N.S. depressants	II C.N.S. stimulants	III C.N.S. hallucinogens *

Mild	1. *Organic solvents*
	e.g. Toluene
	  Acetone
	  Benzene
	  Carbon tetrachloride
	  Ether
	2. *Alcohol*
	e.g. Ethyl alcohol
		1. *Xanthines*
		e.g. Caffeine
		2. *Sympathomimetics*
		e.g. Ephedrine
		  Isoprenaline
			1. Nutmeg (Myristica Fragrans)
			2. Morning Glory Seeds (Convolvulacea)
			3. Cannabis (Cannabis Sativa)

Moderate	(HYPNOTICS–SEDATIVES)
	1. *Barbiturates*
	e.g. Pentobarbitone (s–a)
	  Amylobarbitone (i–a)
	  Phenobarbitone (l–a)
	2. *Miscellaneous*
	e.g. 'Mandrax' = methaqualone &
	  diphenhydramine
	  'Doriden' = glutethimide
	  'Librium' = chlordiazepoxide
	  'Valium' = diazepam
	  'Equanil' = meprobamate
		(ANORECTICS)
		1. *Amphetamines*
		e.g. 'Benzedrine' = amphetamine
		  'Dexedrine' = dexamphetamine
		  'Methedrine' = methylamphetamine
		2. *Miscellaneous*
		e.g. 'Preludin' = phenmetrazine
		  'Ritalin' = methylphenidate
		  'Tenuate' = diethylpropion
			1. Mescaline (Peyote)
			2. Psilocybin (Psilocybe)
			3. 'D.M.T.' = dimethyltryptamine

Severe	OPIATES
	1. *Natural or semi-synthetic*
	e.g. Opium (Papaver somniferum)
	  Morphine
	  Heroin = diacetylmorphine
	2. *Synthetic*
	e.g. Methadone
	  Pethidine
		Cocaine (Erythroxylum Coca or Truxillense)	1. 'L.S.D.' = Lysergic acid diethylamide (Lysergide)
			2. 'S.T.P.' = 4-methyl-2,5-dimethoxy-alpha-methyl phenethylamine

* This word is chosen in preference to others, as it describes the most common manifestation. Other names given to these drugs include:
Psychotomimetics = producing psychotic manifestations.
Psychodysleptics = producing delusional manifestations.

Alcohol will also do both. Tobacco is not included in this classification because of the general uncertainty of its action. While tobacco smoking is undoubtedly a practice to which young people easily become habituated, its essential danger lies not so much in harmful psychological and social effects as in the possible long-term potentiating effect on organic disease.

It is to be pointed out that the drugs which unquestionably cause physical addiction are all listed in the first column and are primarily depressants of the central nervous system. It is also noteworthy that the more powerfully depressant the drug and the more effective it is as an analgesic, the greater is its addictive potential and morbid significance.

4

Drugs Abused by Adolescents

I. THE C.N.S. DEPRESSANTS

1. Organic Solvents

There are many factors which lead an adolescent towards drugs but his age in part determines how he starts.

The use of commercial solvents in particular seems to start among children and the younger adolescents. It has not been reported as occurring to any great extent in the U.K., but there have been many references to it in North America and it has been reported in various other countries. Attention to the problem in the U.K. was first drawn by Merry,[51] who reported on the outcome of a young man who first started glue-sniffing at the age of 20 and who eventually became a heroin addict. He drew attention to the fact that there were over 2000 cases in New York City in the year 1963 and warned that the habit might become popular in the U.K. Individual cases have since been described, such as those of addiction to carbon tetrachloride by Todd,[63] and to a mixture of chlorinatic hydrocarbons in a shoe-cleaning liquid by a group of schoolchildren by Hepple (1968).[33]

The picture in the U.S.A. has been well described by Krug et al.[43] The practice is one of inhalation or 'sniffing' of commercial solvents contained in proprietary preparations sold to anyone and used for quite simple social purposes, such as model and household glues, cleaning fluids, lacquer thinners, fingernail-polish remover, and even lighter fluid and petrol. The material is usually put into a container or a plastic bag, or on a rag or handkerchief, and sniffed until a transient intoxication and accompanying elation, like that of drinking alcohol, results.

The main substances involved are the aromatic hydrocarbons such as benzene and toluene (contained in polystyrene glue); the halogenated hydrocarbons such as carbon tetrachloride (contained in cleaning fluids); the ketones such as acetone (contained in nail-polish remover); and also various esters, alcohols and ether. In fact any volatile organic solvent will produce a state of intoxication from which the young person can derive a thrill.

Unwin[65] has reported an incidence of glue-sniffing in Winnipeg schools in 1967 of between 2 and 5 per cent. His summary of the typical clinical picture of solvent inhalation describes how, within minutes of sniffing the solvent, a pattern of acute intoxication develops and this is occasionally accompanied by visual and auditory hallucinations. This lasts up to one hour and is followed by drowsiness. Much depends on the concentration of vapour inhaled but, if it is considerable, stupor and convulsions may occur. Abnormalities of the electroencephalogram have been reported during the period of intoxication and for several weeks afterwards.

Bozovsky and Winkler[12] reported on nineteen children and adolescent glue-sniffers under the age of 16 admitted to hospital in Brooklyn, N.Y., with a clinical picture of acute brain syndrome with confusion, hallucinations and epileptiform seizures, associated in five cases with severe but reversible electroencephalographic changes.

Press and Done[56] have reviewed the subject at length. They found that most solvent-sniffers were aged between 10 and 15 years, but some start even younger. Boys were far more frequently involved than girls. Tolerance and habituation occurred in many cases, although serious withdrawal symptoms have been rare. The most consistent physical finding was transient urinary abnormalities.

Opinions on the question of permanent brain damage are divided, but there has been one report of cerebellar degeneration by Grabski.[30] Other transient findings of renal and blood pathology and of possible liver damage have been reported by Sokol[61] among teenagers in Los Angeles. Repeated frequent inhalation or ingestion of solvents will lead to local damage to the mucous membranes of the nose and mouth.

Owing to the rapid response and the unpleasant side-effects of these solvents, such as headache, nausea and vomiting, most children soon abandon the habit. Nevertheless a few persist in a truly addictive way. It has been claimed that physical as well as psychological dependence can occur but there is little substantial evidence yet to confirm this. Death has usually occurred as a side-effect with the habit, as for example from suffocation by the plastic bag.

2. Alcohol

Addiction to ethyl alcohol among adults is the largest of all problems of addiction in most countries of the world. Williams[66] estimates that there are some 300 000 'alcoholics' in the U.K. It is difficult, however, to evaluate the problem among adolescents. While it is evident in the last two decades that increasing numbers of adolescents are drinking alcohol, and start to do so progressively earlier in life, the numbers which can be considered as truly addicted remain unknown. It is likely that alcoholism as such does not usually become entrenched until the individual is past the chronological period of adolescence. Nevertheless, cases of adolescent alcoholism are occasionally seen.

Kessel and Walton[42] draw attention to the appearance in the U.K. of teenage drunkenness in the 1950s, but they make no comment on the incidence of alcoholism as such in the under-20 age group. Most authors on the subject only report the incidence of alcoholism in terms of young people under the age of 30. Glatt and Hills[28] have shown a significant increase in the number of admissions to their units of alcoholics of this age group as between the 1950s and the 1960s. Glatt[26] has also shown, from a survey in 1961 of adolescents aged 15–18, that 6 per cent of boys and girls had taken alcohol before the age of 10 years and 90 per cent by the age of 15; and that 40 per cent of the boys and 18 per cent of the girls were regular drinkers by the age of 18. This and other studies by the same author point to the early onset of regular drinking among adolescents. He makes the significant comment, however, that the great majority of young drug addicts in the U.K. are contemptuous of alcohol.

Table II shows the number of offences of drunkenness in England and Wales in the under-18-year-old age group for the years 1958–1968. These figures support the view that adolescents are indulging increasingly in alcohol.

TABLE II

Number of Offences of Drunkenness in the Under-18-year-old Age Group 1958–1968

	1958	1959	1960	1961	1962	1963	1964	1965	1966	1967	1968
Male	941	949	1460	1535	1435	1478	1775	1810	1772	1919	2141
Female	59	59	87	118	88	88	77	97	108	129	163
TOTAL	1000	1008	1547	1653	1523	1566	1852	1907	1880	2048	2304

Source: H.M.S.O. *Offences of Drunkenness 1958–1968 inclusive.*

In the U.S. a study of the alcohol consumption by high school students was undertaken by Maddox and McCall.[48] A total of 1962 youngsters in the 11th and 12th grades were interviewed. All but 8 per cent had occasionally taken or tasted alcohol, 9 per cent were regarded as regular drinkers, 6 per cent as frequently drinking and 23 per cent as occasional drinkers.

Glatt and Hills[28] consider that normal adolescents drink not for 'kicks', but as an aid to social acceptance. This can be seen either in terms of the youngster having to do what others, especially his peers, expect him to do, as a sign of virility and perhaps of adult identification, or in terms of needing a bolster to social courage. On the other hand, the young alcoholic consistently makes the deliberate attempt to achieve the effects of acute intoxication. The same pattern appears to distinguish the majority of young people who use 'pep pills' at the weekend from the minority who become juvenile addicts.

Glatt and Hills suggest certain predisposing socio-pathological factors in juvenile alcoholism which generally mirror those used to account for all forms of addiction, and they conclude that young alcoholics are even more disturbed than their adult counterparts. This would also seem to hold true of the young person who becomes a narcotic addict while still in his adolescence. One perhaps significant point in the background of these youthful alcoholics is the not uncommon finding of heavy drinking by one parent.

3. Hypnotics and Sedatives

It is well recognised that barbiturate drugs are the most widely pre-scribed sedatives. Their use poses a severe problem of addiction in adults. Bewley[5] has suggested that approximately 100 000 persons in the U.K. are dependent on them; and he has also pointed out[6] that in the last ten years there has been a marked increase in all age groups in the use of bar-biturates both in causing accidental deaths and for suicidal purposes. The same applies to non-fatal poisonings. Glatt[27] suggests that the total number of annual cases of barbiturate poisoning probably exceeds 10 000. The actual number of N.H.S. prescriptions in the U.K. for barbiturates has, however, at last begun to decline, probably due to a greater awareness and caution on the part of doctors prescribing them, but in 1968 15·5 million National Health Service prescriptions for barbiturates were pro-vided (Table III).

TABLE III

Numbers (in millions) of National Health Service Prescriptions Provided by Retail Pharmacists in the Years 1965–1968

	1965	1966	1967	1968
Amphetamines	3·8	3·7	3·0	2·4
Barbiturates	17·2	16·8	16·1	15·5
'Mandrax'	0·05	0·6	1·3	2·0

Source: Ministry of Health.

In a British survey conducted in 1963, Adams *et al.*[1] found that out of 407 patients receiving prescriptions for barbiturates in a large general practice of about 10 000 people, only 7 patients (0·6 per cent) were in the age group 10–19. With adolescents the chronic abuse of barbiturates by themselves has already begun to be a serious problem, however, and it would now seem that they are being increasingly used as alternatives to narcotic drugs. In the past they have been used extensively in the form of mixtures with anorectic drugs, e.g. dexamphetamine sulphate with either amylobarbitone (intermediate acting) or phenobarbitone (long acting). The most popular with adolescents is the first mentioned ('Drinamyl') and is known in the U.K. as 'blues', 'French blues' and previously as 'purple hearts'.

It would appear that the sedative component in these combinations prevents the stimulant one from becoming excessive and so suppresses some of the unpleasant experiences of amphetamine intoxication both during and immediately after taking the drug. It may also be the more responsible of the two components in the production of addiction to these preparations.

The adolescent opiate addict will crush hypnotic pills and capsules in water and inject the suspension intravenously. He usually does this when he cannot find sufficient opiate or when he seems particularly impulsive, desperate and self-destructive. Such drugs as methaqualone in combination with diphenhydramine hydrochloride ('Mandrax'), glutethimide ('Doriden') and dichloralphenazone ('Welldorm') have all been experimented with in this way. The first of these has become popular with young drug-users in the U.K., some of whom take it during the daytime to become intoxicated. Youngsters will swallow up to eight or ten tablets often with a stimulant drug, or as a supplement to heroin or methadone. They appear to enjoy the intoxicating results of these drugs which at first give an effect similar to that of over-indulgence in alcohol, but longer-lasting, and which may cause considerable confusion, drowsiness and even coma. What is so astonishing is the ease with which boys of only 15 or 16 can still persuade doctors to prescribe these drugs by using the simple excuse that they are suffering from insomnia! This dangerous habit and the severe inebriation which follows not only places the youth (and others) at immediate risk but also adds further encouragement to him to follow the road to serious drug abuse. Table III shows the increase in prescribing of 'Mandrax' in the last four years, which appears to be replacing barbiturates.

Nyswander[55] described the serious addictive quality of glutethimide, its capacity to cause tolerance and severe withdrawal symptoms, and its popularity with American adolescents. Bewley (1969)[7] comments on the wide abuse of these particular drugs in the U.K. and the U.S., but emphasises that much less is known about them than is known about barbiturates. He notes that overdosage and suicide rates with them have risen and he rightly suggests that probably far more of these compounds are being prescribed than is justified medically. Indeed there can be very little justification in prescribing hypnotics or sedatives to an adolescent unless he is suffering from an emotional or physical illness, and even then such drugs should always be given to a responsible adult to safeguard and control.

There is no evidence of adolescent abuse of chloral hydrate and other similar sedatives, but a word should be added on the subject of tranquillisers. It is remarkable that in this group of drugs reports of addiction do not occur. However, a distinction has been drawn between what have been called the major and the minor tranquillisers in respect of addiction.[50] Addiction, with tolerance and withdrawal syndrome, to meprobamate, chlordiazepoxide and diazepam has been observed, while the phenothiazines themselves appear to be non-addictive. One reason for this difference may lie in the greater similarity in clinical effect of the so-called 'minor tranquillisers' with other hypnotic drugs. Adolescents have been known to find such drugs as chlordiazepoxide extremely gratifying, and have used them for intravenous injections. Commercial preparations containing mixtures of 'minor tranquillisers' and amphetamines are occasionally prescribed to young people by doctors who are unaware of the significance in addictive potential of these medicines and of their tendency to lead youngsters to search for other types of drug-gratification. The phenothiazines on the other hand fail to give that immediate and identifiable response which first attracts the young to abuse a particular drug. Perhaps because of this as well as other reasons they have an important role to play in the treatment of the adolescent addict.

4. Opiates

Although other drugs such as alcohol and the barbiturates provide far the larger numerical problem today in the field of drug addiction, the opiates have always dominated the story. Their use, in the form of opium itself, goes back into the reaches of recorded history, and no other drug has been used to do so much good and so much evil.

The significance of opium and its derivatives probably lies in their capacity to provide the ultimate source of relief from mental as well as physical pain and thus the most effective promise, albeit illusory, of escape from the burdens of man's daily life. For many centuries opium was indeed the panacea offered by the priest to the sorrowful of soul and by the physician to his suffering patient. It also became one of the deadliest of weapons put into man's hands with which to kill himself and others, to capture world trade, to conquer nations and to enslave millions. An excellent account of the history of opium is provided by Scott[58] and is a reminder of the circle of events which have led to the present and tragic backlash of narcotic addiction in the western world, and most recently in the U.K. itself.

A careful national and international control has been imposed on this group of drugs since the turn of the century. In spite of this, however, the problem of opiate addiction is still a very serious one. The two western countries most involved are the U.S. and the U.K., but addiction to the opiates is still a very great problem in certain eastern countries where opium has been chewed and smoked for centuries. Following the western pattern, however, these countries are now also turning towards the use of heroin, and a popular way of using this drug in Hong Kong is known as 'chasing the dragon'.[64]

In the U.K. the abuse of opiate drugs had not posed a major problem until the last decade, and this was in marked contrast to the U.S. For many years the different epidemiological picture between the two countries was attributed to contrary attitudes in treatment in both the social and medical fields. The American approach had become increasingly strict and punitive, and heroin itself was banned completely. When criticising this, many people ignore the fact that at the turn of the century there were some 240 000 opiate addicts in the U.S., a unique situation which probably derived from the excessive use of morphine in the Civil War. This figure was progressively reduced to 43 000 in 1958 by the strenuous efforts made to enforce strict laws. This trend and its subsequent reversal since 1958 has been carefully analysed and well reported by Arthur D. Little Inc.[45]

In the U.K. there was no such vast endemic problem to correct, and until the post-war expansion in the use and abuse of drugs of all kinds, the addict population was extremely small and restricted to adults either therapeutically induced or having professional access to the opiates. In fact the whole epidemiological pattern in the U.S. and in the U.K. in the past has been entirely different. In the U.S. there has been a tremendous smuggling enterprise closely allied to the criminal underworld and affecting many thousands from both the delinquent and immigrant subcultures and those living in the most unfavourable urban conditions, with a strong emphasis on those under the age of 40, and on Negro and other racial minorities. Heroin was the main narcotic used. In the U.K. the problem was almost exclusively one involving a very small number of educated white people of middle age and professional status. Morphine was the drug used by this group. It seems likely that it was not at the time so much a question of specific attitudes towards the opiates that created these marked differences, but the whole question of a vast difference in the historical, evolutionary and cultural characteristics of the two nations. It may well be that the American narcotic problem was also enhanced by that of alcohol and the disastrous years of prohibition from 1919 to 1933, which had no counterpart in the U.K.

In the Little report[45] on the American situation in 1965 it was shown that the number of real known addicts had doubled since 1959 to approximately 34 000. To this figure had to be added the carefully assessed number of 21 400 real but unknown addicts, making a total of 55 700 for 1965, which compared closely with the estimate of 57 199 addicts compiled by the Federal Bureau of Narcotics.

This Bureau, just reconstituted as the Bureau of Narcotics and Dangerous Drugs, has recently presented the latest American statistics (1969)[14] before the sub-committee of the Committee on Appropriations, House of Representatives. The pattern of drug abuse generally was reported as seriously increasing. As far as opiate addiction is concerned, the numbers have increased to over 64 000 in 1968 of which 4·2 per cent were under the age of 21. In the last two years over 20 per cent of the new addicts reported were under the age of 21, a significant departure from the statistics for previous years. Heroin addiction is reported in New York City as the leading cause of death in the 15–35-year age group.

In a statement by the Surgeon General before the same sub-committee[15] it was reported that as at December 31st 1968 93·5 per cent of opiate addiction occurred in only thirteen States, with 50·4 per cent in New York and 12·8 per cent in California.

The figures for opiate addiction in the U.K. during the period 1959–1968 are shown in Table IV. These figures must be interpreted broadly, and are probably an under-estimate of the numbers involved. There was in fact no official or accurate system of registration, and only an index, derived from various sources, was kept by the Home Office.

Until 1967 these sources consisted chiefly of police reports, doctors' reports and the inspection of records of wholesale and retail suppliers. In 1968 the newly introduced system of compulsory notification by doctors has brought some of the hidden addicts to light, and this has been further encouraged by the new provision of physicians specially licensed to prescribe heroin and cocaine. There is no provision for the compulsory surveillance or treatment of opiate addicts in the U.K. and there is no doubt that many are still unknown to the authorities. This especially applies to recent neophytes, teenagers still living at home and fearful of discovery by their parents, and a few others who have preferred to keep their names secret and out of official files.

It is evident from Table IV that there has been a steady overall increase in opiate addiction during the decade. The increase from 1967 to 1968 shows a jump for all addicts of 72 per cent, a figure which has probably been somewhat augmented by the new measures in force. In the under-20 age group this increase is 93 per cent. Even if these increases have to be understood in the light of changed procedures, the general trend of heroin addiction in the U.K. has been very unfavourable, and the most serious aspect of it is the extent to which the teenager is involved. In the U.K. nearly 27 per cent of all opiate addicts are under the age of 20, in the proportion of more than five males to one female; and the great majority, i.e. 92·8 per cent, of this age group are heroin addicts.

Table V shows the breakdown of the numbers of adolescent opiate addicts into the ages from 14 to 19 years over the years 1960–1968. Bearing in mind that the youngest element of this group are the least likely to present themselves for official treatment and so disclose their problem, it is likely that there are youngsters under the age of 15 or even 14 who are presently experimenting with these drugs.

The patterns in both countries, but especially that in the U.K., are changing. In some ways they are drawing closer together. Nevertheless,

Table IV

Opiate Addicts: United Kingdom 1959–1968

		1959	1960	1961	1962	1963	1964	1965	1966	1967	1968
Number taking all opiates (and cocaine)		454	437	470	532	635	753	927	1349	1729	2782
Number taking heroin (alone or in combination)		68	94	132	175	237	342	521	899	1299	2240
Number aged under 20	all opiates	0	1	2	3	17	40	145	329	395	764
	heroin	0	1	2	3	17	40	134	317	381	709
Number aged 20–34	all opiates	50	62	94	132	184	257	347	558	906	1530
	heroin	35	52	87	126	162	219	319	479	827	1390
Number aged 35–49	all opiates	92	91	95	107	128	138	134	162	142	146
	heroin	7	14	19	24	38	61	52	83	66	78
Number aged 50 +	all opiates	278	267	272	274	298	311	291	286	279	260
	heroin	26	27	24	22	20	22	16	20	24	20
Number age unknown	all opiates	34	16	7	16	8	7	10	14	7	82
	heroin	*	*	*	*	*	*	*	*	1	43
Number taking (alone or in combination)	morphine	204	177	168	157	172	162	160	178	158	198
	pethidine	116	98	105	112	107	128	102	131	112	120
	methadone	60	68	59	54	59	62	72	156	243	486
Number taking (alone or in combination)	cocaine	30	52	84	112	171	211	311	443	462	564
Number of all addicts	male	196	195	223	262	339	409	558	886	1262	2161
	female	258	242	247	270	296	344	369	463	467	621
Number of heroin addicts under 20	male	*	*	*	*	*	*	*	*	*	598
	female	*	*	*	*	*	*	*	*	*	111

Source: U.K. Home Office.

certain essential differences remain and these depend at least in part on fundamental attitudes towards heroin as a legitimate drug and towards the recognition of the addict as primarily an invalid.

TABLE V

Breakdown into Separate Age Groups of Opiate Addicts under 20 Years of Age

	Aged 14 years	Aged 15 years	Aged 16 years	Aged 17 years	Aged 18 years	Aged 19 years	Total under 20 years
1960	—	—	—	—	—	1	1
1961	—	—	—	—	1	1	2
1962	—	—	1	—	—	2	3
1963	—	—	2	2	2	11	17
1964	1	—	1	8	11	19	40
1965	—	8	5	19	42	71	145
1966	1	17	26	68	111	106	329
1967	—	3	38	82	100	172	395
1968	—	10	40	141	274	299	764

Source: U.K. Home Office.

Heroin (diacetymorphine hydrochloride) is the opiate choice of the majority of non-therapeutic addicts in both the U.S. and the U.K. It is about three times as powerful as an equivalent dose of morphine although the duration of its action is shorter. Its effect lasts only about two hours, and the addict experiences the early symptoms of withdrawal within four hours. It is generally the opinion of both addicts and doctors that heroin constitutes the most effective opiate available, but this opinion is differently appreciated and expressed. For the youthful proselyte heroin provides the most immediate and gratifying 'buzz', a feeling that has never been adequately described, of immediate pleasure and transient well-being. No other opiate, sedative or stimulant offers the equivalent sensation, and although it is claimed that heroin addicts soon lose this initial effect and persist in drug taking only to avoid withdrawal symptoms, it seems to the writer that it is never entirely lost. Certainly it can be enhanced after a short period of abstinence and it always remains as an urgent thought in the mind of the addict. After the 'buzz' the youngster experiences an interval of unusual peace and tranquillity, which is interrupted a few hours later by a return of tension and worry and the early somatic symptoms derived from these and the organic features of withdrawal.

For full details of all these experiences reference must be made elsewhere. The most commonly seen signs of withdrawal, roughly in sequence of time over a period of several days, include first irritability, anxiety, yawning, lachrymation, sweating, shivering (gooseflesh), flushing, nausea, abdominal cramps, vomiting and diarrhoea, and dilated pupils. Later, fever, variations in blood pressure and respiratory rate, and vasomotor disturbances accompany the above. Finally, insomnia, anorexia, weight loss, blood changes, and other distressing physical and psychological experiences occur before a slow recovery takes place. These symptoms are tabulated by Blachly[9] in a five-stage sequence.

What is important about these events, particularly in the adolescent addict who is on a relatively small dose of opiate, is the ease with which they can be simulated both consciously and unconsciously, so that for example the mere promise of a 'fix' will terminate an attack of vomiting, sweating and other physical features of distress. With the young addict it is often fear and panic that initially determine the clinical picture of withdrawal, and there is nearly always a strong hysterical quality to it. This is not to imply that the distress is not genuine, but to caution those who have to determine when to offer and when to refuse a supplemental dose of opiate, and what quantity of the drug to provide.

Other opiates used by young addicts are always substitutes for heroin when this is unavailable. Methadone, pethidine (meperidine), morphine, hydromorphine, codeine, opium itself and preparations containing opiates such as paragoric and chlorodyne are probably the most popular; although any of the opiates may be used, according to their availability, and they may be taken intravenously even when not manufactured for this intention. Pharmacists should be very cautious indeed when an adolescent presents with a request for a commercial preparation containing even a small fraction of opiate. This can be crushed or evaporated down and the opiate extracted.

Recently in the U.K. the illegal appearance of what is called 'chinese heroin' has complicated the picture. This is a vicious preparation, the product of smuggled heroin, sold as a powder and containing large quantities of adulterants and impurities such as caffeine, in addition to the uncertain amount of heroin which usually constitutes only about 40–50 per cent. It is sold on a black market in London controlled in part by indigenous Chinese, and is offered in paper packets.

In the U.S. all heroin is illicit and it is also mixed with large quantities of adulterants, especially lactose. This accounts to some extent for the fact that the average dose of heroin taken by the American addicts is said to be usually much smaller than that of their British counterparts, who until very recently used only pharmacologically pure heroin obtained from the overprescribing to other addicts already accepted as formal patients by certain doctors.

Bewley[7] reports that the average daily dose of heroin of the New York addict is about 80 mg, compared with 240 mg for the British addict. The latter does, however, does not reflect the adolescent intake in the U.K. which is unlikely to be more than 90–100 mg and is usually less. Many youngsters in treatment, especially those with fairly well-integrated personalities and severe, probably transient, neurotic conflicts as the basis of their disturbance, appear to be able to subsist on as small a dose as 20–30 mg of methadone in place of their original heroin. Yet one finds it extremely difficult to help to release them from this almost token addiction, and if once it is acquired they may require this attachment for a great part of their adolescence.

The physical complications which occur in the course of opiate addiction have been described in full by numerous authors. Helpern[32] has given an excellent description, with particular regard to those leading to a fatal outcome. Bewley et al.[8] have described the complications which they observed in 100 consecutive in-patients. Age groups were not, however, compared in this respect, although there is no reason to imagine that adolescents differ greatly from adults. In Bewley's series 39 out of the 100 addicts had a history of septic complications, 29 of hepatitis, 17 of overdosage, and 12 of 'other' physical complications.

Among the most important complications seen by the writer in the course of treating adolescent opiate addicts are those caused by sepsis, ranging from local abscesses, thrombophlebitis and cellulitis, to septicaemia and the peripheral consequences of this, such as pulmonary infarct, collapse and pneumonia, and endocarditis. Hepatitis is frequently encountered in the very young with marked disturbance of liver function as shown by extremely high serum transaminase figures (some up to 3000) and by other routine liver tests. Acute reactions, such as overdosage, have also been observed, although more frequently these have been due to the intravenous injections of drugs other than the opiate itself. Bewley et al.[8] have suggested five possible causes for the hepatitis: (1) direct hepatotoxic effect of the drugs, (2) contaminant, (3) bacterial, (4) viral and (5) malnutritional.

Louria et al.[47] have listed seven groups of complications. They also noted levels in serum transaminases often in the order of 1000 to 2000 at some time during the course of hepatitis. They state that hepatitis may be a frequent, recurrent, chronic and lethal complication of opiate addiction. They include tetanus and malaria as complications which used to occur in addicts in addition to those already mentioned.

Death is of course a frequent intervention in opiate addiction. Helpern[32] reports that in New York City there were between 300 and 350 deaths from the use of opiates each year from 1962 to 1966, representing about 10 per 1000 of the addict populations, of which 10 per cent occurred in adolescents. James[39] noted in a survey between 1955 and 1965 of heroin addicts known to the British Home Office, that the figures indicated a mortality rate of 22 per 1000, which is approximately twenty times that expected in a population of comparable age distribution. The rate for male addicts was found to be three times that for the females. There is no separate analysis of the mortality rate for adolescents but there have been many individually reported deaths in this age group.

Death may result from any of the complications mentioned above, or as an acute response to an injection and this may be due either to overdosage, intention or accidental, or to a hypersensitivity to the injected material.

II. THE C.N.S. STIMULANTS

1. Caffeine is mentioned in passing not only because of its worldwide use as a mild habit-forming drug but also because of its use in the adulteration of smuggled heroin. It appears to increase the stimulant reaction to this impure heroin and to give a false impression of its strength.

2. Ephedrine and *Isoprenaline* have been included in the overall classification of drugs in the context of adolescent drug abuse because of their therapeutic use in childhood and its possible relationship to drug-taking later on by the teenager. It has been observed that a number of young addicts who have suffered from childhood asthma and allergic disorders, such as hay fever, have become accustomed early in life to the use of preparations containing these drugs. Later this has become a habit in some individual cases, and has continued into adolescence and then extended to other stimulant and sedative drugs and even to the opiates as well. The fact that ephedrine is often combined with a barbiturate or an amphetamine in commercial preparations for treating asthma is perhaps a point which should not be ignored.

3. The Anorectics

This group of drugs has had great significance for adolescents and much has been written about it in many countries, especially the U.K., U.S.A., Japan and Sweden, where young people have indulged in their abuse to an enormous extent.

It is of interest that the amphetamines were originally studied in the search for alternatives to ephedrine and they are chemically and pharmacologically related to the sympathomimetic group of drugs such as adrenaline and ephedrine. The amphetamines, however, generally have a greater stimulating effect on the central nervous system than do these substances and it is this which is significant to the adolescent. Allied to the amphetamines, because of their similarity pharmacologically and to some extent structurally, are phenmetrazine and diethylpropion. All these drugs are comparative newcomers in pharmacology, being first synthesised by Alles in 1927.

The stimulating effect is one of arousal and wakefulness combined with a lessening of fatigue, an increased sense of well-being and self-confidence, and an increase in psychic and motor activity. In addition to these effects, this group of drugs causes an inhibition of appetite which may be either a primary effect or secondary to cerebral stimulation. This inhibition, however, is transient because tolerance develops and as anorectic agents these drugs are of limited value.

Kalant[41] has covered the literature in great detail, with particular attention to the clinical and toxic effects of amphetamines in man. It has been pointed out that overdosage with an amphetamine may imply that of a barbiturate as well. Sedatives should therefore be used with care in treating cases where this occurs. The use of chlorpromazine has been suggested by Hopkin and Jones.[36] Kalant[41] reported that the clinical picture of acute intoxication often consisted of a transitory psychotic reaction and relatively minor physical symptoms. When a psychotic reaction did not occur, the picture was one of over-stimulation of the central and sympathetic nervous systems, with tachycardia, restlessness, excitation, anxiety, headache, dilatation of the pupil, hypertension and respiratory distress. One could add to this list dryness of the mouth, sweating, severe insomnia, fever, convulsions, coma and death in rare cases. Kalant also noted that these drugs can apparently be used for long periods without untoward toxic effects, although there have been some reports of dermatitis and other infrequent complications. What is of serious consequence is the effect on the personality and mental state of the individual who indulges in repeated and excessive amounts of these drugs, and becomes addicted to them. Associated with this is the inevitable danger of a psychotic reaction.

The whole subject of amphetamine psychosis was clinically explored by Connell.[19] He was concerned at the time in differentiating this condition from paranoid schizophrenia. Much has been written about this since, but not a great deal has been added to his findings and conclusions. He gives an excellent description of the clinical picture, which he describes as a paranoid psychosis, with ideas of reference, delusions of persecution and frightening auditory and visual hallucinations. It may be indistinguishable from acute or chronic paranoid schizophrenia or from the mental state in alcoholic withdrawal. It may be diagnosed by a history of drug-taking and the presence of amphetamine in the urine; and if the urine becomes amphetamine-free without recovery of the psychosis, it is probable that amphetamines are not the cause. He suggested that recovery of the psychosis should occur within a week provided there was no further access to the drug.

There has been a good deal of argument about whether the amphetamines merely spark off a latent psychosis or whether they induce a specific psychotic reaction. It seems likely that both may occur and that it would be wrong to infer that only pre-psychotic personalities are at risk to psychosis. It could well occur in normal people. Confusion and violent excitement precede and accompany the psychotic episode, and severe depression may follow its recovery.

Most of the cases of amphetamine psychosis which have been reported have occurred in the young adult age group. Nevertheless, there have been frequent psychotic episodes in adolescents, often quite brief but very frightening, occurring for example in the course of weekend parties, in which hallucinatory and delusional fantasies, usually of a persecutory nature and involving the police, have been experienced. It seems likely that there is no clear division between the confusion and excitement of gross stimulation and the onset of a psychotic experience.

There are no reliable national figures on the amounts of amphetamines being consumed by young people. Table III shows that doctors in the U.K. have been prescribing these drugs with increasing caution in the last few years, but this does not indicate the extent to which such drugs can be stolen and diverted into illicit channels from the source of manufacture, in transportation and storage, and from retail pharmacists. Nor does it indicate how many of them are over-prescribed and so used by those for whom they were not intended. There is no evidence that young people are using the amphetamines less than they have done, although one might expect it to be so since the introduction of The Drugs (Prevention of Misuse) Act 1964 and the increased police surveillance. However, short-term trends in this respect reflect more the cyclical changes in drug vogue than any real departure from the habit. Drugs, like the hems of skirts, will repeatedly rise and fall in popular esteem.

According to Markham[49] there are no useful statistics in the U.S. on this subject, but he notes that the amphetamines, as well as the barbiturates and the hallucinogens, are not limited by region or social class as are the opiates. There is crude evidence to support the generalisation that one-seventh of students across the country use these drugs.

In Japan a severe epidemic of amphetamine abuse occurred between 1946 and 1954 and is described by Nagahama,[54] in which it is estimated that about a million young people, many of whom were adolescents, were addicted to the amphetamines, including intravenous methylamphetamine. This epidemic was apparently well controlled by extremely severe and efficient legal measures.

Goldberg[29] has described the Swedish experience with amphetamines and other drugs in a very thorough survey including a study of over 150 000 school youngsters. The statistics show a remarkably extensive use of all types of drugs especially of the stimulant group among adolescents, with phenmetrazine and methylphenidate greatly outnumbering other amphetamines. Goldberg also describes toxic psychosis as occurring in many chronic phenmetrazine abusers, and he considers that this drug is the most potent of the anorectic group.

Up to 1954 almost no Swedish youngsters under the age of 21 were involved in drug abuse; and while in 1965 only 2 per cent of those arrested for drug offences were juveniles, the figure for 1967 was 28 per cent.

Connell[22] has reported the British pattern of adolescent amphetamine abuse which began about 1961. No figures are available, but he quotes

Scott and Willcox[59] who found that nearly 18 per cent of adolescents admitted to two remand homes had positive results for amphetamines on urine analysis. He concludes from other findings of that report that the drug-taking appeared to be incidental to the youngster's delinquency, although it probably had similar roots in opportunity and predisposition. Connell[23] has also drawn attention to the possibility of brain damage from amphetamine use, and he describes certain early highly suggestive patterns of behaviour typical of, but not exclusive to, amphetamine and amphetamine-barbiturate adolescent drug-takers. These include unexplained absences in the evenings and at weekends, moodiness, irritability, verbal and sometimes physical aggressiveness to parents, usually the mother, especially on return from being out and on the first and second day of the week.

This behaviour was accentuated in young people taking intravenous methylamphetamine and methylphenidate, which began to be a very serious problem in the U.K. from 1966 to 1968. It was clearly allied to heroin addiction, with methylamphetamine often replacing cocaine in many cases, or being used as an alternative to heroin itself when this was unobtainable. It made work in the new treatment centres almost impossible because of the violently agressive behaviour it provoked in these addicts and the destruction and chaos that resulted. The withdrawal in 1968 from British pharmacies of supplies of intravenous methylamphetamine and methylphenidate, by voluntary agreement between the manufacturers and the medical authorities, relieved a situation that was rapidly becoming uncontrollable.

It is difficult to understand why the amphetamines really require to be prescribed, except perhaps in rare cases of narcolepsy and in circulatory collapse (methylamphetamine). It seems doubtful if they are really valuable in helping childhood behaviour problems, epilepsy and Parkinsonism. They are unjustified in the treatment of aggressive psychopaths because of their uncertain response and of the danger of their being abused and disseminated by this group. They are unjustified in the treatment of obesity because their effect as anorectics wears off in about two months. They are not justified in the treatment of depression, or as energisers or to lessen fatigue, and they have no place in the treatment of narcotic poisoning, enuresis and many other minor complaints. Intravenous methylamphetamine is not justified in the diagnosis of schizophrenia, and its true therapeutic value as an abreactive is questionable.

4. Cocaine

This drug is still regarded as the more powerful and the most toxic of this group. It has long been used in conjunction with the opiates, most frequently with heroin. It has been falsely described as a narcotic and is usually included under legislation for the opiates. It is produced as a powder and can be sniffed or injected as a solution intravenously.

It has been taken by addicts for two reasons. One is to produce a 'buzz' or 'flash', an immediate and dramatic state of excitement and elation. The other is to counteract the narcotic effect of the opiate with which it is taken. The similarity of its effect to that of intravenous methylamphetamine is considerable and explains why the latter became so popular.

Cocaine produces considerable tolerance but no marked signs of physical dependence, and its addictive quality is essentially psychological. However, it is an extremely toxic drug and the course of acute poisoning is very rapid.

Among the milder toxic effects are extreme excitement, confusion, headache, nausea and vomiting with abdominal pain. The pupils are dilated and there is often a marked sensation of irritation of the skin and formication. In more severe cases the excitement leads to violence and aggression, and finally to a severe toxic psychosis, with delirium, convulsions and coma supervening. The psychosis is similar to that described for the amphetamines, but Willis[67] states that it is his impression that cocaine is more dangerous than intravenous methylamphetamine. The drug damages local tissues with which it comes into contact, causing ulceration, and it may cause a dermatitis.

Adolescents have used cocaine in the same way as adult addicts, usually in somewhat smaller doses of about 20–40 mg. In the U.K. it has not been a drug easily available to them and it has been the older adolescent who has been chiefly involved. There is no statistical breakdown of cocaine addiction for the under-20-year-old group over the last decade, but Table IV shows the increase in its use generally. In the U.K. in 1967, 89 youngsters under 20 were addicted to cocaine, nearly all in combination with heroin. In 1968 the figure had risen to 127, of which 104 were taking it with heroin and 3 were taking it on its own. Most of these youngsters originally obtained their drug by prescription until the new laws were introduced in 1968. They then switched to methylamphetamine until this too was officially withdrawn.

The present medical use of cocaine is very limited and there is no excuse for prescribing it on psychological grounds. As there is no marked physical addiction to the drug, it should be withdrawn from any addict, within a few days, and no youngster should ever be given a maintenance dose of it.

III. THE HALLUCINOGENS

So much has been written by such a variety of authors on this group of drugs that no attempt can be made to review the vast literature on the subject. It is important to recognise that young people in particular are fascinated and intrigued by these substances for the reasons mentioned earlier, and perhaps because of their already very labile perceptive tendencies. There is a great deal of controversy about some of these drugs. With the opening of the door to their use by both the layman and the professional, it seems likely that their impact on society and on psychiatry could be considerable. Yet in spite of all that has been done in the last twenty years in the way of investigations on these drugs, and of all that has so far been stated, it remains doubtful if any of them offer any medical use of a truly reliable and worthwhile nature. For example, cannabis as a sedative has long been outclassed in safety and effectiveness by other drugs although it is still available in the U.K. as a tincture and an extract. Lysergic acid diethylamide ('L.S.D.'), which has already been used in psychotherapy on several thousands of patients, has as yet proved inconclusive, and it will require much more careful study as a therapeutic agent.

Most of the drugs in this group are being used and abused by adolescents in considerable quantities, but there are no reliable statistics on the numbers of young people regularly taking them.

The classification given in Table I is necessarily incomplete. It lists only those hallucinogens more commonly used by young people and does not attempt to distinguish their chemical characteristics. Jacobsen,[38] however, divides the most important hallucinogens into three convenient pharmacological groups: the cannabis group, the sympathomimetic group and the parasympatholytic group, but this is somewhat limiting. A very comprehensive description of the hallucinogens, excluding cannabis, is given in the excellent monograph by Hoffer and Osmond;[35] while the pharmacology of cannabis has been well described by Wilson and Linken.[68]

1. Nutmeg (myristica fragrans) is a widely distributed plant hallucinogen whose abuse by adolescents is apparently spreading in North American high schools and colleges. Its hallucinogenic ingredient may be myristicin derived from the oil of the seed, and it belongs to the methylenedioxy-amphetamine group of compounds. It can be taken by sniffing the powder or, more usually, by swallowing it in water. It produces a mild variable psychedelic effect not unlike that of Lysergide ('L.S.D.').

2. Morning Glory seeds are really only mentioned because they contain alkaloids of lysergic acid. They produce a very variable and rather disappointing psychedelic response, and had been popular with youngsters in America until apparently sprayed with nauseating chemicals. Probably other drugs such as Lysergide and cannabis have proved much more gratifying, and the vogue for these seeds of the convolvulacea is limited.

3. Cannabis. This is the generic name of Indian Hemp (Cannabis sativa), a plant which varies somewhat in size and appearance depending on the soil and climate where it is grown. That grown in India is known as Cannabis Indica and in North America as Cannabis Americana. It is a plant the fame of which goes back into history like that of the poppy. Bloomquist[10] has written an engaging and useful book on the whole subject of cannabis, and Blum[11] provides a brief history in the first of his two volumes on Drugs.

There is a large variety of names, depending on the geographic locality, for preparations of cannabis, including 'marijuana' for that made from the dried leaves, and 'hashish' for that from the resin of the flowering tops. The most common slang expression for the drug is 'Pot' and the hand-rolled cigarette in which it is usually smoked is called a 'reefer' or a 'joint'. [Lingeman[44] provides an exhaustive dictionary of all drug terms used in the professional, commercial and lay vernacular.]

The active principles of cannabis are the tetrahydrocannabinols. The potency and quality of the effect of smoking the drug, however, depends on a number of additional factors, including its country of origin, its form, and on the person, place and society involved. The effect is often un-predictable.

It is clear from the many descriptions given that the process and ex-perience of intoxication is one which can be very pleasurable, provided the youngster has learnt to overcome any initial nausea, and if he knows the ritual and method of obtaining maximal results from making the reefer and inhaling the smoke.

The effects of one or two smokes may last for several hours. Usually the first effect is one of feeling 'high', a mild sense of intoxication accompanied by a variety of responses depending on the company present. Often the individual will be quiet and introspective if alone, or talkative and hilarious if with others. He becomes less inhibited and more self-confident. Usually most adolescents do not indulge beyond this point, but with more in-tensive smoking the youngster may experience a sense of increased acuity of perception and a rapid flow of thoughts and ideas. Sounds and sights become excitingly vivid. This may be followed by space and time distor-tion. With acute intoxication the individual becomes 'stoned', his judgment and memory become impaired, followed by confusion, disorientation and mood-variation. Finally hallucinatory experiences may occur, which are not usually disturbing. In addition thought-disorder and delusions are sometimes experienced, with disturbances of body image and deperson-alisation. The drug usually produces a mild euphoria in non-toxic doses, with unexpected outbursts of laughter and an associated inappropriate detachment. Drowsiness may also occur. Ames[2] has described both these subjective experiences and behaviour as well as the physical signs of intoxication with cannabis in adults. The only consistent physical signs which she describes are dryness of the mouth, conjunctival suffusion, sinus tachycardia and some mild muscular incoordination and abnormal move-ments. Vomiting and a diuresis sometimes occur.

Murphy[53] made an excellent review of the authoritative psychiatric literature in 1963, and the conclusions he reached are as valid today as they were six years ago. He examined the important earlier work of the Chopras[16] in India, Freedman and Rockmore[24] in the United States, Benabud[4] in

Morocco, Haneveld[31] in the Lebanon, and of many other writers from the areas where cannabis has been used for centuries. He found that: 'Majority opinion appears to be that cannabis is habit-forming, like alcohol, and not addiction-producing like opium. It probably produces a specific psychosis but this must be quite rare, since the prevalence of psychosis in cannabis users is only doubtfully higher than the prevalence in general populations. More important is the mental inertia which its use can produce, leading heavy longterm users to resemble chronic deteriorated alcoholics, though with less aggressiveness. Single doses in correct amount produce euphoria, but in greater amount may produce hallucinations or distortion of perception with hypersensitivity and emotional lability.'

Anyone working in the social and psychiatric fields of the adolescent will acknowledge that cannabis-smoking (in the form of hashish in the U.K.) is clearly becoming a substantial habit. It is an integral part of the adolescent scene of pop music, coffee bars and social life, and it crosses nearly every boundary of race and nation. It would appear to take the place of alcohol, which has less appeal to the young because it is more costly and has less desirable side-effects. In addition, alcohol consumption is essentially an adult custom (largely brought about by licensing laws), and the public house and hotel bar are an almost exclusive venue of adults. Compared with smoking cannabis, alcohol is often felt by youngsters to be clumsy and lacking in refinement. With cannabis, which can so easily be passed from hand to hand unnoticed, the youngster can enjoy his own circle of friends in his own chosen rendezvous. He is not so easily intoxicated by it as he is by alcohol, and it does not make him sick or give him a 'hangover'.

It is true that the adolescent will smoke excessively at times as the adult will drink to excess, but he usually learns to become discreet about this quite quickly. The dangers attached to the adolescent indulging in this habit are similar to, but probably less than, those attached to his drinking alcohol, but it is evident that if he indulges in cannabis more than occasionally he will begin to suffer the results of this at a critical period of his psychosocial development and of his education. School drop-out and subsequent failure to pursue academic studies or a steady occupation may be related to drug abuse, and the inertia produced by cannabis in the young is relevant in this respect.

There is also a potential danger that cannabis may alter interpersonal relationships and the adolescent's developing psychosexual adjustment, although many youngsters will claim that it helps with these. As Wilson and Linken[68] have indicated, such questions are difficult to answer, especially as it is the more unstable youngsters who will probably use these drugs the most. It is an arguable point as to whether it is helpful or harmful for youngsters at times to seek escape in this way from the pressures imposed upon them.

The concept of escalation to other drugs from cannabis is almost certainly a false one if it infers that cannabis will give a relatively normal youngster a taste for drugs which will then lead him to the inevitable danger of addiction to dangerous drugs. The issue is really the other way round. The adolescent opiate addict has the kind of personality which will lead him to heroin whether he has tried cannabis or not, and when other drugs, more easily obtained and taken, have failed him. There is good reason, however, to attempt to separate the different drug cultures from each other so as to protect the potential opiate addict from his more entrenched colleagues. The present laws encourage the identification of all drug-takers into one group, which is clearly undesirable.

TABLE VI

Number of Convictions Involving Drugs Controlled
(a) under The Dangerous Drugs Act 1965,
(b) under The Drugs (Prevention of Misuse) Act 1964

Drug	Offence	Total 1967	Total 1968
a. Opium	Unlawful possession	49	61
	All offences	58	73
Heroin	Unlawful possession	213	391
	All offences	274	539
Other opiates	Unlawful possession	114	197
	All offences	213	449
Cocaine	Unlawful possession	39	56
	All offences	86	111
Cannabis	Unlawful possession	2193	2663
	All offences	2393	3071
b. Amphetamines L.S.D. D.M.T. Mescaline	Unlawful possession	1992	2091
	All offences	2486	2957
a. The longest prison sentence for unlawful possession		7 years	6 years
b. The longest prison sentence for unlawful possession		2 years	2 years

Source: U.K. Home Office.

Table VI shows the number of convictions in the U.K. for cannabis offences in all age groups in 1967 and 1968 under The Dangerous Drugs Act 1965. This is the only statistical information presently available in Britain about cannabis abuse, although similar figures are now being collected for the under- and over-21-year-old age groups. The increase in such convictions in one year is considerable and reflects previous trends. It probably implies that there is both more cannabis being used and greater surveillance by the police. It also suggests that the present laws do not discourage the habit. They may in fact provoke it, as did the prohibition laws in the U.S. with alcohol.

The question of the dangers of cannabis has been repeatedly raised in recent times and it is difficult to judge, from all that has been written, to what extent these dangers have been misrepresented, exaggerated or misinterpreted. The recent report in the U.K. by the Hallucinogens Sub-committee of the Advisory Committee on Drug Dependence 1968 under the chairmanship of Baroness Wootton of Abinger [69] concluded that an increasing number of people, mainly young, are experimenting with cannabis and that substantial numbers are using it for social pleasure. The Committee found that there was no evidence that this was causing violent crime or aggressive antisocial behaviour, or that it produced conditions of dependence or psychosis requiring medical treatment in otherwise normal people.

The Committe agreed that cannabis is a potent drug acting like alcohol, but considered it to be physically less dangerous than the opiates, amphetamines, barbiturates and alcohol; while the implications of its mental effects were much less clear. It concluded that it was necessary to maintain legal restrictions on its availability and use, but stressed that it is difficult to draw a hard-and-fast line between purely self-regarding actions and those that involve wider social consequences. It suggested that the Courts should recognise these distinctions in considering cannabis offences and offenders, because they cannot be written into the law.

The Committee felt that there was a great deal still to know about cannabis before substantial changes in the law should be made to legalise its use, as with alcohol. It did feel, however, that certain changes in the present law were indicated, such as removing cannabis from the legislation governing the opiates and creating separate legislation for it, as well as lowering the present penalties for unlawful possession and supply, which in recent times have been unduly harsh by comparison with the treatment of offenders with other more dangerous drugs.

The Committee has made a number of valuable recommendations on the social, research and legal aspects of cannabis, all of which are logical and reasonable. However, the response to this report of many people in authority, medical and lay, has often been highly critical, and one can but speculate at the extent of this criticism which may well stem from ignorance and fear of drugs and drug users, and the punitive reactions which these provoke in some people.

4. *Psilocybin* (from the Mexican mushroom Psilocybe) and *dimethyltryptamine* ('D.M.T.') are both related to Tryptophan; and there are other hallucinogenic members of this indole group. Mescaline from the Peyote

plant belongs to the group of phenylethylamines. Their use as hallucinogens is not as wide as that of Lysergide ('L.S.D.'), although they have all been used in the U.S. by adolescents for psychedelic purposes. For various reasons, however, they are less effective and less popular. Mescaline has occasionally been brought to Britain by visitors from North America, but like psilocybin it does not present a problem to adolescents in Europe at this time.

Dimethyltryptamine, which is prepared as a liquid and usually smoked with tobacco, or taken by mouth or injection, has a milder and shorter effect than Lysergide, as well as greater autonomic effects. Its popularity is therefore limited.

5. *Lysergic acid diethylamide* or *Lysergide* ('*L.S.D.*') is the most commonly used psychedelic drug. It is derived from Lysergic acid, an alkaloid found in ergot which is present in rye and morning glory. It was discovered by Hofmann who accidentally experienced its hallucinogenic properties in 1943. Its potency has been stated to be 5000 times that of mescaline and 200 times that of psilocybin, and a 'therapeutic' dose is considered to be in the region of 25–50 micrograms. Doses in the region of 100–500 (or more) micrograms have been taken for a 'trip'. It may be prepared either as a colourless liquid or as a soluble powder, and has been distributed in the U.K. adsorbed on to blotting paper or on to a lump of sugar, and more recently in the form of pills.

The symptoms and signs of Lysergide intoxication begin after about thirty minutes and last for about twelve hours. They depend on the dose, the personality of the individual and many other variables. Some of the psychological effects are fairly consistent, such as those of derealisation and depersonalisation, associated with a sense of self-detachment and observation, and visual hallucinations of considerable richness in colour and content. Auditory hallucinations are rare, but hyperacusis occurs. The thought process is altered with a loosening of associations and thought blocking. Confusion of sensory perceptions occurs and time discrimination is lost.

The mood responses vary; anxiety, apprehension and even panic or alternatively elation and ecstasy may occur. Depression or rage may sometimes supervene. The behaviour varies from complete withdrawal and passivity to marked hyperactivity. Transcendental states are said to occur under special conditions.

These reactions have been well documented by Cohen[18] who has also made a useful classification of the complications of the drug[17] which he has described under (1) psychotic disorders, including long term schizophrenic reactions and acute paranoid and depressive states; (2) non-psychotic disorders, including acute panic states and chronic anxiety reactions and antisocial behaviour, and (3) neurological reactions, such as grand mal seizures and possibly brain damage.

In addition to these complications, there have been reports of chromosomal and teratogenic effects with this drug. Smart and Bateman[60] have reviewed the literature and conclude that the evidence for these is very strong during pregnancy. They advise extended studies especially at other times.

Lysergide is potentially a very dangerous drug and should never be used without very careful medical supervision. Yet it is increasingly used by adolescents in the U.S. and it has become popular to a more limited extent in the U.K. and other European countries. Louria[46] reports that in a 16-month period, over 130 patients had been hospitalised at Bellevue Hospital in New York City for severe Lysergide intoxication, and that 38 per cent of these were under the age of 21 years.

The numbers of young people in Britain using Lysergide are probably still relatively small, but there is little concern for its dangers among those already known to experiment with it.

There is another hallucinogen known in North America as 'S.T.P.' (standing for 'Serenity, Tranquillity and Peace'), the formula for which is 4-methyl-2,5-dimethoxy-alpha-methylphenethylamine. It is said to be far more potent than Lysergide and much less consistent. The psychedelic experience lasts for several days, and psychotic and other complications, including death, are much more likely.

5

Legal Controls

The legal controls applied to dangerous drugs are briefly summarised as follows.

On the international side, the Single Convention on Narcotic Drugs 1961 replaces all other international agreements since The Hague Convention of 1912. It lays certain obligations on the signatory nations to maintain adequate national and international controls of the opiates, cocaine and cannabis, and the laws of nearly all countries are based upon it.

In the U.S. the chief Federal laws are still essentially those of the Harrison Act of 1914 and the Marihuana Tax Act of 1937. The interpretation of these treats the 'narcotic' addict primarily as a criminal, even if he may now choose commitment to a civilian hospital for treatment. Depressant and stimulant drugs which are not covered by the Harrison Act are now controlled by the Drug Abuse Control Amendments of 1965.

In the U.K., where the law is kept under review by a Standing Advisory Committee, there have been changes in recent years which have been designed to continue to treat the opiate addict as a sick person while penalising those who traffic in drugs. At the time of writing, the Dangerous Drugs Act 1965 covers the requirements of the Single Convention on the general control of opiates, cocaine and cannabis; and that of 1967 with its attendant Regulations (1968) implements nearly all the recommendations of the second report on drug addiction of the Interdepartmental Committee under the chairmanship of Lord Brain.[13] These include the compulsory notification of narcotic addicts, the licensing of special doctors and the provision of special treatment centres where heroin may be legally prescribed to confirmed addicts. It allows, however, for stricter controls and greater powers to the police to detain and search.

The Drugs (Prevention of Misuse) Act 1964 was brought in to stop the tremendous abuse of the amphetamine drugs (particularly by young people) and later extended to include Lysergic acid diethylamide, dimethyltryptamine, mescaline and certain derivatives of these. Unlawful possession of these drugs is penalised under this Act. The barbiturates, however, are not covered by this Act and their supply is only controlled by The Pharmacy and Poisons Act 1933.

A new Bill before Parliament proposes to rationalise and replace the Acts of 1964, 1965 and 1967. The new Misuse of Drugs Act will give the Home Secretary wider powers than previously, and provide even stronger punitive deterrents for those who sell drugs illicitly. If this new Act also includes the hypnotic drugs in its list of controlled drugs it will have succeeded in correcting one of the serious deficiencies of the present laws. It should be noted that there is no provision in the U.K. for the compulsory treatment of addicts.

6

Personality and Background

On reviewing the literature it is remarkable how little really useful scientific research has been done into the personality characteristics of the drug addict. This may reflect the inherent difficulties involved with this type of patient or perhaps the lack of any appropriate measure.

Hill *et al.*[34] have made comparative M.M.P.I. studies of adults, and from these have shown a high degree of social deviance in adult opiate addicts. Bell and Trethowan[3] could not identify any specific type of personality deviation in their small study of 14 amphetamine-takers. In an older study by Gerard and Kornetsky[25] of 32 male adolescent opiate addicts, they concluded that the addicts showed greater personality deviation than the controls; the results however were marginal. They also attempted to define a syndrome of opiate addiction and to classify addicts according to certain clinical psychiatric categories. They pointed out, however, that the aetiology of addiction lay in a complex of personality structure, life history and family and peer-group interaction.

Although many of the characteristics of the adult are also seen in the adolescent, it is less easy and of even less value to attach labels of a psychopathological kind to the youngster. The tendency to fit the adolescent into some category such as psychopathy or psychosis is rarely justified. At this age psychopathology is seldom well defined or constant and the youngster usually has a long way to go in his development and maturation.

Certain broad features, however, are observed in the opiate-addicted adolescent. He is usually very disturbed indeed, and more so than he at first appears to be. His drug-taking and behaviour are clearly a means both of medicating that disturbance and at the same time of avoiding it, or displacing it elsewhere. Thus, instead of his drug-taking being seen as an expression of a much deeper problem, it is seen as the cause of a problem, and neither the patient nor his family can understand or deal with what is happening.

In fact it is not until the youngster is removed from his environment and studied carefully as an in-patient that the real difficulties begin to emerge. Then one can observe certain consistent features. One is the intense underlying suspicion that often exists in most of these adolescents. They have an abnormal capacity to feel paranoid towards anyone in their environment, especially adults in authority, and this constantly tends to undermine any therapeutic relationship. They are intensely rivalrous with their own age group, particularly when it comes to the need for adult attention, and in consequence they can seldom persist in any peer friendship. Nearly all of them are chronically depressed although this depression is not necessarily always expressed overtly except in certain behaviour patterns. It is related to a profound sense of emptiness and failure, and a deep conviction that they have no power of inner creativity.

These adolescents also have considerable difficulties with their sexual identification. Like the alcoholic, they are often verbally hostile about homosexuality, yet they may associate with homosexuals in their underworld activities, and the male adolescent clearly has a great need for adult masculine attachment. Unlike the alcoholic, they usually handle this difficulty not with an extroverted affability but by a veneer of passivity and submission which, under stress and without the drug, will turn to extreme hostility and destructiveness, often associated with verbal obscenities.

It is of significant importance that the opiates and the whole ritual that goes with their injection, largely replace sexual activity and thereby remove a vast dilemma.

It has been said that these patients have weak egos and weak superego functioning. In fact it is not a lack of superego but a labile reaction to an extremely punitive superego that seems to be present in these cases, and the as yet unformed ego cannot sustain its onslaught. Within this unintegrated ego there lies a great deal of emotional immaturity which seems to display itself at various levels. It allows only a very low tolerance to anxiety and frustration, as well as a tremendous need for instant gratification perhaps to relieve unbearable psychic pain. This can be seen not only in terms of the drug itself but also in many other aspects of the youngster's personal interactions.

The patient's attitude to his drug and his self-injection cannot be discussed at length, but it is evident that, as with all his other attachments, there is extreme ambivalence in this object relationship. The act of 'fixing' is clearly an auto-erotic event, and one which seems to involve both breast and phallus in a highly symbolic fashion. The addict nurtures himself, yet at the same time he is incorporating something bad and destructive.

There have been a number of important psychoanalytic contributions to the understanding of the whole problem. Rosenfeld[57] has reviewed these in an excellent essay. He stresses the significance in addiction of certain factors of orality, narcissism, mania and depression, and of destructive and self-destructive impulses and perversions; and he discusses at length the important contributions by Rado, Simmel and Glover, among many others.

In the addict's family background there always seems to be disturbance. Sometimes it is difficult to know how much preceded and how much followed the onset of addiction. It seems likely that in fact this only brings to the surface conflicts which have for long remained covert. In particular, there seems to be an imbalance in the parental roles, and mothers are often found to be controlling, overprotective and indulgent. They have been described as willing to do anything for their sons but leave them alone. Fathers often seem to be passive and indifferent. These descriptions, however, while pointing out some truths, are too simple and facile an explanation of parental pathology, and a great deal of study needs to be done on the whole of the addict's environment. One very clear pattern of parental failure is that of their inconsistency in attitude and behaviour. This inevitably leads to their seeming unreliable in the eyes of the youngster, and from this stems his deep suspicion and lack of trust in adults.

It is much more difficult to characterise the personality and emotional state of youngsters who abuse the whole range of other drugs. There is a great variety of adolescents who for one reason or another indulge in this way, some of whom have marked emotional disturbance not very different from that described above, while others are much more integrated and mature. It must be presumed that these differences will in large part determine the extent to which a young person becomes involved in drug addiction, although there are certain indefinable qualities about the opiate addict which seem to separate him from other types. It must, however, be pointed out that drug-taking can suddenly take hold in a normal youngster who is passing through a transient emotional or situational crisis. This will happen in particular when the youth finds himself unable to seek appropriate assistance from those who should be close to him.

Connell[21] classifies six groups of adolescent amphetamine-takers, ranging from those who will restrict their activity to an occasional experiment or mild weekend indulgence, to those who rapidly proceed to opiate addiction. He also found that in a group of 36 amphetamine-takers, there was a high incidence of unstable personalities, neurotic traits in childhood, antisocial activities and poor work records. Four adolescents, however, had normal backgrounds and personalities.

The relationship between delinquency and addiction is well recognised. As James[40] has pointed out, estimates of this in the United States with regard to the incidence of delinquency before addiction vary considerably; but he quotes figures contrasting the crimes of violence of 'narcotic' addicts and non-addicts, appearing before the New York Supreme Court in 1960, which would imply that aggressive criminal behaviour is less prevalent among the addict group. In his own controlled study of 50 British heroin adult male addicts in London prisons during 1967 there was no evidence of familial, ethnic or social class predisposition. There was usually a history of personal and social maladjustment dating from adolescence and three-quarters of them had a history of court convictions predating their addiction to opiates. However, only 4 out of 128 of these convictions were for aggressive behaviour. Twenty-two of these addicts had a history of Juvenile Court convictions, which were not for drug offences.

In the writer's experience of 103 adolescent opiate addicts recently seen over a period of sixteen months, 67 have had a history of convictions for non-drug offences, but these have not necessarily predated the drug abuse.

It is clear that both delinquency and addiction share certain predisposing factors in common and become fellow-travellers, perhaps encouraging each other in the process.

7

Diagnosis and Treatment

Detection

It is seldom easy to detect the early signs of drug-taking by young people. Usually this occurs at a time when the adolescent is already concealing many of his thoughts and activities from his family and his teachers. Truancy from school, loss of interest in his studies and sports, disappointing work and general evasiveness may well reflect drug-taking, but could also just be an expression of the upheaval of adolescence. Similarly, at home, when the youngster's habits and mood begin to change noticeably and unaccountably; when he comes in late at night (especially if he has no regular girl friend), or stays out over the weekend; when he is deceptive about his friends and actions, and when he loses his appetite and weight, the same suspicion must arise.

Unusual excitability, restlessness, anxiety, hand tremors, slurred speech, sleeplessness, marked irritability and mood-swings, are all signs that may be found in amphetamine taking. In such cases the early clinical picture of intoxication will be evident, with dilatation of the pupils, tachycardia, nystagmus and weight loss. The condition will have to be differentiated from an anxiety state; but if other aspects of the adolescent's behaviour suggest drug involvement, there is good reason to investigate further.

Frank inebriation can occur with the daytime taking of sedatives. Unusual drowsiness, slight ataxia, sluggishness and lethargy may otherwise result from them. Cannabis will often produce a giggling hilarity, not typical of normal good spirits, and following it, a somewhat lazy vacant look with reddened eyes, sweating and marked pallor. It is less easy to detect a person who is taking Lysergide, because of the few physical symptoms that it produces.

Most of the early behavioural patterns described above will occur in the case of the addict who has taken heroin or some other opiate. His pupils will be pinpointed and he may be incessantly scratching himself. At times of mild withdrawal he may have watery eyes, a runny nose and he may be yawning. He will lose weight and appear preoccupied and neglectful of his person. He may also be found to have lost valuable possessions or got rid of his clothes; and he will become extremely secretive and often moody and hostile. He may be observed concealing the pin-pricks on his arms.

The family doctor, if approached frankly and discreetly by the parents, can see the youngster on general medical grounds and make a careful examination without necessarily revealing what he is looking for. A urine specimen can be taken for analysis in a special laboratory for the opiates, barbiturates, cocaine and the amphetamines. All this is best done on a Monday morning. The detection of drug-taking depends on the history presented, the truthful admission (if possible) of the patient, the clinical appearances, the needle or other distinctive marks, and most importantly a reliable analysis of urine. Urine analysis, however, is not possible for detecting the hallucinogens.

It should be stressed that young people will invariably deny taking drugs if they believe that this will deprive them of the drugs or in some way restrict their freedom; while they will lay false claim to be taking drugs and exaggerate the dose if they believe that thereby they will obtain a prescription. The writer has known boys, who were not addicted, deliberately get themselves injected with an opiate, before coming to the clinic, in order to demonstrate both the needle marks and a positive urine test. This will be done for various reasons including that of selling the 'script' on the black market.

The diagnosis of the youngster as a disturbed person is a matter of full psychiatric assessment, including that of the family dynamics and relationships.

Treatment

There is no specific provision in the U.K., as there is in the U.S., for the compulsory hospital treatment of opiate addicts although under special circumstances a 3-day or 28-day order, under Sections 29 and 25 of The Mental Health Act 1959, could be made if the patient is psychotic or severely intoxicated. For the adolescent it is conceivable also that he could be detained under Section 26 as a 'psychopath', or under Section 60, if convicted of a criminal offence. However, at present there are at least two good reasons why this is seldom desirable. The first is that there are no proper facilities for the compulsory treatment of the severe adolescent addict; and the second is that it remains doubtful if compulsory hospital treatment would be of any long-term value to him. Where a youngster has consistently broken the law in addition to mild drug-taking, compulsory detention in an appropriate corrective school, with close psychiatric supervision, may be a means of helping him to pass through a transient drug phase in the course of his general rehabilitation.

The greatest of all problems in the treatment of any addict is that of his motivation to abandon his dependency on drugs. With the adolescent it is possible to help to create this motivation in certain circumstances.

In terms of the non-opiate drugs, such as the amphetamines and amphetamine-barbiturate mixtures, special out-patient treatment facilities as advocated by Connell[20] offering a full psychiatric and social service, are clearly essential. These should be under the authority of the National Health Service. The opportunity must be there for the youngster to visit a clinic freely and without prejudice and to be given sophisticated attention, including psychotherapy if indicated. Work with the family, or girl friend, and liaison with the local authorities to enable the adolescent to make the necessary shifts in direction in his life, are also necessary. This may include leaving home, changing occupation, special training, hostel accommodation and rehabilitation. Only a few of these youngsters will require to be hospitalised, either to intervene in a crisis at home or for special investigation, or in cases where acute intoxication or some severe psychiatric illness supervenes.

With opiate addiction very special facilities are required for the adolescent. He should, if possible, be treated separately from non-opiate addicts on the one hand, and from adult opiate addicts on the other. For reasons which are obvious he cannot be treated in the ordinary adolescent unit, but the special psychiatric needs of the disturbed youngster apply to the addict just as much as they do to other forms of adolescent disturbance, and addiction adds to his problem a dimension which excludes him from other adolescent psychiatric facilities. In the U.K. one such special facility has recently been started in London in 1968 within the National Health Service scheme of new Treatment Centres, introduced under the provisions of the Dangerous Drugs Act 1967. It provides both an out-patient and in-patient service for youngsters under the age of 18.

The programme it follows is a voluntary one, but attendance in the first place is ensured by the initial need for prescribed drugs. In the course of time a close relationship is built up which helps the adolescent to place his problems where they really belong and to begin to see the desirability of a change in his behaviour. It is only in this way that the youngster will be able to return to the path of his proper development and then, as he succeeds, learn to abandon his dependency on drugs.

The small in-patient section is based on lines similar to those of other open adolescent units, with a programme of individual and group psychotherapy and a variety of occupational and other activities. The whole treatment milieu is that of a model surrogate family, in which insight can be offered to the youngster on the variety of problems and conflicts which emerge in the course of the interaction within the group, both with peers and with adults. Short-term stay is usually unprofitable in this respect, but may be very useful for crisis intervention.

In this project experience has already shown that the rapid withdrawal of opiates is seldom of real therapeutic value, and that the drug can only be abandoned in the much longer context of maturational development, which implies among many things some understanding of the profound role which the drug plays in the emotional life of the young person. The substitution of heroin with methadone over a short period and the immediate transfer from self-administered intravenous injections to staff-administered intramuscular injections are essential parts of the programme. Smuggling of drugs into the unit carries an absolute sanction.

Antidepressant drugs in the course of the general treatment of these adolescents are seldom effective, but chlorpromazine has proved of considerable value in reducing the anxiety and tension that almost invariably arises, especially during critical periods of withdrawal. Care is taken not to provide highly addictive sedatives.

Other forms of treatment have been tried elsewhere with the young addict, including behavioural procedures such as that of Thomson and Rathod [62] involving aversion with suxamethonium chloride. This is a frightening procedure, especially to a young person, and there is no indication of its lasting value.

The use of 'narcotic antagonists' such as cyclazocine and high-dosage methadone are methods which may contain the adult heroin addict and enable him to function better in society; but they are seen at the present time as less relevant to the purpose of treating the very young person in our society who may still have a fair possibility of abandoning his addiction, if adequately helped while his emotional life is still in a developmental stage.

The need for other special facilities for the adolescent, especially with regard to rehabilitation, is most urgent. In the U.K. this subject has been reviewed in a report by the Subcommittee of the Advisory Committee on Drug Dependence under the chairmanship of Arthur Blenkinsop, M.P. [52] This report makes some excellent recommendations among which is that of providing halfway house and after-care accommodation. This is clearly a vital requirement for the adolescent opiate addict and should be an integral part of his specific treatment programme. Ordinary youth hostels will not accept addicts of any kind and special provision must therefore be made.

A final word should be added about the dangers of well-intentioned voluntary agencies attempting to provide understanding and shelter for young drug addicts. There are some very serious pitfalls. Those doing so must avoid over-identification with their charges, or they will unwittingly encourage disregard for proper authority and for the therapeutic discipline essential to this field. The natural inclination of drug addicts is to congregate together and to perpetuate each other's addiction. They are not strong enough to work constructively together of their own accord. It is, therefore, a matter of considerable doubt if the provision of shelter and social facilities is itself therapeutic, unless it forms part of the discipline of the treatment centre, and unless it is properly supervised by a trained team, working together with full knowledge of this complex problem and answerable to rigorous professional ethics.

REFERENCES

1. ADAMS, B. G., HORDER, E. J., HORDER, J. P., MORELL, M., STEEN, C. A. and WIGG, J. W. 1966. Patients receiving barbiturates in an urban general practice. *J. Coll. Gen. Practit.*, **12**, 24.
2. AMES, F. 1958. A clinical and metabolic study of acute intoxication with cannabis sativa, and its role in the model psychoses. *J. ment. Sci.*, **104**, 972.
3. BELL, D. S. and TRETHOWAN, W. H. 1961. Amphetamine addiction. *J. nerv. ment. Dis.*, **133**, 489.
4. BENABUD, A. 1957. Psychopathological aspects of the cannabis situation in Morocco: statistical data for 1956. *U.N. Bull. Narcot.*, **9**, 1–16.
5. BEWLEY, T. H. 1966. Recent changes in the pattern of drug abuse in the United Kingdom. *Bull. Narcot.*, **18**, 1.
6. BEWLEY, T. H. 1968. Recent changes in the pattern of drug abuse in London and the United Kingdom. In *Adolescent drug dependence*, Ed. C. W. M. Wilson. London: Pergamon Press.
7. BEWLEY, T. H. 1969. Drug dependence in the U.S.A. *Bull. Narcot.*, **21**, 13.
8. BEWLEY, T. H., BEN-ARIE, O. and JAMES, I. P. 1968. Morbidity and mortality from heroin dependence. *Brit. med. J.*, **1**, 725.
9. BLACHLY, P. H. 1966. Management of the opiate abstinence syndrome. *Amer. J. Psychiat.*, **122**, 742.
10. BLOOMQUIST, E. R. 1968. *Marihuana.* Beverley Hills: Glencoe Press. London: Collier McMillan.
11. BLUM, R. H. and Associates. 1969. *Society and drugs.* San Francisco: Jossey-Bass.
12. BOZOVSKY, M. and WINKLER, E. G. 1965. Glue-sniffing. *N.Y.St. J. Med.*, **65**, 1984.
13. BRAIN, R. 1965. *Drug addiction.* The Second report of the Interdepartmental Committee, Ministry of Health and Scottish Home and Health Department. London: H.M.S.O.
14. BUREAU OF NARCOTICS AND DANGEROUS DRUGS, U.S.A. Hearings before a Subcommittee of the Committee on Appropriations: House of Representatives Ninety-First Congress. 1969, **1**, 952.
15. BUREAU OF NARCOTICS AND DANGEROUS DRUGS, U.S.A. Hearings before a Subcommittee of the Committee on Appropriations: House of Representatives Ninety-First Congress. 1969, **3**, 526.

16. CHOPRA, R. N. and CHOPRA, G. S. 1939. The present position of hemp-drug addiction in India. *Indian med. Res. Mem.*, No. 31.
17. COHEN, S. 1966. A classification of L.S.D. complications. *Psychosomatics*, **7**, 182.
18. COHEN, S. 1967. Psychotomimetic agents. *Ann. Rev. Pharmacol.*, **7**, 301.
19. CONNELL, P. H. 1958. *Amphetamine psychosis*. London: Chapman & Hall.
20. CONNELL, P. H. 1964. Amphetamine misuse. *Brit. J. Addict.*, **60**, 9.
21. CONNELL, P. H. 1966. Clinical manifestations and treatment of amphetamine type of dependence. *J. Amer. Med. Ass.*, **196**, 718.
22. CONNELL, P. H. 1968. The use and abuse of amphetamines. *The Practitioner*, **200**, 234.
23. CONNELL, P. H. 1968. Clinical aspects of amphetamine dependence. In *Adolescent drug dependence*, Ed. C. W. M. Wilson. London: Pergamon Press.
24. FREEDMAN, H. L. and ROCKMORE, M. J. 1946. Marihuana, factor in personality evaluation and army maladjustment. *J. clin. Psychopath.*, **7**, 765 and **8**, 221.
25. GERARD, D. L. and KORNETSKY, C. 1955. Adolescent opiate addiction: a study of control and addict subjects. *Psychiat. Quart.*, **29**, 457.
26. GLATT, M. M. 1966. 5th Ann. Symp. Med. Off. Hlth., Public Hlth., **130**, 294.
27. GLATT, M. M. 1968. Recent patterns of abuse of and dependence on drugs. *Brit. J. Addict.*, **63**, 111.
28. GLATT, M. M. and HILLS, D. R. 1968. Alcohol abuse and alcoholism in the young. *Brit. J. Addict.*, **63**, 183.
29. GOLDBERG, L. 1968. Drug abuse in Sweden. *U.N. Bull. Narcot.*, **20**, No. 1; *U.N. Bull. on Narcotics*, **20**, No. 2.
30. GRABSKI, D. 1961. Toluene-sniffing producing cerebellar degeneration. *Amer. J. Psychiat.*, **118**, 461.
31. HANEVELD, G. T. 1959. Hashish in Lebanon. *Ned. T. Geneesk.*, **103**, 686. (In Dutch.)
32. HELPERN, M. 1968. Causes of death from drugs of dependence. In *Adolescent drug dependence*, Ed. C. W. M. Wilson. London: Pergamon Press.
33. HEPPLE, N. V. 1968. Sniffing of a shoe cleaner. *Brit. med. J.*, **4**, 387.
34. HILL, H. E., HAERTGEN, C. A. and DAVIS, H. 1962. An M.M.P.I. factor analytical study of alcoholics, narcotic addicts and criminals. *Quart. J. Stud. Alcohol*, **23**, 411.
35. HOFFER, A. and OSMOND, H. 1967. *The hallucinogens*. New York and London: Academic Press.
36. HOPKIN, B. and JONES, C. M. 1956. Dextroamphetamine poisoning. *Brit. med. J.*, **1**, 1044.
37. ISBELL, H. 1967. Meeting a growing menace—drug addiction. In *Narcotics and hallucinogenics*, Ed. John B. Williams. Beverley Hills: The Glencoe Press.
38. JACOBSEN, E. 1968. The hallucinogens. In *Psychopharmacology*, Ed. C. R. B. Joyce. London: Tavistock Publications.
39. JAMES, I. P. 1967. Suicide and mortality amongst heroin addicts in Britain. *Brit. J. Addict.*, **62**, 391.
40. JAMES, I. P. 1969. Delinquency and heroin addiction in Britain. *Brit. J. Crim.*, **409**, 108.
41. KALANT, O. H. 1966. *The amphetamines*. Toronto: University of Toronto Press.
42. KESSEL, N. and WALTON, H. 1965. *Alcoholism*. Harmondsworth: Penguin.
43. KRUG, D. C., SOKOL, J. and NYLANDER, I. 1965. Inhalation of commerical solvents: a form of deviance among adolescents. In *Drug addiction in youth*, Ed. E. Harms. London: Pergamon Press.
44. LINGEMAN, R. R. 1969. *Drugs from A to Z: a dictionary*. London: McGraw-Hill.

45. LITTLE, A. D. (Inc.) 1967. Drug Abuse and Law Enforcement: Report to the President's Commission on Law Enforcement and the Administration of Justice. U.S. Department of Justice.
46. LOURIA, D. B. 1968. Abuse of lysergic acid diethylamide. In *Adolescent drug dependence*, Ed. C. W. M. Wilson. London: Pergamon Press.
47. LOURIA, D. B., HEUSLE, T. and ROSE, J. 1967. The major medical complications of heroin addiction. *Ann. intern. Med.*, **67**, 1.
48. MADDOX, G. L. and McCALL, B. C. 1964. *Drinking among teenagers*. New Haven, Conn: College and University Press.
49. MARKHAM, D. F. 1968. Epidemiological aspects of adolescent drug dependence in the United States. In *Adolescent drug dependence*, Ed. C. W. M. Wilson. London: Pergamon Press.
50. MASON, P. 1965. Drug dependence in drug-induced diseases. *Excerpta Medica Foundation*, **3**, 271.
51. MERRY, J. 1967. Glue-sniffing and heroin abuse. *Brit. med. J.*, **2**, 360.
52. MINISTRY OF HEALTH 1968. *The rehabilitation of drug addicts*. Report of the Advisory Committee on Drug Dependence. H.M.S.O.
53. MURPHY, H. B. M. 1963. The cannabis habit. *U.N. Bull. Narcot.*, **15**, 15.
54. NAGAHAMA, M. 1968. A review of drug abuse and counter measures in Japan since World War II. *U.N. Bull. Narcot.*, **20**, iii, 19.
55. NYSWANDER, M. 1965. The withdrawal treatment of adolescent drug addicts. In *Drug addiction in youth*, Ed. E. Harms. London: Pergamon Press.
56. PRESS, E. and DONE, A. K. 1967. Solvent-sniffing (I) and (II). *Pediatrics*, **39**, 451, and **39**, 611.
57. ROSENFELD, H. A. 1965. Drug addiction and alcoholism in psychotic states—a psychoanalytic approach. In *The International Psychoanalytic Library*, No. 65, Ed. J. D. Sutherland. London: Hogarth Press.
58. SCOTT, J. M. 1969. *The white poppy*. London: Heinemann.
59. SCOTT, P. D. and WILLCOX, D. R. C. 1965. Delinquency and the amphetamines. *Brit. J. Psychiat.*, **111**, 865.
60. SMART, R. G. and BATEMAN, K. 1968. The chromosomal and teratogenic effects of lysergic acid dimethylamide. *Canad. med. Ass. J.*, **99**, 805.
61. SOKOL, J. 1965. Glue-sniffing in Los Angeles. In *Drug addiction in youth*, Ed. E. HARMS. London: Pergamon Press.
62. THOMSON, I. G. and RATHOD, N. H. 1968. Aversion therapy for heroin dependence. *Lancet*, **ii**, 382.
63. TODD, J. 1968. Sniffing and addiction. *Brit. med. J.*, **4**, 255.
64. U.N. *Bulletin on Narcotics*. 1958. Chasing the dragon: the smoking of heroin in Hong Kong. **10**, 6.
65. UNWIN, J. R. 1969. Illicit drug use among Canadian youth. *Canad. med. Ass. J.*, **98**, 402, 450.
66. WILLIAMS, G. P. 1965. *Chronic alcoholics*. Rowntree Social Service Trust.
67. WILLIS, J. H. 1969. *Drug dependence*. London: Faber & Faber.
68. WILSON, C. W. M. and LINKEN, A. 1968. The use of cannabis in relation to the adolescent. In *Adolescent drug dependence*, Ed. C. W. M. Wilson. London: Pergamon Press.
69. WOOTTON OF ABINGER. 1968. *Cannabis*. Report by the Advisory Committee on Drug Dependence. H.M.S.O.
70. W.H.O. 1950. Expert Committee on Drugs Liable to Produce Addiction. Report on the 2nd Session, W.H.O. Tech. rep. ser. 21.
71. W.H.O. 1957. Expert Committee on Addiction-producing Drugs. 7th Report W.H.O. Tech. rep. ser. 116.
72. W.H.O. 1964. Expert Committee on Addiction-producing Drugs. 15th Report W.H.O. Tech. rep. ser. 273.

XIV

THE SYNDROME OF DEREALISATION IN ADOLESCENCE

M. V. Korkina*

D.M.

Prof. and Head of the Course of Psychiatry
Medical Faculty, Patrice Lumumba Peoples' Friendship University
Moscow, U.S.S.R.

1

Introduction

A search of the available literature has revealed a lack of data specifically devoted to the derealisation syndrome in adolescence, although derealisation phenomena in this age group are frequently described in association with depersonalisation, or even under the unifying term of 'depersonalisation'.

Apart from its global effect on the general character of the illness, age plays a definite part in determining a particular clinical picture, and is often intimately involved in the mechanisms of the so-called syndromogenesis. However, we know that the degree to which age affects the formation of sydromes is far from uniform. The derealisation syndrome, although not entirely belonging to those disorders termed 'troubles pubertaires',[76] is nevertheless closely associated with adolescence.

The analysis of data from the literature (investigations specially devoted to depersonalisation–derealisation phenomena in childhood and adolescence,[86, 102, 112, 117] or descriptions of separate observations[16, 57, 142, 143]), as well as our own experience show convincingly that pure derealisation disorders do not appear, with a few exceptions, earlier than at the age of twelve or thirteen years. It seems that only at this stage of ontogenesis are created the conditions which contribute to the appearance of this kind of pathology. (It may be proper here to draw a certain analogy between

* Translated by E. V. Alexandrova.

typical derealisation phenomena and typical paranoid syndromes, which also are seldom present prior to adolescence, because of certain psychological features of childhood.) Disorders encountered at an earlier age are defined as disorders of the sensory syndrome and are caused by organic lesions of the brain. However these disturbances too (described by some authors under the common term of 'derealisation' [42, 62, 102, 137]) usually begin only with the so-called second transitory phase, i.e. the age of seven or eight.

Derealisation disorders in adolescence occur in a pure state—in the proper sense of the word, and in combination with such phenomena as metamorphopsia, dismegalopsia, etc. The latter, depending on the nature of the illness, may also arise in isolation.

Derealisation disorders are often combined with depersonalisation, especially in the form of autodepersonalisation. However, as the purpose of our work is to describe the derealisation phenomena, we will devote our attention to this task without dwelling in greater detail on depersonalisation disorders, although these are not less important.

2

Terminology and Description

The meaning of the term 'derealisation' has been revised many times. For instance, lately it has been recommended[158] that instead of the former terms 'depersonalisation' and 'derealisation', the terms 'derealisation' and 'desanimation' (Krapf) should be used, including under 'derealisation' any alteration in the perception of the inner and outer media, and under 'desanimation' any alteration of 'self'. We should like to emphasise that here we are using the term 'derealisation' in its former, classical meaning, i.e. as expressing the 'disturbance of perception of the surrounding real world'.

This perceptual disorder is usually accompanied by a feeling of alteration, alienation, unnaturalness, 'irreality' of familiar objects of living creatures and of spatial relationships so familiar before. Because of this, patients suffering from derealisation, also known as 'alienation from the perceptual world',[56] in describing their experiences often resort to comparisons, metaphors, hypothetic definitions, using such words as: 'somehow', 'as it were', 'kind of . . .', 'something like . . .', etc. For instance, they say, 'The houses are somehow bleak and far far away . . .', 'Everything appears as if through a frosty haze', 'The trees are as if painted, though I know that they are real', 'Everything seems as if dead', 'Everything is the same and yet not the same, as if seen in a dream', 'People are like ghosts', etc.

Patients who experience these changes in their environment are at a loss when they are asked to give a more or less definite description of their extraordinary experiences. They often use the following phrases: 'I have no words, no images to describe them'; 'I feel that everything is somehow different, but I find nothing to compare it with . . .' When this feeling of altered surroundings is particularly strong the patient may even want to reassure himself that what he sees is real: 'Why, this is my own street, I am quite certain, I am sure it is my street.'

Typical derealisation disorders are usually characterised by the patient himself being aware of the singularity and unnaturalness of his experience and questioning it. This confrontation of new experiences with the data of former experiences, this dissociation between previously acquired knowledge and new sensations distinguishes derealisation disturbances proper from other psychopathological phenomena, such as the symptom of 'substitution of surrounding people', illusory or hallucinatory perception, false recognition in the proper sense of psychopathological phenomena, delusional orientation and delusional interpretation of the environment. Despite this feeling of alteration, the patient perceives his environment adequately (contrary to illusions), without any false perceptions (as in hallucinations), and with no feeling of influence from outside, of interference, of 'made' changes such as are characteristic of the syndrome of Kandinsky–Clerambault.

In derealisation not only may separate images and objects be involved in the perceptual disturbances ('people's faces are changed', 'things are somehow different'), or phenomena and spatial relationships ('everything has retreated somewhere, and has become flat, as if painted'), but there is also a changed perception of time: 'time flows too slowly', 'time is standing still', or, conversely, 'time flies with great speed, it is barely perceptible', 'it seemed to me that during this brief moment centuries passed over my head'.

In derealisation phenomena the milieu is usually perceived as something alien, lifeless, grey, devoid of colour, 'not alive', 'drab', 'ghostly', 'faces are kind of blurred', 'sounds are muffled as if my ears were stopped with cotton wool', 'everything is seen as through a fog', etc. (it is probably this specific feature of the experiences that has led to the coining of the term 'de-realisation'. The Latin prefix 'de' indicates decrease, segregation, removal, cancellation, downward movement).

However, this feeling of alteration in terms of a fading, paling, alien environment does not exhaust the whole variety of derealisation disorders. There are perceptual disorders in which everything, or only separate objects and images, seem extremely bright, sometimes unusually coloured, 'striking', sounds are 'very loud', 'they pierce the ears', everything around seems more vivid, impressive, highly spectacular. Close to this is a state called hyper-realisation, in which in all that is 'old, familiar, already well known, the patient discovers new traits, catches new nuances'.[146] Within the range of derealisation disorders comes also the loss of perceptions, especially visual ones [86, 118, 119, 132, 140] when the patient is unable to summon the well-known images of his nearest relatives, his home, his own photographic picture.

Derealisation, this changed perception of the surrounding world, may affect simultaneously several senses (visual, auditory, tactile, gustatory) or only one of them. Thus, for instance, the patient is unable to determine by touch whether an object is made of wood or of iron; any food seems to him equally tasteless—'everything tastes like grass'. However, in clinical practice and, hence in the descriptions of many authors, the visual and the auditory senses are the most frequently affected.

Allied to derealisation phenomena are the symptoms of 'déjà vu' (seen before), 'déjà éprouvé' (experienced before), 'déjà vécu' (lived before), or, conversely, 'jamais vu' (never seen). Close to the experiences of 'déjà vu' and 'jamais vu' are the states of anovation and hypernovation, but these are simpler in their content, whereas experiences of the 'déjà vu' or 'jamais vu' are far more complex, being characterised 'not only by a feeling of novelty (like anovation and hypernovation) but also by distinct changes in their other feelings, especially the feeling of time.'[145, 146]

Within the framework of derealisation phenomena is usually assigned a peculiar disturbance of spatial orientation—a sudden attack-like disturbance of orientation in the vertical or in the horizontal plane. Faulty orientation in a vertical plane is extremely rare, while disturbances of orientation in a horizontal plane are far more frequent, especially in the form of the sensation that a familiar environment is turning right round by 180° (global derealisation). Less frequent is regional derealisation—the sensation of a turn of 90°. This experience of a 'turn of the environment' is frequently accompanied by derealisation phenomena in the proper, 'pure' sense of the word, when the environment not only seems to turn by 180° but is also perceived as something strange and alien.

There is no unanimous opinion concerning the relationship between derealisation phenomena (with a feeling of an incomprehensible, hardly explicable change of the outside world) and disturbances of the type of metamorphopsia, micropsia, macropsia, dismegalopsia, etc., characterised by more concrete sensations of changes in the size and consistence of surrounding objects, or in their accustomed disposition.

Some investigators consider these phenomena as heterogenous, while others decidedly refer the disturbances of the metamorphopsia type to the domain of derealisation disorders,[34, 38-43, 58-59, 62-63, 128-131, 137] since both are based on a disorder of constancy of perception.[4]

The same relationship seems to exist between derealisation proper and disorders of the metamorphopsia type, as between depersonalisation proper (or autodepersonalisation) and disorders of body-schema (somato-depersonalisation), which are often described together. Pure derealisation is usually a functional disturbance in the modern interpretation of this concept,[17] while disorders of the type of metamorphopsia are symptoms of an organic lesion of the brain.

Derealisation experiences are often accompanied by emotional disorders, such as feelings of fear, anxiety, amazement, perplexity, helplessness and dejection. Less frequent are feelings of happiness, delight and fascination.

Here it must be added that the frequent combination of derealisation and depression requires a most thorough consideration of differential diagnosis. Depressed patients with no derealisation experiences are apt to use in their self-descriptions figures of speech and comparisons which could give the impression that they were suffering not only from depression but also from derealisation. Therefore such expressions as 'everything has lost its meaning', 'the world is grey, featureless', 'everything is uninteresting, dreary, gloomy', 'everything around has lost its significance' and so on, require much questioning and a careful assessment. The necessity of differentiation was recognised as early as in the thirties,[81] and is quite rightly emphasised today.[124] It must be added that such an analysis is most important both in adult and in adolescent clinical practice.

Derealisation may be combined with phenomena of hypopathia,[151] a state characterised by a loss of sensation of external stimuli. Thus, for instance, the patient realises that lemons are acid and sugar is sweet, but the association evokes no sensation, either pleasant or unpleasant. Sometimes, attacks of derealisation are accompanied by dizziness or states approaching faintness.[9, 77, 114, 132]

The above shows that derealisation disturbances are not entirely similar, uniform and homogeneous either in their clinical manifestations, or in combination with other pathological phenomena, usually of an emotional nature. This means that the essence of this pathology is more adequately determined by the term *syndrome* than symptom of derealisation.

3

Historical

In clinical practice, the syndrome of derealisation is often combined with the syndrome of depersonalisation. Derealisation disorders in their pure state, unconnected with depersonalisation phenomena, are less frequent.

When reviewing the literature, one is struck by the fact that in the descriptions of the combination of derealisation and depersonalisation disorders (which should be named depersonalisation–derealisation syndrome[93]) all these disorders are usually defined as depersonalisation only.

The reason for the above seems to lie in the history of the theory of derealisation, when the latter was separated from the so-called disturbances of self-awareness and became independent from the formerly common syndrome of depersonalisation. Because of this, the history of the description of derealisation disturbances is closely connected with the history of the theory of depersonalisation. We do not attempt here to give a complete historical review of the theory of depersonalisation as this is beyond the scope of this work, and moreover other authors have already given a full account,[26, 86, 118, 140] but would merely like to illustrate by some examples the history of the description of derealisation disorders within the framework of the syndrome of depersonalisation.

Derealisation disorders were first described by the otolaryngologist

M. Krishaber [77, 78] in his work on cerebro-cardial neuropathy (1872–1873). Krishaber, who is properly considered to be the founder of the theory of depersonalisation, may be rightly named the founder of the theory of derealisation, since this peculiar perceptual disorder is also vividly described in his clinical observations. The patient described by Krishaber had the feeling of finding himself 'on another planet', of 'being for the first time in the world'. He did not feel the ground under his feet when he walked and was afraid lest he should fall; he lost his ability of orientation and could not recognise by touch the objects placed before him.

L. Dugas, [24] who in 1898 suggested the term 'depersonalisation', also described derealisation together with depersonalisation, although not recognising it terminologically.

P. Janet, [54, 55] who has contributed greatly to the theory of derealisation, considered the disturbance of the function of the real ('loss of the function of the real') as one of the most characteristic features of psychasthenia. With depersonalisation, he has also given an excellent description of derealisation. It is Janet who defined the experiences of patients suffering from a 'loss of feeling of the real' as 'irreal', 'dreamy', 'strange'. In his work, there are also examples of disturbances of feeling of time, characterised by the 'loss of the function of the real', and of the appearance of phenomena of 'déjà vu' and 'jamais vu'. The phenomena of 'déjà vu' Janet describes in greater detail; according to him, 'the essence of "déjà vu" is a negation of the present rather than an affirmation of the past'.[55]

As early as at the beginning of the century, A. Kutzinsky [79] was the first to emphasise the presence of puzzlement in patients with depersonalisation–derealisation disorders and their tendency to use in self-descriptions such expressions as 'somehow', 'as it were', etc.

Noteworthy among subsequent works on derealisation disorders, are the investigations of K. Haug,[46] who employed for this kind of pathology the term 'allopsychical depersonalisation' (from the Greek *allos* meaning 'other', 'different'). The term 'allopsychical depersonalisation' is still frequently used by clinicians as opposite to 'autopsychical depersonalisation' (depersonalisation in the proper sense of the word), and of somato-depersonalisation, which means disturbances of body-schema. As far as we know, the term 'derealisation' as such was suggested in the thirties by W. E. Mapother and W. Mayer-Gross.

Later, with the recognition of the so-called psycho-sensorial syndrome, derealisation disorders have been described in greater detail. In a series of works, M. O. Gurewitch,[38–43] using as examples illnesses with organic brain lesions, described psychosensorial disorders which 'are the consequence of a disturbance of the sensory synthesis, this resulting in a distortion of complex perceptions of the outside world and of one's own body, while the sensations received directly by sense organs remain intact'.[42] Psycho-sensorial disorders (or, rather, simply sensorial, because as rightly observed by A. V. Snezhnevsky,[61] the 'sensorial', the 'sensuous' is always psychical too), comprise together with depersonalisation and body-schema disorders, such phenomena as derealisation proper, disorders of the feeling of time, phenomena of 'déjà vu' and 'jamais vu', disorders of the perception of space, size and shape of surrounding objects.

The works of M. Gurewitch are of special interest from this standpoint, as well as for the purpose of a detailed understanding of all kinds of derealisation disorders, because of his thorough descriptions of these phenomena. Thus, for instance, states are described in which the patients feel that everything around them is strangely changed: the objects seem to have changed their shape (metamorphopsia), to increase in number (polyopia), they become larger or smaller (macropsia, micropsia), are shifting (optical allesthesia), they fall on the patient, squeeze into him, or are in turbulent motion (optical storms). The patients may also feel that the walls of the room draw together, collapse, fall in, or on the contrary, slide apart, the floor undulates, the space is as it were, being torn apart, etc.

Detailed clinical descriptions of different derealisation disorders in the disorders of sensorial synthesis may be found in the works of R. Ya. Golant,[34] D. S. Ozeretskovsky,[104] A. S. Shmaryan,[128-131] N. L. Garkavi,[31] V. V. Shalskaya,[135] R. A. Kharitonov,[62-63] and others. If such a comparison be permitted, it may be said that the so-called psychosensorial syndrome is much the same as the phenomenon to which J. Todd[152] has given the poetical name of 'syndrome of Alice in Wonderland'. Making use of the well-known story of Lewis Carroll, where Alice goes through various transformations—she grows now tiny, now enormous, her neck stretches out, or her legs become extremely long and all her surroundings seem changed to her—Todd unites in this syndrome depersonalisation and derealisation, disorders of body-schema and metamorphopsia. Closely akin to the disturbances of sensorial synthesis are also descriptions of the so-called amorphosynthesis (D. Denny-Brown and B. Banker[18]).

Noteworthy contributions to the description of derealisation disorders were made by authors who did not characterise them as separate but in conjunction with depersonalisation. For instance, P. Schilder[119-120] points out that depersonalisation is not infrequently accompanied by a feeling of alienation from the whole world. B. D. Fridman[29] regards derealisation phenomena as a component of the depersonalisation syndrome. H. Ey[26] writes: 'Or la depersonalisation est aussi une "derealisation".' B. Bird[9] notes that the term depersonalisation is in practice used to depict all forms of the feeling of irreality. In the works of A. A. Megrabyan[86] indications may be found that the concept of depersonalisation comprises in its broad sense derealisation too. D. Salfield[117] uses the definition 'depersonalisation and allied disturbances'. K. Davison[16] speaks of a combination of symptoms named depersonalisation. L. Takas and L. Varga[148] describe depersonalisation as a double syndrome, consisting of depersonalisation in the narrow sense of the word on one hand and derealisation on the other. Detailed characteristics of derealisation

M

disorders, analogous to the examples cited above, may also be found in other investigations, but they are mainly descriptive and the term 'derealisation' is not used at all, or is mentioned only briefly.

Thus it may be seen that since the time of Krishaber a substantial number of works have appeared containing detailed descriptions of derealisation, and that derealisation disorders are dealt with in the literature far more often than may seem from a cursory review, although with no special terminological recognition of this type of perceptual disorder.

Thus the time has come for a clear-cut recognition of the syndromological independence of derealisation disorders, not only because of the specific clinical features inherent in depersonalisation and derealisation (though frequently accompanying one another) but because they differ in their very essence: depersonalisation is a disorder of self-awareness, while derealisation is a form of pathological perception, as has been especially emphasised lately.[82]

4

Derealisation Phenomena in Healthy Adolescents

Transient experiences of derealisation may appear in healthy adolescents under the same conditions as in adults. Since these phenomena have been better studied in adults, let us briefly examine them as they present in this latter age group.

Derealisation phenomena in healthy individuals [11, 21, 46, 47, 71, 72, 80, 86, 89-90, 111, 118, 119, 132, 146] are described with stress, fatigue, anxiety and lack of sleep. Descriptions are found today of derealisation phenomena, with depersonalisation, induced by transient weightlessness.[37]

Certain varieties of derealisation experiences are found in healthy persons as frequently as in the ill; an example is a periodically arising sensation of 'a turn of the environment by 180°'. The author,[72] who has specially studied this phenomenon, has recorded these transient experiences in 235 out of 280 healthy persons, i.e. in 84 per cent of all those examined.

Descriptions of states of alienation produced by emotional experiences, are not infrequent in works of fiction. Some new examples may be added to the earlier cited descriptions given by Chekhov, Dostoevsky, Kipling and Dickens. Thus, besides the well-known excellent description of 'déjà vu' by Charles Dickens, we have also his description of the feeling of derealisation experienced by David Copperfield after the death of Dora and after other misfortunes that befell him. He went about with a 'desolate feeling', 'roamed from place to place . . . seeing all . . . as a dreamer might', 'bearing my painful load through all and hardly conscious of the objects as they fade before me'.[19] In his novel *Little Roque* Guy de Maupassant describes the psychic state of a man who, in his capacity of major, is obliged to assist at the inquest into a murder perpetrated by himself. 'He participated in it as a sleep-walker, seeing persons and objects as if in a dream, as if through a drunken haze, with that feeling of irreality which troubles the mind in the hours of great catastrophes.'[62] Finally, in *The beautiful lady*, a story by Aleksei Tolstoy, the hero, after great emotional stress, experiences a feeling of rest and happiness when everything 'seems a little unreal'.[153]

There are reasons to believe that in healthy adolescents transient episodic derealisation is not a rare phenomenon. A study of alienation phenomena carried out by questionnaires[47, 80] showed that these states are often encountered in pubescent individuals after mental work, and upon acute emotional experiences. It was noted[47] that a tendency to alienation experiences is observed mainly in highly emotional individuals subject to mood-changes and irregular work performance.

It is noteworthy that in the description of alienation phenomena in everyday life,[86] they are most frequently reported in adolescents of pubescent age as episodic transient pathological changes determined by various psychic and somatic factors. This is illustrated by the examples of a fifteen-year-old schoolgirl and a nineteen-year-old student. The episodic occurrence of alienation phenomena is explained in the first case by the endocrine-vegetative changes of pubescence and by a peculiar type of response to physical and emotional stress in the second. It is also worth noticing that episodic experiences of derealisation in adolescents usually appeared in the spring and disappeared later.[86]

Interesting data are found in the description of normal and abnormal depersonalisation.[111] By normal depersonalisation the author means episodic phenomena of depersonalisation and derealisation arising in healthy individuals. The 11 students who, in answering the questionnaire, were able to remember the date of their first experience of alienation, gave the following ages: 1—at age four, 1—at age seven, 3—at age twelve, 3—at age fifteen, 2—at age seventeen and 1—at age nineteen. Thus the overwhelming majority of first episodes of alienation fell within the period of adolescence. Conditions which favoured the appearance of alienation phenomena were states arising from extreme activity and physical or emotional stress.[111] In other words, these phenomena were in response to fatigue.

All authors point out the connection of alienation phenomena in healthy adolescents with fatigue, stress, etc., i.e. the same factors as are operative in adults. It must be emphasised, however, that it is precisely during this transitional period that these factors are most frequent, because the normal psychological factors of adolescence also involve an alternation of outbursts of energy with periods of abatement,[149] when intensive outputs are followed by exhaustion. Thus at this age conditions are favourable for the appearance of derealisation phenomena.

In agreement with this statement is the opinion of those authors[100, 119-120, 148] who think that a characteristic feature of depersonalisation–derealisation phenomena is their appearance at 'critical periods of life',

and in particular in pubescence, as a manifestation of the 'crisis of maturation'.[89] It is not accidental that in the description of episodic derealisation
given by K. Davison (and in the descriptions of this author these attacks
of depersonalisation, recurring with different intensity, are closely inter-
twined with derealisation phenomena) the onset of the first attack in 5 of his
7 observations falls in between the period of ages twelve and seventeen,
and only in 2 cases between the ages of twenty-three and twenty-six.

5

The Derealisation Syndrome in Neuropsychiatric Disorders of Adolescents

As many authors have noted, psychiatric illnesses of adolescents resemble
those of adults more than those of children, although they have certain
features of their own. With a few exceptions, the resemblance of alienation
in adolescents and in adults consists of a similar list of conditions, within
which these experiences are found. Their dissimilarities are determined
firstly by the character of the alienation experiences themselves, and
secondly by a certain peculiarity of their syntropy with other psychopathological phenomena.

Qualitative Peculiarities

Alienation phenomena in adolescents, as compared with analogous disorders in adults, are distinguished by a certain ephemerality, a discreteness,
especially in the first stages of the illness, and by these experiences having a
more marked link with the senses.[112]

Syntropy of the Derealisation Syndrome with other Psychopathological Phenomena

In psychopathology a definite concordance, or conversely a mutual
exclusion, is known to exist between different syndromes, i.e. their relationships may be syntropic, distropic or neutral.

Experiences of derealisation in adolescents, together with depersonalisation or alone, may, just as in adults, occur in combination with compulsive
phenomena, states of altered consciousness and emotional disorders. But
here too certain peculiarities are observed. In adults derealisation is more
often in syntropy with true depression, while in adolescents it is more
frequently associated with restlessness and fear, sometimes with a protracted feeling of apprehension and anxious waiting for another attack.[112]
Attacks of derealisation experiences in adolescents are frequently accompanied by a fear of going mad, and this may be the reason why these
disorders are often obstinately concealed.

Derealisation disorders in adolescents never seem to occur in combination with the symptom of anaesthesia psychica dolorosa, arising against a
background of deep depression.[73] Although this syntropy is frequent in
adults, we have never come across descriptions of it in adolescents or ob-

served it in our own practice. The same applies to ideas of negation of the world. In regard to the syndrome of Kandinsky–Clerambault in its connection with derealisation phenomena, it can be said that the formation of this syndrome in adolescents, as compared with adults, is usually very slow and gradual. Even in cases in which separate early expression of the syndrome of psychical automatism appear simultaneously with the first attack of derealisation ('there is something behind this change of the surroundings', 'all this is done on purpose'), many years may elapse before it becomes possible to recognise the presence of a typical syndrome of Kandinsky–Clerambault.

Special attention should be given to the combination of derealisation phenomena, together with depersonalisation or in isolation, with the syndrome of dismorphophobia–dismorphomania,[70] so characteristic of adolescence, and with the more special phenomena of 'mirror symptom' and 'photography symptom'.

The Derealisation Syndrome and the Syndrome of Dismorphophobia–Dismorphomania

Dismorphophobia, described for the first time at the end of the last century (1886–1894) by E. Morselli,[94-95] has not been given much attention by clinicians for a long time, although this condition is of great importance. Dismorphophobia is often one of the initial manifestations of many psychiatric illnesses. At the same time dismorphophobia phenomena, like derealisation, are also closely allied to the normal reactions of adolescents. Owing to a renewal of interest in dismorphophobia during recent years,[20, 22, 23, 28, 44, 66, 68, 69, 70, 98, 99, 147] many interesting data have been obtained on the clinical characteristics of these disturbances. This syndrome, which in most cases presents a characteristic triad of ideas of physical defect, ideas of reference and depressed mood, is of great diagnostic and clinical importance.[68, 69, 70]

Since ideas of physical defect or even of deformity may bear the character of both obsessive and delusional thoughts, and very persistent at that, it seems better to speak not simply of a syndrome of dismorphophobia but rather of a syndrome of dismorphophobia–dismorphomania, a term which describes more completely these pathological phenomena.

In many cases the term 'dismorphomania' seems more adequate also because patients pathologically convinced of having a physical defect are possessed of an obstinate and passionate desire to remedy this pseudo-defect by any possible means; they may demand a useless cosmetic operation or even inflict severe mutilations upon themselves. The Greek word 'mania', which is sometimes wrongly used as a synonym of 'delusion', means 'ardent, irresistible attraction' to something, in this case to the correction at any price of the imaginary physical defect.

Over many years our observations of patients with a dismorphophobia–dismorphomania syndrome have revealed in many cases a distinct syntropy of this symptom-complex with the depersonalisation–derealisation syndrome. Depersonalisation phenomena were the more evident in some patients, in others derealisation phenomena prevailed. The sequence in which these two syndromes appeared, their duration, and the nature of their progress were found to be widely different.

Without dwelling in detail on the different relationships between depersonalisation phenomena and the delusion of a physical defect, we would like to examine at some length instances where the syndrome of dismorphophobia–dismorphomania is in syntropy with derealisation disorders. Here the following clinical variants could be recognised (possible combinations of transient experiences of derealisation with thoughts of physical defects frequent in healthy adolescents are not touched upon):

1. Phenomena bearing the stamp of derealisation preceded the appearance of ideas of a physical defect. Such a concordance was observed most often when thoughts about one or another physical defect were either obsessive or overvalued, but not very steady, i.e. did not assume the nature of a stable paranoic delusion.

2. Derealisation disorders were secondary to the syndrome of dismorphophobia–dismorphomania, the interval varying from a few months to several years. In no case did we observe the simultaneous appearance of both syndromes. In instances with a secondary addition of derealisation experiences the variants of syntropy, noted only in schizophrenia, were as follows. (1) The experiences appeared only against a background of marked depression, which usually was especially deep, even to the point of suicidal tendencies, in the first stages of the syndrome of dismorphophobia–dismorphomania, and was usually the first to disappear with the regression of this symptom-complex. (2) The syndrome of derealisation, usually combined with depersonalisation phenomena, adding to the syndrome of dismorphophobia–dismorphomania secondarily, gradually susperseded it and established itself with increasing persistence. (3) The derealisation–depersonalisation syndrome joined the delusion of a physical defect, syntropised with it for a long time, until both formations were replaced by the syndrome of Kandinsky–Clerambault.

The *mirror symptom* and the *photography symptom* are secondary, but nevertheless important, symptoms deserving attention, as they may serve as indicators of the concealment of derealisation experiences by adolescents. These symptoms, which almost invariably accompany the syndrome of dismorphophobia–dismorphomania, are also infrequently encountered in derealisation depersonalisation experiences.[70]

The Mirror Symptom

E. Morselli, in describing patients with dismorphophobia, noted that 'all of them stand all day long before a mirror checking whether their face is still exactly the same or whether their nose has shifted, their forehead decreased etc.'[95] Somewhat later, E. Mendel mentioned that when the patient examines himself in a mirror 'the contours of his own body may seem to him to have assumed a different form'.[88]

The first work devoted to this 'signe du miroir' was that describing investigations of P. Abely and A. Delmas, so that it would be appropriate to name this symptom the 'symptom of Abely-Delmas'. Noteworthy is the observation of P. Abely[1] that the symptom of the mirror may appear in connection with disorders or perception and unpleasant sensations caused by imaginary alterations of the body.

Later several works have been devoted to the mirror symptom;[65, 103, 161] in these most of the authors emphasised its special importance for an early diagnosis of schizophrenia. This urge to examine oneself in a mirror is not uncommon in derealisation–depersonalisation phenomena.[16, 86, 114, 134] Experiences of a changed face seen in a mirror are observed both in transient derealisation in healthy persons,[46] and especially in pathological states. The patient perceives his own reflection as something alien; he sees an unknown face, the face of a stranger[109] and he does not recognise it.[89]

This desire to examine oneself in a mirror has great significance for an objective evaluation of the derealisation–depersonalisation syndrome, because of the typical tendency of such patients to conceal their experiences from everybody for fear of being misunderstood or taken for mad.[132] An opposite phenomenon is sometimes observed in patients with derealisation experiences—a kind of negative mirror symptom when patients, experiencing a feeling of the unreality of their environment and afraid to discover that their face may have changed too, carefully avoid not only mirrors, but any reflecting surfaces. Mention of this phenomenon is found in the first work on the mirror symptom:[1] the patient feared to look at his own reflection because of a strong feeling of non-existence. Analogous descriptions are encountered in other works.[86, 114]

Apart from the fear of one's own reflection, the patient may also be afraid to look at the images of other persons on cinema and television screens. Very interesting in this connection are data on patients with a phobic anxiety–depersonalisation syndrome.[114] Although this refers to adults rather than to adolescents, we think it appropriate to mention instances of patients afraid to look at images on the screen because 'they had acquired a sinister, evil aspect, sometimes associated with an illusion of distortion of mouth, nose or eyes'.

The Photography Symptom

Much has been written on the clinical importance of the mirror symptom, but, unfortunately, the same cannot be said of the photography symptom. Unnatural attitudes of patients towards their photographic image in the course of a mental illness are mentioned far less frequently, although the nature of these attitudes[12, 14, 27, 30, 160] is of great practical and theoretical importance in various fields of psychiatry.

According to our observations, an unnatural attitude to one's own photographic image, particularly characteristic of adolescents with a delusion of physical defect, may also develop in prolonged derealisation–depersonalisation experiences. Noticing that their image has 'changed' on the photograph too, the patients will, with different excuses, avoid being photographed, even if this is necessary for some important matter, for instance to obtain a passport. The patients may explain their reluctance to be photographed by other reasons, wishing to conceal their derealisation experiences, which in adolescents are often accompanied by the fear of going mad.

6

The Derealisation Syndrome in Pathological States

In their pathological expression the derealisation disturbances of adolescents are very similar to those of adults. With a few exceptions, these disorders are encountered in the same illnesses and pathological states.

Summing up the material described in the works cited above (see References), it may be said that derealisation disorders, whether in combination with depersonalisation or alone, are described in adolescents under schizophrenia, epilepsy, borderline states, depressions of different types, migraine, infectious diseases of the brain, traumas and tumours of the brain, intoxications, states associated with hypoxia of the brain and states of altered consciousness. Furthermore, derealisation disorders arise together with other disorders under the affect of psychotropic drugs, in particular the best known of them—mescaline, derivatives of lysergic acic (mainly lysergil acid diethylamide) and psilocybin.

Let us now consider some of the diseases and pathological states of adolescence in which derealisation disorders are most obvious.

Schizophrenia

While descriptions of the depersonalisation syndrome are frequently encountered in schizophrenia, many authors regarding these disturbances as one of the earliest manifestations of the disease, few works are devoted to the description of true derealisation. Usually this peculiar perceptual disorder is merely mentioned in descriptions of depersonalisation, whether in schizophrenia of adults or of adolescents. There are some interesting indications which in schizophrenia somato- and autopsychic depersonalisation, i.e. a disorder of body-schema and true depersonalisation, usually appear first and are followed later by allopsychic depersonalisation, or, in other words, by derealisation.[64]

Derealisation disorders, like true depersonalisation are a common phenomenon in adolescent schizophrenia, but with one peculiarity: they are very often concealed. This is the reason why these disturbances, which sometimes arise in the earliest stages of the schizophrenic process, are recognised less frequently than they occur in reality. By taking a special interest in derealisation phenomena, we were able to discover these disorders retrospectively by active questioning of patients, who first became ill as adolescents, although there was often no mention of derealisation experiences in their case-histories. In this respect the derealisation syndrome has much in common with the syndrome of dismorphophobia–dismorphomania, which is often concealed by adolescents and remains hidden from the psychiatrist.

Patients in a premorbid state, who are most likely to have depersonalisation–derealisation disorders, are described as having 'diffident' personalities, with a tendency to depressive reaction,[123] touchy and timorous,[112] although not necessarily so.

Analysis of the literature and our own observations allow us to recognise in adolescent schizophrenia the following variants, often in combination with depersonalisation and, less frequently, in isolation.

First manifestation: derealisation phenomena which arise as a separate episode, or several episodes, long before the obvious stage. It is not quite clear, however, whether these episodes should be regarded as the onset of the process or as a display of reactions usual in adolescence, except of course the instances where episodes of derealisation are accompanied by other symptoms suggestive of schizophrenia.

Second manifestation: derealisation phenomena, which at first arise transitorily, but later last for a more or less prolonged time among other 'little symptoms' appearing in the clinical picture with a greater or lesser degree of clearness. Derealisation disorders are often in syntropy with compulsive phenomena. Frequent too are combinations of the syndrome of dismorphophobia–dismorphomania, with one peculiarity, namely a secondary addition of derealisation, or derealisation–depersonalisation disorders, with ideas of a physical defect, especially when bearing the stamp of a stable paranoic delusion is seen only within the framework of schizophrenic processes with a favourable course. A definite concordance is also observed between the initial psychopathoform symptoms, especially with psychasthenoform changes, and increasing failure.

Third manifestation: derealisation, or derealisation–depersonalisation disturbances which arise as a stage of transition in the formation of a delusion of persecution. These disturbances are here a component of a 'delusional mood' (Wahnstimmung), and are involved in the phenomenon to which K. Conrad[15] gives the name of 'anophenia of the outer space', when the patients experience the outside world 'strangely' and 'otherwise'.

A special feature of the derealisation disorders themselves in adolescent schizophrenia is their ephemerality, their discreteness in the first stages of the illness.[112] This agrees with data indicating that the development of this disease as a whole is characterised essentially by a lack of continuity.[49]

Pronounced derealisation disorders, usually in combination with depersonalisation, are described in schizophrenia with a sluggish course [96, 127, 155] and early onset—just in the adolescence period, when these disturbances often occupy an important place in the course of the initial period of the illness.[155] Derealisation disorders may form a characteristic syndrome in the psychopathological picture of an acute onset of schizophrenia,[143] especially in cases when this acute onset coincides with a violent period of pubescence.[136]

Derealisation–depersonalisation disorders are also described in the course of attacks of periodical schizophrenia in adolescence. Depending on the stage of development of oneiroid cloudiness of consciousness,[110] the dynamics of derealisation–depersonalisation phenomena arising against an oneiroid background may assume the form of affective–delusional derealisation and depersonalisation, fantastic affective–delusional derealisation and depersonalisation and, finally, illusory–fantastic derealisation and depersonalisation.

But whichever course is taken by the process in which the derealisation disorders are described, their presence is usually observed in the most favourable variants and for this reason they have great prognostic value. Like asthenic, affective, obsessive states, derealisation–depersonalisation disorders correlate with the least pronounced negative symptoms.[127]

Epilepsy

In contrast to schizophrenia where true derealisation disorders are frequent and disturbances of the type of metamorphopsia[39] are rare and of a somewhat peculiar kind,[31, 74] epilepsy is characterised by a great variety of derealisation disorders. Moreover, derealisation phenomena encountered in this illness range from experiences of true alienation and phenomena of the type of 'déjà vu', to numerous disorders of sensory synthesis associated with disorders of perception of subject reality, local spatial relationships, etc.

In the epilepsy of children and adolescents appear two particular variants of the spatial depersonalisation–derealisation syndrome, which have been described.[62] Patients, simultaneously with the sensation that their hands are increasing or decreasing in size, experience the feeling that the surrounding objects are getting bigger and are approaching them in the first case (propopsia), or are diminishing and retreating in the second type (porropsia).

Optical spatial disorders are encountered in epilepsy of adolescents in the form of a paroxysmal feeling of the turn of a familiar environment by 90° or, more often, by 180°.

It is known that various paroxysmal psychosensorial disorders may occur in childhood too, but they too are confined to definite age-periods.[3, 4] Thus the most typical alienation phenomena do not usually appear before pubescence.[102] This is why in adolescence, along with disturbances of the perception of local subject reality, subtle experiences of alienated surroundings may also occur. Thus the list of derealisation disorders during this period is far more varied than at earlier ages.

Derealisation phenomena in adolescent epilepsy occur as some varieties of aura and as the content of psychic equivalents. They may also arise in patients emerging from states of altered consciousness after a seizure. Derealisation experiences are closely allied to the 'dreamy states' of Jackson and the 'peculiar states' of Gurewitch. The 'dreamy states' described by Jackson and thoroughly investigated by Penfield and his colleagues,[106-107, 108] include, besides states of altered consciousness and hallucinations, also various experiences belonging to the domain of derealisation. The patients experience an 'illusion of alienation',[106] i.e. a sudden feeling of a strangeness, an unreality of the outside world, of 'déjà vu', of increasing and decreasing objects, etc. M. O. Gurewitch, who goes so far as to use the term 'psychosensorial epilepsy',[40] describes 'peculiar states' consisting of seizure-like disorders of consciousness, changes in thinking and affectiveness, and particularly vivid psychosensorial disorders not followed by amnesia.

Psychosensorial paroxysms usually arise in focal lesions of the parietal, occipital and temporal regions. The latter, in particular, are characterised by experiences of the type of 'déjà vu' and metamorphopsia. Experiences of a turn of the environment by 90° and 180° are associated with disturbances of the optical and vestibular systems. However, although recognising the importance of topical diagnosis, it must be said that not all varieties of derealisation disorders are caused by local lesions. The most subtle alienation experiences, with their special character of reality-reflection, owe their origin solely to functional changes. The origin of cases where alienation phenomena occur in combination with typical psychosensorial disturbances may be probably explained by general functional changes, general functional shiftings, because local paroxysmal disturbances do not exist outside a unity with general cerebral disorder.[1]

In conclusion, although psychosensorial paroxysms are characteristic of certain forms of epilepsy, it would not be justified to consider the appearance of these paroxysms as mere manifestations of epilepsy.[35, 63] In adolescents these attacks may be the expression of neuroallergic disorders,[2] or of a psychosensorial form of brain rheumatism,[91] etc.

Borderline States

Apart from the experiences of unreality inherent in psychasthenic personalities, particularly in connection with over-fatigue or lack of sleep, pronounced derealisation disorders may arise in adolescence against a background of reactive depression, especially if the depression is attended by somatic weakness. Derealisation disorders may also take place in phobic anxiety–depersonalisation syndromes of a neurotic nature.[114]

The overwhelming majority of patients described by Roth were middle-aged individuals, but among them were also a schoolgirl of fourteen, and a young girl whose case-history is given in greater detail. The experiences of this 'emotionally immature' girl after breaking her engagement consisted of anxiety, phobias, depersonalisation, hypochondrial complaints, together with derealisation phenomena.

Psychotomimetic Drugs

The numerous psychic disorders induced by mescaline, LSD and psilocybin include various disorders of perception of the outside world experienced by adults and by adolescents alike.

Although most of the references given here are to general works,[49, 51, 121, 123, 139] since there are numerous specific investigations of this problem, we think it useful to mention the description of the Swiss chemist A. Hofmann, who in 1943 obtained a preparation of LSD and studied its effects on himself.

Apart from other disorders induced by this drug, Hofmann experienced a disorder of feeling of time, the faces of people and the shape of objects around him appeared as if seen in a 'distorting mirror' and were unnaturally coloured, and the floor and the walls seemed to be rocking.

Mescaline, psilocybin and, especially, LSD induce both phenomena of true derealisation, when all the surroundings, including people, seem alien, gloomy, lifeless, drab; and disturbances of the type of metamorphopsia: the objects seem distorted—enlarged, or, less frequently—diminished; they lose their usual relationships, appear sometimes extremely bright, vivid, unnaturally coloured. Perspective is disturbed, distances between objects are misjudged, plane surfaces, such as floor and ceiling, seem raised, undulating or merging.

A thorough study of the neurophysiological and biochemical basis of these disturbances, which arise so vividly in healthy people under the effect of psychotomimetic drugs, will greatly advance the study of the pathogenesis of derealisation phenomena.

7

Neurophysiological Aspects of Derealisation Phenomena

The main purpose of this chapter is to give a clinical description of derealisation disorders, without digressing into their different theoretical interpretations, which are rather varied, especially if their historical aspect is taken into account. But it would be equally wrong to ignore this question entirely, because examination of the theoretical explanations of derealisation phenomena, especially as studied today, may help to reach an explanation of these phenomena in adolescence.

As already mentioned, P. Janet, the first to describe psychoasthenia, regarded the loss of feeling of the real as one of its basic features. It was Janet, who introduced the concept of psycholepsy, which means 'falling of psychic stress'. I. P. Pavlov, describing the psychasthenic personality from the viewpoint of a physiologist, wrote: 'In the psychasthenic the general weakness will again naturally fall upon the basic foundation of the relationships of the organism with its environment, the first signal system and the emotional fund. Hence an absence of feeling of the real, a constant sensation of incompleteness of life. . . .'[105] Thus there is weakness of the first signal system and of the 'emotional fund', i.e. of the very systems which constitute 'the basic foundation of the relationships of the organism with its environment'.

Since Pavlov viewed the pathophysiological basis of psychasthenic phenomena as a 'sharply expressed morbid prevalence of cortical activity over the subcortical, and of the second signal system over the first',[52] it is logical to infer that similar disturbances of higher nervous activity may take place in one of the basic symptoms of psychasthenia—impaired feeling of reality. Interesting too is the typological description of psychasthenic personality; Pavlov defines it as 'some intensification, some extreme variation of the meditating type'.[53] (The meditating type, according to Pavlov, is a purely human type of higher nervous activity, in which the second signal system is prevailing over the first one.)

Subsequent research, now devoted entirely to the study of the pathophysiological basis of the derealisation–depersonalisation syndrome,[59, 138] has revealed, in particular, a pronounced tendency towards the development of passive inhibition which lowers the organising role of the second signalling system. In other words, derealisation and depersonalisation phenomena are found to be related to disturbances in the interactions of the second signal system with other parts of the brain. It is also emphasised that derealisation–depersonalisation disorders arise against a background of hypnotic phases, especially the paradoxical and the equalisation phase; this 'changes the intensity relationships and makes the different analysers accessible to the penetration of stimuli inadequate to them in force and in quality'.[59]

It is worth noting that periodic deepening of the inhibitory state in the cortex was also observed in electroencephalographic investigations of patients with depersonalisation–derealisation disorders.[87] The change in the functional parameters was expressed in changes in the duration of consecutive visual images and a lessening of the functional mobility of cortical neurons, as well as in a periodical change in the clearness of consciousness caused by this periodically deepening inhibitory state.

In order to gain a better insight into the neurophysiological foundation of derealisation phenomena, it is necessary to study the cortical–subcortical relationships, especially because of the present renewal of interest in the relation of the derealisation syndrome to emotional disorders.[125, 126]

Following the well-known investigations of H. W. Magoun and J. Moruzzi, many interesting works have appeared, including those dealing with the use of psychopharmacological drugs, aiming to clarify the role of non-specific systems of the brain, their potentiating or relaxing action. Although the evidence of these investigations indicates that the non-specific systems of the brain participate in the realisation of sensory functions, our knowledge of the role and relative importance of each of these systems (reticular formation, posterior hypothalamus, non-specific nuclei of the thalamus) is still inadequate.[154]

Great attention should be attached to the opinion of such investigators of emotions and emotional disorders as E. Gellhorn and G. N. Loofbourrow.[32] According to their data, the process of recognition may be explained by an extension of the irradiation of discharges of cortical neurons upon activation of the posterior hypothalamus, which in its turn facilitates the establishment of a connection between the acting stimulus and the preceding sensory experience.

Very interesting are investigations of derealisation and depersonalisation phenomena in patients with disorders of the diencephalic region.[60] In recognising different variants in the manifestation of derealisation and depersonalisation and characterising their pathophysiological foundation, this author adheres in general to the modern principle that derealisation phenomena are caused by disturbances of functional interrelationships between three anatomical–physiological registers: sensory (temporal–parietal–occipital) cortex, allocortex and thalamus. In other words, it is the functional-dynamic unity of these structures that determines an adequate perception of the surrounding world and of one's own personality.

The nature of derealisation disorders, the appearance of one or another variety of these disorders is in a great measure determined by the relationships between disturbances of sensory, affective and intellectual mechanisms.[2] This in its turn depends considerably on the level of development, on the conditions prevailing at definite age-periods. Obviously, certain conditions have to be present and a certain level of psychic activity has to be reached for the appearance of such a perceptual disorder as the experience of the unreality of the surrounding world.

Many years ago I. M. Sechenov[122] stated that even the 'simplest of all psychic acts, the recognition of objects, cannot be performed without the participation of thought'. 'Recognition has, after all, elements of rational reasoning, so far as the process resembles deductive acts.'[122] More recent experimental data,[6] show that it is just the comprehensiveness of perception that ensures the clarity of the perception of an object. According to these data, the participation of active speech in the process of spatial perception lowers thresholds, while the impossibility of verbal identification of perceptual images renders them vague and amorphous, and excludes them from their habitual relationships with other objects. In other words, the comprehensiveness of perception, the participation of active speech in the perceptual act contributes to a more clear-cut, more definite structuration of the image, while the inclusion of life experience by means of words imparts to perception a stable character, conforming to the nature of things.[33]

Perception, as well as other higher forms of cognition, is a social form of reflecting reality; this is characterised firstly by the fact that the subject-content of perception is determined by social-practical rather than by biological activity, and secondly, by the world being reflected by man through the prism of meanings fixed in words.[33] Thus perception in man is mediated by social experience and has a comprehensive character.

Let us now consider the peculiarities of the transitional age of adolescence, which make this period of man's life at once difficult and important. At this age there is a powerful reconstruction of the neurohumoral and endocrine system, a characteristic intellectual progression expressed in the development of conceptual thinking and a different type of information processing as a result of the increasing role of the second signal system. It is also noteworthy that at this time takes place the transition from individual to social consciousness.[156]

It is natural that at such an important stage of life as adolescence the most vulnerable structures and systems are those which, at this critical age, are subjected to greatest stress. One of these systems is the central nervous system. Of great importance are emotional maturation, which takes place during this period, the establishment of correct relationships between cortical and subcortical activity, and the corresponding interrelationships between the second signal system and other instances of the brain. N. I. Krasnogorsky,[75] who devoted many years to the study of physiological and pathophysiological activity of the brain in children, wrote: 'During the juvenile period the functional organisation of the brain and its analyser-synthetising activity reach their full development, and the type of nervous system, strength of cortical control, direction of the basic interests with which the young man enters the mature period of his life are definitely determined.'[75]

We have already presented some data on the disturbance of regular cortical–subcortical relationships in depersonalisation–derealisation disorders, the pronounced prevalence of the second signal systems observed in a number of cases, and at the same time the marked tendency towards development of passive inhibition within this system, which lowers its organising role. Such conditions may occur in adolescence, if only in response to fatigue[149] following stress or extra concentration. The fact that derealisation phenomena are caused by transitory (response to fatigue), or protracted (in psychasthenic personalities) disturbances of the relationships between different systems (including a pathological prevalence of the second signal system) provides a theoretical basis which substantiates the data indicating that this kind of disturbance is more frequent in personalities intellectually developed, but emotionally immature,[132] or with a tendency towards reflection,[111] as well as the observation that in derealisation experiences the state of the patient 'improves with the improvement of the emotional sphere'.[86]

It is probably the part played by the second signal system in the appearance of derealisation disorders that accounts for the fact that true derealisation phenomena are almost never described in childhood, nor are they encountered in oligophrenes and dement epileptics.[46, 92, 102] Considering all that has been said above, it is hardly possible to disagree with the authors [71, 72, 146] who point out the protective role of derealisation disorders and, in particular, compare derealisation to pain as a signal of 'trouble in the act of perception'. 'It is possible to speak of the biological effectiveness of derealisation in the same way as this question is posed in regard to pain.'[71] Indeed the periods of derealisation occurring periodically in healthy adolescents should probably be regarded as a protective response to fatigue.

I. P. Pavlov in his study of the higher nervous system repeatedly pointed out the importance of differentiating in the picture of mental illnesses the direct manifestations of pathology from the protective reactions of the organism, which at first may seem to be pathological symptoms too. According to Pavlov, these protective reactions of the organism are associated with the development of inhibition, which protects the nervous cells from over-stress. It seems that this inhibition, in particular in the form of phasic states, develops in the central nervous system of healthy adolescents upon fatigue, not to speak of the probability of its development as a response to pathogenic factors.

REFERENCES

1. ABELY, P. 1930. Le signe du miroir dans les psychoses et plus spécialement dans la demance précoce. *Ann. méd.-psychol.*, **1**, 28–36.
2. ABRAMOVICH, G. B. 1963. Data of the examination of a neuroallergic family. *J. Neuropath. Psychiat.*, **5**, 752–761.
3. ABRAMOVICH, G. B. 1964. The role of the age factor in the clinical differences of epileptic fits. In *Problems of the psychoneurology of childhood*, pp. 375–384. Moscow.
4. ABRAMOVICH, G. B., ADAMOVICH, V. A. and KHARITONOV, R. A. 1967. Clinico-psychopathological and electro-encephalographical investigations of focal cortical epilepsy in children and adults. In *Localisation problems in psychoneurology*, pp. 49–144. Leningrad.
5. ACKNER, B., 1954. Depersonalization, *J. ment. Sci.*, **100**, 858–872.
6. ALEXANDROVA, M. D. 1957. The question of spatial thresholds in visual perception. (*Conference on psychology. Moscow, 1955.*) Moscow: Academy Press.
7. ALEXANDROVSKY, A. B. 1934. Self-control in mescaline intoxication. *J. Neuropath., Psychiat., Psychol.*, **3**, 44–51.
8. ANTONI, N. 1946. Dreamy states, epileptic aura, depersonalization and psychasthenic fits. *Acta Psychiat. Neurol.*, **21**, 1–20.
9. BIRD, B. 1958. Depersonalization, *Arch. Neurol. Psychiat.*, **80**, 467–476.
10. BLEULER, E. 1920. *Manual on psychiatry* (Russian trans.). Berlin.
11. BLISS, E. L., CLARK, L. D. and WEST, C. D. 1959. Studies of sleep deprivation-relationship to schizophrenia. *Arch. Neurol. Psychiat.*, **71**, 348–359.

12. BURTON, A. and ADKINS, J. 1961. Perceived size of self-image body parts in schizophrenia. *General psychiatry*, **5**, 131–140.

13. CHAPMAN, J. 1966. The early symptoms of schizophrenia. *Brit. J. Psychiat.*, **112**, 225–251.

14. CLEVELAND, S. E., FISCHER, S., REITMAN, E. E. and KOTHAUS, P. 1962. Perception of body size in schizophrenia. *Arch. gen. Psychiat.*, **7**, 277–285.

15. CONRAD, K. 1958. *Die beginnende Schizophrenie (Versuch einer Gestaltunganalyse des Wahns)*. Stuttgart: Georg Thieme Verlag.

16. DAVISON, K. 1964. Episodic depersonalization observations on seven patients. *Brit. J. Psychiat.*, **110**, 467.

17. DAVYDOVSKY, I. V. 1969. *General pathology of man* (2nd edition). Moscow: Meditsina.

18. DENNY-BRCWN, D. and BANKER, B. Q. 1954. Amorphosynthesis from left pariental lesion. *Arch. Neurol. Psychiat.*, **71**, 302–313.

19. DICKENS, C. 1850. *David Copperfield*. (Russian trans. 1955.)

20. DIETRICH, H. 1962. Über Dysmorphophobie (Misgestaltfurcht). *Arch. Psychiatr. Nervenkr.*, **203**, 511–518.

21. DIXON, J. C. 1963. Depersonalization phenomena in a sample population of college students, *Brit. J. Psychiat.*, **109**, 371–375.

22. DOSUZHKOV, F. N. 1962. The question of dismorphophobia. *J. Neuropath. Psychiat.*, **1**, 132.

23. DOSUZKOVA, B. and DOSUZKOV, B. 1947. Prispevek ke studiu bludu v dysmorfofobii. *Cas. Lek. ces. Phara*, **86**, 576.

24. DUGAS, L. 1933. Sur la dépersonalisation. *J. Psychol. norm. path.*, **33**, 276.

25. DZHAGAROV, M. A. 1935. Observation and self-observation in atropine intoxication. *J. Sov. Neuropath.*, **2**, 53–60.

26. EY HENRI. 1954. *Études psychiatriques*, Vol. III. Paris: Desclee De Brouwer.

27. FAURE, H. 1956. L'invertissement délirant de l'image de soi. *Evolut. psychiat.*, **3**, 545–583.

28. FINKELSTEIN, B. A. 1963. *Dis. nerv. Syst.*, **24**, 365–370.

29. FRIDMAN, B. D. 1934. On the theory of depersonalisation. *Transactions (Trudy) Psychiatr. Clinic I, Moscow Med. Inst.*, **4**, 48–60. Moscow: Biomedgyz.

30. GALLWITZ, A. 1963. Versuch einer experimentalen Erfassung des body image bei weiblichen Magersuchtigen. *Anorexia nervosa Symposium*, 24/25 April, in Göttingen.

31. GARKAVI, N. L. 1946. Psychosensory disorders in endogenous psychoses. Master's thesis. Moscow.

32. GELLHORN, E. and LOOFBOURROW, G. N. 1963. *Emotions and emotional disorders. A neurophysiological study*. (Russian trans. 1966.) Moscow: MIR.

33. GEORGIEV, F. I., DUBOVSKY, V. I., KORZHUNOV, A. M. and MIKHAILOVA, I. B. 1965. *Sensuous cognition*. Moscow: Moscow State Univ. Press.

34. GOLANT, R. Y. 1941. Depersonalisation and derealisation syndromes and their localisation. *Kharkov Psychoneurol. Conference*, **5**.

35. GOLNITZ, G. 1958. Über Auraerlebnisse atypisch verlaufender epileptischer Manifestationen. *Psychiat., Neurol. med. Psychol.*, **10**, 299–312.

36. GOPPERT, H. 1960. *Zwangskrankheit und Depersonalization*. Basel: N. V. Karger.

37. GORBOV, F. D., KUSNETSOV, O. N. and LEBEDEV, V. I. 1966. The modelling of psychosensory disorders under conditions of short-time weightlessness. *J. Neuropath. Psychiat.*, **1**, 81–88.

38. GUREWITCH, M. O. 1933. Disturbance of body-scheme associated with psychosensory disorders in psychic illnesses. *J. Sov. Neuropath. Psychiat., Psychol.*, **2**, 1–11.

39. GUREWITCH, M. O. 1933. Pathophysiological investigation of syndromes and symptoms in schizophrenia. *Modern problems of schizophrenia*. Moscow: Medgyz.
40. GUREWITCH, M. O. 1938. Psychosensory epilepsy. In *Problems of theoretical and practical medicine* (pp. 147–158). Moscow: TSIU Press.
41. GUREWITCH, M. O. 1948. *Nervous and psychic disorders associated with closed traumas of the skull* (2nd edition). Moscow: U.S.S.R. Acad. Med. Sci.
42. GUREWITCH, M. O. 1949. *Psychiatry*, pp. 45–47. Moscow: Medgyz.
43. GUREWITCH, M. O. 1950. The physiological foundations of psychopathology. *Proc. 3rd All-Union Congr. Neuropathology and Psychiatry*, pp. 43–54. Moscow: Medgyz.
44. HANAU, R. 1963. A propos du problème diagnostique de la dysmorphophobie. *Ann. méd.-psychol.*, 1, 856.
45. HARPER, M. and ROTH, M., 1962. Temporal lobe epilepsy and the phobic anxiety-depersonalization syndrome. I. A comparative study. *Comp. Psychiat.*, 3, 129–151.
46. HAUG, L. K. 1939. Depersonalization und verwandte Erscheinungen. *Handb. Geisteskr. Erganz.*, 1, 134–204.
47. HAYMANNS, G. 1904. Eine Enquette über die Depersonalization. *Z. Psych. d. Sinnerorg.*, 36, 321–343. (Quoted by Megrabyan.)
48. HEUYR, G., DURANTON, P. and LAROCHE, G. 1959. La schizophrenie de l'adolescence et de l'enfance. Aspects cliniques. II. *Intern. Kong. Psychiatr. Congress Report*, 10, 104–109. Zurich.
49. HOFMANN, A., HEIM, R., BRACK, A. and KOBEL, H. 1958. Psilocybin, ein psychotroper Wirkstoff aus dem mexicanischen Rauschpilz. (Psilosybe mexicana Heim). *Experimentia*, 14, 107–109.
50. HOFMANN, A., HEIM, R. and BRACK, A., Coll. 1959. Psilocybin und Psilocin, zwei psychotrope Wirkstoffe aus mexikanischen Rauschpilren. *Helv. chim. Acta*, 42, 1557–1572.
51. HOFMANN, A. 1960. Psychotomimetica. Chemische, pharmakologische und medizinische Aspekte. *Svensk. Kemisk. Tidskrift.*, 72, 723–747.
52. ISAEV, D. N. 1964. Asthenic confusion in adolescents. In *Problems of the psychoneurology of childhood*, Vol. 41, pp. 254–262. Moscow: Institute of Psychiatry of Russian Federation.
53. IVANOV-SMOLENSKY, A. R. 1952. *Essays on the pathophysiology of the higher nervous system*. Moscow: Medgyz.
54. JANET, P. 1908. *Les obsessions et la psychasthénie*. Paris.
55. JANET, P. 1911. *Neuroses*. (Russian trans.) Moscow: Kosmos.
56. JASPERS, K. 1962. *General psychopathology*. (Trans.) (7th edition). Manchester: Manchester University Press.
57. KANNER, L. 1948. *Child Psychiatry*. Oxford: Blackwell.
58. KASHKAROVA, T. K. 1957. The pathophysiological essence of the syndrome of depersonalisation. In *The practice of psychiatry and the pathology of higher nervous activity* (pp. 172–188). Leningrad.
59. KASHKAROVA, T. K. 1959. Disturbance of the sensory synthesis and its clinical significance. In *The practice of psychiatry and the pathology of higher nervous activity* (pp. 22–52). Leningrad.
60. KATKOVNIKOV, A. I. 1964. The structure of some psychopathological syndromes in lesions of the diencephalon. In *Problems of localisation and pathophysiology in neurology and psychiatry*. Kiev: Zdorov'e.
61. KERBIKOV, O. V., KORKINA, M. V., NADZHAROV, R. A. and SNEZHNEVSKY, A. V. 1968. *Psychiatry*. Moscow: Meditsina.
62. KHARITONOV, R. A. 1967. Epilepsy with focal lesions of the temporal and

occipital regions of the brain in children. In *The problem of localisation in psychoneurology* (pp. 55–67). Leningrad.

63. KHARITONOV, R. A. 1967. Pecularities of epilepsy with foci in the temporal lobe in children. In *The problem of localisation in psychoneurology* (pp. 145–154). Leningrad.

64. KLAGES, W. 1959. Depersonalizationserscheinungen bei hirnorganischen Kranken und Schizophrenen. *Arch. Psychiat. Nervenkr.*, **199**, 266–273.

65. KNOOS, H. 1937. The mirror sign. A rather neglected symptom in certain mental diseases. *Acta psychiatr. neurol. scand.*, **12**, 155–171.

66. KOHLMEYER, K. 1964. Dysmorphophobie als unspezifisches klinisches Syndrom. *Med. Welt*, **3**, 137–139.

67. KOLOMETS, L. V. 1969. Somatogenic psychic disturbances associated with thyroid pathology under conditions of a focus of endemic goitre on the Urals. Master's thesis. Sverdlovsk.

68. KORKINA, M. V. 1959. The clinical significance of the syndrome of dismorpho-phobia. I. The phenomenological substance of the syndrome of dismorpho-phobia. *J. Neuropath. Psychiat.*, **8**, 994–1000.

69. KORKINA, M. V. 1961. The prognostical significance of the syndrome of dismorphophobia. In *Schizophrenia, neuroses, reactive conditions and the organisation of psychiatric aid* (pp. 27–31). Moscow.

70. KORKINA, M. V. 1968. Dismorphophobic disorders (Syndromological and nosological analysis). Doctor's thesis. Moscow.

71. KOROLENOK, K. KH. 1946. Derealisation. In *Problems of general psycho-pathology* (pp. 111–130). Irkutsk.

72. KOROLENOK, K. KH. 1948. Classification of delusions of orientation in space and conditions of their appearance. In *Problems of clinical psychiatry* (pp. 33–50). Irkutsk.

73. KORSAKOV, S. S. 1901. *Course of psychiatry*. I. (pp. 217, 235–236) (2nd edition). Moscow: V. Rikhter.

74. KRAITS, S. V. 1936. Psychosensory disorders in schizophrenia. *J. Neuropath., Psychiat. Psychohyg.*, **5**, 615–639.

75. KRASNOGORSKY, N. I. 1954. *Transactions on the study of higher nervous activity in man and animals.* **1**, 423. Moscow: Medgyz.

76. KREVELEN, A. VAN, 1966. La clinique des troubles pubertaires et des troubles pendant la puberte. *Acta paedopsychiat.*, **33**, 175–182.

77. KRISHABER, M. 1872. De la névropathic cérebro-cardiaque. *Gaz. Sci. med.* Bordeaux. (Quoted by Storring.)

78. KRISHABER, M. 1873. *La Génesthopathie cérebrocardiaque*. Paris. (Quoted by H. Ey.)

79. KUTZINSKI, A. 1913. Über das Fremdheitsigefuhl. *Zschr. Psych. Neurol.*, **34**, 301.

80. LEROY, B., 1898. Sur l'illusion dite dépersonalisation et fausse reconnaissance. *Rev. Philosoph.*, **157**. (Quoted by Megrabyan.)

81. LEWIS, A. J. 1934. Melancholia. A clinical survey of depressive states. *J. ment. Sci.*, **30**, 277–378.

82. MALKIN, P. F. 1966. Some methodological problems of the pathology of consciousness. In *Problems of consciousness* (pp. 450–453). Moscow: Proceedings of Symposium.

83. MAUPASSANT, GUY DE. 1958. *La petite roque*. (Russian trans.) Moscow: Pravda.

84. MAYER-GROSS, W. 1935. On depersonalization. *Brit. J. med. Psychol.*, **15**, 103.

85. MAYER-GROSS, W., SLATER, E. and ROTH, M. 1960. *Clinical Psychiatry*. London: Cassell.

86. MEGRABYAN, A. A. 1962. Depersonalization. Armgosizdat, Yerevan, **19**.

87. MEGRABYAN, A. A. and ARUTUNYAN, R. K. 1964. Electroencephalographic picture of the syndrome of depersonalization. *J. Exp. Clin. Med.*, 5, 17–20.
88. MENDEL, E. 1904. *Brief manual of psychiatry* (Russian trans.). Sankt-Peterburg: Practical Medicine.
89. MEYER, J.-E. 1959. *Die Entfremdungserlebnisse über Herkunft und Entstehungsweisen der Depersonalization.* Stuttgart: Georg Thieme Verlag.
90. MEYER, J. S. 1956. Studien zur Depersonalization. I. Über die Abgrenzung der Depersonalization und Derealization von schizophrenen Ich-Störungen. *Zschr. Psych. Neurol.* 132, 221–232.
91. MISIKOVA, I. Z. 1962. Peculiarities in the course of the vestibular and psychosensory form of cerebral rheumatism in children and adolescents (according to the data of a catamnestic examination). *J. Neuropath. Psychiat.*, 7, 1067–1071.
92. MNUKHIN, S. S. 1964. On the pecularities of the pictures, course and prognosis of epilepsy in children. In *Problems of psychoneurology in childhood*, vol. 41 (pp. 385–399). Moscow: Institute of Psychiatry of Russian Federation.
93. MOROZOV, V. M. 1958. Derealisation. *Great Med. Encyclop.*, vol. 8, pp. 1078–1080. Moscow.
94. MORSELLI, E. 1886. Sulla dismorfofobia e sulla tafefobia. *Boll. della K. Accad. med. di Geneva*, 6.
95. MORSELLI, E. 1894. *Manuale di Semiotica delle Malattie mentali*, vol. II. Milan: F. Vallardi.
96. NADZHAROV, R. A. 1955. Slow schizophrenia. Master's thesis. Moscow.
97. NEVSKY, M. P. 1962. Derealisation and depersonalisation in remote results of brain lesions. *Diagnostics and therapy of psychic and nervous diseases* (pp. 251–256). Cheliabinsk.
98. NIKOLAEV, YU. S. 1945. Sensitive delusion of a physical defect and its nosological substance. Master's thesis. Moscow.
99. NOVLYANSKAYA, K. A. 1960. One of the forms of protracted pathological reactions in pubescence (syndrome of dismorphophobia). *J. Neuropath. Psychiat.*, 60, 891.
100. NYIRO, G. 1961. *Psychiatria*. Budapest.
101. OBERNDORF, C. P. 1936. Feelings of unreality. *Arch. Neurol. Psychiat.*, 36, 322–330.
102. OSERETSKY, N. I. 1940. The desintegration of psychosensory functions in epilepsy in children and adolescents. *J. Neuropath. Psychiat.*, 9, 66–74.
103. OSTANKOV, P. A. 1934. The mirror symptoms in dementia praecox. *J. Sov. Psychoneurol.*, 106, 123–125.
104. OZERETSKOVSKY, D. S. 1936. The connection between psychosensory decay and compulsive phenomena. *J. Sov. Psychoneurol.*, 2, 41–45.
105. PAVLOV, I. P. 1951. Types of higher nervous activity in connection with neuroses, psychoses and the physiological mechanism of neurotic and psychotic symptoms. In *Twenty-year experience of objective study of the higher nervous activity (behaviour) of animals* (7th edition) (pp. 464–465). Moscow: Medgyz.
106. PENFIELD, W. and ERICKSON, T. S. 1941. *Epilepsy and brain localisation.* (Russian trans. 1949.) Moscow: Medgyz.
107. PENFIELD, W. and JASPER, H. *Epilepsy and the functional anatomy of the human brain.* (Russian trans. 1958.) Moscow: Foreign Literature.
108. PENFIELD, W. and ROBERTS, L. 1959. *Speech and brain mechanisms.* Princeton, New Jersey: Princeton University Press.
109. PERELMAN, A. A. 1927. Depersonalisation phenomena. *Azerbaijan State Univ. Press, Sect. Natural Sci. and Medicine*, 6, 1–11. Baku.

110. POPADOPULOS, T. F. 1967. Psychopathology of attacks of periodical schizophrenia. Doctor's thesis. Moscow.
111. ROBERTS, W. W. 1960. Normal and abnormal depersonalization. *J. ment. Sci.*, **105**, 478–493.
112. ROMANOV, A. S. 1967. Zur Frage der Depersonalization-erscheinungen bei der Schizophrenie Jugendlicher. *Psychiat. Neurol. med. Psychol.*, **2**, 41–46.
113. RONCHEVSKY, S. P. and SKALSKAYA, V. V. 1935. Perceptual delusions in children. *J. Neuropath. Psychiat. Psychohyg.* **4**, 221–232.
114. ROTH, M. 1959. The phobic anxiety–depersonalization syndrome. *Proc. Roy. Soc. Med.*, **52**, 589–95.
115. ROTH, M. and HARPER, M. 1962. Temporal lobe epilepsy and the phobic anxiety–depersonalization syndrome. II. Practical and theoretical considerations. *Comp. Psychiat.*, **3**, 15–228.
116. SALDINA, L. P. 1962. Psychoses in acrichine intoxications of children suffering from lambliasis. *J. Neuropath. Psychiat.*, **7**, 1072–1076.
117. SALFIELD, D. J. 1958. Depersonalization and allied disturbances in childhood. *J. ment. Sci.*, **104**, 472–476.
118. SAPERSTEIN, J. Z. 1949. The phenomena of depersonalization. *J. nerv. ment. Dis.*, **110**, 236–251.
119. SCHILDER, P. 1914. *Selbstbewusstsein und Persönlichkeitsbewusstsein.* Berlin.
120. SCHILDER, P. 1923. *Das Körperschema.* Berlin: Springer.
121. SCHWARZ, C. J. 1968. The complications of LSD: a review of the literature. *J. nerv. ment. Dis.*, **146**, 174–186.
122. SECHENOV, I. M. 1908. *Elements of thought.* Complete works, vol. 2, pp. 272–416, 343. Moscow: Moscow Imperial University.
123. SEDMAN, G. and KENNA, J. C. 1963. Depersonalization and mood changes in schizophrenia. *Brit. J. Psychiat.*, **109**, 669–73.
124. SEDMAN, G. and REED, G. F. 1963. Depersonalization phenomena in obsessional personalities and in depression. *Brit. J. Psychiat.*, **109**, 376–379.
125. SHINGAROV, G. KH. 1966. Consciousness and emotions. In *Problems of consciousness* (pp. 158–169). Moscow: Proceedings of Symposium.
126. SHINGAROV, G. KH. 1966. Emotions as a form of reality reflection (a medical-psychological aspect). In *Philosophic and social problems of medicine.* Moscow: Meditsina.
127. SHMAONOVA, L. M. 1968. Slow schizophrenia, according to data of remote catamnesis. Doctor's thesis. Moscow.
128. SHMARYAN, A. S. 1934. The psychophysiological patterns of depersonalization. *J. Sov. Neuropath. Psychiat. Psychohyg.*, **6**, 67–96.
129. SHMARYAN, A. S. 1935. The pathophysiology of optical psychosensory disorders. *J. Sov. Neuropath. Psychiat. Psychohyg.*, **5**, 23–36.
130. SHMARYAN, A. S. 1940. *Psychopathological syndromes in lesions of the temporal lobe.* Moscow: Medgyz.
131. SHMARYAN, A. S. 1949. *Pathology of the brain and psychiatry.* Moscow: Medgyz.
132. SHORVON, H. J., HILL, J. D. N., BURKITT, E. and HALSTEAD, H. 1946. The depersonalization syndrome. *Proc. Roy. Soc. Med.*, **39**, 779–792.
133. SHREIDER, N. I. 1950. The syndrome of depersonalisation in schizophrenia and other psychoses. In *Trans. Moscow Regional Psychiatric Clinic. Problems of social and clinical psychoneurology* (pp. 136–147), **10**.
134. SIMSON, T. P. and KUDRYAVTSEVA, V. P. 1959. Clinical aspects, etiology and pathogenesis of schizophrenia in children and adolescents. In *Schizophrenia in children and adolescents* (pp. 11–52). Moscow: Medgyz.
135. SKALSKAYA, V. V. 1945. Clinical investigation of psychosensory disturbances in mental patients (adults and children). Master's thesis. Leningrad.

136. SKANAVI, E. E. 1964. Clinical peculiarities of schizophrenia in adolescents with endocrine disorders. In *Problems of psychoneurology of childhood*, vol. 41 (pp. 17–28). Moscow: Institute of Psychiatry of Russian Federation.

137. SLUCHEVSKY, I. F. 1957. *Psychiatry*. Leningrad: Medgyz.

138. SLUCHEVSKY, I. F. 1957. Psychopathological syndromes and their patho-physiological foundation. In *The practice of psychiatry and problems of the pathology of higher nervous activity*, vol. 2 (pp. 12–24). Leningrad: Gosizdat.

139. STOLYAROV, G. V. 1964. *Model psychoses and psychotomimetic drugs*. Moscow: Meditsina.

140. STORRING, E. 1933. Die Depersonalization (eine psychopathologische Unter-suchung). *Arch. Psychiat. Nervenkr.*, 98, 462–545.

141. SUKHAREVA, G. E. 1938. Epilepsy in children and adolescents. In *Problems of theoretical and practical medicine* (pp. 234–261). Vol. 8, *Epilepsy*. Moscow: TSIU Press.

142. SUKHAREVA, G. E. 1955. *Clinical lectures on the psychiatry of childhood*. Moscow: Medgyz.

143. SUKHAREVA, G. E. 1962. Influence of age on the clinical picture of schizo-phrenia in children and adolescents. In *The psychiatry of childhood* (pp. 67–75). Moscow.

144. SUKHAREVA, G. E. and PERSKAYA, S. S. 1936. Clinico-psychopathological peculiarities of a certain original form of acute schizophrenia on a pubescent material. *J. Neuropath. Psychiat. Psychohyg.*, 4, 567–579.

145. SUMBAEV, I. S. 1948. The disturbance of self-consciousness in schizophrenia. In *Problems of clinical psychiatry* (pp. 132–150). Irkutsk.

146. SUMBAEV, I. S. 1958. The psychopathology and clinical aspects of depersonali-zation. In *Problems of general psychopathology*, 6. Irkutsk.

147. SZYDIK, H. and HRYNKIEWIC, L. 1954. Dysmorfofobie. *Neurol. Neurochir. Psychiat. pol.*, 4, 563–567.

148. TAKAS, L. and VARGA, L. 1967. Angaben zur Rolle der Depersonalization-serscheinungen. *Nervenarzt*, 38, 24–29.

149. TEICHER, J. 1956. Normal psychological changes in adolescence. *Calif. Med.*, 85, 171–176.

150. TEICHER, J. 1964. The occurrence of depersonalization phenomena under L.S.D. *Psychiatr. Neurol.*, 147, 129–137.

151. TIMOFEEV, N. N. 1945. The disturbance of the feeling of reality. In *Problems of war psychiatry* (p. 193). Moscow: Medgyz.

152. TODD, J. 1955. The syndrome of Alice in Wonderland. *Canad. med. Ass. J.*, 73, 701–704.

153. TOLSTOY, A. 1958, *Complete works*, vol. 2, p. 462. Moscow: Gikhl.

154. TRAUGOTT, N. N., BAGROV, YA. YU., BALONOV, L. YA., DYAGLIN, V. L., KAUFMAN, D. S. and LICHKO, A. E. 1968. *Essays on the psychopharmacology of man*. Leningrad: Nauka.

155. TSIVILKO, M. A. 1967. Neurosoformic onset of schizophrenia. Master's thesis. Moscow.

156. USHAKOV, G. K. 1966. Essay on the ontogenesis of levels of consciousness. In *Problems of consciousness*. Moscow: Proceedings of Symposium.

157. VAGINA, G. S. 1966. The syndrome of dismorphophobia in schizophrenia. *J. Neuropath. Psychiat.*, 1228–1233.

158. VELLA, G., 1965. Depersonalization somatopsychique et troubles du schema corporel. *Evolut. Psychiat.*, 30, 147–160.

159. VIKKER, YA. YA. 1933. A peculiar disturbance of spatial orientation (turn of the environment by 180°). *J. Sov. Neuropath. Psychiat. Psychohyg.*, 2, 101.

160. WECKOWICZ, T. E. and SOMMER, K. 1960. Body image and self-concept in schizophrenia. *J. ment. Sci.*, **106**, 17–39.

161. ZAITSEV, A. A. and PAPLIAN, M. E. 1951. The diagnostic significance of the mirror syndrome in the delusional form of schizophrenia. *J. Neuropath. Psychiat.*, **20**, 70–72.

162. ZYUZIN, M. K. 1943. Paroxysmal psychosensory disturbances in commotions and concussions of the brain. *J. Neuropath. Psychiat.*, **12**, 21–23.

XV

DEPRESSION IN ADOLESCENTS

JAMES M. TOOLAN
M.D.

Director of Medical Services
United Counseling Service of Bennington County, Vermont
Psychiatric Consultant to Bennington College and Marlboro College
Assistant Professor of Clinical Psychiatry
University of Vermont, College of Medicine
U.S.A.

1

Introduction

Depression is one of the most frequently encountered clinical syndromes in psychiatry and general medicine, yet it is poorly understood and, until very recently, seldom studied. As Grinker[19] has pointed out, 'It is a curious phenomenon that, although depressions are so frequent, not only in hospital practice but also among ambulatory patients seeking clinic and private office care, very few investigations have been made on this syndrome as contrasted with the intensive work carried out on schizophrenic, psychosomatic and other psychiatric conditions . . . it seems as if the psychiatric profession has taken for granted that all that can be known about depressions has already been discovered and thoroughly described. As a matter of fact one finds . . . that clinically relatively little new has been added to the description of depressions in general since antiquity. Textbook descriptions of this entity are stereotyped accounts which have been copied from book to book and repeated from generation to generation. . . . This is all the more strange since the term "depression" is a description of a predominating affect and gives no clue to the underlying processes, the nature of the patient's problems, the predisposing factors, or the precipitating causes. As an affect which may dominate the mood of individual patients, depression may be a symptom of a wide variety of psychological problems and accompany almost any clinical nosological entity. Furthermore the mood of depression which leads one to make a diagnosis of this entity is not so easy to determine. It may be hidden and masked by a wide variety of behavioral and psychological defences. Many patients cover up depressive feelings with smiling, gay and joking exteriors. Others deny primary sadness but attribute worry to single symptoms such as insomnia, gastro-intestinal distress, headaches, etc., or complain of boredom or fatigue. Still others present compulsive doubts or hypochondriacal preoccupations, dissociated states or paranoid delusions.'

Yet, as Lehmann[26] writes, 'There has always been agreement among clinicians about the phenomena that characterize the psychiatric condition which we call depression or sometimes melancholia. The characteristic symptoms are: a sad, despairing mood; decrease of mental productivity and reduction of drive; retardation or agitation in the field of expressive motor responses. These might be called the primary symptoms of depression. There are also secondary symptoms . . . feelings of helplessness; hypochondriacal preoccupations; feelings of depersonalization; obsessive–compulsive behavior; ideas of self-accusation and self-depreciation; nihilistic delusions; paranoid delusions; hallucinations; suicidal ruminations and tendencies.'

Similar clinical pictures are rarely encountered in children and pre-adolescents. Kanner[21] in his text *Child psychiatry* (1960) and Pearson[29] in *Emotional disorders of children* (1949) do not include the term in the indices. Several authors have concluded on clinical or theoretical grounds that depression does not exist in children. Rie[30] after a critical review of the literature on depression in childhood states, 'An examination of the implications for child psychopathology of the dynamics of adult depression, including the roles of aggression, orality, and self-esteem, generates serious doubt about the wisdom of applying the concept of depression to children.' He adds, 'There may be room to believe that the fully differentiated and generalized primary affect characterizing depression, namely despair or hopelessness, is one of which children—perhaps prior to the end of the latency years—are incapable.' Rochlin,[31] on purely theoretical grounds, concludes that 'Clinical depression, a superego phenomenon, as we psychoanalytically understand the disorder, does not occur in child-hood.'

However, a number of authors, particularly in the past few years, have come to the opposite conclusion. They argue, as does Toolan[38] that 'We have to cease thinking in terms of adult psychiatry and instead become accustomed to recognizing the various manifestations by which depression may be represented in younger people.'

2

Symptomatology

Infantile Depression

Spitz and Wolf[35] were the first to describe infantile depression, which they called anaclitic depression. They noted a group of infants in an institution who exhibited withdrawal, weeping, insomnia, loss of weight and retardation of development. These symptoms often continued on to stupor and death. The authors related this reaction to the child's separation from the mother between the sixth to eighth month, for at least a three-month period. They further added that the reaction was more severe when the mother–child relationship had been a good one. Goldfarb,[18] also working with a special group of institutional children, ascribed their intellectual and social retardation to deprivation—though he did not use the term depression.

Engel and Reichsman[13] report on a case of spontaneous and experimentally induced depression in an infant with a gastric fistula. Upon recovering from a severe depression and marasmus, the infant would react with a depression–withdrawal reaction when confronted with a stranger, and recover when united with a familiar person. The authors felt that the child was reacting to loss of the mother and an awareness of its state of helplessness. This conclusion is similar to the explanation of childhood depression offered by Sandler and Joffe.[32] Bowlby,[8] who has written extensively on the effect of maternal separation upon the infant's psyche, describes three stages the child goes through when separated from its mother: Protest, Despair and Detachment. He calls this process 'mourning'. It is somewhat unclear just how he differentiates mourning from depression.

Latency Years Depression

In a somewhat older age group, Despert[12] described 26 out of 400 treated children as having 'depressive moods and/or evidenced preoccupation with suicide or expressed realistic suicide threats'. She writes, 'Depression in children is not so uncommon as a survey of the literature would indicate. It is rarely associated with suicidal preoccupation. Suicide in children is predominately of an impulsive character.'

Keeler[24] reported eleven children who reacted to the death of a parent with mourning or depression. He noted that children often mask these feelings, which can be readily determined from psychological testing.

Bierman et al.[6] carefully described a severe depression in a six-year-old boy with acute poliomyelitis. Their description is closely similar to that seen in adult depressions—'He looked sad and depressed, so much so that the interviewer was prompted to record that he had at times what one would call in an adult a *melancholic facies*. He talked in a low, weak, sad voice.' He continued depressed for two months following his hospitalization. It is interesting, as the authors state, that 'James said very little directly about his disability, but in his doll play and psychological test performance a great deal was revealed which bears on the topic of body damage and hence on the narcissistic injury. The extent and severity of the perceived damage far surpass those of the disability as objectively measured.' The authors also noted a lowered self-esteem as comparable with that seen in adult melancholies.

Harrington and Hassan[20] described seven depressed girls out of a group of fourteen in an eight- to eleven-year-old age group treated in a child outpatient clinic. They found 'a common syndrome of weeping bouts, some flatness of affect, fears of death for self or parents, irritability, somatic complaints, loss of appetite and energy, and varying degrees of difficulty in school adjustment.' They compared the syndrome to a depressive neurosis in adults, and related the depression to ego weakness and self-depreciation secondary to faults in early identifications.

Agras[2] has discussed the relationship of school phobia to childhood depressions in case studies of seven children from six to twelve years of age. He uses the term 'depressive constellation' to denote a tendency towards depression in the mother and child, and states: 'It is suggested that these children show a syndrome comprising depressive anxiety, mania, somatic complaints, phobia and paranoid ideation. This syndrome is close phenomenologically to the depressive disorders of adults.' Campbell,[10] writing on manic–depressive disorders in children, has also suggested that many children with school phobias are actually cases of an endogenous depression. Statten[36] described homesickness in children as 'a symptom complex, usually associated with separation from home, which reflects an underlying depressive state, to which a child is attempting to adjust'.

Sperling[34] speaks of equivalents of depression in children. She maintains, as does Toolan,[38] that the overt manifestations of depression are usually different from those observed in adults, and she emphasizes that anorexia, ulcerative colitis and insomnia may be such equivalents.

Toolan[38] mentions gastrointestinal disturbances and insomnia in infants as a manifestation of depression and notes, as did Sperling,[34] that mothers of children with such symptoms are frequently depressed. He describes the latency-aged child as displacing depressive feelings with behavioral disorders such as 'temper tantrums; disobedience; truancy; running away from home; accident proneness; masochism, as indicated by the child who manages to get beaten up by the other children; and self-destructive behavior. The youngster is convinced that he is bad, evil, unacceptable. Such feelings lead him into anti-social behavior, which in turn only further reinforces his belief that he is no good. The youngster will often feel inferior to other children, that he is ugly and stupid. All of the above-described symptoms should be considered as evidence of depression.'

Case history

Joe, a nine-year-old boy, can be cited as a good example. He was described as disobedient at home and school, antagonistic to his parents, and frequently involved in fights with other children. Previously a good student, he now showed little interest in his school work and had begun to truant. Joe's parents had been divorced about two years before he was seen and he had been living with his mother. Both parents stated that Joe had changed markedly since the divorce. Previously they described him as a happy, outgoing child with many interests who got along well with everyone. Since the break-up of the home, they both felt he was angry with them, and was expressing his anger by his unacceptable behavior. It was true that Joe was angry with his parents, and he expressed such feelings easily at the beginning of therapy. He resented both his parents and believed that they had deserted him. As treatment progressed, other feelings emerged. Joe began to speak of being unloved by his parents, whereas previously, as an only child, he had felt himself to be the center of his parents' universe. Even though they had carefully explained that the divorce was due to their inability to live together without constant discord, Joe suspected otherwise. He was convinced that his father wouldn't have left the house if he really loved him. It was only when these feelings were expressed and resolved that Joe's behavior began to improve.

Early Adolescence Depression

In preadolescence and early adolescence we continue to see a similar picture to that described for the latency-age group. Boys often find it very difficult to face and express their true feelings, especially if they regard them as evidence of weakness. Youngsters will often utilize denial as a mechanism for avoiding depressive feelings. The following two cases described by Toolan[38] are characteristic of such adolescents.

Case history 1

A twelve-year-old boy was seen at the request of his mother. She complained that he was obese, a compulsive eater, enuretic, fecally incontinent and troublesome at home, as he constantly picked on his two younger sisters. She added that he was very disturbed in his relationships with other children. He refused to participate in their activities and, a student of superior talents, he would always point out their inadequacies in the scholastic area.

When seen, Michael was a sullen, negativistic fat boy who stoically maintained he had no problems and didn't wish to see me. At the mother's insistence, however, he continued in therapy. For weeks the sessions consisted of brief recitals of the superficial events of the week, always phrased in the most optimistic terms: 'Everything was fine.' Chess was our only avenue of contact. Very gradually he began to reveal himself. He really didn't have any friends, he would like to compete in sports but he wasn't good enough. Each forward step would be followed by two steps backward in his usual fashion of denying all difficulties. He realized he was overweight but couldn't control his appetite. Maybe he wet his bed and soiled his pants but not often and less than before (a bare-faced fabrication). Eventually he could discuss his great shame over such infantile behavior, how horrible he felt when everyone called him 'Stinky'. As time passed, he began to mention that he had never been like the other fellows; he never remembered being happy. He often fantasied being dead and everyone being sorry for their behavior toward him.

Then, for the first time, he began to talk of his parents; how close he was to his mother, how he could get anything he desired from her. Slowly his attitudes to his father emerged. The latter, a successful dentist, was a cold, aloof, distant, hostile person who seldom was at home and on these occasions constantly berated his wife and son. He called the latter lazy, fat, incompetent, a baby. He would beat him, bribe him—all to no avail. Eventually the boy's hostile, angry feelings, which had been so long repressed, emerged. He would like to kill the father but was terrified of him. Why couldn't he and mother live by themselves? As these feelings were explored the youngster changed dramatically. He lost 25 pounds, ceased wetting and soiling, began to relate to his peers, and for the first time tried out for a team which he made, much to his amazement. That summer at camp (which incidentally accepted him back only at the urgent request of the therapist) he surprised everyone by his friendly, outgoing behavior and received a citation as the most improved camper.

Case history 2

A thirteen-year-old came to the attention of the Children's Court because of repeated truancy, fighting with other children, and running away from home. When interviewed, he appeared to be a tough, callused, belligerent youngster, indifferent to the feelings of others. He was the youngest child of a large family whose father was a chronic alcoholic, the mother a prematurely tired, discouraged woman overwhelmed by her problems. Initial attempts to involve the boy in a therapeutic relationship seemed futile, but it was noticed that despite his apparent negativistic attitude he continued to attend his sessions faithfully. He constantly tested the therapist by belligerent, provocative statements, as though desiring to be rejected. One of the aides on the ward noticed that he was a capable athlete, especially proficient at boxing. When this was mentioned to him his eyes lit up, and for the first time he appeared alert and interested. Then he shrugged it off with, 'What's the use? I'd never get anywhere.' It soon became evident that he felt doomed to be a failure like his father, that he regarded himself as no good. He expressed this as follows: 'Im just a bastard. I have no feelings for anyone. Sometimes when I've been in a gang fight I wish I could get shot or stabbed to death—get it over quickly. It would serve me right.'

He spoke initially with affection of his mother, how hard-working and noble she was. Gradually, however, other feelings emerged. 'She should have left my father. She said she stayed for us kids. Some joke. How did his drinking and beatings help us?' It then became clear that his running away from home was an attempt to let his mother know how unhappy he was and also to punish her. 'That was the only time she showed any interest. But in a few days she forgot about it and then everything was the same as before.' Therapy revealed that his intensely angry feelings against his parents led him to regard himself as bad and evil. Such an attitude would propel him into aggressive, antisocial behavior, which in turn made him feel more evil and guilty. Assisted by therapy, Fred was able to return home and to school, where for the first time he ceased being troublesome and turned his interests to sports—joining the school basketball team.

The younger adolescent often presents, rather than a frank picture of depression, a set of symptoms that I prefer to label 'depressive equivalents': boredom, restlessness, a frantic seeking of new activities, a reluctance to be alone. Even though all adolescents exhibit some of these symptoms, the persistence of such traits indicates pathology. The feelings of emptiness, isolation and alienation so often described by teenagers can be indicative of depression. Many so-called 'hippies', by banding together, hope to find support and relief from these distressing feelings from which they further attempt to escape by the excessive use of drugs such as marijuana, mescaline, amphetamines and LSD. Sexual promiscuity, especially on the part of the female, is often a thinly disguised attempt to avoid feelings of depression, loneliness and helplessness. Illegitimate pregnancies are often sought either consciously or unconsciously for the same reason. The following case is only too typical (Toolan[38]).

Case history

A fifteen-year-old female was admitted to the hospital on her own request because of suicidal fears. An attractive youngster, she appeared several years older than her age. History revealed that she had been a behavioral problem since the age of seven. She had had frequent fights with other children, was truant from school, and disobedient at home. A bright child, her academic record was very erratic. At fourteen she ran away from home to live in Greenwich Village. There she enjoyed a Beatnik existence for a short period of time, indulged in long talking sessions, mood sessions, and poetry readings. Constantly dissatisfied, she attempted also to find satisfaction by promiscuous sexual activity. As time passed she became increasingly depressed. Marijuana was attempted but provided only temporary relief. Suicide appeared the only solution, but she decided, upon the advice of friends, to give psychotherapy a trial before making a final decision. In interviews with her therapist she became aware of a deep sense of loneliness, depression and despair. She realized that she had had occasional awareness of these feelings before but had, until recently, been able to ward them off by her frenetic behavior. As therapy progressed, she was able to give up her pseudosophisticated façade and behave more as a normal fifteen-year-old.

As Toolan[38] has described: 'Hand in hand with boredom, the teenager frequently complains of fatigue. He alternates between overwhelming fatigue and inexhaustible energy. Undoubtedly some of this fatigue is physiological, being the result of the very rapid growth processes taking place at this time. We should always be suspicious, however, when the fatigue in a physically healthy youngster appears out of proportion to his activity and when it interferes with his normal activity. It is also noteworthy when the adolescent complains of being excessively tired upon awakening in the morning after an adequate amount of sleep. We are all accustomed to observing this symptom in adult patients suffering from depression. Hypochondriasis and bodily preoccupation have also frequently to be considered as evidence of depression, as is also the case in many involutional depressions.

Case history

Simon, aged twelve, was seen in consultation at the suggestion of his pediatrician. The latter was concerned because the youngster was constantly complaining of various physical ailments, which after examination proved to be either grossly exaggerated or totally imaginary. A slender, frail child, he came eagerly to the interview, desirous of discussing his problems. He stated that he had been worried about his health for the past two or three years. Initially he would become frightened whenever he had a minor physical illness, such as an upper respiratory infection. He felt that he would become seriously ill and die. As time passed he began to worry over trivial matters such as a muscle cramp or slight feelings of fatigue. During the past month he had been very alarmed, believing that he had leukemia. This fear had begun after a class in biology at school in which the teacher described the symptoms of leukemia. He related that since that time he had had trouble falling asleep and felt anxious most of the day.

History revealed that he was an only child, whose father had been killed in an airplane accident shortly after his birth. He lived with his mother, who had never remarried and remained constantly attached to the image of her dead husband. The youngster grew up closely attached to the mother and also preoccupied with the image of the dead father. He had no close friends, although he maintained a superficial acquaintance with one or two boys younger than himself. As therapy progressed, it became evident that this youngster had introjected the image of a dead father whom he both idolized and hated for deserting him. Strong incestuous ties to the mother gave rise to guilt feelings. He realized during therapy that he had seldom been happy, that he had always expected to die young (obvious identification with the dead father). As treatment progressed, the somatic preoccupation was displaced by a frank depressive reaction which could then be handled directly.

Many depressed youngsters complain of difficulty in concentration. In fact, this is one of the chief presenting complaints to the school physician and should always be taken seriously, else within a very short time an otherwise capable student may fail in school, to the amazement of parents and faculty alike. Confronted with such a problem, the conscientious student will often spend long hours on his studies with little benefit. He will see others achieving better grades with much less effort and will soon become convinced that he isn't capable enough to master his work. Discouraged, he will then cease working, go frequently to the movies, spend hours watching television and often end up by being accused of failing because he was a playboy.

Delinquency and Depression

Denial and acting out are frequently encountered in adolescents. In such youngsters acting out may lead to serious delinquent behavior. Kaufman[23] has written that 'a crucial determinant (in delinquency) is an unresolved depression, which is the result of the trauma which these children have experienced'. He adds, 'We consider the delinquent acts of taking and doing forbidden things or expressing resentment and hostility to the depriving world, as the child's pathologic method of coping with his depressive nucleus.' Burks and Harrison[6] view aggressive behavior on the part of many delinquents as a method of avoiding feelings of depression. Kaufman[23] has also emphasized that delinquents suffer from a severely impoverished self-image and a profound emptiness of ego comparable to the emptiness of the schizophrenic ego. The following case is an example of such delinquent activity masking a depression (Toolan[38]).

Case history

Richard, a sixteen-year-old boy, was seen at the urgent request of his parents, who had become alarmed at evidence of increasingly delinquent behavior on his part. This had recently culminated in his suspension from school following an incident during which he struck a teacher. The boy, the elder of two children, came from a comfortable middle-class family in a suburb of New York City. He had always been somewhat small for his age—a matter of deep concern to him. A poor athlete, he tended to shun all competitive sports. He was extremely shy and frightened in the presence of girls, whom he avoided despite obvious interest in them. The parents noted that about six months previously he had lost all interest in his school work and in his usual friends, and had begun to associate with a delinquent street gang from a distant neighborhood. At this time he evidenced a distinct personality change. He appeared cocky and self-assured, while all previous signs of anxiety disappeared. His parents had recently become aware that he had engaged in several gang fights during one of which he had been stabbed with a knife.

When first seen, Richard looked like a typical hoodlum, cigarette hanging out of the corner of his mouth, black leather jacket, tight-fitting black dungarees. He was glib and expressed his disinterest in the whole procedure. He had no problems, except his parents, who were prejudiced against his new friends. The only help he needed was to get them to leave him alone. He hated school and was happy that he had been suspended. He was pleased to converse about his gang, bragging about their delinquent activities and his own prowess in fighting. I asked him if he ever became frightened during such fights and was surprised when after much hesitation he replied, 'Yes, I'm afraid I will lose control and kill someone.' He went on to explain that he was losing his temper with increasing frequency and that he had not intended to strike the teacher but the latter had pushed him and then he lost his head. I remarked that perhaps this was important and also that it would obviously interfere with his plans to pursue a career in the Navy as he had intended for several years.

As therapy progressed, it was readily apparent that this patient was a frightened, anxious, chronically depressed youngster. He recalled how unhappy he had been prior to joining his gang, how inferior he had felt compared to other fellows, how scared he had been in the presence of girls, how stupid he had appeared at school, how worried that he would never amount to anything. Following his entry into the gang and by means of a vicarious identification with their supposed strength, he had felt different. 'For the first time in my life I felt alive. I was a different person. I no longer worried, wasn't afraid of anyone.' He began to go out with girls and felt equal to the challenge in that area. As therapy continued, a crucial period occurred when he became aware of the significance of the gang in relieving his previous depressions. He wanted to give them up but was afraid of the consequences, namely, that he would again become depressed. He finally was able to do so, but only at the expense of a return of his previous feelings until these could be properly handled.

In many adolescents and adults we encounter sexual acting out as a method of relieving their depressive feelings. Such a person frenetically seeks contact with another human being by means of sexual intercourse, the only method of relating that he knows. Quite often, as in the case of the alcoholic, this activity produces only further depression and guilt, which once again he attempts to relieve by further sexual acting out.

Mid- and Late Adolescence Depression

By mid-adolescence one not infrequently encounters a picture of actual classical depression. This I believe is much more the case than has been recognized. The depressed adolescent frequently exhibits a confused self-identity, a feature not often encountered in adult depressives. He feels unworthy and unlovable; he often complains of feeling isolated. He often resents his parents yet is overly dependent upon them—as his emancipation from them is viewed as a further loss of love. The following case histories are illustrative.

Case history 1

Charlie was a fourteen-year-old boy who made a serious suicide attempt by swallowing a bottle of medicine. He left a note indicating that he wished to die and was discovered only when he became physically ill. When interviewed he appeared markedly depressed. His speech was slow and underproductive. He stated that he wanted to die as life no longer held any meaning for him. For the previous six months he had felt unhappy and depressed. He had lost interest in his school work and found it increasingly difficult to concentrate upon it. His marks, which previously had been excellent, declined. He began to complain of abdominal pain. An exploratory laparotomy revealed no pathology. The weekend of the suicide attempt he felt desperate and decided to kill himself. In therapy several important events emerged. The mother had experienced a serious depression and received ECT when the patient was two to three years old. She had made a fairly good recovery but had devoted herself to a musical career. This often necessitated her being away from home, as she had been on the weekend of the suicidal attempt. About six months previously, Charlie had been involved in a homosexual experience with an older man which had terrified him. He began to doubt his masculinity. When a girl in whom he was interested refused to become his girl-friend he felt completely devastated, and the depressive symptoms ensued.

N

Case history 2

Ella, a seventeen-year-old girl, made a suicidal attempt shortly after graduation from high school. The only child of two professional people, she had been very close to her father until his death when she was ten years of age. The father, who was ill and unable to work for several years before his death, took care of the child while the mother supported the family. The girl was very devoted to the father. They would often spend hours talking quietly together. After the father's death the mother continued to work and the girl was sent to a boarding school. Ella did not react strongly to her father's death; in fact, she wondered why she was so little troubled by her loss. At school she worked diligently at her studies but felt completely alone. She began to doubt her scholastic abilities, despite a fine academic record. She matured early physically, but this only made her feel different from the other girls. She continued to withdraw even more from contact with the other students. While at preparatory school she felt attached to the institution. With her excellent academic record, she was accepted by an outstanding woman's college. The summer following graduation was spent with her mother. She noted that she was becoming more depressed, and would spend hours alone in her room, brooding and crying. One day, convinced that life was worthless, she decided upon suicide. At first Ella found it difficult to understand why she had become so depressed. She was eager to enter college and had been thrilled upon being accepted by the college of her choice. Gradually she was able to understand the factors leading to her depression and suicidal attempt. The loss of her father had been a serious blow—so severe indeed that she had been forced to repress her feelings completely. During her prep school days, although she had been lonely and isolated, she had been able to feel that she belonged, that she had a home. Following graduation she felt lost. The repressed reaction to her father's death came to the surface and overwhelmed her. 'I'm no good. Why should I live while others die?' was a frequent thought.

Case history 3

Connie was a nineteen-year-old female college student who requested psychiatric assistance when she became very depressed upon her boy-friend's deserting her for another girl. Connie had had a very tumultuous history since she was fifteen years old. Previously a good student, her marks became erratic. She became rebellious both at home and school. She would sneak out of the house at night to meet her semi-delinquent friends and was sexually promiscuous. After her expulsion from the public high school she was attending, she was sent by her parents to a private boarding academy where her behavior continued essentially unchanged. She was almost expelled shortly before graduation. She did, however, manage to enter the college of her choice. The non-restrictive atmosphere of this college enabled her to diminish her rebelliousness. Her sexual promiscuity, however, continued. During her second year she became deeply attached to a young man. When he deserted her for another girl she became profoundly depressed. She developed anorexia, insomnia and difficulty in concentration; and lost interest in her usual activities. During therapy, Connie related that she had always felt different from other girls and that somehow she didn't belong. Furthermore she felt a stranger in her own home. She would make attempts to be close to her parents but only felt rejected by them. This was followed by antisocial behavior on her part to punish them, which only alienated them further. She sought solace in sexual activity but beneath a veneer of sophistication believed that she was a 'tramp'. Her love affairs inevitably ended in disappointment. She believed that she was always rejected. Yet closer inspection to these relationships revealed that she would usually maneuver the boy into rejecting her. For example she had arranged a date for her boy-friend with a girl she knew because she herself had school work to do. Much to her surprise and anger the boy-friend preferred the other girl.

Case history 4

Debbie was a tall, well-developed fifteen-year-old girl who was referred for therapy after a serious suicidal attempt while at preparatory school. Initially, she claimed that she couldn't understand why she had done so. 'A sudden impulse overcame me,' she stated. As she described the events leading up to the attempt, it became evident that she had been depressed for a long time. At eighteen months of age she had lost two-thirds of her right ring-finger following an accident. Excessively self-conscious, she considered herself mutilated and disfigured. In addition, she was slightly obese, which only added to her feelings of low self-esteem. She was a good student but never attained any real satisfaction from her school work. For the past year she had been extremely promiscuous, at times engaging in sexual intercourse with several boys in one evening. This would produce severe guilt feelings, yet she felt compelled to continue because 'It proves that boys think I'm attractive'. Since entering boarding school her sexual activity was markedly limited, but her guilt feelings and depression increased. On several occasions prior to her suicide attempt she became very much disturbed while gazing at her hands, believing that she saw the stigmata upon them.

Case history 5

Edward, a nineteen-year-old college sophomore, was referred for therapy by the school physician who was treating him for a duodenal ulcer, and who recognized his frank depression. Edward was the eldest of four children and had always been a shy, quiet, sensitive child. At age fifteen, accompanied by another youngster, he engaged in a sudden, unprovoked outburst of vandalism which caused several thousand dollars' worth of damage. Shortly afterwards he was sent to a boarding school. There he was an outstanding student but felt alienated from the other students. He spent almost all of his time at his studies. While Edward was in his freshman year at college his father died suddenly of a heart attack. Edward noticed that he was gradually becoming depressed. During his sophomore year he was diagnosed as having a duodenal ulcer. In addition he developed anorexia, and severe insomnia; and he lost interest in his studies. He felt that he was ugly, a disgrace, a failure. He believed that no one could care for him if they truly knew how horrible he was. He would make occasional attempts to date girls but was always convinced that they found him repulsive. He often contemplated suicide. His only pleasure in life was driving his expensive sports car. Edward's father, an extremely successful businessman, had always berated him for not being good enough. Terrified of his father, he had, nonetheless, greatly admired him for his accomplishments in business. He had a series of repetitive dreams in which the father would appear before him and castigate him for being such a failure.

Case history 6

Mary was fifteen years of age when she entered therapy after being expelled from boarding school for repeated violations of the school rules. A small, stocky, yet attractive girl, she was the daughter of professional parents. She had been a serious behavior problem from an early age. She resented her siblings, especially her younger brother whom she frequently tormented. She was sent to boarding school in an attempt to end her rebelliousness at home, but the same behavior continued at school. She was eager for therapy, as she had not wished to leave her school and had begun to recognize that she always managed to antagonize the people she cared for. She had a most ambivalent relationship with her mother. Although she deeply loved and admired her, she would mercilessly provoke her. Mary had always felt that she was an outsider; yet it was she who would antagonize the other children and cause them to reject her. During her second year of therapy she became involved with a boy several years her senior. This young man, a school drop-out at sixteen years of age, had a long criminal record. Their relationship was very stormy. Her parents strenuously objected to him but she managed to see him surreptitiously. He was an inadequate individual who became very dependent upon her and often threatened to harm himself if she stopped seeing him. Finally convinced that the relationship was destructive, she decided to end it. This decision produced a serious depression in Mary, followed by a suicide attempt. Although it had been her decision to end the relationship she couldn't face the loneliness that this loss produced.

The cases cited all illustrate youngsters who manifested a depression entirely similar to that of adults. Many of them did exhibit behavioral difficulties prior to the onset of their depressive symptoms that the author previously labeled as 'depressive equivalents'. This would appear to verify the thesis that such symptoms are manifestations of depression in younger individuals. The youngest patient in this series is fourteen years of age. The majority, however, were over sixteen years of age before they developed such frank symptoms of depression. It should be noted that the behavioral manifestations of depression usually ceased before a true picture of depression developed.

There seems to be general agreement on the low incidence of manic-depressive psychosis in children and young adolescents. Kanner[21] in the 1960 edition of his text *Child psychiatry* does not mention the term in the index. Kasanin and Kaufman[22] described only four affective psychoses before sixteen years of age. All four cases presented initial symptoms after fourteen years of age. Anthony and Scott[4] have completed an exhaustive review of the literature on the topic from 1884 to 1954. They discovered three cases in late childhood that fit the criteria for the diagnosis, and added one case of their own in considerable detail in which the initial symptoms occurred at twelve years of age. Campbell[10] has been one of the few authors to describe the illness as not uncommon in childhood, but his views have not been generally accepted. Manic-like behavior is frequently described in children and adolescents, but careful study and observation almost invariably indicates either a hyperactive, organic, brain-damaged child or an excited schizophrenic.

3

Diagnosis

The diagnostic classification of childhood disorders is quite unsatisfactory. The new classification of the American Psychiatric Association DSM–II[3] has enlarged the categories relating to children, but it is still far from adequate. It does not mention depression. Faux and Rowley[15] have proposed the following categories of depressions of childhood:

Grief response (functional depression),

> Overt depression manifested by feelings of futility, guilt, unworthiness, or self-destruction.
> Depression masked by manipulative expression.
> Depression masked by denial.
> Depression masked by hostility.
> Depression associated with withdrawal and fantasy.

Endogenous depressive diathesis (a term that implies an idiopathic constitutional tendency; possibly the early manic-depressive should be so categorized).

Depression associated with cultural deprivation (a circumstance in which there is insufficient stimulation, which results in listlessness and apathy).

Depression associated with physical incapacity (medical disorders: diabetes, polio, muscular dystrophy, etc. Mutilation: amputations, burns, etc.).

Drug-induced pseudo-depression (a type of reaction that occasionally occurs when hypnotics, anticonvulsants, or sedatives are used in the treatment of emotional or physical disorders).

Like Grinker,[19] we view depression as an affect that can be present in any diagnostic category—adjustment reaction, neurosis, psychosis, and organic brain damage.

The recognition of a depression in children and adolescents can be facilitated by the study of dreams and fantasy material. The dreams of depressed children will often refer to dead persons beckoning them to join the dead person in the other world. Often their dreams picture them as being attacked and injured. On other occasions their dreams will depict bodily emptiness or dissolution and loss of either inner or outer parts of the body. We interpret the latter, as does Kaufman,[23] to imply a loss of a significant relationship, rather than castration anxiety. Depressed young-sters often relate fantasies of being unloved and unwanted. They find it difficult to identify with members of their family and fantasize belonging to another family. Fantasies of running away are very common and fantasies of being dead are far from uncommon. Associated with both of the latter fantasies is the thought that someone (usually the parents) will be sorry for having treated them so unkindly.

Psychological testing can be of great assistance in recognizing depressive reactions in children and adolescents. The psychodiagnostic picture tends, however, to differ from that shown by adult depressives. Anger is often prominently displayed and openly expressed, while depressive feelings tend to be overshadowed—the reverse of the picture usually seen in adult depressives. On the Rorschach there is a diminution of the color response as well as detailing of dark, shadowy colors. In addition, the Rorschach protocol reveals many images of body emptiness as well as angry, aggressive, sadistic images. The Wechsler scale usually shows a higher performance than verbal score, also the reverse of that seen in adult depression. The patterning may at times be similar to that shown by psychopaths; perhaps this is related to a tendency towards acting out, previously described in the clinical picture.

The important topic of suicide will not be discussed here, as it has been adequately covered by Connell[11] in 'Suicidal attempts in childhood and adolescence' in *Modern perspectives in child psychiatry* (1965).

4

Therapy

The treatment of children and adolescents is complex, and would require considerable space were it to be adequately covered. But a few comments of particular import to the therapy of depressed children and adolescents are essential.

Treatment must, of course, be influenced by the age of the patient, his circumstances, the clinical picture presented, facilities available, etc. Groups of infants suffering from infantile or anaclitic depression require changes in their living arrangements. They need the attention of one significant person, hopefully the mother. As Spitz[35] has reminded us, time is of the essence. Many such children will not recover if the condition continues longer than three months. More important than the treatment of such infants is the prevention of such reactions. Children should not be separated from their mothers, unless absolutely necessary. If they require hospitalization, mothers should be allowed to visit daily, to spend several hours with the infant and help feed and care for it. Those infants living in institutions should have one person assigned to give them special attention.

The group of latency, preadolescent and early adolescent-aged children who present behavioral problems require an approach suitable for acting-out youngsters in general. These children seldom recognize that they need therapy and unfortunately their parents and others may not do so either. Frequently school officials or other authorities will urge the child and parents to seek help. If the child is living at home it is imperative that the parents be included in the treatment program, as they must be helped to understand the child's feelings of depression, pain, loneliness and helplessness, and, even more important, to change themselves in order to give the child the type of relationship he needs. Psychotherapy of such youngsters is often difficult. Not only do they seldom recognize the need but their use of denial and projection as mechanisms of avoiding facing their painful feelings requires judicious therapeutic skill. They will invariably test the therapist to see whether he really cares for them. The therapist must never lose sight of the fact that, though these youngsters appear to desperately need a close relationship to another human being, they often become anxious and frightened when they achieve such closeness as it makes them only too aware of the losses they have experienced in their lives. Great patience is required. Premature interpretation must be avoided lest the youngster discontinue treatment. The therapist must realize that it may require considerable time before the youngster is even able to talk about his painful feelings. Michael (p. 362) is a good example. Many weeks elapsed before he was able to get beyond a simple recital of the events of the week, and then only in a censored version. In working with many youngsters it must also be borne in mind that they are not accustomed to discuss their feelings even with those closest to them. If therapy is successful within this group, the therapist can expect to encounter overt depressive feelings which obviously require a different technical approach.

Therapy with an overtly depressed patient poses other therapeutic problems. Many therapists become bored and impatient in dealing with depressed patients—they want movement and progress—not a repetition of sad, hurt feelings. Other therapists may become frightened of the possible suicidal risk and recommend hospitalization prematurely.

Evaluation of suicidal risk is never easy at best. If a very depressed adolescent is seen for the first time, especially following a suicidal attempt, it is wise to insist upon a period of evaluation in a hospital setting. This can often be arranged in the pediatric service of a general hospital. Such a period of hospitalization not only allows for a period of observation but also interrupts the conflict that may be going on between the child and its parents.

Whether psychotherapy is conducted on an in- or out-patient basis, the relationship to the therapist is the main support for the patient. He must be able to trust and rely on the therapist in order to have the strength to face and explore his painful feelings. Here too we must bear in mind that the depressed adolescent will often appear almost insatiable in his demands upon the therapist. He will oscillate between trust and distrust for long periods of time before accepting the fact that the therapist will not desert him. Many depressed patients feel so unworthy that they find it almost impossible to believe that anyone can truly care for them. In one respect, at least, the therapist's task is easier with the adolescent than with the younger child who is manifesting depression by behavioral symptoms, as the depressed adolescent recognizes that he is troubled and ordinarily is eager to obtain help. As a general rule treatment of depression in adolescents requires intensive therapy. Simple techniques such as environmental manipulation, support, suggestion and reassurance may appear to resolve the problem but usually the gains are temporary at best.

At the present time various methods of group and family therapy are being attempted with adolescent patients. Though it is too early to evaluate thoroughly the results of these newer techniques, family therapy would appear to be of great value, as the basic feeling of loss of love that adolescent patients experience can often be fruitfully worked with in family groups.

The question of medication for depressive children and adolescents is difficult to assess. Most workers have reported negative results with anti-depressive medication. Perhaps the younger patient metabolizes these compounds differently than does the older depressed patient in whom they frequently produce beneficial effects.

Frommer[17] reports favorably on the use of phenelzine in depressed children from nine to fifteen years of age. Connell[11] also mentions the use of this drug in treating suicidal depressions in children.

There are very few reports in the recent literature on the use of ECT in depressive reactions of children and adolescents. Many clinics have dis-continued its use even with adult depressions, except following an un-successful trial of anti-depressant medication or where the suicidal risk is considered especially serious. Most child psychiatrists do not use ECT at the present time. We would suggest that this procedure be used only as a last resort in adolescent patients who present a clinical picture of overt depression, when psychotherapy and medication have proven ineffective.

The recognition and proper management of depressive reactions in adolescence are of the utmost importance. The suicide rate of the fifteen to nineteen age group in the U.S.A. has doubled over the past ten years. Even more important, however, is the deleterious effect that depression has upon the functioning of the adolescent, especially in his school work. Many youngsters troubled by difficulty in concentration do poorly academically and drop out of school, altering their entire future. We have, as yet, little information as to the effect of depression during the adolescent years upon future psychic functioning. While some might spontaneously overcome such feelings, it is likely that many will continue as depressed adults. One can only wonder what influence depressive feelings during the adolescent years have upon the psychotic depressions of the involutional years.

5

Psychopathology

At this point one can conclude that adolescents from fourteen years on do show depressive reactions quite similar to those seen in adults. Younger children do not. The question, as already indicated, is whether children younger than fourteen do not become depressed or whether they manifest depression in a different fashion. There is to date no agreement on this point, but it would appear on careful study that the latter is the case.

Such a situation should not be surprising. Child psychiatrists, and especially child analysts, argued for many years over the question whether schizophrenia occurred in children. Many, especially those of an analytic persuasion, argued on theoretical grounds that it was impossible for children to become schizophrenic. It is now generally accepted that children can become schizophrenic and that the clinical picture is quite different from that seen in adults. It is noteworthy that at about fourteen years of age the clinical picture in schizophrenia begins to resemble that seen in adults. I propose that a similar situation occurs with depressive reactions.

Child psychiatrists must not lose sight of the fact that we are applying a diagnosis to a developing organism—the child—and must therefore expect that the clinical picture would vary with the psychic maturation of the child.

As Boulanger[7] has written: 'A psychoanalyst may very well be reluctant to perceive in a child the equivalent of an adult's melancholia, for he is besieged at once by all the points of theory which are unsettled and passionately disputed within the school: the organization and functions of the ego, superego, and object relationships, the origins of the Oedipus complex and the complexities of the instinctual development, the purpose of masochism, and the validity of the death instinct.'

Many theories have been advanced to explain the genesis of depression in adults. The classical studies of Abraham[1] and Freud[16] theorized that depression resulted from aggression and hostility turned inwards against the self through the mechanism of a harsh superego. The depressed person identifies with the ambivalently loved object which has been lost. One must be cautious, however, about applying to the depression of children a theory that may be valid for middle-aged melancholics. Both Abraham[1] and Freud[16] stressed the oral introjection of depression. Klein[25] has emphasized this point of view in her work on the depressive position of childhood, which she views as a normal developmental stage for all infants.

Almost all psychoanalysts have postulated that depression follows the loss of a significant love-object, whether the loss is in reality or in fantasy.

Bibring[5] has offered an intriguing theory: 'Depression can be defined as the emotional expression of a state of helplessness and powerlessness of the ego, irrespective of what may have caused the breakdown of the mechanism which established his self-esteem. He adds that the basic mechanism is 'the ego's shocking awareness of its helplessness in regard to its aspirations'.

The issue of self-esteem has begun to assume a nodal position in all theories of depression. This has led Rie[30] to question 'at which point in the child's life such an experience develops with sufficient intensity to constitute what has been called low self-esteem'. Citing Erikson[14] and Loevinger,[28] Rie[30] concludes that 'It may be no accident that this level of ego identity, or ability to conceptualize one's self, and the typical adult manifestations of depression are both generally agreed to occur at the earliest during adolescence.' Rie[30] goes farther in stating that an affect of helplessness is essential for the development of depression. Quoting Schmale[33] and Lichtenberg[27] he concludes: 'There may be reason to believe that the fully differentiated and generalized primary affect characterizing depression, namely despair or helplessness, is one of which children, perhaps prior to the end of the latency years, are incapable.'

Sandler and Joffe[32] have modified Bibring's[5] view of the concept of self-esteem as regards depressive reactions in children. They 'stress rather the basic biological nature of the depressive reaction, related to pain (and its opposite, "well-being") rather than the psychologically more elaborate concept of "self-esteem" '. In our opinion this modification answers the objections raised above by Rie.[30]

Sandler and Joffe[32] make the significant point that depression 'can best be viewed as a basic psychobiological affective reaction which, like anxiety, becomes abnormal when it occurs in inappropriate circumstances, when it persists for an undue length of time, and when the child is unable to make a developmentally appropriate adaptation to it'. Sandler and Joffe[32] modify the concept of the significance of the loss of the desired love-object: 'While what is lost may be an object, it may equally well be the loss of a previous state of the self. Indeed we would place emphasis on the latter rather than on the fact of the object-loss *per se*. When a love-object is lost, what is really lost is, we believe, the state of well-being implicit, both psychologically and biologically, in the relationship with the object. The young infant who suffers physical or psychological deprivation in the phase before object-representations have been adequately structured may show a depressive response to the loss of psychophysical well-being. Even an older child, who can distinguish adequately between self and object-representation, may react with depression to the birth of a sibling—a reaction which in our view is not an object-loss but rather a feeling of having been deprived of an ideal state, the vehicle of which was the sole possession of the mother. . . . If his response is characterized by a feeling of helplessness, and he shows a passive resignation in his behavior, we can consider him to be depressed.' They note that as the child grows older the object-loss becomes more important than the loss of the state of well-being embodied in the relationship to the object. In brief, they view depression 'as a state of helpless resignation in the face of pain, together with an inhibition both of drive discharge and ego functions'. Some children, they add, will make strenuous efforts to restore the missing state, others may react with angry protests and aggression; some may regress to an earlier phase.

If we accept the thesis that depression is a reaction to loss either of an object or a state of well-being, with a feeling of diminished self-esteem and hopelessness, we can better understand the vicissitudes of depressive reactions at various ages. It is true, of course, that not every child reacts to loss with a depressive reaction. But certainly we are aware that individuals vary considerably in their abilities to tolerate pain or discomfort of any sort, whether it be physical or mental. The end result of any object-loss will depend upon the developmental level at which it first makes its effect felt. In general, the younger the child the more serious the consequences. In infants ego-development may be profoundly disturbed. There may be a lack of ego-development or even profound regression. The infant and young child may find it difficult or impossible to form adequate object-relationships. This naturally will affect his whole future psychic development. It will seriously impair his ability to identify with the significant figures in his life. Disturbances in identification will of necessity affect the formation of the ego-ideal and superego and consequently the future personality structure. In some infants and children the impairment of ego-development will seriously hinder their intellectual potential.

Where the loss arises during the latency and early adolescent years, it will often cause the child to react with anger and hostility toward the love-object who he feels has deserted and betrayed him. By reacting with anger and aggression he can ward off the painful feelings of impotence and helplessness. Such hostile feelings can often lead to serious acting-out and delinquent behavior. Unfortunately such defensive operations seldom prove successful and lead to serious conflict with parents and drive them farther away at the time the child still needs their love and support. Ironically, the more neglected the child is, the more he needs his parents' love and affection. The child will often inhibit the expression of this anger in the hope that his parents may once again love him if he should be good. He often turns the anger and hostility against himself, believing that he is evil and has been deserted for that reason. Such an evil self-image can only lead to evil acts—the frequent acting-out so often seen in depressed children. Such behavior, of course, can only reinforce the child's image of himself as an evil, horrible person, which will lower his self-esteem even farther and increase his depressive feelings.

The child and adolescent will utilize many defensive operations to ward off the pain of depressive feelings. In addition to regression already mentioned, denial, repression, and projection are commonly employed.

During adolescence displacement onto somatic symptoms is often attempted. Occasionally we may encounter youngsters who utilize a reversal of affect.

As the child approaches mid-adolescence his ego, especially its aspect of reality-testing, develops significantly. He finds it increasingly difficult to use denial as a defense. He begins to recognize the role of his parents in the object-loss he has suffered and as a result his hostility toward them increases, but so too do his guilt feelings. The hostility previously directed toward the parents is now directed toward their introjects within the child. As described by Toolan[37] the superego does not reach maximum development until mid or late adolescence. This, plus the further realization that reality will not change, reinforces his feelings of lowered self-esteem and helplessness and leads to the clinical picture of depression described for older adolescents.

We must not overlook another important factor in the formation of depression in adolescence. The reactivation of the oedipal complex and its resolution at this period cause a definite sense of loss leading to depressive feelings. This will often reinforce feelings of loss from an earlier age.

6

Conclusion

A review of the pertinent literature indicates that there is controversy as to whether children under twelve years of age do become depressed. The author concludes that they can and do, and he describes clinical pictures of depressive manifestations in children. Adolescents from fourteen to sixteen years of age often exhibit adult depressive symptoms.

A theoretical discussion is offered pertaining to the dynamics of depression, especially as it relates to the child and adolescent, and an explanation based on growth developmental phases is provided for the varying clinical pictures.

REFERENCES

1. ABRAHAM, K. 1911. Notes on the psychoanalytic investigation and treatment of manic-depressive insanity and allied conditions. *Selected Papers, 1927.* London: Hogarth Press.
2. AGRAS, S. 1959. The relationship of school phobia to childhood depression. *Amer. J. Psychiat.,* **116**, 533.
3. American Psychiatric Association. 1968. *Diagnostic and statistical manual of mental disorders* (2nd edition). Washington, D.C.
4. ANTHONY, J. and SCOTT, P. 1960. Manic-depressive psychosis in childhood. *J. Child Psychol. Psychiat.,* **1**, 53.
5. BIBRING, E. 1953. The mechanism of depression. In *Affective disorders*, Ed. P. Greenacre. New York: International Universities Press.

6. BIERMAN, J., SILVERSTEIN, A. and FINESINGER, J. 1958. A depression in a six-year-old boy with acute poliomyelitis. *The psychoanalytic study of the child*, **13**, 430. New York: International Universities Press.

7. BOULANGER, J. B. 1966. Depression in childhood. *Canad. psychiat. Ass. J.*, **11**, S 309.

8. BOWLBY, J. 1960. Childhood mourning and its implications for psychiatry. *Amer. J. Psychiat.*, **118**, 481.

9. BURKS, H. L. and HARRISON, S. L. 1962. Aggressive behavior as a means of avoiding depression. *Amer. J. Orthopsychiat.*, **32**, 416.

10. CAMPBELL, J. D. 1955. Manic-depressive disease in children. *J.A.M.A.*, **158**, 154.

11. CONNELL, P. 1965. Suicidal attempts in childhood and adolescence. In *Modern perspectives in child psychiatry*, Ed. J. G. Howells. Edinburgh: Oliver & Boyd.

12. DESPERT, J. L. 1952. Suicide and depression in children. *Nerv. Child*, **9**, 378.

13. ENGEL, G. L. and REICHSMAN, F. 1956. Spontaneous and experimentally induced depressions in an infant with a gastric fistula. *J. Amer. Psychoanal. Ass.*, **4**, 428.

14. ERIKSON, E. H. 1950. Growth and crisis of the 'healthy personality'. In *Symposium on the Healthy Personality*, Ed. M. J. E. Senn. New York: Josiah Mary Jr. Foundation.

15. FAUX, E. J. and ROWLEY, C. M. 1967. Detecting depressions in childhood. *Hosp. Community Psychiat.*, **18**, 31.

16. FREUD, S. 1917. *Mourning and melancholia*. Standard Edition **14**. London: Hogarth Press.

17. FROMMER, E. A. 1967. Treatment of childhood depression with anti-depressant drugs. *Brit. med. J.*, **i**, 729.

18. GOLDFARB, W. 1946. Effects of psychological deprivation in infancy and subsequent stimulation. *Amer. J. Psychiat.*, **102**, 18.

19. GRINKER, R., MILLER, J., SABSHIN, M., NUNN, R. and NUNALLY, J. 1961. *The phenomena of depressions*. New York: Hoeber.

20. HARRINGTON, M. and HASSAN, J. 1958. Depression in girls during latency. *Brit. J. med. Psychol.*, **31**, 43.

21. KANNER, L. 1960. *Child psychiatry*. Springfield: Thomas.

22. KASANIN, J. and KAUFMAN, M. R. 1929. A study of the functional psychoses in childhood. *Amer. J. Psychiat.*, **9**, 307.

23. KAUFMAN, I. and HEIMS, L. 1958. The body image of the juvenile delinquent. *Amer. J. Orthopsychiat.*, **28**, 146.

24. KEELER, W. R. 1954. Children's reaction to the death of a parent. In *Depression*, Eds. P. HOCH and J. ZUBIN. New York: Grune and Stratton.

25. KLEIN, M. 1935. A contribution to the psychogenesis of manic-depressive states. In *Contributions to psychoanalysis*, 1948. London: Hogarth Press.

26. LEHMANN, H. E. 1959. Psychiatric concepts of depression: nomenclature and classification. *Canad. psychiat. Ass. J.*, Sup. **4**: S1.

27. LICHTENBERG, P. 1957. A definition and analysis of depression. *A.M.A. Arch. Neurol. Psychiat.*, **77**, 519.

28. LOEVINGER, J. 1959. A theory of test response. In *Invitational conference on testing problems*. Princeton: Educational Testing Service.

29. PEARSON, G. H. J. 1949. *Emotional disorders of children*. New York: Norton.

30. RIE, H. E. 1967. Depression in childhood—a survey of some pertinent contributions. *J. Amer. Acad. Child Psychiat.*, **5**, 653.

31. ROCHLIN, G. 1959. The loss complex. *J. Amer. Psychoanal. Ass.*, **7**, 299.

32. SANDLER, J. and JOFFE, W. G. 1965. Notes on childhood depression. *Int. J. Psychoanal.*, **46**, 88.

33. SCHMALE, A. 1964. A genetic view of affects with special reference to the genesis of helplessness and hopelessness. *The psychoanalytic study of the child*, **19**, 287. New York: International Universities Press.

34. SPERLING, M. 1959. Equivalents of depression in children. *J. Hillside Hosp.*, **8**, 138.

35. SPITZ, R. and WOLF, K. M. 1946. Anaclitic depression; an inquiry into the genesis of psychiatric conditions in early childhood. *The psychoanalytic study of the child*, **2**, 313. New York: International Universities Press.

36. STATTEN, T. 1961. Depressive anxieties and their defences in childhood. *Canad. Med. Ass. J.*, **84**, 824.

37. TOOLAN, J. M. 1960. Changes in personality structure during adolescence. In *Science and psychoanalysis*, Ed. J. H. MASSERMAN. New York: Grune and Stratton.

38. TOOLAN, J. M. 1962. Depression in children and adolescents. *Amer. J. Ortho-psychiat.*, **32**, 404.

XVI

PSYCHOSES IN ADOLESCENCE

D. Arn. van Krevelen

*Lecturer in Child Psychiatry at the University of Leiden
Director, Stichting Medisch-Psychologische Kinderkliniek
Oegstgeest, The Netherlands*

1

Introduction

To the student of adolescents' psychoses two main problems present themselves: (1) Are there psychoses unique to adolescence? (2) To what extent do psychoses during adolescence differ from those in childhood and adulthood? These two questions will be discussed separately.

The Problem of Psychoses Unique to Adolescence

In 1871 Hecker,[18] describing a psychical disorder during puberty, termed it *hebephrenia* (or 'Jugendirresein' = adolescent psychosis), thus expressing his view that this clinical picture is related to the age-period of adolescence. The concept became associated not only with the symptomatology, suggestive of exaggerated adolescent behaviour, but also with the pathogenesis, which Hecker believed to arise from a disturbance of sexual maturation. After him, Kraepelin[26] denied a causal relationship between what he called a sub-group of dementia praecox and puberty, stating that the majority of cases follow the conclusion of sexual development. However, he agreed that the inevitable course of the process means complete mental disintegration.

In time it was found that some cases did not have such a fatal course, and this caused a reaction to the views previously held. Schizophrenia was diagnosed only in patients with a poor prognosis, whose illness led to mental disintegration. Hence patients presenting an atypical picture, with a reasonably fair prognosis, were considered cases of borderline psychoses (Kleist[23, 24]) and were assigned to a nosological category of their own. As a subcategory of this group might be considered those psychoses, appearing during puberty and having a good prognosis, in which puberty—in the sense of somatic *and* mental maturation—is a pathogenetic factor.

It is interesting that students of *normal* adolescence (Charlotte Bühler,[6] Spranger,[51] Stern,[54] Leta Hollingworth[19]) came to similar conclusions. They pointed out not that psychosis resembles adolescence, but the reverse—that adolescence shows certain features of a psychosis. Hutter,[20,21] a Dutch psychiatrist, described adolescence as a period 'in which normally abnormalities so often happen, whereas it is abnormal that everything passes normally'.

In our era the emphasis is upon development. Added to environmental factors, modern child psychiatry pays attention to *developmental* noxae. Concepts like 'developmental psychopathy' and 'developmental psychosis' are terms used nowadays which imply that development *per se* may exert a noxious influence. Thus the view that psychoses specific to adolescence do exist becomes new again. The problem is reduced to the question whether adolescence may have a real pathogenetic significance or whether it gives a specific colouring to the picture, which would mean that its influence is merely pathoplastic. It follows that the essential criterion for the diagnosis of adolescent psychosis is complete recovery, or as stated by Adriana de Leeuw-Aalbers:[34] 'If a psychosis appears during the years of adolescence whereas later psychotic symptoms are completely absent and the person in question is able to remain efficiently in his profession, his family and in society, one has a right to think of the possibility of a psychosis related to the developmental disturbances, which may accompany the adolescent years.'

Hence it is important to be aware of the fact that the qualifying addition of 'developmental' or 'adolescent' influences our prognosis; the important criteria should be that adolescent psychoses vanish during or towards the end of this developmental stage. It is obvious that in some cases it would be possible to make a diagnosis with certainty only after the course of the illness is known. It is an academic question how far the course and the issue of a morbid process may rank as diagnostic criteria.

The follow-up investigation carried out by Adriana de Leeuw-Aalbers[34] in the Valerius Hospital at Amsterdam provides interesting data. This follow-up refers to 63 cases of unclear and atypical psychoses during adolescence, for whom no precise diagnosis could be made at the time of admission. The longest period of follow-up was thirty-eight years, the shortest interval was one year. No fewer than 20 patients had completely recovered and had been able to live successfully in society for many years (twenty years and longer). This worker demonstrated the absence of uniform syndrome that might be called characteristic for adolescence. Yet she divided the patients into four groups:

(*a*) Depressive states, not belonging to the group of manic-depressive psychoses. These states presented in patients who either had a hereditary taint or had shown a neurotic development during puberty. These disorders had their beginning in the last years of adolescence.

(b) Disinhibitory (impulsive) states, occurring after normal puberty development. There was no hereditary taint. However, a serious psychical trauma was found in the history of these patients.

(c) Hysteriform or paranoid psychoses, in the pathogenesis of which constitution, neurotic development, and more or less serious trauma, played a role.

(d) Schizophreniform pictures, confusional states and katatoniform syndromes. In the majority of cases hereditary transmission was obvious.

Among the case histories related in the above study one finds mentioned a seventeen-year-old girl, who reacted upon the first coition with impulses and hysterical symptoms. Years later the same patient developed an hysterical aphonia following the birth of her first (legitimate) child. This case is presented by the author as a characteristic adolescent psychosis. Although it is possible to agree with the author that in the genesis of the first hysterical condition adolescence means a pathogenetic factor, this is no longer valid in regard to the aphonia of a later date. Hence it becomes doubtful whether the concept of adolescent psychoses has been rightly applied. It is also strange that the depressive psychoses did not appear before the age of eighteen. Because of this finding, the author concluded that the most unstable stage of adolescence is around the eighteenth year. This, however, is at complete variance with what is known of the psychology of adolescence. In all cases, moreover, other factors could be demonstrated, which might likewise have pathogenetic significance. Viewed in the light of the facts presented by the follow-up, adolescence has a pathoplastic, not a pathogenetic, importance. If it is not justified to state that adolescence acts in a pathogenetic sense, the diagnosis 'adolescent psychosis' is utterly unfounded.

Even if one would accept that a definite developmental stage like adolescence has a particular psychopathological significance, to the extent that deviations from the norm may come more easily into being than in an earlier or a later life stage, various possibilities must be considered:

1. A pathological predisposition needs a certain time before it can manifest itself. An example is juvenile paresis.

2. Disorders revealing themselves during puberty have nothing to do with the developmental stage as such, but merely become obvious as the child becomes older. These disorders are due to the increasing discrepancy between the development of the individual's faculties and the relatively higher demands from society. To assess correctly this kind of disturbance, it is necessary to consider the importance of sociological factors, community tasks and traditions, which differ from country to country and from social stratum to social stratum.

3. Adolescence may be considered as a period during which the individual is more susceptible. Noxious factors get more influence, in so far as they affect an organism which is more vulnerable than before. Among the pathogenic factors psychical trauma comes first and foremost. This means that this category of disorders may be counted among psychogenic reactions.

4. Morbid conditions, which are not reactions to noxious factors from outside, appear autochthonously, their origin being somatic or psychic. This group of disorders depends immediately on adolescent characteristics. Examples of this group are: *adolescent neurasthenia*, characterised by irritability and fatiguability; *individuation depression* founded upon extreme mother-fixation; *hypochondriacal reactions* to masturbation and to changes of body image; *dysmorphophobia*, characterised by the individual's doubt of the normality of his bodily evolution and resulting in anxiety. It is to be noted that these conditions, not psychotic *per se*, may be initial phenomena of a schizophrenic process.

5. Discrepancies between somatic and psychic growth may involve disintegration of personality and hence adjustment disorders, in the origin of which the environment plays an important role; but here the emphasis is on growth inconsistencies.

All kinds of combinations of mental and physical development may be noted; there is no parallelism. The rhythm of maturation may be accelerated or retarded; mental development may precede physical growth and vice versa; certain elements of the psychical structure may develop sooner than others, endangering the adolescent's integration. Thereby follow adjustment disorders, particularly in the middle of adolescence and towards its end. If the acceleration or retardation is disharmonious, which means that it only concerns some facets of the total evolution, the consequences may be far-reaching. A striking example is that of a twelve-year-old girl, physically and sexually six years ahead of her age, who on entering a new class was mistaken for a colleague by her young male teacher. Any disruption of maturation creates its specific problems. It is noteworthy that in German literature much attention is paid to the observation that modern youth matures earlier than previously, which is of considerable consequence for adolescent psychiatry and jurisprudence.

The question arises whether we are not mistaking disorders *during* adolescence for disturbances *of* adolescence. How often it happens that the concepts of pre-adolescence and adolescence are included in the diagnostic description, without taking into account that beyond the period of adolescence occur morbid conditions which do not essentially differ from those which come to manifestation during puberty. It seems as if the qualifying addition of the term 'adolescence' implies an explanation, or even an etiology, which in reality does not exist.

It is essential, therefore, to distinguish between disorders during adolescence and those which have their origin in adolescent development. This view is based on the experience that adolescence is not the critical stage of development which it is usually assumed to be. It is often forgotten that there are not only revolutionary adolescents, but also evolutionary youths (Nÿssen[39]). By comparing children's disorders with those of adolescents, I have come to the conclusion that the critical character of adolescence cannot be rigidly maintained. It would be impossible to demonstrate the opposite by looking for an increase in the frequency of referrals during the stage of adolescence, because in fact there is no such peak. Quite rightly Fleming[16] has inverted the view of Stanley Hall[17] by stating: 'Development is gradual rather than saltatory in character'.

The Problem of the Specificity of Disorders during Adolescence

How far do processes during adolescence assume a specific quality, clearly different from that of childhood and adult disorders? May one take it for granted that adolescence has a pathoplastic influence, as a result of which adolescent psychoses present stage-bound characteristics? This may be true, as there are many examples in literature of typical disease pictures which would not conform to patterns of disease occurring before or after the stage of adolescence.

An example of this is the syndrome of *mania phantastica infantilis*, described for the first time by Rümke,[43, 44] then by Hutter,[20, 21] Adriana de Leeuw-Aalbers[34] and the author.[28, 29] As publications on the subject are rare and have appeared only in the Netherlands, it may be doubted whether this psychotic condition is as frequent as it appeared to its first recorder. Rümke's patients were nine, eleven, fourteen (2) and sixteen years of age, those of Mrs de Leeuw-Aalbers fifteen and seventeen years old. A follow-up was possible for one of Rümke's patients, whose disease was suggestive of a schizophrenic process.

The girl, whose case is briefly reproduced here is a typical example of what Rümke[43, 44] has called the 'juvenile psychosis par excellence'.

She was fourteen years old when admitted to the child psychiatric in-patient department, because of her excessive temper tantrums, which made her unmanageable at home. She had lived with an aunt, under whose care the parents had put her a year before, when they returned to Indonesia after their leave. At first the girl was well behaved in the environment of her relative to whom she had been attached from the age of five, but soon she manifested fits of passion. She gave expression to her fear her aunt might abandon her. She started to run away, as if she wanted to beg the question.

The patient's aunt gave the following information: The girl behaves very childishly, sucks her fingers, bites her nails. She is unable to mix with children of her own age, but she is very fond of little children, and may romp with them as if she were a toddler herself. Towards adults she is somewhat shy at first, but she shows forced affection towards men. She revels in phantasies in which men play a role. Recently she said that she walked out with the milkman. She has no hobbies, reads rarely and, if she reads, prefers books for small children. She is very passive. She is fussy, jumps from one thing to another. Usually she is in high spirits, though her cheeriness seems forced.

Her development was not retarded. She had no illnesses of importance. She had attended several schools, and her school records were good. She was often teased by the other pupils and was considered 'a baby'.

Outwardly she is—still according to the aunt—the counterpart of her mother, who is pictured as an easy-going, cheerful, but short-tempered person, inclined to seek pleasure, who gives her children insufficient affection. The father, because of his profession, is often away from home, has little patience with his children, and expects them to behave like adults. Presumably the girl has experienced many frustrations in her original environment. On the other hand, the aunt appears to have a warm personality and a good understanding of the girl. It is only on account of her own insecurity that she has found it necessary to send her niece to the hospital.

The data concerning other relatives are not significant. The father's youngest sister is in a mental hospital because of a meningoencephalitis.

The girl's appearance is characterised by the contrast between childish facial expression and gestures and the body configuration of an adult woman. Her motor behaviour is that of a very young child; she averts her face, sucks her fingers and speaks in a childlike voice. Her behaviour in the group gives a different picture; there she is noisy and boisterous, without any reason screams with laughter, which then stops as suddenly as it started. Her jokes are at a primitive level and find little response. Her state of mind is extremely variable; her habitual hypomania culminates in crying fits and temper tantrums. Apart from these sudden outbursts at the slightest provocation, there are periodical emotional crises of a psychotic character, which leave a mark for days after. The patient is then beside herself, starts panting, her head in an oblique position, her eyes turn upwards, so that the white of the eye is visible, her mouth is distorted. Then she talks louder and louder until she is shouting at the top of her voice, her speech unarticulated turning to unintelligible jabber. She becomes more and more excited, tears her clothes, tramples upon her spectacles, knocks a pane of glass to pieces and attacks the nurses, particularly her favourite nurse, in unrestrained aggressiveness. During these crises she is impervious to reason, but afterwards she remembers everything and is remorseful in a childlike way. She wants to hear again and again that nobody is angry with her and everybody is as fond of her as before.

Very briefly, the findings of the psychological and medical examination were as follows. Her intelligence is slightly below the norm. The girl feels uncertain about her capacities. Her frustration tolerance is minimal. She feels emotionally deprived, but then the question arises whether her excessive need of affection could ever have been satisfied. Physically the girl has entered puberty. Her bodily configuration is dysplastic. She has erythrocyanosis crurum. Neurological examination does not reveal any abnormalities.

It is obvious that we are confronted with a multitude of life problems.

The girl is aware of her plumpness and accentuates it by her untidiness in clothing and coarseness in her choice of words. Her unharmonious development impedes her adjustment to other children. Her increased need of attaching herself to adults clashes with her incapacity to make contact. This is related to the unsuccessful resolution of oedipal fixations, to the unsolved oedipal conflict. Uncertainty concerning the readiness of adults to protect her goes with the inner urge for protection. From this conflict spring the provocations of mother images.

Despite this the question arises of how much is the patient herself living through her problems, however obvious they are to us. For that which characterises her nature is the *form*, by which her problems find expression. Strictly speaking, the content of the girl's inner life is hypothetical, because it originates from the observer's attempts at entering into the life history of the girl. But the girl herself is elusive, she lacks the ability—directly or indirectly, during the interview or the testing—to communicate her former or existing conflicts, and that is precisely the disturbance of the patient. In other words, the patient strikes us not by her attitude to life, but by the antithesis of her womanlike body and her primitive childlike mind.

One of the characteristic features of the patient suffering from *mania phantastica infantilis* is *immaturity* and unripeness of personality. Superficiality, playfulness, credulity, naïveté, lack of seriousness and lack of profundity are salient traits in the framework of the maturation disorder, which is characteristic of the patient described above. In the middle of an earnest talk she may, without any reason, burst into loud laughter. This has so much the appearance of an acted part, that it looks as if the girl is making fun of the adults in her environment.

Another feature bears the stamp of a disturbance of *temperament*, namely a shift to the maniacal pole. Maniacal traits predominate in the manifestation of the syndrome to such an extent (increased rate of speed of all mental functions and internal experiences, episodical course) that the condition seems akin to maniacal psychoses of adults. Excitement, noisy behaviour, restlessness, lack of attention and concentration, flight of ideas—these are the symptoms, the concomitance of which is due to the underlying temperamental disorder.

A fragment of a letter written by the above-mentioned patient to her aunt reads as follows:

'Dear aunt, I am sitting upon my bed writing a letter. Mr P. who lives at A. has dropped in today for a while. Thanks for the school-bag. When you were here, I lay in bed. Has your menstruation started already? Today I received the parcel. . . .'

A behavioural trait which occupies a central place is the inclination to confabulate. One of Rümke's patients, for instance, fabricated stories about Indonesia, where he purportedly was born, inventing about his having joined in a tiger hunt and the way his father shot at a tiger. The confabulations of my patient related to pretended sexual adventures.

Her bodily development—the start of puberty—fostered the contents of her confabulations: she was preoccupied with sexual fantasies. There is no doubt that in her confabulations she found a compensation for her feelings of inferiority. Though the contents of the confabulations may be understood in this way, it is obvious that the confabulatory behaviour as such finds no explanation in the life history of the girl. The inclination to fancy and fantasy is, according to Rümke, proper to children; I would prefer to say, proper to the stage of beginning puberty.

The same may be said with respect to the impressive symptom of running away. Fugue and confabulation are related phenomena, as we are reminded by the 'fables en marche' described by Dupré.[11, 12] It may be seen that running away is fostered by and associated with imaginative faculties and tendency to fancy, a special category of the 'fugueurs' are the 'mythomanes infantiles migrateurs'. Obviously the 'contents' of the fugue, the fantasy interwoven with it, is to be found in the personal history of the patients. In the case we reported here the cause of the girl's running away is her basic insecurity, the lack of reliable mother figure. The form of the symptom, the running away as such, is due to the pathoplastic influence of the developmental stage.

Immaturity, maniacal exaltation states, tendency to confabulations and fantasies, increased self-esteem, better expressed overcompensation of inferiority feelings—all these phenomena add up to the syndrome of *mania phantastica infantilis*: *mania* because of the basic disorder, *infantilis* because of the stage in which the syndrome occurs or the retardation of maturation, *phantastica* on account of the conspicuous behaviour, the confabulations and the running away.

Whereas Rümke[43, 44] preferred to consider the syndrome as an entity, which ought to be differentiated from manic-depressive psychoses—the manic traits should be explained in the light of a general predisposition of adults and children to respond to a noxious agent in a manic or depressive way—I am inclined to regard *mania phantastica infantilis* as the juvenile form of manic psychosis, or as a mania in immature human beings, i.e. pubescents and immature personalities.

From a five-years follow-up of my patient it emerged that manic episodes had so far not recurred, but the patient is unable to assert her independence. She has changed her simple jobs several times. She is still without friends and even within the family she is an outsider. Though it is evident that she has not much gained in maturity, she is more preoccupied by her parents' indifference ('You surely don't love me!'). It appears that her infantilism is her greatest handicap, whereas the predisposition to mania up to now has not realised itself, maybe because she lives in the sheltered atmosphere of her home. The tendency to indulge herself in confabulated adventures with boys is still noticeable.

It would seem that pathoplastic influences of some developmental stage may be established only when a comparison can be made between analogous pathogenicity in different stages. However, our psychiatric knowledge, particularly of adolescents, has not yet reached the point when such analogies can be determined. For this reason, I have preferred to present an example of a syndrome which not only by part of its contents (sexual fantasies), but also by part of its form (confabulation, running away) gives evidence of maturational, i.e. puberal, influences.

It becomes evident from the follow-up that the phenomena caused by the patient's retardation of maturation are still present. The psychogenic influences are still active; the conflicts have not yet been solved. Only the features which depended directly on the manic phase have disappeared, and it is precisely these which led to hospitalisation. The pathoplastic factor of adolescence is still operative, the maturation has made little progress, as it is shown by the tendency to confabulate.

2

Adolescent Schizophrenias

Symptomatology

A discussion of the characteristic of adolescent schizophrenic processes may be preceded by the following case history.

> A fifteen-year-old boy of middle class environment is admitted to our in-patient department because of tendency to withdrawal, inactivity and stereotyped movements (scratching). His passivity is held responsible for his poor school achievements, his intelligence being superior. In the department the boy adapts himself neither to the members of his group nor to the nurses, towards whom he behaves disrespectfully. His total behaviour bears the mark of insolence. After running away a few times, he finally leaves the department before any treatment could be established.
>
> On account of his ungainly behaviour, his clumsy movements, his way of speech (between his teeth) and his lack of naturalness, the differential diagnosis of hebephrenia was considered. It is worth noticing that the patient did not give any evidence of loss of contact with reality, nor of incoherence of thoughts. His behaviour of perpetual opposition was to a certain extent even suitable to his age. A psychiatrist, who had treated him with psychotherapy for the two years previous to his admission, had diagnosed a neurosis in a schizoid personality.
>
> The parents, who with the patient and his elder sister led an apparently harmonious family life, *had observed a change of behaviour from the age of five*, when from an amiable and cheerful child he had become more and more solitary. When the boy was three years old, the father had been imprisoned for three weeks by the occupation forces. The father confesses that he neglected his son. The mother, however, has protected him. Between mother and son there has always been a profound attachment, which has probably interfered with the patient's development of independence.
>
> Certainly the revival of oedipal conflicts and the resulting feelings of

ambivalence and defence mechanisms in the context of adolescent development, have largely contributed to the disturbed behaviour.

On the heredity side, in the father's family can be seen traits of self-centred attitude towards society and life in general. One of the father's brothers started a retired and asocial life at exactly the same age as his nephew is now. He had the good fortune to find employment in a small drug store. This uncle is said to be a sociable person nowadays.

At the age of twenty-three the patient had to be admitted into a mental hospital. The diagnosis of hebephrenia could not be doubted any more.

The case quoted is interesting, as it shows that a beginning schizophrenic process was first suspected in the child psychiatric department. The parents themselves, however, had observed a gradual change in the behaviour of their son from his fifth year on. The manifestation of pathology—the development of the process—has taken many years; moreover, adolescence has scarcely functioned as a decisive and provoking factor, it has only added a special flavour to the clinical picture.

The process may require such a long period of time before it comes to full manifestation, that even seventeen years may not be enough. It appears that the beginning of the pathologic process goes back to pre-school years. The conclusion is that the source of schizophrenic disease during adolescence may be found elsewhere. This causes confusion, as hitherto it has been usual to regard as adolescent schizophrenias those schizophrenic psychoses which become manifest during adolescence. In reality adolescent schizophrenias belong to two groups, one with onset during adolescence, the other with a source in a far earlier period.

Here should be mentioned the work of the Russian psychiatrist Ushakov.[62, 63, 64, 65] This investigator has repeatedly insisted on the necessity of paying attention to the *developmental* aspects of schizophrenic processes. Distinction must be made between the beginning of the illness and the appearance of unmistakable symptoms, or—as Ushakov puts it—between the 'state' (which is the process in its prime), and the initial stage. The latter must not be confused with the premorbid condition, which is the condition of the organism in the period *prior* to the appearance of initial symptoms. Ushakov has also pointed out that the acute or subacute forms of adolescent schizophrenia may reach back to the eleventh year of age, whereas the beginning of the forms which are characterised by insidious onset and slow progress is to be sought in children of pre-school age or during the first years of elementary school.

The initial changes to be observed have been discussed at length by Ushakov, hence a brief summary only will be given here. The first manifestation of the initial period is *autism*, not to be confused with early infantile autism, as the patients in their premorbid phase until the beginning of the initial period were vivacious, active, affectionate and sociable. The change in the relationship of the child with his environment usually follows psychogenic influences, hence the high frequency (84 per cent) of such factors in the material of Ushakov.

A second characteristic of the initial stage is the decrease of potential energy (Conrad[8, 9]). The child, previously active, full of interest and initiative, loses his spirit and increasingly slows down. The patients themselves are aware of these changes, as proved by expressions like 'my head is not fresh', 'it is difficult to think', 'I read and I feel as if I did not read', etc. This may even result in 'school phobia'; hence a need to bear in mind the possibility of *psychotic* school refusal.

The third disorder which is characteristic of the initial stage is complete dissociation of the patient's personality reactions. Adequate and harmonious reactions give way to discordant responses. Achievements, interests and judgments are so arbitrary that the personality presents an agglomeration of contradictions. To this are added disturbances of motor behaviour: mannerisms, grimaces, loss of grace and of suppleness.

The symptoms which complete the clinical picture may, for the greater part, be considered as secondary phenomena, or pathoplastic supplements, due to adolescent developmental influences. This is made clear by the list given by Ushakov: obsessions, instability of mood, ambivalent attitudes, coenesthetic sensations. All additional phenomena should be analysed, as they may be distributed into different categories. They may be signs of deterioration, due to the diffusion of the process; they may be reactions of a vulnerable organism to psychological trauma (psychoplastic factors); they may give expression to defence mechanisms originating from healthy personality components; they may be directly related to 'phase' conditions, dependent on the maturation level (pathoplastic factors).

Ushakov rightly states that only comparative studies in children of different ages may contribute to our understanding of the nature of the schizophrenias. (The present author does not agree with Ushakov's assertion that schizophrenia is a pathological entity.) Such a study has been made by Gruñia Ssucharewa,[52, 53] who by applying the criteria *onset* (acute or slow) and *course* (continuous or by crises (Schub)) came to distinguish three groups, adopted by Ushakov. These groups are:

(1) Forms with insidious onset and slow progress (52·4 per cent of Ushakov's material, characterised by a heavy hereditary load (73·7 per cent)).

(2) Forms with an acute onset and a course by jumps, showing exacerbations and remissions.

(3) Intermediate forms, in which after a rather long phase of continuity the course becomes 'jumpy', deterioration, however, being the outcome.

For each type of course the importance of age was taken into consideration. For the purpose, the symptoms were divided into negative (elimination of functions) and positive (productive) phenomena. The data which have a bearing on adolescence will be briefly discussed. In children suffering from (1) above, the negative symptoms predominate but they are less obvious in adolescent patients. Of greater importance, however, is the qualitative difference between pre-adolescents and adolescents. The schizophrenic adolescent is characterised by apathy, asthenia, decrease of energy, but he may also manifest acting-out impulsive and aggressive behaviour (inadequately termed 'psychopathic-like'), sexual attacks, vagrancy (already described by Wilmanns[66]) and aggressive acts. The patient is particularly hostile to those he has very much loved in the past. In this context, Ssucharewa mentions the 'delusion of the strange parents'. Again experience suggests that these forms may have their beginning in the pre-school period.

As a characteristic cluster of positive (in the sense of productive) symptoms Ssucharewa considers the following: (1) fears and obsessions, (2) morbid indulgence in fancies, (3) depersonalisation. The characteristics of development phase manifest themselves in the degree of elaboration. In adolescents the diversity of fears is remarkable; moreover, they are complex in character. They include fear of contagion and of death, preoccupations with one's own health, dysmorphophobia, and fear of insanity. Fantasies have a guilt content. Fears and fancies gradually become delusive ideas (of reference, of being influenced, of persecution), which means that the influence of self-criticism decreases. Eggers[13,14] observed more or less elaborate outlines of a beginning of ideational systematisation in intelligent pre-adolescent children (from twelve to fourteen years of age). In later years the autonomy of the delusion increases. Depersonalisation phenomena culminate in adolescence, leading to the assumption that they might be connected with the identity problems of the normal adolescent. Whereas depersonalisation in young children has a playful character, in adolescents, whose obsessional ideas often are accompanied by uncontrollable anxiety, it is lived through.

Hallucinations in children are rare, but in adolescents they occur in great variety, although not so pronounced as in adult patients. Katatonic symptoms may be observed in young children in the form of bizarre movements, general restlessness, purposeless circling and also as speech and language disorders (mutism, echolalia, verbigeration). With advancing years the katatonic movements become more complicated and diverse, reaching their full development in adolescence.

It has been established that the positive (productive) symptoms occur in greater variety than the negative ones and that they are also more liable to changes according to age. The older the patient at the time of the beginning of the process, the more complicated and various they are. This is the cardinal difference between childhood and adolescent schizophrenia: the symptomatology of childhood schizophrenia is poor in comparison with the polymorph clinical picture found in adolescents.

On the other hand, the schizophrenic manifestations in adolescents clearly differ from those in adult patients. According to Ushakov,[62, 63, 64, 65] the main characteristic of incipient adolescent schizophrenia is the episodic, transitory, fragmentary nature of the symptoms. May we not say the same with reference to the adolescent himself? His own inner life is made up of particles, still awaiting restructuring, his reactions are contradictory, his feelings ambivalent. Is it not as if the disintegrating process finds unconsolidated soil, in which it may flourish?

By the time the 'state' has become established, the symptomatology resembles that of adult schizophrenia; but there are still some differences. The symptoms, though the same as in adults (paranoid, delusional) are more transitory and rudimentary, less pronounced and less continuous. The formation of clusters makes little progress. Modifications may be seen because of pathoplastic influences, manifesting themselves in learning difficulties, delinquent behaviour and so on.

In his monograph on the subject Spiel[50] has studied 23 acute cases (7 males, 16 females) in the age range of ten to fourteen, and 29 slowly progressive cases (19 males, 10 females) from eleven to fourteen years of age. His findings are not completely in agreement with those of Ssucharewa and Ushakov, although there is no doubt that he started from the same concept of schizophrenia. Even in the cases with slow progress, the impact of heredity was negligible. In one-third of each group noxious environmental factors were demonstrated. The most striking difference is in the interval between the time of onset and that of manifestation: in 3 cases only, the slowly developing processes began when the patient was four to seven years old; in the majority of cases, the difference between onset and manifestation was one year or less. My own findings support those of the Russian authors. As Ushakov rightly observes, the child psychiatrist usually has his first contact with patients, whose process has already reached the 'established state'; hence he is dependent on the parents' discernment in determining the initial phase.

Spiel's findings on symptomatology correspond for the most part with those of the Russian workers. One of the most interesting aspects of symptomatology is the occurrence of thought disturbances in the older group instead of the speech disorders characteristic of the younger group, e.g. incoherence of thoughts, bizarre ideas, confusion and derailment of thoughts, delusional state of mind. Also in agreement with the Russian findings is the observation that motor behaviour is seriously disturbed (grimaces, bizarre attitudes, 'hypererethism'). Electroencephalography does not throw light on the basic disturbance; only in 4 cases was the EEG abnormal.

Spiel has made an effort to find an explanation for the fact that the acute forms show a preponderance of girls over boys. He concludes that, as he found in manic-depressive psychoses, hormonal influences play a role. This may be true, but it does not explain the fact that in the slowly progressive forms a reverse proportion is found. The difference in sex distribution furnishes incontestable proof that the two forms of schizophrenic processes are fundamentally different, giving support to the belief that there is not merely *one* schizophrenia, but at least two.

An example of the group of schizophrenias could be that described by Spiel separately, because of its particular characteristics. The prevailing symptom is obsession (arithmomania, compulsion to pray, to wash hands incessantly); and also the absurdity of its characteristic contents. For instance, one of Spiel's patients became panic-stricken any time she heard the sound 'S'. Apart from the obsessional ideas there were no thought disturbances. The differences from the other forms of schizophrenia were: (1) evidence of heredity of schizophrenia and schizoid traits, (2) evidence of obsessional traits in the family environment (obsessional environment), (3) probability of disturbed cerebral function (in half of the cases abnormal EEG), (4) evidence of year-long behaviour anomalies (loss of contact, eccentric behaviour). In all cases a complete deterioration of personality was the end of the process.

Differential Diagnosis

The problems of differential diagnosis have been summed up by Ushakov[64] by their slow progress; the insidious forms may also suggest the existence of a neurotic development, or a psychopathic condition. Ushakov uses the terms *pseudoneurotic* and *pseudopsychopathic schizophrenia*. Abortive forms of paranoid schizophrenia may be mistaken for paranoid syndromes rooted in a paranoid personality. Catatonic attacks may be confused with acute exogenous psychoses. The differentiation between schizophrenia and episodic psychoses in mentally defectives or encephalopaths may present problems. Recently, Eggers and Stutte[15] have pointed out the difficulties of diagnosis and classification.

Prognosis

Many investigators have found that the insidious forms, which may be traced back to the pre-school or early school years, have the poorest prognosis. Relatively the best prognosis is for acute cases with a 'simplex' course, which have their beginning in the period of adolescence (Lutz,[36] Spiel[50]). This is easily understood. The younger the child in the initial phase of the process, the more vulnerable is his organism in general and his cerebrum in particular. The process, operating at any early age, may paralyse further mental development. In adolescence the situation is different. Growth energies and defence mechanisms may constitute adequate counter-influences; furthermore mental development has reached a certain level. The outcome is the result of an interaction. Grunia Ssucharewa[53] points out that the prognosis must take into account the interaction of two tendencies, on the one side the destructive forces dependent on the intensity of the noxae, on the other side the progressive powers, which depend on the inherent developmental strives.

The prognosis of the schizophrenias is usually very poor. According to Stutte[58] more than half of all the patients need institutionalisation. Spiel[50] is of the same opinion. He divides the half, which remains in or returns to society, into three equal parts. One-third never gets beyond the level of a defective personality, with permanent defects in the intellectual and emotional sphere. The second third belongs to the group of odd, eccentric, 'pseudopsychopathic' characters. The rest, only one-sixth of all the patients, recovers.

Therapy

The shortest chapter on schizophrenia is that on therapy. The data on prognosis have included results of all methods of treatment, which show that therapeutic efforts have hitherto been unsuccessful. Spiel[50] gives a survey of the treatment methods employed in the University Psychiatric Hospital of Vienna. His conclusions may be summarised as follows. Electroshock and insulin shock had dubious results. Insulin shocks, though producing a remission in the beginning, do not arrest the process in its fatal progress. The efficacy of drugs has not yet been thoroughly tested, which, in some hospitals, leads to the prescription of complex compounds. Psychotherapy, in whatever form, is of great importance, in so far as it aims at enabling the patient to live with his defects and to exploit the healthy part of his personality. However, it is an open question whether psychotherapy (analysis) will ever be able to cure the basic disorder.

Another question is whether better therapeutic results would be obtained if the disease was treated in its initial phase. Here we are confronted with iatrogenic damage. The initial stage is so often ignored mostly because of the physician's unwillingness to make a diagnosis of schizophrenia in a young child—a diagnosis which even today is a sentence of psychical death. Yet from the point of view of effective (secondary) prevention, early diagnosis is a matter of paramount importance.

3

Manic-depressive Psychosis

The occurrence of manic-depressive psychoses before adolescence is in general contested; according to Shirley,[49] usually they are not diagnosed until early adulthood. A thorough analysis of the anamneses of manic-depressive patients, who were diagnosed as such during or after adolescence, shows clearly that typical fluctuations of mood may begin at an early age (Stutte [60, 61]). Nevertheless, the frequency of manic-depressive psychoses in children is remarkably lower than that of schizophrenia, low as the latter is.

The reasons why manic-depressive psychoses in childhood so often escape the clinician's notice have been enumerated by Stutte. As they primarily affect the vital strata of the infantile personality (drives, instincts, mood and vegetative processes), the manic-depressive psychoses do not cause radical and lasting personality alterations, which might give cause for concern. They are often mistaken for mischievous behaviour or crises of maturation. Their periodicity may be overlooked because of the relatively short duration of the phases (from days to hours even), which readily alternate.

Several authors underline the difficulties inherent in the diagnosis. Adriana de Leeuw-Aalbers[34] warns against mistaking the first stage of a schizophrenic process for a mania; Lutz[36] maintains the same with regard to a depressive state of mind; Von Stockert[57] states the contrary, pointing out the error of considering the first maniacal phase as a hebephrenia.

It can be concluded that differential diagnosis between manic-depressive and schizophrenic psychoses poses many problems.

Genuine adolescent mania is characterised by the primary symptoms: manic disposition, flight of ideas and motor restlessness. If to this rather simple picture there are added symptoms such as confusion of thoughts or paranoid ideas, the suspicion of a schizophrenic process is justified. The symptomatology of the depressive phase is, by the description of Spiel,[50] lack of initiative, languor, weariness, proneness to cry, sometimes tendency to withdrawal and introversion, and particularly school failure, which makes the family and the school think that the child is lazy. Consequently the depression may be intensified through the interference of an environmental factor. In nearly all cases Spiel found anxiety, stupor and abstention from food.

The contents of thought is determined by phase-specific interests, conflicts and instinctual needs (masturbation conflicts). Stutte[59, 60, 61] draws attention to the fact that the depressive contents closely resemble those of adult depressive patients. 'One is again and again surprised, when an infantile depression presents reproaches, delusional self-accusations, ideas of sinfulness and nihilistic scruples similar to those of a female patient with climacterial depression' (Stutte[61]).

Stutte could demonstrate in the majority of his cases (5 girls and 8 boys under the age of ten), homologous heredity (circular psychoses, suicide, cycloid temperament). In the cases of Spiel[50] the hereditary load was indistinct in the age group between ten and fourteen years, as compared with the younger age group. This author found in 3 cases (out of 12) also a link with menstruation. In one of Mrs de Leeuw-Aalbers[34] cases, a connection with the menarche could be established. One is inclined to associate the beginning of the psychosis with physical, i.e. endocrine alterations. This would also explain the preponderance of girls in Spiel's material.[50]

Bilikiewicz[5] holds the view that a pathogenetic factor must be sought in the metabolism of catecholamines. Reserpine, ethionamide and other compounds can provoke an endogenous depression. A psychic trauma may bring about biochemical changes. Here mention must be made of the effect of lithiumcarbonate in maniacal patients.[33] This will be demonstrated by a case history.

A fourteen-years-old boy was admitted into our in-patient department. A few months previously he had suddenly changed. He manifested various fears: of being alone, of thieves. He had become depressed, he cried much and lacked appetite. After some weeks there was a sudden change: he took money away, became aggressive, ate like a wolf and smoked incessantly. Such phases, lasting some weeks, continued to alternate, each excitation state lasting longer than a depressive state.

The patient is the fourth of five children. His father was a well-to-do farmer, who died four years before the patient was admitted. His mother (assisted by her family) took over the management of the farm. She was uncertain and too indulgent toward her son.

Heredity: nothing significant. Pregnancy and birth without complications. Normal motor development, only retarded speech. Until his sixth year, enuresis. His school performance was poor; he did not like school. The sudden death of his father was a great trauma for him. He did not accept the new management of the farm. After passing through elementary school, he went to an agricultural school, which turned out to be too difficult for him. He refused to attend, wanted to take over the management of the farm. Because his relatives feared him, he often succeeded in having his own way.

At the time of admittance he showed an uncontrolled behaviour, which could be sedated successfully only by injections of morphine-scopolamine. He was overactive, hypererethic, dangerous to others. Some weeks after admission, the picture changed: in the course of a few days he changed from an uncompromising savage into a pitiful bungler.

This condition lasted for a week, then he awoke to fresh activity, his restlessness returned. He responded when addressed, but he could not control his violent behaviour, though he felt sorry about it. In the evening he became frightened, on one occasion he thought that his bed was electrically charged and that holes were drilled in the wall in order to watch him.

This case is characterised by the predominance of pronounced alternations of mood of short duration and by a periodical course. It may be seen that the manic phases lasted longer and were more intense than the depressive states. The patient was dull. His concept of reality was seriously disturbed. Clinical examination, the cerebrospinal fluid analysis, and EEG produced negative neurological findings. Some responses in the Rorschach Test were suggestive of a schizophrenia.

It was interesting to note the immediate favourable effect of lithium carbonate (four times a day 300 mg combined with natrium bicarbonate in equal doses). Its efficacy is so striking that it suggests that manic states could be caused by lithium deficiency. Another view is that lithium interferes with kalium metabolism. The experience is that lithium salts have a specific effect in manic conditions.

Moreover this case shows the difficulty of different diagnosis, already referred to. As long as the patient took lithium carbonate his condition remained satisfactory. Two years later, however, owing to pressure of work, the boy failed to take his medicine for a few weeks and the manic symptoms recurred. Recovery started on the day the medicine was taken again. Nevertheless the ultimate results were disappointing. Four and a half years after his first manic manifestation the patient had to be hospitalised. He was diagnosed as of borderline intelligence with an evolutive schizophrenic process in the foreground in spite of the sudden changes of mood of a cyclic character.

Opinions differ as to the question whether there is a strict dividing line between manic-depressive psychoses and constitutional tendency to mood changes (Kurt Schneider[47]) or whether there are rather smooth transitions between both conditions (Stutte,[60, 61] Spiel[50]).

Atypical manic-depressive psychoses have been described by Nagy, Kleininger and Lipák[38] of the Debrecen Psychiatric Hospital. The pneumoencephalogram showed subcortical cerebral atrophy. EEG-alterations were suggestive of a diencephalic disorder. Brain damage together with adolescence was considered as a pathoplastic influence. These cases recall those described by Elfriede Albert;[1] two patients shortly before the onset of puberty developed psychotic pictures resembling manic-depressive psychoses, but the abrupt change of the phases together with the absence of hereditary taint and the presence of somatic complaints pointed to organic genesis. Both children were suffering from damage of the brain, i.e. a diencephalic process in the first period of life. According to Elfriede Albert the significance of adolescence might rest on the fact that a certain maturation of distinct parts of the brain stem is needed in order to allow the manifestation of psychotic pictures. She arrives at the hypothesis that the so-called endogenous manic-depressive psychoses also have their origin in disturbed function of the brain stem.

There are many other kinds of 'atypical' manic-depressive psychoses, in all of which the phasic course is the essential feature. Various forms are to be distinguished: impulsive states and signs of distressing aggressiveness (Bürger-Prinz[7]), silly behaviour suggestive of hebephrenia, obsessional (Von Stockert[57]), oneiroid, delirious and amentia-like states. Care should be taken to avoid expanding the concept of manic-depressive psychoses by continually adding clinical pictures, just because of their manifesting a cycloid course. Anyway, there are clinicians who distinguish manic-depressive psychoses from cycloid psychoses (Janse de Jonge[22]) and these again from episodic psychoses.

Obviously there is a connection between manic-depressive psychoses and suicide. It appears, however, that the majority of suicidal attempts do not fit in with the category of endogenous psychoses. Hence the publications on suicide in adolescents rarely refer to psychiatric categories (Duché,[10] Otto[40]). Mention must be made of the favourable result of electroshock therapy in adolescent depressions, which makes it a useful clinical tool.

4

Juvenile Paresis

Whereas in earlier textbooks much space has been devoted to the chapter of juvenile paresis, the topic is almost neglected in recent works. A clear picture of the situation is obtained by comparing Lutz's chapter in the well-known manual of Benjamin (1938[3]) and the omission of any mention by the same author in his own later textbook (1961, 1964, 1968[36]). The reason is obvious: the majority of investigators underline the extreme rareness of the disease, owing to the efficacy of preventive measures (treatment of the syphilitic pregnant woman) and the penicillin therapy of the child (Beucher,[4] Shirley[49]).

The designation of juvenile paresis would suggest a relation between adolescence and the disease. Still in 1917 Ziehen[68] described the age at onset to coincide most often with puberty. But the classical investigation of Schmidt-Kraepelin[46] had already shown the highest frequency of onset lies in school age (eight to ten years for boys, ten to twelve years for girls). This, as well as the fact that there are even cases of earlier manifestation —a four-year-old girl in the material of Schmidt-Kraepelin and two six-year-old patients (Marr,[37] Zappert[67])—proves that the interval between the parental luetic infection and the manifestation in the child—in average twenty years—is the real point.

Consequently, juvenile paresis is not an adolescent psychosis in a narrow sense; it may be a psychosis *during* adolescence. If the age at onset falls in the adolescent period, adolescence functions as a pathoplastic factor: delusions (of grandeur) tinged with simplicity ('niaiserie'), and also hallucinations of a daydream character, predominate (Babonneix,[2] Schachter[45]). If the age at onset is earlier, however, mental deterioration is the outstanding clinical feature, overshadowing pathoplastic characteristics.

The present-day decrease in the frequency of juvenile paresis implies the risk of disregarding the diagnosis—Kolle[25] illustrated this by a striking example—which may also happen in the case of a 'Pfropfparalyse' (juvenile paresis on the basis of mental deficiency) or when the initial picture is marked by a gradual decline in school performance.

5

Exogenous Psychoses

It is almost needless to mention that exogenous (traumatic, infectious, metabolic, toxic, neoplastic) cerebral affections may occur at any period of human development; so the influence of adolescence is merely pathoplastic. It may sometimes be difficult to discriminate between the 'exogenous reaction type' and a schizophrenic process, but the occurrence of disturbances of consciousness may be helpful. Nevertheless one must reckon

o

with the possibility of the exogenous affection acting as a provocative factor in the genesis of schizophrenia.

Perhaps the only typical symptomatic psychosis is that which is caused by atropine intoxication. In connection with psychoses during adolescence it is worth mentioning, as it may come about after wilful misuse (an example is given by Spiel[50]). The same is to be said with regard to LSD psychoses, the incidence of which is probably highest among modern youth (Ludwig and Levine,[35] Robbins et al.,[41] Rosenthal[42]).

6

Conclusion

Adolescence is a period of life, which by its disintegrative character may seem a psychosis in itself. This makes it difficult to discern in this stage a pathological process from normal development. If, however, a psychosis comes to manifestation, it appears that the initial symptoms often are to be found in the years of childhood. It is, therefore, necessary to discriminate psychoses which occur *during* adolescence and *adolescent psychosis*. Manic-depressive psychoses generally do not manifest before puberty. From this one may conclude that the breakthrough of the psychosis needs a soil of disintegration. This would hold particularly true in the case of diencephalic manic psychoses. Considering the problem in this light, adolescence implies a *provocative* factor.

The *contents* of the psychosis is also determined by the features of adolescence. Psychoses in children are characterised by simplicity, with growing age the contents become richer, more varied, more complicated even. The content of psychoses during adolescence is nearer to that of adults' psychoses than to the substance of children's psychoses. Here, then, the influence of adolescence is *pathoplastic*.

The author considered five different adolescental influences:

1. A pathological predisposition or damage passes a period of latency before manifesting itself (*time factor*).

2. Pathology is dependent on the disproportion between the demands of society and the individual's capacities (*age factor*).

3. Adolescence is a period of increased vulnerability (*provocative factor*).

4. Adolescence, as a delimitated psychological (psychopathological) period, produces an impact on disorders appearing in this period, whatever their origin may be (*pathoplastic factor*).

5. Adolescence *per se* is at the root of the disturbance (*pathogenetic factor*). This group, if it exists at all, is smaller than has formerly been supposed.

REFERENCES

1. ALBERT, E. 1952–3. Organisch bedingte affektive und psychomotorische Psychosen bei Kindern. *A Criança Portuguesa*, **12**, 67–112.
2. BABONNEIX, L. 1906. Les idées de grandeur dans la paralysie générale du jeune âge. *Rev. mens. Mal. Enf.*, **24**, 97–112.
3. BENJAMIN, E. 1938. *Lehrbuch der Psychopathologie des Kindesalters für Ärzte und Erzieher*. Erlenbach-Zürich, Rotapfel Verlag.
4. BEUCHER, M. 1965. Troubles de l'intelligence. In *Psychiatrie infantile*, by L. Michaux (3rd edition). Paris: Pr. Univ. de France.
5. BILIKIEWICZ, T. 1968. Psychopathologie des Pubertätsalters. In Göllnitz. G. and Rösler, H. D. II. *Symposium der Arbeitsgruppe von Kinder- und Jugendpsychiatern sozialistischer Länder*, Rostock.
6. BÜHLER, C. 1929. *Das Seelenleben des Jugendlichen* (5th edition). Jena: G. Fischer.
7. BÜRGER-PRINZ, H. 1935. Der Beginn der Erbpsychosen. *Nervenarzt*, **8**, 617–624.
8. CONRAD, K. 1958. *Die beginnende Schizophrenie*. Stuttgart: G. Thieme.
9. CONRAD, K. 1959. Das Problem der 'nosologischen Einheit' in der Psychiatrie. *Nervenarzt*, **30**, 488–494.
10. DUCHÉ, D. J. 1968. Les tentatives de suicide chez l'enfant et l'adolescent. *Acta paedopsychiat.*, **35**, 345–373.
11. DUPRÉ, E. 1909. Mythomanie infantile. Un cas de fugue suivie de fabulation avec déclaration mensongère. *Encéphale*, **4**, 117–126.
12. DUPRÉ, E. 1925. *Pathologie de l'imagination et de l'émotivité*. Paris: Payot.
13. EGGERS, CHR. 1967. *Prognose und Verlauf kindlicher und präpuberaler Schizophrenien*. Marburg: Diss.
14. EGGERS, CHR. 1967. Wahninhalte kindlicher und präpuberaler Schizophrenien. *Acta paedopsychiat.*, **34**, 326–340.
15. EGGERS, CHR. and STUTTE, H. 1969. Zur nosologischen Umgrenzung der kindlichen und präpuberalen Schizophrenie aus katamnestischer Sicht. *Fortschr. Neurol. Psychiat.*, **37**, 305–318.
16. FLEMING, C. M. 1949. *Adolescence, its social psychology: with an introduction to recent findings from the fields of anthropology, physiology, medicine, psychometrics and sociometry*. New York: International Universities Press.
17. HALL, G. S. 1904. *Adolescence, its psychology and its relation to physiology, anthropology, sociology, sex, crime, religion and education.* (Vols I and II.) New York: D. Appleton and Co.
18. HECKER, E. 1871. Die Hebephrenie. *Virchows Arch. Path. Anat.*, **52**, 394–429.
19. HOLLINGWORTH, L. S. 1928. *The psychology of the adolescent*. New York: D. Appleton and Co.
20. HUTTER, A. 1934. Endogene en functionele Psychoses bij Kinderen in de Puberteitsjaren. *Ned. T. Geneesk.*, **78/II**, 2565–2577.
21. HUTTER, A. 1938. Endogene und funktionelle Psychosen bei Kindern in den Pubertätsjahren. *Z. Kinderpsychiat.*, **5**, 97–102.
22. JANSE DE JONGE, A. L. 1964. Cycloide psychose in de jeugd. *Ned. T. Geneesk.*, **108/II**, 2206–2211.
23. KLEIST, K. 1921. Autochtone Degenerationspsychosen. *Z. Neurol. Psychiat.*, **69**, 1–11.
24. KLEIST, K. 1926. Über Zykloide Degenerationspsychosen besonders Verwirrtheits und Motilitätspsychosen. *Arch. Psych.*, **78**, 416–420.
25. KOLLE, K. 1967. *Psychiatrie* (6th edition). Stuttgart: Georg Thieme.

26. KRAEPELIN, E. 1913. *Psychiatrie, ein Lehrbuch für Studierende und Ärzte* (Vol. 3, part 2 (8th edition)). Leipzig: J. Ambrosius Barth.

27. KREVELEN, D. ARN. VAN. 1955. Der Einfluss der Präpubertät auf die Entwicklung des Kindes. *Mschr. f. Kinderheilk*, **103**, 48–53.

28. KREVELEN, D. ARN. VAN. 1961. Mania phantastica infantilis. *Ned. T. Geneesk.*, **105**, 1177–1181.

29. KREVELEN, D. ARN. VAN. 1962. La manie fantastique des enfants. *Rev. Neuropsychiat. infant.*, **10**, 133–138.

30. KREVELEN, D. ARN. VAN. 1966. La clinique des troubles pubertaires et des troubles pendant la puberté. *Acta paedopsychiat.*, **33**, 175–182.

31. KREVELEN, D. ARN. VAN. 1967. Prognosis of childhood neuroses and psychoses, *Acta paedopsychiat.*, **34**, 104–111.

32. KREVELEN, D. ARN. VAN. 1968. Prognosis of childhood neuroses and psychoses; *Proceedings Fourth World Congress of Psychiatry* Part 1: Plenary Sessions/Symposia (Ed. J. J. Lopez Ibor). *Excerpta Medica Found. Int. Congr. Ser. No. 150*, pp. 85–90.

33. KREVELEN, D. ARN. VAN. and VOORST, J. A. VAN. 1959. Lithium in der Behandlung einer Psychose unklarer Genese bei einem Jugendlichen. *Acta Paedopsychiat.*, **26**, 148–152.

34. LEEUW-AALBERS, A. J. DE. 1947. *Psychosen in de Puberteit*, '*Een Klinische Studie*' (Diss.). Oud Beijerland: W. Hoogwerf.

35. LUDWIG, A. M. and LEVINE, J. 1965. Patterns of hallucinogenic drug abuse, *JAMA*, **191**, 92–96.

36. LUTZ, J. 1961, 1964, 1968. *Kinderpsychiatrie* (1st, 2nd, 3rd editions). Zürich and Stuttgart: Rotapfel.

37. MARR, H. 1899. Notes, clinical and pathological, of a case of general paralysis of the insane occurring in early life. *Lancet*, 838–839.

38. NAGY, T. A., KLEININGER, O. and LIPÁK, J. 1967. Atypische manischdepressive Psychosen in der Pubertät. In *Symposion über psychiatrische Probleme in der Pubertät*. II. Symposion der Arbeitsgruppe von Kinder- und Jugendpsychiatern sozialistischer Länder. Rostock.

39. NŸSSEN, R. 1942. *Leerboek der Kinderpsychiatrie en der heilopvoedkundige behandeling*. Leiden: H. E. Stenfert Kroese.

40. OTTO, U. 1964. Suicidal attempts in adolescence and childhood. States of mental illness and personality variables. *Acta Paedopsychiat.*, **31**, 397–411.

41. ROBBINS, E., FROSCH, W. A. and STERN, M. 1967. Further observations on untoward reactions to LSD. *Amer. J. Psychiat.*, **124**, 393–395.

42. ROSENTHAL, S. H. 1964. Persistent hallucinosis following repeated administration of hallucinogenic drugs. *Amer. J. Psychiat.*, **121**, 238–244.

43. RÜMKE, H. C. 1927. Over Psychosen bij kinderen, *Geneesk. Bladen* 25e *reeks*, 319–358.

44. RÜMKE, H. C. 1928. Über Psychosen bei Kindern in Zusammenhang mit einigen Problemen der klinischen Psychiatrie betrachtet. *Z. Neurol. Psychiat.*, **114**, 113–151.

45. SCHACHTER, M. 1959. Étude clinique psychiatrique d'un cas de paralysie générale juvenile chez une débile mentale. *G. Psichiat. Neuropat.*, **87**, II.

46. SCHMIDT-KRAEPELIN. T. 1920. *Über die juvenile Paralyse*. Berlin: Springer.

47. SCHNEIDER, K. 1943. *Die psychopathischen Persönlichkeiten*. Vienna: Deuticke.

48. SCHNEIDER, K. 1946. *Beiträge Zur Psychologie. Pathopsychologie der Gefühle und Triebe in Grundriss*. Stuttgart: Thieme.

49. SHIRLEY, H. F. 1963. *Pediatric psychiatry*. Cambridge, Mass.: Harvard University Press.

50. SPIEL, W. 1961. *Die endogenen Psychosen des Kindes- und Jugendalters*. Basel and New York: S. Karger.

51. SPRANGER, E. 1949. *Psychologie des Jugendalters* (19th edition). Leipzig: Quelle & Meyer.

52. SSUCHAREWA, G. E. 1932. Über den Verlauf der Schizophrenien im Kindesalter. *Z. ges. Neurol. Psychiat.*, **142**, 309–321.

53. SSUCHAREWA, G. E. 1967. Die Bedeutung der vergleichenden Berücksichtigung des Lebensalters für die Untersuchung der Verlaufsgesetzmäszigkeiten der Schizophrenie bei Kindern und Jugendlichen. *Acta Paedopsychiat.*, **34**, 307–320.

54. STERN, W. 1929. *Anfänge der Reifezeit. Ein Knabentagesbuch in psychologischer Bearbeitung* (2nd edition). Leipzig: Quelle & Meyer.

55. STOCKERT, F. G. VON. 1942. Die Psychopathologie der Erziehungsschwierigkeiten im Lichte der Reifungsphasen. *Z. Kinderforsch.*, **49**, 155–160.

56. STOCKERT, F. G. VON. 1956. Psychosen im Kindesalter. In *Jahrb. Jugendpsychiat.* (Ed. W. VILLINGER), **1**, 223–232. Bern and Stuttgart: H. Huber.

57. STOCKERT, F. G. VON. 1967. *Einführung in die Psychopathologie des Jugendalters* (4th edition). Munich, Berlin and Vienna: Urban & Schwarzenberg.

58. STUTTE, H. 1959. Die Prognose der Schizophrenien des Kindes- und Jugendalters. In *Kongressbericht II. Int. Kongr. Psychiat.*, **1**, 328–333. Zürich.

59. STUTTE, H. 1960. Kinder- und Jugendpsychiatrie. In *Psychiatrie der Gegenwart*, Vol. II. Klinische Psychiatrie. Berlin, Göttingen and Heidelberg: Springer.

60. STUTTE, H. 1963. Endogen-phasische Psychosen des Kindesalters. *Acta Paedopsychiat.*, **30**, 34–42.

61. STUTTE, H. 1963. Psychotische und psychoseverdächtige Zustände im Kindesalter. *Päd. Fortb.*, **9**, 29–46.

62. USHAKOV, G. K. 1965. Symptomatologie der Initialperiode der im Kindes-oder Jugendalter beginnenden Schizophrenie. *Psychiatrie (Leipzig)* **17**, 41–47.

63. USHAKOV, G. K. 1965. Contribution à l'étude des stéréotypes de développement de la psychose chez les enfants et les adolescents. *Psychiat. Enf.*, **8**, 1–56.

64. USHAKOV, G. K. 1966. Problems of diagnosing schizophrenia in adolescents. In *Psychiatric approaches to adolescence (l'Abord psychiatrique de l'adolescence)* (Eds G. Caplan and S. Lebovici). *Exc. Med. Found.*, pp. 75–80 (165–170).

65. USHAKOV, G. K. 1969. Trends in the investigation of clinical problems in child psychiatry. In *Modern Perspectives in International Child Psychiatry* (Ed. J. G. Howells). Edinburgh: Oliver & Boyd.

66. WILMANNS, K. 1906. *Zur Psychopathologie des Landstreichers*. Leipzig: J. Ambrosius Barth.

67. ZAPPERT, J. 1905. Mitt. Ges. inn. Med. Kinderheilk. *Wien. klin. Wschr.*, **18**, 649.

68. ZIEHEN, TH. 1917. *Die Geisteskrankheiten des Kindesalters*. Berlin: Reuther & Reichard.

XVII

FAMILY GROUP THERAPY

JOHN G. HOWELLS

Director, The Institute of Family Psychiatry
The Ipswich Hospital, Ipswich, England

Gentle bakers, make good bread!
(The Dyetary of Health. Andrew Boarde. c. 1490–1549)

1

Introduction

In the short history of family group therapy, families with adolescents have been the commonest subject for this new therapeutic technique. There are two main reasons for this: firstly, as the adolescent is a near adult, a group with adolescents, rather than with young children, is the easiest family group to handle in therapy; secondly, because the commonest target of family group therapy has been the adolescent schizophrenic. Thus it is appropriate to consider family group therapy in a work devoted to adolescence.

Family group therapy with many adherents, and diverse techniques has now a vast literature, which has been reviewed elsewhere.[1] This chapter is a personal account of one approach. The art and science of family group therapy cannot be taught in one brief communication, and this therefore can only be an introduction. The place of family group therapy in family psychiatry will be apparent from the brief review of the latter that follows.

2

Family Psychiatry

Definition

Family psychiatry is based on the principle that the family, not the individual, is the unit in clinical practice. It asserts the existence of a group psyche, or 'collective psyche', of the family; the family collective psyche is as real an entity as the psyche of an individual. In family psychiatry, the procedures of investigation are aimed at exposing the collective family psyche; the processes of treatment have as their target the repair of dysfunctioning in the collective family psyche. Thus, throughout, family psychiatry is concerned with the 'group psyche'. It starts with the whole, but may proceed to the analysis of the whole, if that serves the purpose of adding to its understanding or improvement of the *group psyche*. This analysis may in turn be followed by resynthesis.

Family psychiatry should not be confused with a related but different approach, the psychiatry of the family. This starts at the opposite pole; it starts with the individual and, to understand or improve him, is prepared to add other elements of the family to its procedures. Thus it encourages family studies of many kinds in order to find means of controlling the family milieu for the betterment of the psyche of one individual. An example of the latter approach is the vast and valuable literature, representing a large proportion of family studies, on the treatment of an individual schizophrenic through family group therapy. The aim in this case is the improvement of one individual; and thus it is not family psychiatry, which aims to improve the collective group psyche of the family.

Family psychiatry, then, in its clinical application, is an approach which takes the family as the unit for the organisation of practice. Taking the family as the unit, in the author's system, applies to the referral plan, to the explanation of symptomatology, to the procedures of investigation (Family Diagnosis) to the recording of data, and to the processes of therapy (Family Therapy). The family is the focus of endeavour throughout; the aim is to produce a harmonious, healthy and well-adjusted family.

The presenting member, irrespective of age or clinical condition, is regarded merely as an indicator of family psychopathology. Thus, after accepting the presenting member, all the remaining family members are investigated and later treated—the aim is to produce an emotionally healthy family.

Family Diagnosis

Family diagnosis aims to present a picture of the functioning and dysfunctioning of the family group. It proceeds through techniques such as individual interviews, dyadic interviews, family group diagnoses and special techniques such as the Family Relations Indicator.

Family group diagnosis is a procedure whereby all the members of the family who are meaningful in the family's situation at the moment of referral are interviewed together. This may involve two or three generations. It may include nannies, lodgers, etc., present in the family at that time. The aim is to get a first-hand picture of the dynamics of the family. Family group diagnosis is a procedure of such value that it is certain that it will have an established place in psychiatric practice, and indeed should rarely be overlooked in the exploration of the family dynamics. However, the true situation in the family will not usually emerge until after a few interviews.

Family group diagnosis should not be confused with family group therapy. Many family group procedures are termed therapeutic, when in fact they merely undertake an exploration of the family dynamics. At the same time, diagnosis may sometimes lead to family therapy. Furthermore, family group diagnosis may be an essential first step in vector therapy and run parallel with it.

Family Therapy

Within family psychiatry, the term *family therapy*, treatment of the family, embraces any procedure employed to improve the family's health.

Three main procedures are available in family therapy:

1. Family psychotherapy which seeks, by various techniques, a direct change in the individual, the dyadic or the family group psyche.

2. Vector therapy, which seeks to produce a more harmonious pattern of emotional forces within the life space of the family.

3. Producing a salutiferous society, which creates the optimum emotional environment for the family.

Sometimes there is an emphasis on one, rather than another, but all forms of therapy can exist together; in the ideal case all three forms are in use. The treatment programme must at all times be flexible to meet the ever-changing demands of the family situation. This applies to the choice of individual, the dyadic, or the family group approach in psychotherapy, and to the decision whether psychotherapy or vector therapy should be the approach to be employed at that moment.

1. *Family psychotherapy* means treatment of the collective psyche of the family. Family psychotherapy can be practised with an individual (in divi-dual therapy), a dyad (dyadic therapy or joint therapy of two people), or a whole family (family group therapy or conjoint family therapy), a number of families treated together (multiple family therapy), and a non-family group (group therapy). Multiple Impact Psychotherapy describes an intensive approach developed by the Galveston group of workers in the U.S.A. In view of the attention given to the new technique of family group therapy, it should be emphasised that it is only one of the procedures of family psychotherapy, which itself is only one section of family therapy; its exclusive use leads to gross limitation of family therapy.

2. *Vector therapy*. A vector denotes a quantity which has directions. Force, including emotional force, is a quantity with direction and therefore can be represented by a vector. Furthermore, as direction is a property of a vector and direction implies movement, it results in a dynamic situation.

Vector therapy effects a change of the emotional forces within the life space to bring improvement to the family within the life space.

The forces in the life space can be thought of in terms of fields of force. Within these fields there are potent forces, continually bearing, for good or ill, on families. These forces, if positive, harmonious and constructive, promote well being; but, if negative, disharmonious and destructive, they must be removed or counterbalanced. These fields of force are: (*i*) within the individual, (*ii*) outside the individual and within the family, (*iii*) outside the individual and the family and within society.

Vector therapy can involve:

(1) A change in the magnitude of the emotional force; e.g. father's aggression may be diminished.

(2) A change in the direction of the emotional force with no change in its magnitude; e.g. father abuses mother instead of child.

(3) A change in the length of time during which the emotional force operates; e.g. father works away from home, spends less time at home and his aggression has less duration.

(4) A change in the quality of the emotional force when one force replaces another; e.g. father treats his son with kindness instead of with aggression.

3. *A salutiferous society*. The third approach to family therapy calls for consideration of the author's concept of a salutiferous, health-promoting society. In the long term this is the most effective help in the service of society, the family and the individual.

The author sees society as a vast field of forces in which elements are loosely defined—culture, community, neighbourhood, family, individual; these elements are indivisible and each element has essentially equal significance. The emotional forces within the life space produce degrees of well-being or harm, and they can be re-patterned to promote either. Understanding of the re-patterning of emotional forces is a step forward towards bringing well-being to society and to the elements within it. Thus a re-shaping over the generations of the emotional strata of society has great opportunities for society's emotional self-improvement. This is the ultimate goal of vector psychiatry, of which family psychiatry is a part.

Thus a vast study of society is required, embracing every aspect of its functioning—organisations, institutions, roles, standards and aims. Every one of its multitudinous facets should be examined to assess its value in promoting emotional health. Over the generations increasing improvements will result in a salutiferous society, which will supply optimum conditions for emotional health in itself and its elements—culture, community, neighbourhood, family and individual.

Schizophrenia and the Family

The quest for the factors responsible for schizophrenia has focused attention on family psychopathology as the possible causal agent. There is such interest in this aspect of family psychopathology that it might be thought to be the whole of family psychiatry. It has led to prominence being given to the management of this one clinical condition in family practice and to overlooking the value of family psychiatry in the management of a wide variety of other clinical conditions. Indeed, there is controversy as to the contribution of family psychopathology to schizophrenia and as to the efficacy of resolving family psychopathology in its treatment. Whatever contribution family psychiatry has to make in schizophrenia, it has a more certain place in the management of the far commoner and equally destructive condition of emotion disorder, or neurosis.

The lack of an adequate definition of schizophrenia* nullifies much of the research in this field. But Langfeldt's concept of 'process' and 'non-process' schizophrenia is apposite. The former is incapable of explanation in terms of family psychopathology: the latter, like all neuroses, is a product of disruption of the family psyche. The former, 'process' schizophrenia, has been described as a 'split mind'; in fact it is a 'split family mind'. The organically determined perceptual anomalies of the schizophrenic make him unresponsive to the group psyche. Just as a fighting-ship put out of action cannot communicate signals to the fleet or respond to the signals from the fleet, but remains an element in the fleet although communication is lost, so does the schizophrenic remain an element in the family, but communication is depleted or lost. He remains a responsibility; the family must perforce adjust to him, but he is lost as an active element in the family psyche.

Conclusion

Family group therapy (treatment of the family as a group) is then a part of family psychotherapy, in turn an element of family therapy, which in its turn is an element of family psychiatry. Family group therapy is at its most effective when practised as a part of the total approach of family psychiatry. Before moving to the entity that we wish to change—the family—a brief account of the family group, this most significant and potent small group in society, will be a helpful introduction.

3

The Family Group

Definition

Humanity flowing in a stream from the Past, through the Present into the Future, might appear at first glance to be made up of a multitude of unrelated individuals. Closer observation, however, shows that they coalesce into groups. These groups, the families, expand, individuals split off and new groups are formed. But for the coalescing groups, the families, the flow of humanity would stop; through these groups humanity

* See also 'Classification of Psychiatric Disorders', this volume, Chapter IX.

propagates itself and nurtures and trains its new members. Hence the family is the most significant unit in society. In his life span the individual usually experiences two groups, his family of origin as a child, and the family he creates later. Such groups, family groups, are so tightly formed and have such a continuous history that they can claim to be the basis on which society is built.

The nuclear family, sometimes termed the 'immediate family', or the 'elementary family', can be defined as a sub-system of the social system, consisting of two adults of different sexes who undertake a parenting role to one or more children. Hereafter, the 'nuclear family' will be referred to as the 'family'. The 'family of orientation' is often used to designate the nuclear family in which a person has, or has had, the status of a child, and the term 'family of procreation' denotes that in which a person has, or has had, the status of a parent. The term 'extended family' is used to refer to any grouping related by descent, marriage or adoption, which is broader than the nuclear family. 'Lateral' extension would embrace uncles, aunts, cousins, etc., while 'vertical' extension would embrace two or more generations.

A family exists for a particular purpose in the social context in which it finds itself, and is shaped by this fact. The unit may be a small or large nuclear family, a nuclear family extended laterally or vertically or both, an extended family large enough to merit the term 'clan', or it may melt into a community that regards itself as the effective unit.

In psychiatry, concern should be with individuals who have emotional significance as a group. This is, most commonly, the family. But a blood tie is of secondary importance to an emotional tie, e.g. a servant given intimate care of the children may have more significance for them than the natural parents. Thus, in clinical practice, the concept of the family may have to be widened to take account of this.

It is usually agreed that the functions of the family are: (*i*) the satisfaction of the affectional needs of the family members; (*ii*) the satisfaction of sexual needs by reproduction; (*iii*) the protection, upbringing and socialisation of children; (*iv*) the material maintenance of the members of the family; (*v*) other, normally subsidiary, functions that may have a political, ritual or religious connotation. The emphasis given to each function is not only a matter of variation amongst individual families, but is influenced also by class, community and cultural considerations. The family is a flexible unit.

Description

These coalescing groups, the families, need description. They are complex. Categorisation is essential, so that an understandable description can be communicated to others. To be able to encompass them calls for some frame of reference, which should take account of the separate functioning parts of the family and the family as a whole.

Furthermore, the family is an ever-changing, flowing dynamic entity.

To grasp change is usually beyond our conceptualisation. Therefore, we freeze the family process at one moment in time, usually our first contact with the family, and describe what we see. We must be careful to add dynamism to this static picture.

Life development is not smooth, nor is human development—hence pain, anguish and incompetence. For the clinician, description is more than a theoretical exercise. For sick families, he needs a conceptual framework that will allow assessments to be made, therapy to be planned, and the outcome to be predicted.

Labelling of families by clinical or other categories is to be avoided. It has the disadvantage of concentrating upon one element, which by chance has come into focus, and thus of giving that element disproportionate attention. In individual psychiatry, for instance, such labels as anxiety neurosis, obsessional neurosis, depression, etc., have focused upon the presenting symptom in the individual, and have led to a situation where the symptom itself is regarded as the illness, and scant attention is given to the rest of the psychopathological processes within the individual. Such labels limit description. It is the whole process in individual, family and society which has to be understood and described and then re-patterned to bring health, efficiency and competence to the individual, family and social system.

It is suggested that the needs of an adequate description can be satisfied in the fifteen-dimensional approach to the family. Five dimensions are each described at three consecutive time periods, the Past, the Present and the Future. The five are those of the Individual Dimension, the Relationship Dimension, the Group Properties Dimension, the Material Circumstances Dimension, the Family–Community Interaction Dimension.

Usually, a family description starts with the Present in its five dimensions. To understand the Present in the light of what has gone on before requires a description of the Past in five dimensions. Ideally, it should be completed with a description of the Future in its five dimensions; in our present stage of knowledge this is only predictable within crude limits, e.g. that a university career is possible, a marriage breakdown likely or financial difficulties probable.

Phases of Development

Every family is the product of two previous families, the families of orientation of the parents. Families begat families—a fundamental truth in family psychiatry. Moving to the past takes one to the group psyche of the past family—each parent is an element in the collective psyche of the family of his childhood—and this is a most potent factor in controlling his contribution in the collective psyche of his present family.

Emerging from his own family, the individual meets another from a different family and the courtship starts. This period of coalescence of one individual with another and that of his family with the family of another is a phase without children and it ends when the first child arrives. The child-bearing and child-rearing period ends when the last child leaves home. An age of greater maturity follows with no children, more independence and, usually, less contact of the one partner with the other. Lastly comes retirement, which usually brings prolonged contact between the partners. Each phase has its characteristics, its potential for gain or loss for the participant.

Therapy may start in any phase and must always take account of what went on before.

Communication within Families

The interaction between individuals has not received the same degree of attention from psychopathologists as have the intrapersonal processes of the individual. Interaction includes consideration of relationships and of communication.

Relationship is the standing of one person to another. In psychological and psychiatric work special attention is given to the kind of feeling between people; a qualitative judgement is involved, e.g. is the relationship hostile, dependent, etc?

Communication, in the psychological and psychiatric field, is concerned with the process of connection between persons. It includes: (i) study of the means for the passage of information, and (ii) the meaning or message passed between persons; i.e. how it is passed and what is passed.

The interaction starts and ends with the persons involved having standing to one another, i.e. a relationship. Persons start with standing to one another, a meaning to be passed is formulated, the meaning is passed through the process of conveyance, the meaning is received, the standing between the persons is altered. Thus three elements are involved, the standing (relationship), the meaning (message) and the process of conveyance.

In common usage, the term 'relationship' is often employed to cover the whole interaction, the standing and the conveyance. In the following discussion the two terms are distinct.

While the standing between individuals and the meanings conveyed between them have received some attention from psychopathologists, although less so than the intrapsychic life of the individual, less attention has been given to the process of conveying meaning between people. Also, there has been even less interest in non-verbal, as against verbal, communication.

Communication denotes conveyance between people. It includes consideration of (1) the meaning, message or information that is conveyed, and (2) the process of conveyance, the apparatus, the channels. It applies in a conveyance between one person and another (e.g. adolescent to father), one person and group (e.g. adolescent to family), group and group (e.g. family and community). It need not be restricted to interaction, but what is said is relevant to consideration of communication in the family group, which amounts to transaction between many rather than the interaction between two people.

The purpose of communication is to influence others, to react to the present situation, to gain security by mutual support, and to receive from others all those elements essential to maturation, existence and security.

The process of communication involves emission, transmission and admission. In sequence there is a stimulus, sensation, percept, memory, thought, motor expression and feedback (which allows opportunity for correction and clarification). Many elements are employed—physical, nervous, humoral and chemical; one form may change into another, e.g. physical sound into the chemistry of a neuron. Proprioception is concerned with stimuli arising within the individual or the group, enteroception with stimuli arising outside the individual or the group. In communication, in addition to a message, instructions for its interpretation are conveyed; the part of communication which deals with interpretation is termed meta-communication.

We may expect meaning to be conveyed through the five senses (auditory, visual, olfactory, tactile and gustatory), or through extra senses not yet defined, or through the combination of a number of senses.

More knowledge is required about the capacity of the individual for communication; there must be limits. A person, subject to hurt for long enough, ceases to cry when the point of exhaustion has been reached. It may explain spontaneous recovery from, for example, depression, when the mechanisms for its expression become exhausted.

Study must pay increasing attention to the time factor in communication. Possibly, rarely, an overwhelming stress acting over a short period of time may have permanent ill effects—the nuclear incident so significant in outmoded psychotherapy. Stress acting over long periods of time may be a commoner situation and have more permanent ill effects.

To understand negative communication in families is as important as to understand the positive. The steps not taken, the unuttered words, the movements not made, the unsent messages, are as important as positive actions. The family member finds it difficult to define this negative communication and calls it an 'atmosphere'. When the atmosphere threatens to explode he calls it 'tension'.

The Family as a System

A family may consist of two people—a dyad in dyadic communication. A child brings triadic communication. Beyond the triadic there is tetradic and beyond that the polyadic communication pattern of the whole family. The whole has many properties of its own and is more than the sum of its parts. Even polyadic communication added to the elements of the individuals together make up only part of the group psyche.

Starting from the total family psyche and going on to a consideration of its parts emphasises the need to replace interactional with polydynamic concepts. In a polydynamic system there is an active network of mutually dependent communication processes. The family is such a system and has a number of possible communications. (1) A simple triad (F, Father; M, Mother; C, Child) can be thought of in terms of three communications between dyads in the group, Father–Mother, Mother–Child, Father–Child. (2) Each communication is reciprocal, making three interactions of six communications, F–M and M–F, M–C and C–M, and F–C and C–F. (3) Furthermore, each pair of family members acts as a small 'collective psyche' and communicates reciprocally with the remaining member: FM–C and C–FM; MC–F and F–MC; FC–M and M–FC. In large families the coalitions can extend to three, four, five or more people who interact not only with individuals but also with other coalitions. (4) Each element in the family is capable of *simultaneous* reciprocal communication with a number of other elements. (5) Lastly, communication within the family group can be indirect; for example, through mother to father, who in turn influences the child. Thus, the group psyche has a complex polydynamic system. Whoever, investigator or therapist, enters this system is incorporated by it and changes it—like an extra ship entering the fleet. Not to be lost in the family group is a tribute to the clinician's personal computer, which has the great advantage of having been brought up from birth on group situations.

Systems theory, linked with cybernetics, communication theory and field theory, has a useful place in the understanding of family functioning— sometimes as a reality and sometimes in producing worthwhile analogues. It also has its limitations; its judgements are quantitative rather than qualitative. If, for example, father shouts at the child, and with equal force mother soothes the child, the child does not remain neutral; he avoids his father and clings to his mother, i.e. he does not behave along the resultant of these forces, since the two cannot be compounded. To base therapy on mechanical principles is useful, but limited. Vigilance must guard against changing mere mechanical properties and producing a new situation with a different complexion, but equally unhealthy.

The Sick Family

An emotional symptom is always the expression of the psychopathology of the whole family. Symptomatology for which obscure and symbolic explanations have been given becomes startlingly comprehensible when seen in the context of the family. The following example will help to make this clear. A boy of twelve suffers from anorexia; for the first few years of his life he was brought up by two grandmothers who lived with his family. The maternal grandmother was permissive and did not believe that a child should be forced to eat. The other held equally firmly that a child should eat what was put before it. The strict grandmother forced the child to rebel against her, the other grandmother offered him a way to express his rebellion. So the child refused to eat. When the strict paternal grandmother left the family, her son, the boy's father, inherited her role and tried to force the child to eat the food he did not like. Thus his symptoms continued. A family creates the emotional stress, the emotional disorder and the particular manifestation of the disorder—the choice of symptoms.

The instance just related concerns a symptom, a manifestation of dysfunction, in an individual. But, as surely, symptoms can show in any facet of the family. By tradition, interest has been focused on the individual. Stress may arise in the family in any of its dimensions and at any point in a dimension. As clouds gather in the sky due to a complex of variables, so do stresses within the family. Thus symptomatology can appear in any or all of the five dimensions of the family—the individual, the relationship, the group, the material circumstances, and the family–community inter-action. Careful examination may show that they invariably appear in all. It should not be overlooked that the family–community interaction dimension is a frequent source of stress, and least under the control of the family. However, a family group may not manifest dysfunction equally throughout its system. One dimension, or one aspect of it, may show disproportionate dysfunction due to the 'set' of the emotional events at that time.

The choice of symptom is a reflection of family dysfunctioning. The individual's choice is dictated by his life experience in the family, e.g. anorexia in an adolescent may be dictated by a continuing family ex-perience wherein father disciplines him by sending him from the table and after his return demanding that he eat. The choice of expression in a relationship is similarly determined, e.g. physical hostility may be taboo and verbal hostility alone possible in that family. Again, the material changes in the family can take place only within the limits set by its condition. Group manifestations may be a family expression, e.g. sulking may be an expression of hostility in a particular family. The community interaction may determine symptomatology, e.g. that fear be controlled by obsessional ritual or that sexual taboos be imposed. Not only do present events dictate choice of symptomatology but so do those from the past.

After this brief consideration of the family group we can now turn to its therapy; the aims of family group therapy merit discussing first.

4

The Aims of Family Group Therapy

The general aim of family group therapy, as in all forms of family therapy, is to produce a harmoniously functioning family in the situation within which it lives. What is harmonious in one situation may not be in another. The standards in relation to 'harmony' depend on what is regarded as harmonious or healthy at the present time. Today's average family may well be regarded as 'unhealthy' by future standards. However, most therapists are satisfied to bring the family to the average standard of today.

The 'collective group psyche' of the family is the target for therapy. It is easier to understand the psychopathology of the family, and the means of its improvement, by looking at the historical development of the collective group psyche of the family. Each family is the product of two previous families, the families of orientation of each marriage partner. Each marriage partner has been habituated to act in the way he or she does by the dictates of his or her family. Thus each carries its own imprint * of its family life in the past into the family of procreation in the present. Harmony results from the capacity of the two families, as represented by their member, to integrate. A clash produces disharmony.

As part of his imprint each person carries: (1) a way of life and attitudes capable, or not capable, of adjusting to the way of life of the other partner; (2) the tendency or otherwise to neuroticism, dictated by past experiences, largely in the previous family; (3) sensitivity to general stresses because of past experiences, largely in the previous family; (4) sensitivity to *particular* stresses because of past experiences, largely in the previous family; (5) a tendency to react to stress by the development of particular signs and symptoms because of the dictates of the family of orientation.

The 'past' in the life of an adult family member may be reinforced or changed by continuing interaction with the family of orientation. In therapy this reinforcement or change may be encouraged or discouraged. It is relevant to mention that changes, sometimes dramatic, occur spontaneously as the result of the demise of a member of the family of orientation. The change, beneficial or damaging, may wrongly be credited to coincidental therapy.

The liabilities brought to the family of procreation by an adult member may be overt or covert, either to the member who brings them or to the other family members. To add to the problems of assessment by each other, standards of conduct will be judged by the family imprint of each; and its standards may deviate not only from the average standards in the community but also from those of the other family members.

The imprint produces needs which may or may not be satisfied by the imprint of the partner, e.g. an individual because of experiences in the family of orientation may react by hostility if ignored. The partner's imprint may be able to deploy assets and allow him or her to contain this. Thus harmony results. An inability to contain brings disharmony. Harmony may be possible by *building defences* to the imprint deficiencies of the other. These defences are possible if the antagonist's family imprint allows of it, e.g. to withdraw when hurt and refuse retaliation. Another mechanism insufficiently exploited in therapy is *circumvention*; a deficiency in the partner is accepted, and the way of life of the family of procreation is then

* The term 'imprint' is used not in a special ethological sense but in its ordinary usage of 'stamp' or 'mark'.

planned so that the deficiency has little or no opportunity for expression. Therapy must employ all these natural procedures in a systematic fashion —deploying assets, building defences and circumventing deficiencies. The great advantage of family group therapy over individual therapy is the possibility of enlisting not only the aid of assets possessed by the therapist but also that of the family members themselves. Success will largely depend, given the best of all therapists, upon the qualities of the imprints facing one another; there are occasions when they allow no resolution.

While the imprints from the family of orientation are of basic importance, it must not be ignored that the family of procreation is also developing a course which is superimposing an imprint on the fused imprints of the marriage partners. Again, children of the marriage are in the process of 'imprinting' in the present. The collective group psyche at first composed of two fused imprints expands as it embraces the children and all the new experiences it meets. The past impressions of the parents however are always paramount, even if hidden, simply because they resulted from a long-lasting experience in the families of orientation.

A family group with adult members imprinted with gross deficiencies does not necessarily collapse. The deficiencies may be complementary, e.g. an excessive need to be mothered in one partner may satisfy an excessive need to mother by the other partner. Again, deficiencies in an adult family member may produce marital clash but not be inconsistent with excellent qualities as a parent. Indeed occasionally a parent may 'wall off' himself or herself with the children in an enclave that protects them from the onslaught of the family imprint of the other partner.

Family group therapy is a contrived situation whereby the collective group psyche meets with a therapist who by his skill reveals as much of the strengths and deficiencies of the imprints of the family of orientation as it is necessary for the task on hand. He deploys assets, builds defences (without destroying existing ones) and circumvents difficulties. It must be noted that the mere meeting together of a family to talk with a therapist is not necessarily beneficial; it can equally be damaging. The difference is made by the skill, experience and personal qualities of the therapist. Furthermore, it must be emphasised again, to reveal psychopathology is not of itself therapeutic; a beneficial *change* must result for therapy to be achieved.

Therapeutic goals vary from family to family. In general, targets can be set at levels: (1) Situations created by stresses in the present. These may be mild or serious in extent. Family group therapy should here take place hand in hand with vector therapy; re-patterning of forces may be very rewarding. (2) Situations arising from the past, i.e. the families of orientation. Here family group therapy in conjunction with a flexible use of individual therapy to deal with situations in that person's family of orientation, may bring considerable benefit. Not only can individual therapy go on simultaneously, but in addition the family of orientation can also join the individual for therapy and even join the family of pro-creation for joint therapy. There are instances when both families of orientation can join the family of procreation.

A complete change, or a complete stabilisation of the family members, may not be required to effect a considerable improvement in a family situation. For example, as the result of free discussion in family group therapy a highly disturbed, rigid, obsessional father, with a highly ab-normal attitude towards sexual matters, finds himself able to see that his son should be free to leave the family, and to adopt the values of the community rather than the values of the father. Father's personality is not changed, but the release of his son lets the son gain immeasurably in his own emotional life.

How the aims can be achieved will become apparent in the discussion that follows on the organisation of therapy, the therapist and elements of strategy in therapy.

5

Organisation of Family Group Therapy

Comparison with Individual Therapy

Family group therapy has some features in common with individual therapy, e.g. transference, counter-transference, development of resistances, catharsis, etc. But in family group therapy the number of relationships is greater, the therapist is part of a web of communication and he addresses himself to the 'collective group psyche' of the family. The great advantage of family group therapy is that in the group there is a built-in corrective to misinformation by an individual by the sifting and re-evaluation of the others. Furthermore, it is possible to deploy assets not only in the therapist, but also in the family itself.

Comparisons with Group Therapy

Group therapy treats together a number of individuals from different families. Groups may be male, female or mixed. They may meet formally for intensive therapy, or informally in a club setting. One or more therapists may be employed, and the clinical material is interpreted according to the school of thought of the therapists. The aim is to bring profit to the *individual*.

The family group has a strong identity, which reaches from the past and extends into the future. It existed as a group before therapy, and will go on after it. It is a heterogenic group of both sexes and of all age groups. It is subject to strong influences from the extended family group. Its members have learnt rigid patterns of behaviour in relation to one another. Each member of the family has strong meaning for the others. Powerful emotions can be aroused in it, for good or ill. The aim of therapy is to change the *collective group psyche* of the family. Yet the family group has features in common with any other small group, and thus its therapy has some elements in common with group therapy.

Flexibility in Therapy

It must be emphasised that family group therapy is but one procedure of family psychotherapy, which in turn is only one part of family therapy. The use of family group therapy alone seriously limits the treatment of the family.

Family psychotherapy, vector therapy and preventive psychiatry are complementary, and the most effective family therapy employs all these procedures simultaneously. The therapeutic needs at a given moment can be met by a flexible approach ready to utilise whatever is appropriate. Thus individual and family group psychotherapeutic procedures may be employed together, or family group therapy and vector therapy, or family group therapy and dyadic therapy, etc. Whenever possible, the whole family must be involved in the treatment process; this does not mean just for family group therapy alone, but applies to all the therapies appropriate to the task at that time. Treatment may have to proceed with an individual, or with only a part of the family; this may be so because of inability to involve the whole family, or because of the dictates of the treatment situation at that moment. But if only a part of a family is under treatment, the rest of the family is not overlooked, and the aim does not change; to adjust the whole family is still the target.

With the consent of the family group, family members can see the therapist alone, but with the understanding that, whenever possible, material relevant to family life must be reintroduced to the group. The therapist applies no pressure; he concentrates on producing a sense of security, which makes revelation possible to the rest of the family. The therapist of course does not allow himself to be used against the family, or to show special favour to one member. Whenever misunderstanding threatens, it pays to subject the situation to the scrutiny of family discussion; capacity to understand is often greater than imagined. There is no doubt that an experienced family therapist is more comfortable in family therapy than in individual or dyadic therapy, where there is always anxiety lest unseen family members are not taken into account.

Selection of Families

Few units are so well staffed as to be able to apply family group therapy to all their families. Thus selection becomes necessary. In general, units deploy their facilities to give optimum value. Therefore the families selected are those with a degree of disturbance likely to respond, in a reasonable period of time, to the treatment offered by the facilities available. Families with young children have a degree of priority. They have young parents; young parents have not been emotionally ill so long as older people, and

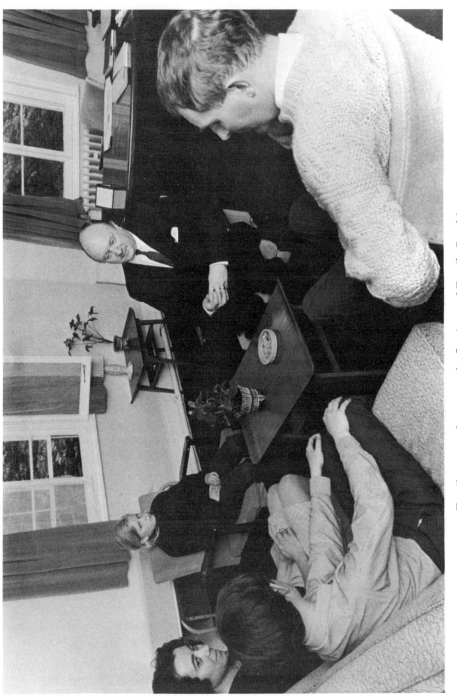

Family group therapy at the Institute of Family Psychiatry

thus respond more readily to treatment. The younger the children when treatment is established, the more they profit. The number of children in the family is a factor in selection; the greater their number, the greater the benefit that will accrue to society by improving their emotional health. In all families, whatever the degree of disturbance, efforts should always be made to bring relief to the children, the younger generation and the generators of new families.

Home or Clinic Setting

Family therapy usually takes place in an out-patient clinic; few clinics offer a service in the family's home. It is held by some that therapy in the clinic is a less artificial situation than therapy in the home, where it creates embarrassment to the family by provoking the interest of the neighbours, and where distractions are many. Therapists feel safer in their own clinic setting, and claim that it offers a controlled environment which makes diagnosis easier. Others claim that the home, as the family's natural setting, is more revealing, that it is easier to collect family members together there, and that it offers less distractions than a clinic. Probably the main determining factor in choice of setting is time; it saves therapeutic time to bring the family to the clinic.

The Clinic Setting

The family group usually meets in the clinic setting. They can meet informally in a comfortable circle of chairs, or seated round a table. All members of the family of any age group, including infancy, are present. Less than $1\frac{1}{2}$ hours is unlikely to be worth while, and more than $2\frac{1}{2}$ hours is likely to be exhausting. About 2 hours is the average period for a group meeting. Family groups should, if possible, meet once a week and not less frequently than once a fortnight. There are occasions when a longer meeting may be indicated—even a whole day, with rest pauses. These longer sessions are useful when a crisis has to be dealt with, or when the family has reached a point where it feels able to resolve a particularly difficult situation.

The room should be restful and quiet. Lighting, while subdued and not harsh or revealing, should allow easy visibility. All the chairs should be of equal height and size; the therapist claims no privilege chair. There should be playing material and reading material for the children, who also need access to a toilet. A profitable arrangement can be to hold evening clinics for families unable to get together during the day.

Size of Group

It is not always clear what constitutes a family group. The family group in therapy should consist of those who are involved together in an emotionally significant way. Thus the functional, rather than the physical, group is important, e.g. in a particular set of circumstances a lodger may be a more important father-figure for the family than a husband; a nanny may be a more important mother-figure than the natural mother. Thus, added to the nuclear family, there may be grandparents, siblings, neighbours, friends, servants, etc. Always, the approach should be flexible—in the course of therapy the group may need to shrink or expand.

Confidentiality

This applies at two points. Firstly, retaining information in the family group, and, secondly, dealing with confidences as they concern one family member within the group.

Families need to be assured that information will be kept confidential. Information must be assumed to belong to the person who gives it. It is imparted because only in so doing can the help needed be received. If it is communicated to others, it must be with the clear understanding and permission of the family. Thus any tape-recording must be made by their permission and with protection of the anonymity of the family. To fail means poor communication and ineffective therapy.

Within the family group, an individual may have information he wishes to impart to the therapist only. Similar 'special information' relationships develop naturally within the family. While this right to communicate alone with the therapist must be maintained, its handicapping effect on therapy must be pointed out. With increasing confidence, more and more information is thrown into the common pool by the family members. Especially in early interviews, the family group cannot produce complete security and thus complete communication. To force it beyond what the relationship in the group can stand only creates greater insecurity and impedes progress.

Recording Information

Given the agreement of the family, the interview can be recorded by sound or video tape. This is either for purposes of teaching or to have material that can be played back to the family during the course of therapy. As a means of expediting day-to-day therapy, recording has a limited part to play. Seldom does a therapist have time to consult a two-hour tape before engaging on another session. Its value is in research and teaching. In our experience, neck microphones offer the best means of recording sound.

Communication

The prime channel of communication within the family group is speech. However, much more occurs which has meaning to the family. The seating arrangements can reflect divisions and combinations in the family. Posture and gesture may convey what is felt and perhaps what an individual might wish to do or how he would like to be regarded, his aspirations, and his defences. At first the therapist may find it difficult to understand both the verbal and the non-verbal communications as families have idiosyncracies.

One or Several Therapists

Another matter of organisation is that concerning the choice of one therapist or several. Sometimes economy dictates the choice of one only. At first, therapists new to the field have difficulty in shifting loyalty from one person to a group. Yet, all have had experience of such a loyalty within their own families; such a shift is possible once the group idea is grasped and habit given time to work. Having a number of therapists carries the danger of each forming an attachment to an individual family member and setting up rivalries. On the other hand, if more therapists are introduced there is more dilution of family disturbance. It has been argued that a number of therapists are collectively wiser and more skilled. But an experienced individual therapist should have the skill to manage alone. The greatest problem in having multiple therapists, and the final argument in favour of one therapist, is maintaining adequate communication between a group of therapists; one therapist is usually of one mind.

The In-patient Setting

With the hospitalised patient, whether accompanied by his family or not, no evaluation is made or procedure undertaken without relating it to the context of his family. This does not mean that the individual must always remain in contact with his family. His particular need may be to escape from it. But this manipulation will be undertaken more effectively if evaluated in terms of the total situation of his family. It leads to a flexible use of hospital facilities—sometimes for an individual, a dyad, a part, or the whole of the family. The admission procedures involve a family evaluation, as do the ward regime and discharge procedures. The out-patient and in-patient management should be a continuous whole. Members of the family are not mere 'visitors', they are participants in the clinical process. Thus a family may join a member who is a hospital in-patient for therapy at stated intervals.

6

The Therapist

Personality

The right personality is more important than training for an effective therapist. The greatest enrichment of personality comes from a happy, warm, constructive benevolent experience in the family of orientation. This creates security and a capacity to relate to other families. The absence of this experience tends to lead to a need to exploit others for the improvement and betterment of the therapist's own personality. Fortunate also is the therapist who, because of the secure platform of his own childhood, has been able to move into other families and gain a wide experience of life.

In addition to his own personal qualities, an added requisite is a wide experience of a therapeutic process, preferably as an apprentice to a successful therapist. A number of therapists fail because they are constantly at war with the family under therapy; there is a need to outwit, manipulate, score off, feel omnipotent towards or crush with hostility. This reflects the therapist's experience in his family of orientation.

In the therapist one looks for qualities such as tolerance, the capacity to understand and be charitable to a wide range of human failings; the ability to be unbiased and unprovoked by the less beautiful aspects of life; a capacity not to blame or moralise. The therapist must be friendly, kindly, understanding. He must be able to make warm relationships with a great variety of people. Indeed, the greater his adjustment the wider his spectrum of affectivity. His attitude must be relaxed and expectant, his very expectation provoking output from the family; his constant attitude conveys a desire to resolve the family's emotional handicaps.

The therapist should aim not at a sentimental approach to others, but rather he should be a detached craftsman who uses his own personal warmth as an effective and affective tool in his task.

Main Role

The therapist's main task is to reveal to the family its collective group psyche based on the family imprint from the past. This is analysis only. Reconstruction must follow. Thus he then, as mentioned previously, has to mobilise the assets in the family to overcome its liabilities. He needs to build defences and he needs to find ways of circumventing deficiencies produced by the families of orientation. For this task he must be a benevolent parent. Handicapped family members have usually experienced unhappy family relationships in the past; now they are in touch with a benevolent family figure. This figure, however, exercises no control or power. Indeed, one of the lessons he has to teach the family is not to use force, power or authority. He aims to create a situation of security, wherein the family can reveal itself, work towards resolution and thus change. Barriers to success are sarcasm, aggression, force or cynicism on the part of the therapist. An academic dissection of events takes one nowhere; a benevolent dissection can be a beginning, if it is used as a precursor to a period of reconstruction.

Chairman and Convener

The therapist has the task not only of convening the meeting but also in general terms of directing its efforts. After all, the family has come for therapy, not for a pleasant afternoon's discussion of contemporary social events. Thus, his presence or his words must continually remind the family group of the task on hand. He must be sensitive to the topics that the family needs to discuss and furthermore can discuss at that moment; sometimes, the family has not, as yet, the capacity to tolerate a topic. He must give everyone in the family the right to speak and the security to speak when one wishes to.

Catalyst and Releaser

Expectation, and sometimes silence, provoke the family towards a discussion of events which are embarrassing, hurtful or painful to them, matters which they would wish to avoid. The therapist provokes an exchange where necessary. On the other hand, he teaches the family members that an interchange can take place without aggression, hostility or fury. He himself indicates and teaches that rational discussion can bring about the resolution of problems. Above everything, he is expectant.

Community Representative

The healthy therapist brings with him the values and the opinions of the community. The family may not conform to the attitudes and principles in the community outside, but can acquire these from the therapist. Explanation may sometimes be called for. However, no formal advice is given; the therapist inculcates an attitude by example rather than by direct teaching. It behoves the therapist to have adequate community values of his own.

Conciliator

The attitude of the therapist is always that of conciliator when faced with hostility or aggression of one family member to another. His aim is to create a climate where constructive work can go on. He is not a judge but a conciliator. He should avoid taking sides. Indeed, he has loyalty to all, and this will be tested time and time again. He must truly be a benevolent, security-giving figure to every member of the family.

Protector

No one within the family group should, if possible, be hurt through the family discussion. Thus, the therapist to some extent is a protector. This is particularly true in relation to the younger or weaker members of the family. In the eyes of the therapist, everyone is equal, everyone deserves support, everyone has equal rights. His loyalty is to the family group, and thus to all.

Diluter

Even if he does nothing else, the therapist, by bringing a healthy attitude into the family group, quantitatively dilutes the psychopathology of the group. The only effective argument for having more than one therapist is that the dilution process is even greater. However, as has already been said, this can have disadvantages.

Expiator

Embarrassing, belittling, hurtful attitudes and experiences are exposed within the family discussion. The toleration of the therapist removes the sting from all these experiences; in particular guilt is expiated.

7

Elements of Strategy

The Warming-up Period

In every course of therapy, there is an initial phase of warming-up, which may extend for a few minutes or up to several hours. This is inevitable, as the therapist and the family have to get to know one another. The family has to go through a period of convincing itself that it can allow the therapist to join the family, that it can trust him, have confidence in him, and confide in him as an equal partner. To some extent, every interview starts with a warming-up period. The therapist must be sensitive to this requirement of a warming-up period.

Explanation

It is valuable at the start of therapy to explain to the family the course of action in general terms. It is possible also to explain to them in outline the aims of therapy, as stated above. Furthermore, it is wise to point out some of the rules under which the family is meeting; for instance, that every member of the family has equal voice, whether it be child or grandparent. Not all these working rules will be acceptable at first. Again, the family will go through a testing-out period; but the attitude of the therapist continually reminds the family of the working rules.

Interpretation

Interpretation in family group therapy is in a sense a contradiction in terms. The only truth is the truth of an event within the life experience of that family member or that family itself. The event does not need interpretation; it is a fact. Thus, a therapist enslaved by interpretation theory may be less effective. If interpretation is fact, then it is only the family who knows the facts. The therapist may occasionally, by his knowledge of the probable patterns of events, arrive at the truth before the family. He should hold back or, at best, guide them to the truth. When the truth has been reached, it can be emphasised by repetition.

It can be educative to hear three experts discussing information conveyed by a patient. They can radically disagree amongst themselves, but the only true meaning of the information is that given by the fourth person, the patient himself. Broadly, people's experiences follow the same pattern, but the significance of events is unique to each person. Stereotyped interpretations have little significance. The therapist must constantly be on guard against assuming that other people's life experiences are like his own and have to be interpreted in the same context.

Insight

Insight is the understanding by the family of the mechanisms of the emotions. The greater the disturbance in the family, the less the insight. The developing understanding of the significance of emotional events takes longer with a more disturbed family, but this time spent on insight is essential. Understanding, however, is not therapy. Once the course of events has been seen, it is essential to reconstruct by re-enacting the situations and causing the family to react now to them in a healthy fashion, or to build defences around the situations that cannot be resolved, or to circumvent such situations.

Re-experience

Within the family group therapy, the family can re-enact disagreement, dissension and hostility, and learn not to be enslaved by these wrong attitudes. Having seen and then having acted correctly, the family may then need to have the learnt reaction continually reinforced.

Silence

The family has to learn that silence on the part of the therapist gives them an opportunity to talk. The 'ideal' interview for the family is one at which the therapist does all the talking; this is the easiest interview but the least worthwhile. The greater the security of the family, the more silent their therapist can be; the greater the skill of the therapist, the more silent also will he be. Silence is the biggest, and yet gentlest, pressure that the therapist can put upon the family to get it to work. For the family, however, to be silent from time to time may be a necessity. During such a silent period it is working in contemplation, and it may be necessary to allow this; for a true move forward in the family's affairs may result from it.

Resistances

These occur as in individual therapy. The family is late, or is absent, or is abusive, or will even exclude some of its own members, etc.

Interruption

The aim should always be to interrupt as little as possible; interruptions result in a break, an artificial break, in the flow of the family's thinking; the wrong comment or question may cause it to go off on a line of thought of less significance, or may give it an opportunity to avoid discussing something which is relevant. Direct questions very rarely bring profitable results. Far better to ask indirect questions, which will inevitably lead to the area being discussed; e.g. it is of little value asking an individual, 'How did you as a child get on with your mother?' It would be much more profitable to ask questions which will inevitably throw light on the relationship between mother and daughter; e.g. 'What did your mother talk to you about on the first day she took you to school?' or, 'What did you talk to your mother about when she washed your hair?' or, 'When you were five, what would be the three wishes that you would most want to come true?'

Family Swings

During the course of therapy, the mood of various family members will change; as one improves, another deteriorates, and so forth. These swings are to be expected in the course of therapy.

Family 'Imprints'

The family moves through certain levels of experience in the course of therapy. At first its concern is with superficial matters of the moment, then it moves to transactions in this family of procreation, then it moves back to its experiences from its early days as a family, and then, lastly, it moves to the families of orientation. The most fundamental therapy takes place at the last level.

Family Events

Much profit comes from getting a family to re-enact actual instances in its own immediate life experience and, as time goes on, in its past life experiences. In this way, a far more factual picture is obtained of real family events and its reactions to them.

Closure

Therapy ceases when the aim outlined at the start has been achieved. Usually there is a weaning-off period, which may last for either a few minutes or several hours of therapy, depending upon the family, its needs, and its degree of disturbance and thus of dependence.

8

Prognosis

The effectiveness of family group therapy is dependent on a number of factors. (a) The less the degree of family disturbance, the more rewarding, of course, is the therapy; with our present knowledge, even the best therapists may have difficulty in resolving a severe degree of family emotional disorder. (b) Problems of the Present resolve very satisfactorily; problems with deep roots in the Past are resistant. (c) In general, the younger the family members the more effective the therapy is. (d) Recent acute situations resolve more easily than long-standing, chronic, situations.

Even in the most resistant families, family group therapy can be a valuable technique in conjunction with vector therapy; insight can develop to the point when the family can accept adjustment which will favourably change the pattern of intra- and extra-family dynamics.

Equally good results can be obtained with all clinical categories, including the neurotic, psychopath, the alcoholic and the delinquent. In the writer's experience, family group therapy is not a profitable procedure for 'process' schizophrenia.

A routine follow-up contact with the family can reinforce previous procedures, offer continuing support, and may, with the detachment of time, allow a realistic appraisal of the extent and technique of clinical effort. There are few good follow-up studies of family group therapy. Problems of evaluation, which are considerable in individual psychotherapy, are even greater in family psychotherapy. Often family group therapy amounts to an evaluation of family dynamics without any clear benefit to the family; i.e. analysis without reconstruction.

Careful research could show that family group therapy not only is the most potent form of therapy, but also has in most situations a clear advantage over individual therapy. The need for research is evident.

9

Conclusion

Family group therapy has been presented as one technique in family psychotherapy, which is one aspect of family therapy, a part of family psychiatry. Following a brief general introduction to family psychiatry and the group properties of the family, the following features of family group therapy were outlined—aims, organisation, the role of therapist, some elements in strategy of therapy, and prognosis.

REFERENCE

1. HOWELLS, J. G. 1968. *Theory and practice of family psychiatry.* Edinburgh: Oliver & Boyd.

XVIII

THERAPEUTIC PROCESSES IN AN INSTITUTION FOR DISTURBED ADOLESCENTS—A GERMAN REPORT*

KARL KLÜWER

M.D.

Therapeutic director of the 'Haus Sommerberg'
Hoffnungsthal, near Cologne
Germany

1

Introduction

This chapter describes experiences with neurotic, dissocial boys between the ages of fifteen and twenty-one in the 'Haus Sommerberg'. In this institution, part of the Workers Welfare Organisation for psychotherapy and social group work, 48 boys live in four groups of 12, with 2 group workers, who are trained social workers. Details about the development and working methods of the institution have been published elsewhere.[13, 14, 15, 16, 17, 18, 20]

Psychotherapy in an institution differs from the usual work in an analyst's office because of several difficulties. The patients do not live in their normal social environment but in an institution, where most of their day to day contacts are with other patients. This type of communal living brings many restrictions in their daily life. The treatment is so expensive that the boys are not able to pay for it unaided, and thus they are financially dependent on anonymous social organisations and juvenile boards and they often find this situation difficult to accept.

On the other hand, therapy in an institution has advantages. The patients live in a type of moratorium,[7] in which for a short time the expectations of society regarding their independence and work responsibilities are reduced. It is a basic necessity for an institution, in which young people should find a

* Translated by Ronald Jantzen, Hoffnungsthal Bez. Köln.

better way to overcome their social difficulties, that it does not put them under an authoritarian system; this would only force them into an outward adaption. Nobody is able to work out his difficulties when he is not even allowed to show that he has some, and to experience the reactions which they bring with them. Society expects to see an immediate change in behaviour, and this is impossible. The amount of risk that can be carried is dependent on the trust placed by the person, the institution and society in each other.

Young people need more than just a therapeutic 'sanatorium situation'; this age group also needs practical and theoretical teaching and training.[22] The teaching, as well as the therapeutic work, can be done only when the special conditions needed for both are fulfilled. If one of the parts is given too much attention, the work will be hindered or even become impossible. Experiences in other homes have proved this.[11] It is necessary that both areas—pedagogic and therapeutic—work together to keep a united approach. This entanglement makes it rather difficult to describe a single element in more detail.

Once a week the juvenile patients have five hours of creative therapy[23] in groups of five, one hour of psychoanalytic group therapy[24] in groups of seven, and one to three hours of individual therapy.

Our boys normally live two years together. They are poor partners. Each one of them waits for everyone else to meet his special needs. This brings them into conflict with one another.

Our experiences will be discussed under three headings:

I. Psychopathology of our special patients.
II. Role of the staff in the group process.
III. Group processes in the total institution.

2

Psychopathology

Sommerberg House accepts boys whose dissocial behaviour has developed from neurotic conflicts. A few of the boys have been borderline cases. Boys with serious neuro-psychiatric disturbances are not accepted; we do, however, have boys who have sometimes become disturbed after ascertained brain injuries so that they are prone to fear or aggressive behaviour.

In the past we have had a few boys who have been brought up in such an inconsistent manner that they finally had become asocial, with no steady standards and a weak character. Our methods usually proved inadequate for this special group.

The asocial and antisocial activities of our 'acting out' neurotic dissocial youth are not direct outlets for primary instinctive drives. The psychic background to all their pseudo-instinctive patterns of behaviour is much more of a compulsive and contraphobic nature. Up to now we have become thoroughly acquainted with 150 boys, none of whom led us to believe that a superego did not exist. On the contrary, after achieving a deep understanding of the psychological processes of each boy, we found that the superego was not only stronger but more cruel than one normally finds in neurotic patients.[10, 21] Because it is impossible to live under the pressure of such a murderous conscience, the efficiency of such a conscience must usually be hindered by all possible defence mechanisms. The assumption that for many of these patients one can speak of two consciences[4] has greatly helped us to understand them. The power of their conscience is so strong because of its special structure. With the normal superego co-exists a second 'superego with contrary values', so that it could be called a 'Tomboy conscience'. The following behaviour patterns are examples:

One day a boy, Henry, made a bet that he would run head first through a veranda window. In his next group therapy session, this much admired act was the centre of attention. During individual therapy it became evident that he had severe guilt feelings and knew perfectly well that it was wrong to break the window. But a type of conscience, that represents a special form of the ego-ideal, had told him that to run head first through the window would be a heroic deed.

Between the demands of these two consciences Henry often lived in agonising tension. In many situations, including the therapy group, he became unable to participate because he could not find a way to solve the conflict between his 'two consciences'—his very strict superego and the herostratically* oriented ego-ideal. Whenever he was inclined to take part in the group, his ego-ideal would ridicule him; if he wanted to perturb the group, his superego would condemn him. In such cases, he would usually withdraw his attention and produce drawings of little men, equipped with deadly weapons who ended up being caught and hung on the gallows. This was his way out of unbearable tension, in which none of his impulses could escape criticism, and he would have an apparently primitive outburst of 'instinctive action', which, on closer scrutiny, proved to be a compromise between drive tendencies and defence mechanisms, similar to other psychoneurotic symptoms.

The asocial impulsive actions of our patients are similar to contraphobic and compulsory symptoms and to the perversions.[5] But a particular characteristic of their behaviour is that this 'alloplastic acting out' represents at the same time a false apprehension of reality.

In the delinquent acting out one can recognise tendencies of a character neurosis with strong narcissistic feelings for these defence mechanisms. The point made by the example of Henry's behaviour could equally well apply to all our boys to a greater or smaller extent.

Anna Freud[10] has given a vivid explanation of the origin of this psychic structure, but it might be helpful to describe how the elements of the

---

* Herostratos was the Greek hero who destroyed one of the seven 'wonders of the world' because he was unable to build an eighth one.

developed structure can be used as a defence system. The more rigidly a sadistic superego hems in a passive feminine-oriented and masochistic ego, the more the ego-ideal requires a compensating moment of herostratically oriented nature. It is quite common for the boys to escape into fantasies of grandeur in order to defend themselves from destructive narcissistic breakdowns; often delinquent acts are performed in the 'ecstasy' of such fantasies of grandeur.[6]

In most instances the patients are unaware of the influence of this ego-ideal in the form of an 'unconscious megalomania'[5] and it does not become clear to them until after a careful working through of their resistances. Some behaviour patterns which are at first incomprehensible can be explained in this way. For example, there was a boy who would refer to going round the corner of a house, as going round a 'gorge in the Grand Canyon'; or another who could not pass a group of boys without thinking that they were the 'black riders' who would immediately follow him, and whom he then outwitted by acting out his fantasy and hiding in adventurous places; or yet another, who imagined that instead of entering the therapy room he entered an assembly of generals, carrying under his arm a bear-like little dog which he then set down in the middle of the table in defiance of the generals, to protest against the 'rigidity of the old men'. There are many similar examples. Time and again it was observed that when such fantasies were made conscious a noticeable stabilisation in the ego began to take place and a more normal confrontation with reality became possible.

This special ego-ideal that should resist a sadistic superego, often makes therapy very difficult, because it gives the patient a feeling of might and superiority. In spite of the fact that this narcissistic increase of self-reliance originated from a defence against feelings of impotence and fear of the representatives of the superego, the boys 'make a virtue of necessity' by reversing passive helplessness into active fantasies of power. This impedes the necessary therapeutic moderation of the pathological superego. An example should again make this clear.

When Bob came to us, his behaviour irritated both the boys and the staff workers. Almost always he spoke as if he were his own father. With his nose in the air he looked down upon the others and with a sonorous tone made statements like: 'Shut up, please, when I talk with you.' This attitude towards his companions soon made him socially unpopular. Through group and individual therapy the compulsiveness of his attitude soon became clear to him. He strove for a better adjustment, but at the same time developed fantasies of magic power which appeared almost psychotic. On one occasion during group therapy some of the boys mentioned that they wished some group workers dead, and Bob immediately felt that he could raise the dead from the grave if he so wanted.

In the course of individual therapy Bob produced an abundance of childhood material which explained how, in a hopeless oedipal rivalry, he

P

developed a passive attitude to his father, while at the same time his sadistic superego was established. This became the basis for a career as the passive partner for homosexuals. In his secret acquaintances with men he felt as if he was being loved by his father while being at the same time the exploiter of his father. He used the condemnation of his superego for these passive anal acts, which destroyed his self-esteem, to 'get away from himself' and to transfer his feeling of being condemned to the feeling of being the condemner. By means of this self-condemnation, he gained the feeling of being vastly superior to his own bad actions. In this way he could expose his long-guarded secrets during therapy without this being a heavy burden for his self-pride; he could do so because this unacceptable behaviour did not have anything to do with his 'superior ego', but rather with the 'nincompoop ego' which was not able to perform the intentions of his superior being. As in examples given by Le Coultre, the communication of his memories could not offer much help in changing Bob's actions. This weak and despicable chap just deserved to be humiliated through continual street-walker situations.

It is evident that a remedial change in his psychic economy could not take place as long as the narcissistic gain, coming from the imaginary superiority over himself, did not become fully conscious. After this had happened, he discovered in a transference situation during a session of individual therapy that he had been trying to defend himself against a terrible fear of his father. In a great rage he played with his pocket knife, and the therapist felt no doubt that life or death was at stake. Before he could release this pressure by crying, he had to be sure that the therapist would not deliver him into a new violent situation. After the herostratically orientated ego-ideal position became conscious to him (in which many traits of early childhood fantasies of omnipotence were again aroused), the boy became slowly able to take advantage of the therapeutic reduction of the superego's might, which until then had served him as a jumping board to catapult himself into the feeling of superiority. In this phase of the treatment it became possible for him to find a new psycho-social integration. He was now able to co-operate in the training programme, as well as being able for the first time to learn something in school or in the workshop. Previously he was always the superior one, and this had made it impossible for him to accept something from others. The ability to learn enhanced his taste for work and his increased rooting in reality stabilised his ego. From then onwards the problems in his treatment conformed increasingly to those normally met in the treatment of a neurotic.

A special technical difficulty in the treatment of narcissistic character neurosis is often connected with the fact that in the development of the narcissistic manhood ideals (which represses and overcompensates the passive trends in the ego) certain behaviour patterns of the father or of similar power figures were incorporated as symbols of power without questioning their usefulness. These behaviour patterns can seldom be understood from the dynamics in the individual alone, because they do not originate in him, but rather are inherited or copied. The boys finally use them without realising their origin. In accordance to the character of the narcissistic defences, these are often behaviour patterns against which, as children, they felt powerless, and which therefore, being incorporated, would give them the feeling of being powerful. Such a way of acting becomes a characteristic in the person and is no longer conscious, but it may nevertheless carry a high degree of narcissistic satisfaction. For this reason the boy would not feel ready to take part in the treatment before he had experienced a kind of estrangement from such patterns.[22] It must become clear to him that such things happen automatically, irrespective of their necessity, suitability or practicability in a given situation, in other words that these behaviour patterns function independently of reality testing. It is only after this discovery that these behaviour patterns become accessible to therapy.

In many cases creative therapy is especially helpful, as it offers opportunities to identify and to make such patterns conscious. Creative therapy can also help the boy to realise that he cannot simply do without these behaviour patterns, although he may have consciously recognised their inadequacy.[23] The following is an example:

> At the beginning of William's first creative therapy session, the therapist said to him, 'Here you have wood, clay, paper and paints. All these things are at your disposal. You can use them just as you wish. What would you like to make?' William looked around and then said, 'Yes, I would like to make a lamp.' The therapist accepted the suggestion and asked, 'And what should the lamp look like?' William became uncertain and replied, 'Ah, I would rather make a bookshelf.' The therapist again agreed and asked, 'How high and how wide should it be?' And obtained the same reaction from William, who was again evasive, 'Hmm, I would much rather make a wastepaper basket.'
>
> Before William came to us, he had repeatedly tried without success to complete an apprenticeship; in his experience, he was a failure. Now for the first time, he began to realise how these failures came about. It was his pattern of behaviour to withdraw as soon as there was need to advance from vague ideas to clear planning.

With progressing treatment the patient becomes slowly aware of the previously unconscious fantasies and is finally led to the production of concrete images which begin to take shape and have a meaning. It is at this point that creative therapy can be of significant help in combating the fears arising from these fantasies. We have often found a boy's areas of conflict are reflected in his drawing and working.[23] Besides that, creative therapy helps the boys to acquire a feeling of achievement when doing manual work.[8] Experiences during creative therapy allow a boy to find new incentives to go deeper in the verbal psychotherapy. In this way the prerequisites of his ability to work are developed and form a basis on which a boy can build in the workshop and later in his occupation.

3

Role of Staff

Some of the difficulties of social group work and the co-operation between group workers and psychoanalytically orientated therapists will first be discussed. An illustration will expose some of the issues.

One of our groups was led by a young couple, who had just had their first baby. The young man had a very good, close relationship to the boys in his group; he was not authoritarian, but rather acted as an older brother. The boys were fond of his pretty wife, in fact they adored her, and this gave her a good feeling.

Tom, one of the boys in the group, passionately fought to stand out among the others. This becomes understandable, if we consider his childhood. Until he was ten, Tom was the only child in the family and then two younger siblings were born. He could not overcome this dethronement; he began to wet his bed again and his behaviour became increasingly socially unacceptable—he ran away, he stole.

His friend and greatest rival in the group was Henry. Henry was not so big and strong as Tom, but was wilder and more cruel in his fighting tactics. The fourth of seven children, his home life had been dominated by his oldest brother, who had often won prizes in boxing and tyrannised the parents and children. The second child had aimed his interest towards intellectual pursuits and was successfully employed in a field which required intellectual inclinations. The third child had revolted furiously against the oldest brother and had become his rival. In doing so he used Henry, the fourth child, as a sparring partner. Until adolescence, Henry had been a lovable little boy, the sunshine of the family, always laughing. He had had to take much battering from his older brother. When he was hurt in these sessions of boxing practice, his brother would give him a biscuit or a sweet to console him. Eventually, during the period of pre-puberty Henry exchanged his passive role to one of wild terrorising behaviour.

Tom and Henry were the ringleaders of the group. It began innocently: 'People in love tease each other.' The female worker was often greeted with silly jokes when she came into the group, 'Hush, hush, the pretty fairy is coming,' or, 'Well, young lady, what are you doing here?' After a while this game became aggressive. Tom made cutting remarks, 'If you can cook watered down soups only, you will become a good-for-nothing.' This game began to offend her increasingly. She could not do anything in the group without being attacked from someone. During the night the boys, who lived in the room above her apartment, often made disturbing noises. Tom bet Henry that he would smack her, whereupon she would become so mad that she would slap him.

The group worker felt she was under growing pressure; as long as she made a joke of the teasing, she was able to endure it. It was not too bad, as long as she could defend herself. But as soon as she began to withdraw and to avoid Tom, he became aggressive. The situation reached the point when at mealtime he would give her only half a portion of meat, whilst taking a piece and a half for himself. Once he went so far as to put a worm on top of her trifle.

Eventually the worker presented the problem to the group workers' meeting, the so called 'experience group' (E-group).

In the E-group meeting, which takes place once a week, all the social group workers and the psychotherapists meet for two hours. (The leaders of the work groups have a similar meeting on a different day.) The participants discuss situations arising in the boys' groups and any material related to them. The therapeutic leader acts as moderator of the group. This procedure is similar to the 'sensitivity training groups in dynamic social-psychology[19] and has the same characteristics of the 'Balint groups'.[2]

To describe the behaviour of another person, one must more or less identify with the emotions of that person. Hence, after a while, in the dynamic realm of the E-group meeting, a situation usually arises which reflects the corresponding emotional constellations among the boys with similar transference and counter-transference. A new term has been coined for this process—'the induced spontaneous phenomenon in the group'.[1]

When the group worker who had been teased by Tom came into the meeting she stated with some feeling that in her group there was a boy whose provocative behaviour had so irritated her, that she had the feeling that she was going to slap him. She could not go on like this. The other people in the meeting immediately asked what had happened, and she told them the whole story as related above. This brought the group into activity. A lively discussion developed, unwittingly provoked by the group worker. Evidently the teasing had first flattered her, said one person. Another person had heard from the boys that she had ordered Henry to do something and had actually slapped him when he had thrown a dish on the floor in defiance. One of the participants became angry and said, 'If you were to handle my friend in that way, I would probably act in the same way as Tom!' Immediately someone else intervened and said that he could well understand the group worker, and he tried to take her side. Another one warned against too much vehemence, holding the opinion that the whole thing was critical and dangerous and he wanted to mediate. In this way the situation became 'alive'. The operative emotional attitude could be clearly seen, and the participants were made aware of these processes. Because the group workers had the opportunity to repeat the boys' behaviour and to experience the feelings and defence mechanisms which influenced the boys' actions, they could understand better their own actions.

Of course these phenomena are not always resolved so easily, but, as in other groups, defences and resistance sometimes become overruling. The experienced group worker and the director of the home, through their work in the dynamic field of the boys' groups, usually come to know relevant events, of a difficult situation, not later than two or three days after the boys have related them to their therapists. If this does not happen, one must presume that there is resistance among the group workers. This resistance must be cleared up. The therapists can use their own knowledge of the boys and of their situation in therapy in order to make clear the processes in the E-group meeting for the group workers, without having to disclose information gained during therapy. In this way the group workers can recognise the processes in their own group, as well as their own emotional reactions to specific topics. This helps them to understand their group better than would have been possible through long theoretical explanations.

This is exactly what happened with our group worker. She became once more able to maintain the necessary professional attitude to the group, she lost her fear that her hand would strike out, or that the whole group would attack her as one man. She knew which boys would be on her side. With this newly won balance, she could set herself an imaginary goal, to prepare the group for 'the slap' that might be administered in the near future. She began by using in the group the insight gained in the meeting, by having conversations in the sense of a 'life-space-interview'[22] with individual boys, as the opportunity arose.

Soon she found that almost half of the group was interested in working with her constructively. It relieved her to know that she no longer needed to submit to Tom's provocation, but was again able to do her job as a social worker with confidence. She took back the half portions of meat or exchanged plates. She used discussions, which arose from these events, in further talks with the boys. Finally in a group meeting with all the boys present, these problems were discussed openly. The boys recognised the difference between their wish to live peacefully together and what they had made out of the situation. The awaited slap in the face did not materialise. On the contrary, the situation in the group became harmonious.

This example is taken from the time when we had not yet analysed the subconscious fantasies of the group with the group workers. It shows that this genuine process can begin to function without being initiated by analytic interpretation.

As the population of the house increased from 24 boys and 8 staff members to 48 boys and 16 staff members, we had to change our method. Today we try to analyse and interpret the arising subconscious fantasies in the E-group meeting,[9] so that the group leaders can meaningfully use this information when working with their group.

In our example the boys acted as if they shared one general fantasy; they were a large family whose oldest brother had just married. They behaved in the way common to all adolescents, when they begin to show interest in the girl-friends of their older brothers, uncles or friends, because they reached the stage when infantile relationships to the family are left behind and replaced by more mature relationships. The adolescents are led by their emotions to feel more interested in girls of their own age, while their fantasy still retains elements of love, rivalry, jealousy and reparation left over from their infantile object relations. Invariably, each individual in the group experiences feelings in accordance with his personality and his unconscious conditions.

The method employed by the group social worker with each of the boys in the different group situations can best be explained through the concepts of the 'life-space-interview'.[22] This method is based on field theory which regards each daily event as resulting from the environmental and the historical conditions in the field of the group, as well as from the conscious and unconscious factors of each individual in the actual dynamic field of the group. The factors in the individuals are influenced by their personal experiences in the past, as well as by their expectations and fears of present and future events. In this way the interview relates to daily events, which are then clinically evaluated. Each time when it became possible to use the unconscious group fantasy (understood through combined efforts with the group workers), the fascination which had increasingly clung to and grown from these fantasies dissolves, and the roles and functions in the group interaction can change to more mature patterns. Often our social group work is aimed not only at classifying group fantasies but at keeping the group processes in motion and thus presenting the boys with learning experiences in concrete group situations.

The following example demonstrates how a group worker takes the opportunity to start a life-space-interview.

> One evening the group worker came into the smoking-room and found five or six boys passionately discussing whether it is possible to split an atom. Two of the boys were particularly involved in the debate. One was Bill, who had the most explosive nature in the group. He made a big show of defending his knowledge of the modern way to split the atom. The other one, Otto, always lived in fear that the normal flow of life could be upset. He tried to prove that the atom from the very meaning of the term is an indivisible substance, which logically cannot be divided. The situation was such that the other boys already mocked the defender of the atom unity by calling him, 'atom Otto'. In such a situation the group worker could limit himself to an objective explanation of how an atom can be split, on the other hand he could go further and ask the boys why they got so excited about this subject. In this way is stimulated a discussion, which can bring the deeper motivations to the conscious ego, and can be continued at a later occasion with individuals or with the whole group.

The following example demonstrates how the whole group can sometimes be the patient, who must be taken care of and who needs help against the provocation of an individual.

> The boys in a group house were having dinner together with a group worker. But Bill, instead of coming down to dinner, had stayed in his room. After being repeatedly called by one of the other boys, he burst noisily

through the door and banged down on the dinner-table a bottle containing his tonsils preserved in alcohol, a memento of his recent tonsillectomy. This bottle was a sign of his superiority over the fear of the operation, and he was saying: 'The tonsils were taken away from the others. I still have mine!' In his anger he was compelling the whole group to take notice of the situation. For the boys this was too much, and some felt sick, others angry.

This situation demands the ability of the group worker to help the boys to come to terms with their anger, panic and guilt feelings. It would have been senseless to tell Bill that his tonsils did not belong on the table. He knew that himself. The worker could only confirm the significance of Bill's behaviour. 'Boy, that was something! The world can see how angry you are.' Bill now had achieved his ends and was satisfied. As the worker took the bottle away, Bill only blustered a bit—he owed himself this final re-action. By this time the other boys began to make trouble; they were so grieved and angry that they could have killed Bill. The worker separated Bill from the group and sent him back to his room. He then allowed the anger of the group and their reproach to be aimed at himself. This had a cathartic effect, and he was then able to start a discussion on what had brought about this situation. Incidentally, at the time this particular group was keen to prove that it was the most progressive in the home. All feelings of hate were projected on to Bill and he fought, although with wrong weapons, against the growing danger of becoming a scapegoat. On the following days the group worker had to expend much energy to keep the means of communication open between Bill and the group.

How much energy is sometimes needed to avoid the deterioration of communication within the group, is shown in the following episode.

After a short outburst of fruitless anger, Hans lost all emotional contact with the others. He became depressed and resentful and retreated to bed. His group worker could do nothing more than sit by his bed while the boy kept repeating, 'Go away! I said, go away!' This continued for about two hours until he finally said, 'You know, up to now I have kept saying that you should go away—but inside I was praying that you would stay. It is very late and your wife will be waiting and I think that now you can really go.' In this way a conversation began, in which Hans was able to talk of his annihilating anger and destructive grief, which had taken away his ability to function.

These examples show the complexity of the emotional relationships in an institution. They also demonstrate how a theoretical training alone is not enough to develop the necessary skills of a group worker. Practical experience together with the gradual acquisition of sensitivity in supervision can impart the skills which enable the worker to recognise in the group and the individual those signs which indicate growing tension leading to acting out behaviour. The earlier the deeper reasons for the interaction in the relationships are understood and deliberately brought into conversation, the less the boys will need to act out, and they will be all the more able to work out their difficulties through their understanding. Constant group supervision in the E-group meetings, regular discussions of our theoretical and practical concepts in comparison of our work with that of others through the literature have become necessary tools in our work.

4

Group Processes

During adolescence boys tend to avoid intensive relationships and frequently change their friends in order to try out various types of regressive and progressive relationships.[3] Because of this, they prefer contacts with a group, in which they tend to act out. If the young patients are in constant contact with each other, which cannot be prevented in a home, the process of working out their difficulties cannot be confined to the meeting in the therapy room. In residential treatment these interactions must be included in the therapeutic programme.

Again, the processes in the E-group meetings are different from the processes in groups like the Balint-groups, because the group workers are confronted with and dependent upon the behaviour of their patients in their daily life. The fantasies arising during therapy have an effect upon the home community, and above all depend to a great extent upon the theme dominating the whole home. Hence the development of the theme in group and individual therapy cannot lead to transference neurosis, as we know it in psychoanalysis. The development of these processes of transference in the group or in individual therapy have the characteristics of episodes. In the home society, we see how the waves of tension and harmony form unconscious group fantasies, which we call 'home theme'.

The atmosphere in the home community is often very emotional. Anything can precipitate specific emotional attitudes and the formation of an unconscious fantasy. When this happens, the whole home is involved in this dynamic phenomenon.

Once the typical pre-adolescent fears of the powerful, active, pre-oedipal mother arose, all the groups and more or less all the boys became involved in this theme. It turned up in conversations about the family, girl-friends, female staff members, etc. Each group had its character and each boy tried to apply his personal means of problem solving and defences in working out the situation. Statements like the following were common: 'She is always after me.'—'If you give her an inch, she takes a mile.'— 'She is never satisfied.'—'She always demands something, but does not believe I can do it.'

Staff members too experienced the same problems and fears and aimed their aggression towards a woman worker: 'One cannot talk to her.'— 'If one doesn't acknowledge her, she runs away and cries.'—'I cannot stand that woman any more.' The interpretation of the fantasy in the group therapy, the analysis of the individual defence mechanisms in the combined individual therapy and the work in the E-group meeting crystallised and explained this theme, which, once brought into the consciousness of the staff members and boys lost is fascination. This phase of fear of the 'pre-oedipal mother' lasted about six to eight weeks. During this time the positive father types were idealised and called upon to help: 'You know you can rely on men.'—'With him (the male group worker) the object becomes tangible.' This positive attitude of transference between the boys and male staff workers continued until and during the period of peace, which always follows a period of tension. An example of the turning-point in this peaceful phase was brought about by the impending departure of a student who had finished his practical training in the home, and of a male group worker, who had said that he was planning to leave the home soon in order to become director of another home. One heard from the boys, 'It would be better if the "old woman" would go, instead of these good men.'

The loss of the good (negative-oedipal) father with all the sorrows pertaining to it could be called the essence of the period thereafter. For example, one of our seventeen-year-olds acted out his ferocious hate against his father, who had left him and his mother. Bill provoked the male group leader and the pedagogic director until they scolded him; he then ran away from the home to avoid the danger of really injuring these hated father figures. At the same time he intended to seek his real father in order to hit him in the face and shatter his jawbone. He stayed away for a while and then returned of his own accord to continue his treatment and his education.

To illustrate our considerations the following comparison is not too far-fetched: in the dynamic realm of the home community with the involvement of almost eighty persons, the basic feelings of love and hate are always present, with their spectrum of possible emotional attitudes. These feelings are always changing. The forming and crystallising of the fantasies through the analytical work lead to reflection upon the events in the co-ordinate system of the social basic model of the oedipus situation. Due to this reflection the development of the home is like a 'dynamic kaleido-scope'; the changes in the emotional attitudes could be compared to the changing of the images in a slowly rotating kaleidoscope. We came to this comparison through the help of the dynamic 'whirlpools' which Eissler[6] and Hermann[12] used to describe the inner psychic processes.

The changes in the group dynamics always lead to new constellations, until some event causes a strong emotional reaction to the constellation just formed. This momentarily stops the rotation of the social-dynamic kaleidoscope. In this way that constellation gains in importance. The provocative effect of this again intensifies the corresponding emotional attitudes in the psycho-social realm. Again the meaning of the imaginary scene is intensified, until finally a *Gestalt* in the sense of an unconscious fantasy becomes manifest and accessible to the perception and inter-pretation.

REFERENCES

1. ARGELANDER, H. 1967. Das Erstinterview. Teil III. *Psyche, XXI. Jg.*, 7, 473–511.
2. BALINT, M. 1964. *The doctor, his patient and the illness.* London: Pitman Medical Publishing Co.
3. BLOS, P. 1962. Intensive psychotherapy in relation to the various phases of the adolescent period. *Amer. J. Orthopsychiat.*, 32, 901–910.
4. LE COULTRE, R. 1948. Probleme bei der Behandlung des Narzissmus. Unpublished paper.
5. LE COULTRE, R. 1968. Splijting van het Ik als centraal Neuroseverschijnsel. In *Hoofdstucken uit de hedendagse Psychoanalyse* Eds P. J. van der Leeuw *et al.* Slaterus, Arnhem: van Loghum.
6. EISSLER, K. R. 1949. Some problems of delinquency. *Searchlights on delinquency.* New York: International Universities Press.
7. ERIKSON, E. H. 1955. New perspectives for research on juvenile delinquency. In *A report of a conference 1955 Ministry for Health, Education and Welfare*, Ed. H. L. Witmer, Washington.
8. ERIKSON, E. H. 1959. Identity and the life cycle. *Psychological issues*, 82–88. New York: International Universities Press.
9. EZRIEL, H. 1950. A psycho-analytic approach to group treatment. *Brit. J. med. Psychol.*, 59–74.
10. FREUD, A. 1949. Certain types and stages of social maladjustment. *Searchlights on delinquency*, 193–204. New York: International Universities Press.
11. HEIGL, F. 1963. Die analytische Gruppenpsychotherapie in Heim. *Prax. Kinderpsychol.*, 4, 115–122.
12. HERMANN, IMRE. 1963. *Die Psychoanalyse als Methode.* Cologne and Opladen: Westdeutscher Verlag.
13. KAPPELER, M. and KAUNE, W. 1964. Ist eine Tätigkeit im Heim für den Sozial arbeiter noch interessant? *Unsere Jugend*, 16, 565–568.
14. KLÜWER, K. 1962. Das therapeutisch-pädagogische Jugendheim 'Haus Sommerberg'. *Neues Beginnen*, 1.
15. KLÜWER, K. 1964–5. Das therapeutisch-pädagogische Jugendheim 'Haus Sommerberg'. *Jahrbuch der Arbeiterwohlfahrt*, Bonn.
16. KLÜWER, K. 1965. Dissoziale Jugendliche in der Industriegesellschaft. *Prax. Kinderpsychol.*, 14, 113–117.
17. KÜNZEL, E. 1965. Aufnahmekriterien und erste Behandlungsergebnisse (Haus Sommerberg). *Prax. Kinderpsychol.*, 14, 214–215.
18. KÜNZEL, E. 1968. Resozialisierung konfliktgestörter Jugendlicher mit psychotherapeutischen und heilpädagogischen Mitteln. *Prax. Kinderpsychol.*, 7.
19. LEAVITT, H. J. 1958. *Managerial psychology.* Chicago: University of Chicago Press.
20. MOSER, T. and KÜNZEL, E. 1969. *Gespräche mit Eingeschlossenen.* Edition Suhrkamp 375, Suhrkamp Verlag: Frankfurt am Main.
21. PARIN, P. 1961. Die Abwehrmechanismen der Psychopathen. *Psyche, XIV. Jg.*, 1, 322–329.
22. REDL, F. 1958. Strategy and technique of the life space interview. National Institute of Mental Health. U.S. Department of Health, Education and Welfare.
23. WAGNER, H. 1969. Über Werktherapie. Unpublished paper.
24. STOCK WHITAKER, D. and LIEBERMANN, M. A. 1965. *Psychotherapy through the group process.* London: Tavistock Publications.

XIX

RESIDENTIAL TREATMENT OF ADOLESCENTS — A DUTCH REPORT

Professor L. N. J. KAMP and Dr J. A. M. SCHOUTEN

Child Psychiatry Department
University of Utrecht, The Netherlands

1

Introduction

Residential treatment is a drastic procedure for children, adolescents and adults. The decision to resort to it can only be motivated by severe mental disturbance or maladjustment.

Treatment in a residential setting is a complicated process. Various treatment-approaches can be integrated in the total process. It would seem adequate to focus in this chapter upon problems of residential treatment typical for the adolescent phase of life. First, however, we shall go into more or less established rules and existing uncertainties regarding residential treatment in general. We shall try to point out similarities and differences between various approaches and styles in residential treatment. Planned treatment-approaches or strategies will be discussed, and this asks for a certain amount of detachment from the author's personal predilections.

In this way we hope to establish a framework for the second part of this chapter, in which the focus is on psychotherapy in the institution. There we shall try to be more specific. Convictions and choices become a primary concern and we draw heavily on our daily practice in a small open residential unit for adolescent boys, which was set up more than a decade ago.

2

Problems of Organisation and Administration

Some Differences between Residential Institutions

If a child enters an institution, this means that further development in a family setting is no longer possible. The reason for this may be the family's material or psychological qualities. In this case the child may have reasonable possibilities for adjustment in more favourable circumstances. In other cases the motive for placement is mainly found in the child's abnormal behaviour. More often than not this is intensively interwoven with the psychopathology of other family members, notably of the parents, or of the family as a whole.

Keeping this in mind, we may subdivide residential institutions into the following three categories:

A. Homes for children in whom maladjustment is only slight or altogether absent. A living situation is offered, that has as many normal elements as possible. Occasional conflicts or signs of pathology are ignored or treated either with common-sense discipline or with other procedures, without bothering much about the reasons for, or the background of, the particular specimen of unusual behaviour. In these homes no pretence at treatment in a strict sense of the word is found and this approach can best be characterized as *residential care*.

B. Institutions, where abnormal behaviour is one of the motives for taking in children or youth. If problems arise during the child's stay, the significance of signs of pathology is scrutinized with the help of consultant-specialists. Often special modifications in educational approach are made, or maybe even case work or psychotherapy is initiated. In general, however, the staff's energy is mainly expended in appealing to the more healthy aspects of the children's personalities and in reinforcing well adjusted behaviour: *treatment homes*.

C. In this category severely disturbed children are taken in. Major efforts through the physical environment, daily programmes and special approaches relating to the children are attuned to their psychopathology and aimed at modifying it. Symptoms are of great interest, the ideal being a 24-hour treatment plan focused on the disturbance of the child: *psychiatric treatment institution*.

Cultural Factors

In judging therapeutic methods it is important not to forget the cultural matrix in which the institution is placed, either through its locality, or the composition of its staff, or the influence of a central person (Redl[21]) who can function as the managing director, the supervisor of psychotherapy or someone else (Polsky[20]).

Among the historical roots of residential treatment in the Netherlands the following are of importance: orphanages dating partly from the Middle Ages; charitable institutions founded during the first technological revolution in the nineteenth century; laws for the protection of minors, which were passed at the very beginning of the twentieth century.

There has always been an antithesis (either material or psychological) between the child's experiences before entering the institution and the 'good life' to which the adult workers in the institution try to guide the child by means of educational attitudes and other ways and means, consciously planned or taken for granted on the basis of traditional, culturally determined convictions.

Roughly schematizing, we can say that in the Netherlands the main accent in 'helping' these children towards a favourable future is on what is called 'the first milieu', i.e. that part of daily life in which children and adults are together informally. The first milieu comprises meals, getting up, going to bed, some activity programmes, guidance with home-work and involving the pupils in household chores.

Schooling and working at a job are indicated as the second milieu, and leisure as the third milieu.

In England (Kamp[15]) one of us has observed a treatment home (B) where most therapeutic endeavours were concentrated on the second milieu. The teachers of the school, which was part of the institution, had small classes; they had individual contacts with many of their pupils, sometimes supervised by higher staff or specialists. The first milieu was organized along rather strict lines, even to the extent of talking being forbidden during meals. The third milieu was characterized by 'freedom', that is lack of concern on the part of the staff.

During an exchange of thought it became clear that the English institution considered as the rationale of their efforts: the child's relation to his family was improved by his better table manners; the schoolroom offered the best available opportunity for individual contact with the child, and teachers were considered relatively best qualified and motivated for this work.

The Dutch approach through the first milieu is usually explained as reasonable since many behaviour disorders arise from tensions in the family. The first milieu is considered the best ground to reactivate these conflicts and make attempts at solving them.

We shall not enlarge upon the advantages of one system over the other, nor are we inclined to generalize regarding the points of view mentioned above. Our only aim is to draw attention to the differences of treatment-approaches in different countries, which seem to be connected with cultural patterns.

These also seem to play a part in the training of child-care workers. Again the following example only serves as an illustration. Surveys needed for a well-founded appraisal seem to be lacking at the moment. In several residential institutions (B and C) in the United States we find adult workers from three levels of training: the house-parents (active mainly in the realm of the first milieu), the case-workers and group-workers (active in the first and third milieu), and specialists from administrators to psychotherapists. The same levels seem to be found in hospitals: aides, nurses and specialists. This presentation is of course too schematic.

Presenting the Dutch situation in the same simplified form we find only two levels of professionally trained staff. Child-care workers have a more specific training than house-parents. The former can co-operate with the specialists on the basis of some understanding of the problems in the institution. They seldom reach the sophisticated level of the methodical work of the case- or group-workers, however. Household work is done mainly by maids, who can be considered even less as discussion partners on the issues at hand than house-parents or aides.

We do not claim that other arrangements never occur in the United States or that case- and group-workers have not entered to some extent into the field of residential treatment in the Netherlands. We only want to stress once again how national differences in the local way of life and work affect the form of residential treatment.

Treatment Approaches

It has been declared that the organization of a psychiatric residential treatment institution (C) would be ideal if the treatment and education of the patient were the central concern during twenty-four hours of the day. For delinquent adolescents this would mean for instance: personnel familiar with the type of disturbance the youngsters suffer from; skilled staff available, not only during the day but also during the night (breaking out to commit burglaries, to steal, or to go joyriding; sexual acting out, etc.); intensive contacts with parents, schools, jobs; individual and group psychotherapy; recreational programmes with a wide variety of facilities, including well-managed 'inbetween times' (Bettelheim[1]).

The difficulties inherent in such 'total treatment' programmes in terms of money and personnel are evident. There are, however, problems of another nature as well. One of these is the optimal size of the institution. To have optimal (which is not necessarily synonymous with maximal) communication among the staff members, the unit should not be much larger than 20 to 30 patients. For such a relatively small number it is impossible to have recreational facilities for a wide divergence of the children's—often fleeting—interests.

If several units are to be combined to form one organization, so that more recreational facilities would become feasible, we are faced with the problem of homogeneity of population and contagion of pathological behaviour among the patients (Redl[22]).

Children, and certainly adolescents, have a tendency to gang together. In a way this is an age-adequate and healthy trend. In an institution of manageable size (20–30 children living in 3 or 4 groups) one can by means of selection and grouping keep some contagion problems more or less in check, like for instance breaking out at night, homosexual activities, running away, etc. In larger institutions this is much more difficult, unless the units are kept quite separate, but then the recreational facilities can hardly be shared by members of different units.

Larger institutions can generally afford more specialized staff like full-time child psychiatrists, well-trained administrators, in-service training, group therapy, etc.

While touching upon the problem of composing (selecting) groups of young patients, it does not seem clear which rules have been found most useful for the time being. In some 'top institutions', notably in the United States, the focus is on a specific kind of mental disturbance, usually on the basis of strong research interests. Even if diagnostic and etiological problems are hardly ever satisfactorily clear, the behaviour disturbances of the children admitted to these institutions (which specialize for psychotic children; hyper-aggressive children, etc.) are more or less homogeneous. This has the advantage that the facilities can be geared to the reactions and initiatives expected from this special group of children. The main aim of this type of institution is, more often than not, research, which implies generous—if not unlimited—finances. For institutions of lesser means, more limitations have to be set for staff and facilities.

Our adolescent unit 'Zandwijk' at Amersfoort (Kamp,[16] Schouten[28]) is part of the Child Psychiatric Department of the University of Utrecht.

This implies that both training and research are major objectives apart from our curative efforts. Twenty boys (aged 14–20 years) have been living there since 1957 in spacious grounds on the fringe of a provincial town in a rather dilapidated building. We admit a mixture of psychiatric disturbances, from schizoid character disorders to acting-out delinquents.

The ingredients of our therapeutic programme can be grouped roughly under the following three headings:

I. *Methods applied more or less outside daily life in the institution.* Individual and group therapy, psychoanalytically oriented.

The interconnection between these processes and the occurrences in the daily life of the institution will be discussed further in the third part of this chapter.

Family therapy has been added more recently (Blankstein[3]), while it seems sensible to consider behaviour therapy in some cases (Kamp[18]).

II. *Methods integrated in the institution's daily life.* Living together in a small group under constant supervision of trained child-care workers is considered an important chapter of life in the institution. Individual pathology and group dynamics are points of orientation for the adult workers.

In the case of crises in the group or critical incidents with a patient, life-space interviews (Redl[24]) are held either by the managing director, the administrative psychiatrist, or the group leader himself (or herself).

Two case-workers work with the parents, often on the occasion of the boy's frequent visits to their homes. The after-care and foster-home placement also belong to the task of these case-workers. Our experiments with case work in the institution (regular individual contact of a case-worker with one of the pupils) somehow did not turn out very well; but this was the results of complications beyond our control rather than of this method as such being inadequate.

Our attempts at active participation of the boys in the responsibility for the daily management of the home have not been a major factor until now. Very often a boy himself is present at the conference where his problems are discussed by the staff.

III. *Methods pertaining indirectly to the approach of the patient.* By this we mean the phenomena usually referred to as staff-interaction. A great deal goes on informally, and we can distinguish overt or official staff interaction from informal and often hidden staff interaction.

As to the latter, some studies (Stanton and Schwarz,[30] Caudill,[4] Polsky[20]) have described how tensions between patients and an increase of symptomatology may have their source in organizational arrangements, which are not sufficiently—if at all—taken into account.

Tensions among staff members may have a deleterious effect on treatment efforts. One of the unexplored areas in this respect is the personality of the director of the institution. Even if he does not necessarily have to be the 'central person' (Redl[21]), he or she seems to represent an important centre in the network of interactions, and also an easily available screen for the projection of unrealistic experiences by staff members and children. In many instances the director stands for the 'philosophy' of the treatment centre, but it has not been studied in how far his explicit views are connected with culturally determined character traits or with personal experiences contributing smoothly or neurotically to a preference for specific treatment approaches, and styles in administrative procedure.

In every institution for psychiatric patients, where intensive treatment is attempted, an elaborate system of communication has to be established. The staff, who share daily life with a group of patients, should meet frequently. Usually these unit-conferences have two separate, though connected, objectives:

(*a*) evaluation of group life, incidents and crises; planning how these facts will modify future action;

(*b*) evaluation of the treatment plan of one particular patient over a longer stretch of time; changing treatment goals in connection with progress made or failure to achieve this. Sometimes it is useful for a greater diversity of workers (therapists, director, clinical psychologist, etc.) to participate in the (*b*) conferences.

Several other contacts are necessary for a co-ordination of efforts based on optimal communication.

Highly trained staff should be available for daily consultation on problems that are liable to arise. We characterize these contacts as 'sharing responsibility in co-operation' (the literal translation of the Dutch term 'work companionship'), rather than supervision. Supervision in the more restricted sense of the term is used only for regular interviews between a supervisee and a person with more experience and/or more training. Here the subject-matter is still the work with patients (daily care or psychotherapy), but the aim is to increase the professional skill of the supervisee.

We shall discuss neither the reasons why supervision i.s.s. is useful for some and not for other staff members, nor the advantages and disadvantages of supervisors being staff members or persons who are not connected with the institution.

Sometimes a need for psychotherapy for the supervisee comes to light. This is then realized outside the realm of the institution and does not belong to the field of staff interaction as such. Obviously therapy of the workers may have repercussions on their work and consequently on the institution.

We consider in-service training an important device to achieve optimal treatment. Training on the job can take different forms, and supervision can be considered one of these. Other ways to increase the staff's standards are: the giving of courses, usually theoretical introductions, followed by discussions; literature seminars; psychodrama sessions with discussion, etc. Conferences on household matters, planning for holidays, festivities, etc., add considerably to the pattern of communication.

These remarks on the organization of staff interaction might mistakenly give the impression that clarity of role and aim can be achieved in all contacts. This of course is neither possible nor desirable, as flexibility and improvisation are also essential features of institutional life at its best.

Each of the approaches mentioned under I, II and III would require a chapter to do justice to its importance, but this would go beyond the limits set for this chapter.

Individual psychotherapy in a residential setting, however, will be described in some more detail further on. Before going into that subject, some remarks are made on treatment planning and on administrative problems.

Treatment Planning

In thinking about treatment planning we are concerned with the phenomenological characteristics of the patient's devious behaviour and with the factors which might have contributed to the development of his condition. The very fact that child and adolescent psychiatry is a young science makes for differences of terminology and for theoretical frames of reference varying with countries, institutions and researchers.

Even if we find a more or less fitting set of models (organo-physiological model; psychogenetic or cathexis model; psychosocial model; learning theory model and many others) to account for the psychopathological syndrome, this does not necessarily mean that a treatment plan can be brought into practice, if it is based upon these data (Craft *et al.*,[6] Dumont[7]).

Ideally the psychiatric theory and model are rationally connected with the theory of treatment and the strategies involved. One of the outstanding qualities of the classic study by Redl and Wineman[26, 27] on hyper-aggressive children is the separation of theoretical explanations of pathological behaviour from strategies to influence the behaviour in question, though an attempt is made to connect the two aspects (explanation and action) in a sensible way. At the present stage of our knowledge it cannot be stressed enough that there is a need for scientific evaluation of treatment strategies in their own right. If an explanatory model can be integrated in such studies, so much the better. The study of the effect of a certain treatment-approach is a worthy subject in its own right, irrespective of the explanatory theories and models, which gave rise to the approach (method) or seem to contradict it. It is self-evident that research of this sort cannot be accomplished without more well-run institutions and more well-trained staff.

For those therapeutically active in the field it is only natural to stress in their studies certain elements in their strategy which seem of special importance to them. To give an example: some have stressed the work with parents, almost implying that inventiveness and energy aimed at improving the parents' attitudes are more important to the child than other treatment skills, even when he is treated in a residential setting. Others (Bettelheim,[2] Kamp[17]) consider it of great importance that the child in a residential setting may be temporarily protected from unfavourable influences from the side of the parents. For this reason some of the parents should not become too closely involved in the treatment process during long parts of the child's stay. How to do this in a hygienic way cannot be described in a few sentences.

This is clearly not an 'either or' issue. The character of the illness, the involvement of the parents in the child's disturbance, the severity of the illness, etc., have to be considered. Here also the child's age is an important factor. In the case of adolescents with clearly pathogenic parents we shall be more inclined to reduce the parents' influence. In this case the explanatory model (psychopathology closely connected with, if not caused by, family interaction) does not form the basis for a causal treatment strategy, i.e. intensive case-work with the parents.

Administrative Technique

The duties of an administrator of a treatment home (in the sense of manager of the institution) call for as many skills as any other job. Specifically designed training programmes for this job are non-existent. Delegating tasks to others in a clear and psychologically clean way may be one of the most important assets, since this contributes greatly to role-clarity and creates a climate of co-operation. Often the responsibility for taking decisions cannot be delegated to others. The administrator trained as a child psychiatrist or in another profession is more often confronted with too many data, too great a variety of information, too many sources (people) that contribute.

Of the many points of view from which a treatment decision can be reached, two will be mentioned. In the first case the patient as an entity is focused on; later we apply the same train of thought to the institution as a whole.

Traditionally, in deciding upon a future course to be chosen, the patient as an entity is focused upon. Ideally the treatment situation should touch both upon the patient's strong points and upon his vulnerable spots, so that he can work on his problems in a fruitful way and mental growth and stabilization will arise. In other words, his ego-functions should be activated, but not overtaxed. We refer to this state of affairs as 'the optimal level of conflict (or anxiety) for the patient'. If a patient is very ill indeed and everybody involved agrees that supportive measures are called for, the situation can be characterized as: 'The patient's level of conflict is too high.' Then the environment has to function as an auxiliary ego in an attempt to diminish the conflicting forces in the patient's basic psychopathology.

On the other hand, some patients in residential treatment go through periods in which little seems to happen. The symptoms persist, the patient's behaviour shows few changes. The suspicion then arises that the treatment situation does not tax the patient heavily enough. Insufficient incentives to ego-activity seem to exist. If this is the case, we may then characterize the situation as: 'The patient's level of conflict (or anxiety) is too low.'

The introduction of the quasi-quantitative concept 'individual level of conflict' may help to integrate heterogeneous data from different sources, when decisions have to be made. Often it is relatively easy for a team to agree whether the patient's level of conflict is too high or too low. After that it is also relatively easy to find a basis for choosing adequate measures to attain a more optimal level; easier in fact than when we start off by choosing between opposing alternatives, the merits of which can be advocated depending on one's point of view.

The following example (Kamp[15]) may illustrate the foregoing discussion:

John, aged 15, passive and withdrawn, refuses to attend school. He is intelligent and has no learning disturbance, but he complains about the many school rules and states that he is not understood at school. He wants to start practical work 'to be more independent'. Group leader I reports: 'John is generally more unmanageable; he incites unrest in the group; what is to become of the boy if he has not even got a school certificate?'

Group leader II is himself not active nor domineering; he is less worried by

John's unrest, shows some doubts, but tends to support group leader I in his advice to force John to attend school by pedagogical pressure, persuasion, stimulation and, if necessary, by sanctions.

The occupational therapist finds John more active than previously. John's attitude reveals a search for protection and support; his manual work yields more finished products. He seems more creative. These findings are reported at the conference of head leaders and specialists. The group therapist adds: John seems preoccupied and not always attentive, but sometimes he flares up and is remarkably fierce. No life-space interviews have been held recently with John. The psychotherapist reports: At the moment John shows considerable uncertainty about his orientation in the female or the male direction. A preference for female identification, which arose under the pressure of family tensions, is occasionally interrupted by attempts at more assertive behaviour. There are indications that the refusal to attend school is an expression of his inclination to reach a more active attitude, although it is also a flight from the consequences of conflicts at school. Forcing him to attend school might have the regrettable result of impairing elaboration of the problems of this rebellious initiative.

According to the social worker, the parents adopt an injured attitude, both towards John (in whom they condemn really everything) and towards Zandwijk, which does not sufficiently take into account the parents' wishes. It is even contended that the parents were insufficiently informed about John's transfer to Zandwijk (from another institution), although this is not in accordance with established facts. John's failure to attend school will be interpreted by the parents as the acme of mismanagement, and the social worker finds herself unable to render this acceptable to the parents.

In the staff discussion it was concluded that John's development showed signs of progress. There was no aggravation of his inhibitions and withdrawal (*vide* group therapy, occupational therapy, psychotherapy). His 'misbehaviour' in the group seemed to be a search for a new pattern of behaviour. So his ego does not seem to be overburdened.

In other words his level of conflict is not too high. Too much increase of the level of conflict did not seem desirable, since he had to cope with many tensions already. On the other hand, if some strategy would involve the risk for such a rise of conflict level, some leeway for this could still be supposed to be present.

With regard to possible measures, it must be borne in mind that forcing him to attend school would lower his level of conflict: he might relapse into the previous pattern of passive resistance and no further discussion with the parents would be required because their wish would be fulfilled. Tolerance for his refusal to attend school is liable to raise John's level of conflict, although superficially it might seem that in this way no demands are made and consequently his conflict level would be lowered. In this case, however, John would be forced to dwell on the consequences of his more active initiatives (refusal to go to school).

It was decided that he would be allowed to stay away from school if he wished to, although he was informed of our opinion that it would be better if he continued to attend school. He will not be assisted in finding work, nor will he be hampered in trying to achieve this. As a result, John will have a chance to remain in his more active oppositional attitude. Our policy will be discussed with him by the deputy director. A discussion in the style of a life-space interview is considered too disruptive at this stage of his psychotherapy.

The supervisor of group leader I will discuss the situation with him, with special reference to the group leader's own authoritative tendencies and his difficulty in tolerating conflicts of authority such as those with John.

The steps essential to John at this period would seem to lie in his psychotherapeutic hours. Confrontation of his rebellious initiatives with his parents can hardly be expected to be very constructive (it might easily raise his level of conflict too much) in view of his parent's inflexibility and irreconcilable attitude. John's powers of growth should remain concentrated in Zandwijk. The social worker will attempt to keep the parents from interfering. For the time being, there is little promise of an essential change in their attitudes. In the presence of these conflicts, it seems undesirable to allow John to visit his home. The parents may be able to accept this, regarding it as 'a punishment for John'.

The main help we have derived from using the concept 'level of conflict' has been to find a common coinage in evaluating heterogeneous information. This goes for the data concerning the actual state of the patient as well as for the various suggestions from heterogeneous sources (staff members) as to the choice of strategy.

A similar way of reasoning can be of use when problems arise concerning the institution as a whole. Occasionally the institution shows increased malfunctioning (to be compared with individual psychopathology): increased acting-out of patients, which disrupts the treatment process; illness of staff members; less intensive participation of patients and staff in programmed activities; staff members planning to leave; indications of increased 'informal staff interaction' of a gossipy nature, etc.

Strategically this calls for supportive measures to lower the institution's conflict level: giving more opportunity for letting off steam in staff contacts; organizing a visit to another institution to increase staff cohesion; increased in-service activity, etc.; discharge of a patient who seems to overtax whatever resilience his fellow-patients, educators and therapists may be able to muster.

Indications that the level of conflict of the institution is too low are sometimes the same as those enumerated above, although the staff discussions tend to be less heated; disease and drop out of the staff does not increase. One of the activities to move to a more favourable level of conflict may be the active planning of new treatment programmes; other possible remedies are the pointing out and working through slackness in routine with more intensity and strictness; considering removal of staff members who cannot or will not function within the framework of the institution, etc.

These remarks on administrative procedures are too schematic to have any pretence of doing justice to the complexities of life in a treatment institution. Administrative duties can, however, constitute a fascinating task even for a well-trained psychiatrist. In any case there is more to it than being a doctor who knows the answers or who reassures people when he doesn't know them.

3

Treatment Plan

In 1927 Anna Freud, in her *Einführung in die Technik der Kinderanalyse* described how some of her young patients could not sufficiently benefit from her therapeutic efforts because of the adverse influence of the parental milieu. She stressed the need to create children's homes, in which the life conditions would be geared to psychoanalytic principles. In the following decades many such treatment homes were created, each with its own style, and emphasizing either the individual psychotherapy or the 'milieu' treatment (Cotter Hirschberg,[5] Bettelheim,[2] Redl[23]). During the same period, many of the numerous existing homes for neglected and disturbed children—including offenders—recognized the need for psychiatric support, and invited psychotherapists to participate in their work.

In both types of institutions one is confronted with the problem of the optimal relationship between the individual psychotherapy and the milieu-treatment part of the programme. Should psychotherapy in such institutions have the same isolated position as is characteristic for the prevalent method in the treatment on an 'out-patient' basis? Should, accordingly, the psychotherapist keep himself aloof and shrink from any interaction with the significant persons in the patient's life milieu? Or should therapy be integrated in the total treatment programme of the institution?

In the treatment centre 'Zandwijk' we have opted for the second alternative (de Levita[19]). During its ten years' existence we have been working out programmes of interaction and communication to promote the integration of the individual psychotherapy in the total treatment design. In the next paragraphs we shall describe why we choose to do so, and what the practical implications of such a combined treatment programme are.

Limiting Conditions

Before proceeding we might first mention some of the patients' characteristics and the situations they live in, as far as these characteristics have a special bearing on the topic concerned.

1. Our patients are *adolescent boys*, 14–18 years of age. The specific resistances to psychotherapy of this particular age group are well known and described in detail by Anna Freud[12] and Selma Fraiberg.[11] We may mention a few: the resistance to develop an intimate relationship with an adult, which would remind the youngster of his early infantile ties with his parents; the ensuing resistance against the recollection of the past. Both trends seem to be adverse to the process of a classical analysis.

2. Our patients are not only adolescents but *emotionally disturbed adolescents*. Most of them belong to the category usually labelled 'neurotically acting-out' patients. They show a preference for specific mechanisms

to cope with their anxieties and depressive feelings. We frequently see for instance: a tendency to deny the feelings of anxiety and sorrow, any 'soft' feelings in general; a tendency to overcome those feelings with bravado; a tendency to fight the inner anxieties with externalized ones, which produces the need for thrilling experiences (i.e. delinquent activities) (Schouten[28]). It is obvious that these specific defences do not facilitate the possibilities of a psychotherapeutic approach, the more so when the 'tough guy' attitude is part of the subculture of the peer group they live in.

3. *The impact of institutional life.* Although each boy before admission has agreed to a one- or two-years' stay in the treatment home, some come to feel their stay as compulsory in the course of time, and, as most of them have been sent by children's courts, as a punishment. The judge, and the staff of the institution, including the psychotherapist may be regarded as a group of overpowering adults, the patients being at the mercy of the manipulation of these powers.

These negative feelings may be increased by the restriction of freedom that the institution imposes upon the patients, a restriction necessitated partly by the inevitable rules and regulations that any community organisation needs, partly by the need to set limits to the patients' symptoms: stealing, car theft, burglary, sexual aberrations involving young children, etc.

They go out to schools and jobs in the neighbourhood, but they are expected to be on the premises for the rest of the time (except for organised outings, special courses, sport events, etc.). No matter how reasonable these limitations are, adolescents may regard them as major infractions upon their freedom.

These notions of being punished, manipulated and contained may considerably endanger any successful treatment effort, since they create reactions of apathy and dependence, and/or passive and active resistance. These reactions have a blurring effect on the diagnostic evaluation of the patient's behaviour, since his original problems tend to blend with the situationally determined reactions. Then it becomes hard to tell what is the patient's 'personal neurosis' and what is his 'institutional neurosis'!

4. *The impact of group life in the institution.* (*a*) The small group (composed of not more than 6 or 7 boys) guided by 3 counsellors (2 male, 1 female) resembles in certain respects a family group. The continuous living with counsellors and fellow-patients with its numerous interactions, calls for intensive and sometimes intimate relationships. Since counsellors take over definite parental functions, the patients will tend to feel for them both love and hatred, at least partly determined by earlier experiences in their families. It naturally follows that it is much more likely that they will invest their strongest emotional reactions in the counsellors and the fellow-patients than in the therapist.

(*b*) Groups of these boys sometimes develop a 'delinquent' climate; delinquent activities are in high esteem, the 'tough guy' ideal is strongly enforced, a trustful relationship with adults is considered a sign of weakness. As in all groups, boys of this type invest much energy in the struggle for power in the group. A rigid pecking order may develop, with clearly defined roles for each member of the group. Since in most cases the kind of role that one gets assigned by the others is related to one's original pathology, a structure of rigid role assignments will usually perpetuate deviant attitudes and prevent progress (Polsky [20]).

5. *The impact of parental influence.* In cases where the patients' deviant behaviour seems to be highly related to specific pathogenic influences of their parents, just the physical removal from home does not stop this influence.

Some patients may profit from this 'vacation' of too intense, energy-consuming, daily conflicts at home. In other cases, both parents and patients seem to continue their old mutual perceptions and attitudes because of the lack of sufficient interaction. More interaction, painful as it would be, would possibly open up new ways of looking at each other.

Summing up the conditions under which individual psychotherapy of delinquent adolescents in a residential setting is to take place, we come up with an impressive list of items which seem to be adverse to the goals of psychotherapy. Adolescents do not easily enter into an intimate relationship with an adult; they dislike talking about the past; delinquent adolescents tend to deny feelings of anxiety and depression; the institutional life itself is the cause of additional conflicts, which are not always easily separated from the original ones; the patients are likely to develop relationships with people connected with the life milieu, rather than with the therapist. A delinquent subculture of the group threatens the development of a trusting relationship with the therapist; a rigid role-structure in the group may prevent members from experimenting with new attitudes.

When conditions seem to be so unfavourable, how can we still effect treatment with some success?

It seems obvious that a great deal of our efforts should be aimed at improving these conditions. This entails:

—an effort to model institutional life so as to meet the needs of adolescents;

—an effort to adapt the therapist's attitude to the age-specific defenses and anxieties;

—an effort to have psychotherapy supported, by any other persons and means available in the institution;

—an effort to support the treatment-approaches in the life milieu by whatever insights are gained from the individual psychotherapy.

Ideally this would result in an integrated treatment strategy, which would promote the full employment of the many resources that a residential treatment centre should have at its disposal.

Life Conditions in the Institution

It is of no use to try individual psychotherapy when the life situation in the institution is characterized by standardized, repressive regulations of a mass of people.

Although it is very hard to abolish all the disadvantages of institutional life, it is possible, at least in small institutions, to limit mass regulations and standardized procedures (concerning, for instance, rewards and punishments) to a great extent. In 'Zandwijk' each boy has his own programme for schooling, job-training and recreational activities, geared to his individual capacities and interests. This individual-oriented programme, together with the architectural arrangement (bedrooms for one or two boys, each boy keeping the key of his own room) facilitates sufficient possibilities for the privacy which adolescents need badly. Constant group-living would make it very hard for them to build up, or maintain, an ego-identity; their weak egos would yield easily to the more powerful group-ego.

Reactions of passive resistance, created by the feeling of being manipulated by the overpowering adult establishment can largely be dealt with when patients can actively participate in their own treatment programme.

Our recently developed policy of inviting the boys to staff meetings concerning their programme proved to have a corrective effect on the distorted and paranoid ideas regarding the staff and the contents of their meetings.

The detrimental effect of a persisting delinquent climate in a group has been mentioned above. Training programmes carried out by a group therapist help counsellors and staff to deal with this problem. Insight in the dynamics of role-assignment and role-taking in groups and the techniques of undoing rigid role-structures will free group members to experiment with different, diversified roles with the ultimate goal of finding their true selves as individuals whose behaviour is not simply defined by the group.

The restriction of freedom and of the scope of the patients' circle of social interactions remains a knotty problem. We improved the situation by assigning the role of 'boarder' to those boys who seem to be approaching the end of their stay in the centre. This status gives them much more freedom and also more responsibility concerning the way they spend both their time and money.

If an institution does not take adequate measures to counteract the detrimental effects characteristic of the massive, standardized approach of large institutions, the inmates will use their 'therapeutic' sessions for an endless recounting of the situationally determined frustrations, leaving the therapist with the embarrassing alternative whether or not to take sides against the staff of the institution.

Adaption of Therapy-content to the Patients' Actual Institutional Life

From our description of the impact of the institution and group life on the patients' behaviour it follows that we cannot look at the institutionalized patient as a person who simply lives under a different roof and will neatly present the internal problems of his pre-admission period.

Since the situational change seems to be of vital importance, the therapist should be well aware of the sequence of phases that patients go through when admitted to an institution. During the first few months of the patients' stay it does not seem wise to focus too much on the earlier problems, since most of the boys have quite an amount of problems in getting adjusted to the new situation. We may mention for instance:

1. The state of mourning, caused by the factual separation from their parents, no matter how ambivalent the relation with them may have been.

2. The state of confusion about norms and values, which is caused by the ideology of the institution. In 'progressive' institutions the system of values may be very different from the family ideology, some actions (even delinquent actions) seem to be taken for granted by the staff in the eyes of the newcomer, whereas the open communication between patients and staff may be equally unfamiliar to him.

3. The newcomer also experiences a great deal of anxiety because of the threat that emanates from the group of peers. The struggle as to who controls whom is very fierce in groups like ours. It is not so much a physical threat as a psychological one, but therefore not less vital to the newcomer. He has to expend a great deal of energy in order to survive in the group. Since some of our patients are only poorly equipped with the needed survival mechanisms, they have to learn it the hard and long way.

In this adjustment phase it is commonly observed that the original symptoms subside. This is a sign that the original internal conflicts have been superseded by the current conflicts of adjustment to the new situation. The therapist might therefore as well focus his attention on the current rather than on the earlier problems. If the therapist is sufficiently acquainted with the vicissitudes of daily life in the institution, he may give the boy active and effective support. Consequently the patient gets proof of the fact that his therapist may be of real importance to him. This, again, favours the development of the next stages of therapy.

When, in the next phase, the patient is adjusted to the new environment, he usually relapses into his earlier symptoms and also into his earlier patterns of relationship. His attitude towards counsellors and fellows increasingly shows the characteristics of his former attitude towards members of his family. When, in the course of sessions, the patient brings up his interactions with counsellors and fellow-patients, many details show the projective nature of the perception of the environment. The therapist can elaborate extensively on the vicissitudes of the here-and-now situation and in the second place relate them to the patient's life-history, elucidating the projective quality of his attitudes and the repetitive nature of his behaviour.

It must be recognized that the transference of emotions on to a counsellor is bound to be less lucid than in classical therapy, due to his active, daily interaction with the patient, which brings an equal share of the counsellor's personality to the fore. If the therapist is fully integrated in the life of the institution and knows the counsellors well, he may be able to separate the patient's realistic reactions to the environment from the ones originating in distorted perceptions. As far as counter-transferential feelings on the part of the counsellors seem to play a part, this calls for training and supervision programmes.

Although it was stated above that the emotional investment of the patient is likely to be strongest in the daily life environment, it is obvious that the therapist will also come in for his share in the projections of anxiety and aggression. Like everyone else in the small community, he is assigned a role that fits into the total pattern of familiar relationships carried over to the institution.

We have observed how a patient tends to assign contrary roles to the therapist and the director, respectively, thereby creating an atmosphere of conflict between the two, which he tries to exploit for his own benefit, sometimes successfully, as he used to do with his ever-quarrelling parents. This example shows that the concept of transference should neither be limited to feelings regarding a therapist, nor to those regarding any other single person in the institution, but that we have to look for the carry-over of more complicated patterns of relationships. It also follows that the handling of these phenomena should not be limited to the therapeutic sessions, but should be extended to the life milieu as well. This calls for extensive communication between staff members, lest they fall victims to the various ambushes set up for them.

Mutual Support of Psychotherapy and Life-milieu Approaches

Being aware of the number of factors inimical to therapy, we would do better by looking for approaches that may be supportive to individual psychotherapy. The fact that the individual psychotherapy is situated in a residential centre, provides possibilities for these supportive techniques: the pedagogical staff, group therapists, counsellors and social workers may all contribute to these efforts.

This is advisable, for instance, in cases where sufficient motivation is lacking. The director, or someone else, then enters into a series of talks with the boy, explaining the necessity of change in particular aspects of his behaviour. These sessions may be useful in helping the boy to realize what exactly is unacceptable about his behaviour, or to explain what makes his behaviour ineffective for reaching the goals he attempts to reach. Also, if the boy keeps blaming other people for all his disturbing behaviour, he should be made aware of this 'Evaporation of self-contributed links in the causal chain', as Redl calls it. Especially in the 'hard' cases it is of great importance to give these reality-oriented comments on the patients' behaviour right on the spot.

Fritz Redl has reported extensively on these 'marginal interviews', later called Life-Space-Interviews (Redl[24]). They play an important part in the milieu treatment and have a beneficial effect in themselves, but they may also stimulate the psychotherapeutic process. The purpose of these interviews is to build up an observing ego, which is a necessary implement of the reflective attitude, needed in psychotherapy. This part of the work can best be done by the people who actually live with the patients, because they are on the spot when the disturbed behaviour manifests itself.

Individual psychotherapy, when carried out in a residential centre, can make use of the fact that the daily vicissitudes of the patients in the institution are within the reach of the therapist. If the therapists are fully involved in staff meetings at all levels, they get an abundance of detailed information about behaviour aspects of their patients that would never spontaneously show up during any therapeutic hour. Even though they may not always use the factual contents of this information in their sessions, the therapists may at least apply it to attain a better understanding of the patient and to be able to realize quickly the significance of minor clues, brought up by the patients.

One day, it was reported that a patient was busy digging rectangular holes. Upon questioning him it seemed that the purpose of this was unknown to him. Later in the course of that day he threw a crucifix out of the window, without knowing why. When—at the next session—the therapist led the conversation to these incidents, they proved to be highly relevant to important therapeutic topics: the boy could be made aware of his depression and terrifying guilt-feelings, that seemed to exist on an unconscious level until then. This illustrates the point that minor incidents in daily life may have a significance, equivalent to the classical source of unconscious material: dreams and free associations. Since this last mentioned source is usually lacking in therapy with adolescents, the first mentioned may at least partially make up for the loss.

We may now summarize the resulting characteristics of this kind of individual psychotherapy. Since hardly any dreams or free association material are available, much of the contents centres around ego-psychological phenomena. The shortcomings of ego-functioning are detected as the distortion of reality and the inability to postpone gratifications. The patients can be made aware of these shortcomings by the therapist's repeated anticipation of the troubles into which these shortcomings may lead him, and by the offering of alternative coping techniques.

Another aspect concerns the patient's distorted relationship with his immediate environment. The therapist relates this to the patient's earlier experiences in his family, and unveils with him the repetitive nature of this phenomenon with the ultimate purpose of helping him to perceive people as they really are and relate to them accordingly.

Another aspect focuses on the dynamics of defences. The therapist can show the patient how his bravado and his addiction to thrilling experiences originate in the need to cover up his feelings of depression and rejection, which—in turn—may stem from the (emotional) loss of significant persons in his early life.

Two comments are to be made in this connection:

1. The core of the kind of therapy described here seems to consist of ego-support and the promotion of insight on the part of the patient. Since a full transference towards the therapist does not usually develop, the corrective emotional experience needed is lacking in most cases. This experiential correction, however, may be produced effectively in the life milieu, if we consider it as the goal of milieu treatment and gear our programme to attain this goal.

2. If we should break through the defences that mask the underlying depressive feelings (from which many of these adolescents suffer), we may produce a full-blown depression with the concomitant danger of suicide. The uncovering of the depression, which the patient tries to ward off, should therefore be accompanied by the building up of new resources in terms of new experiences, achievements and relations in the daily life in the institution; the tie with the therapist, however helpful it may be, is insufficient in a case of life and death.

These two comments bring us to the topic of the next paragraph.

The Therapist's Attitudes and Techniques

In the course of time we came to favour the following attitudes as most helpful to overcome the adolescents' resistances to therapy. Considering the adolescent's fear of an intimate relationship with an adult, therapists do not explicitly encourage the boy 'to tell everything that comes to his mind' with the reassurance 'that everything will be kept between the two of us'. We found that comments like these are not reassuring at all but instead apt to arouse great anxiety, not only because they stress a close intimacy but also because the patient feels this as a downright attempt at intruding into his secret fantasy life.

Many adolescents regard a psychiatrist as a spying adult, and attribute to him magic abilities. They endow him with the power of mind-reading and the power of changing their personality against their will. Since the fear of losing one's identity is very strong in adolescents (Erikson[9] described this phenomenon as 'identity-resistance'), therapists should avoid anything in their appearance and attitude that would support this distorted view. Selma Fraiberg[11] recommends the therapist 'to negate his image of the omnipotent psychiatrist by being quite simply human, open, unmysterious and not too clever'. In a residential centre we can reduce our mysteriousness by occasionally participating in social meetings with the boys, such as having tea, playing soccer, joining sailing trips. Therapists in 'Zandwijk' have been participating in summer camps abroad, organized for the boys.

Since most adolescents, when starting psychotherapeutic sessions, are in a state of tension, which prevents them from speaking freely, the therapist should introduce tension-reducing devices such as bringing up conflict-free topics. Long silences should be avoided, since they are unbearable for most adolescents. It is clear that the above-mentioned recommendations circumvent the interpretation of the resistances which is the chosen method in classical analysis. We feel, however, that direct interpretation of these resistances would be very threatening and could have the effect of increasing resistance.

Many adolescents' therapies wither because of the lack of emotionally significant material. The patients, although they know it is their 'own fault', resent this increasingly and may decide to terminate sessions. Therapists in 'Zandwijk' do not refrain from actively introducing certain topics concerning incidents or relational problems occurring in the institution. Although this may be embarrassing for the patient, it seems to be advisable, at least in those cases where valuable material does not appear for quite a long time.

Total Treatment: a Joint effort of Individual Psychotherapy and Other Treatment Approaches

In trying to define the goals of treatment (for our particular type of patients) we may—with inevitable oversimplification—mention the following:

1. Gradually breaking down the inadequate regulatory (defence-) mechanisms, replacing them by more adequate ones.
2. Helping them to overcome the depressive feelings which subsequently come to the fore, and which led to the inadequate behaviour in the first place, by providing emotional experiences that negate their feelings of being rejected and of not being respected.
3. Changing the self-concept, which entails the increase of self-esteem. As the concept of self is largely shaped by the role one gets assigned by one's environment, this calls for the assignment of a new and more healthy role by the new environment.

Individual psychotherapy can undoubtedly contribute to attaining these objectives. Since adolescents usually do not 'cathect' their therapist to a high degree, and the situation in an institution forces them to 'cathect' the adults and the group constituting their immediate environment instead, the necessary corrective emotional experience should be provided by other treatment approaches.

We shall consider the above mentioned treatment goals one by one and try to illustrate the respective contributions of individual psychotherapy and other treatment approaches in attaining these goals.

1. *Handling the Defences*

(*a*) *The need for thrill.* We adhere to the assumption that defences have an adaptive function and are meant to maintain some sort of equilibrium in the patient. Consequently we should not try to abolish these defensive needs all at once; especially—as is the case with the need for thrill—when they seem to be related to the specific needs of adolescents.

When the relationship between the therapist and the patient has been firmly established, it can certainly be discussed with the patient that he is so much involved in the excitement of scheming and carrying out delinquent activities, in order not to think too much about his failures at school and about the rejection by his parents. As long as these feelings are unbearable for him, and as long as his group of peers stimulates these thrill-producing activities we may as well count on their continuation. In a residential centre we may attack or even use these needs in a different way.

In the past years our group therapist (Hirsch[13]) has been experimenting with activity groups of 'Zandwijk'-boys, in which the activities were mainly centred round the production of a film. They were taught to handle the equipment, asked to compose a plot, and to play the parts. The discussions leading to the choice of a plot provided an abundance of delinquent fantasies, bringing the delinquent subculture into the open and within the reach of the therapist. The actual producing of the film asked for a high level of constructive co-operation between the boys. The films invariably turned out to be 'thrillers'. This method made use of the need for thrill, kept the delinquent tendencies on a fantasy level and provided the patients with a new experience: that a constructive, socialized action can produce both excitement and the satisfaction of having accomplished something 'great', i.e. that rewarding activities do not necessarily have to be delinquent ones.

(*b*) *The tendency to deny 'soft feelings'.* The individual case-histories of our patients report that they have been quite sensitive in their early years. Subsequent traumatic experiences, too hard to be borne, caused a gradual de-sensitization, and a warding-off of softer feelings. Some of them, when psychotherapy was already fairly well under way, have explained when and why they decided to 'harden' themselves in order to be able to cope with life. This psychological 'callousness' has obviously the same protective function as its physical equivalent. Individual psychotherapy is the chosen method for gradually peeling off the hard layers and bringing the weak and painful spots into the open. That adolescents (and other patients as well) resist this process is natural enough. In adolescents living in a group, resistance to this process may be forcefully heightened by their alliance to the standards of the group, which is likely to adhere strongly to the 'tough-guy' attitude. Fritz Redl[25] phrases this phenomenon as 'the gang under the couch'.

In a residential centre one is in the advantageous position of having that gang, to which one's patient belongs, operating on one's own premises. In any table discussion this 'tough-guy' attitude may come up. Depending on the counsellor's knowledge and skill he may succeed—usually with the help of a few members of the group—in breaking up this group code. It must be said, however, that changing the code of the group culture is one of the hardest jobs in the total programme of residential treatment.

2. *The State of Depression*

It has already been mentioned that breaking down the defences may result in the development of a depression. When discussing therapy in regard with children, Irene Josselyn[14] states: 'To tell a child that he behaves the way he does because he is angry while his mother does not love him, is only to define a vacuum; it leaves the child with the same problem of facing a world fraught with danger for him unless he *is* loved and protected'. The same is true for adolescents. If we simply interpret the patient's deviant behaviour as the result of his being unloved and unrespected, he would have a choice between fanatically denying it and yielding to it whereupon he would find himself in a terrible void, unless he has found in the institution a few people to whom he can relate with some mutual sympathy and respect. It may be wise to guide the 'depth' of therapeutic interpretation on the basis of the establishment of at least the beginning of a stable relationship, either with the therapist or with someone else in the institution.

3. *The Self Concept*

A 'lack of love' has usually its concomitant in a 'lack of self-esteem' (Fenichel[10]). In psychotherapy the irrealistic, neurotic grounds for the patient's self-depreciation may be uncovered and discussed. This, in combination with the atmosphere of respect and authenticity that should pervade the basic attitude of the therapist and other members of the staff, can help to heighten the patient's self-esteem. There are, however, some realistic grounds for their low self-esteem. Robert White[31] considers a healthy self-esteem to be the result of cumulative experiences of having accomplished something as well as of the ensuing confidence that one is competent for tasks to come, which confidence is endorsed by positive expectations on the part of the environment. Many of our 'Zandwijk'-boys can look back only at a cumulation of failures. They consequently lack any confidence in future achievements, which is one of the reasons why they commit themselves to delinquent careers. It is our experience that, unless we get them to accomplish something worth while, treatment is bound to fail. Therefore we desperately search for some signs of hidden interests and talents that might provide them with the satisfaction necessary to support the self-esteem.

We have been experimenting with a year-round activity programme, centred round a summer camp abroad. Going far away appealed to their

Q

adventurous natures and motivated them to enter into a variety of activities to prepare them for the great journey ahead, such as learning foreign languages, car repair, filming, first-aid and the like (Eijer[8]).

A number of our patients, although intellectually quite gifted, have been constantly failing at schools. For them we have a small classroom, where a teacher, by whatever unorthodox methods, gets them to absorb small units of scholastic knowledge. The number, as well as the standard of the tasks has to be very modest, and the time set to master them very short. Within a couple of months, when success is guaranteed beyond reasonable doubt, they take an official examination. (A special educational system, called IVIO provides for such possibilities in the Netherlands.) The small success arouses some hope in them, and greater achievements may follow. In some cases we managed to free them of their paralysing fear of failure, whereupon they could attend a normal school.

The distorted self-concepts, from which many of these boys suffer, may have their roots in the early history of the family, where, for whatever reasons, a certain image emerged, e.g. 'the naughty one', 'the stupid one', 'the crazy one', or more complicated images such as 'the one who, by virtue of his brilliance and vigour, would make up for the ever-failing, incompetent father'. The self-image of the boy is modelled to a great extent after these expectations of him harboured by his environment; he behaves in accordance with the role assigned to him. When the patient comes to the institution he will probably continue in this acquired role. In individual psychotherapy, the simple recounting of a few incidents in the interaction with counsellors and group may provide a number of clues that show the qualities of this specific role. It may be the role of the passive victim, or of the tyrant-killer, always trying to emasculate the male adults and take their envied places, or the role of the detached observer who functions as an umpire in the group.

These role aspects of their behaviour can be intellectually clarified during the sessions. Furthermore, when these attitudes also show themselves in the relation to the therapist, he can interpret them while at the same time refusing to play the complementary role that the patient tends to assign to him, in order to make both roles fit, which would enable the patient to perpetuate his own.

In some cases, the historical roots of the distorted self-concept and the role, related to this concept, may be touched upon. It then becomes clear to what extent the patient's role is influenced by parental attitudes and expectations. The patient may become aware that he is still regarding his future development in terms of yielding to, or defying, parental expectations, rather than seeking, as an independent individual, the routes that lead to a unique self-realization.

The problem with adolescents is that they, unlike adult patients, *are* factually dependent on their parents to a great extent, both financially and otherwise.

Even when our patients are in the institution, parents still have an enormous impact on the adolescents' perception of themselves and their mutual relationship. They may continue to ventilate their highly ambitious prospects of the boys' future development, or show down-right rejection again and again.

The logical consequence of this problem is that parents should be helped to change their way of looking at the boy. To that end two social workers of our institution have regular counselling contacts with the parents. In incidental cases, where the particular role assignment of the 'deviant' member seems to be intricately interwoven with the total family pathology, family therapy is undertaken (Blankstein[3]).

In a residential centre there are more possibilities to change fixed role patterns of patients. In individual psychotherapy, the therapist can contribute to clarify, intellectually and emotionally, the patient's role for him. The beneficial effect of these weekly sessions may, however, easily be undone by the impact of the patient's life in the group where the patterns of interactions between members may be rigidly fixed. This is specially the case when the respective pathological tendencies of patients seem to complement each other accurately.

A striking illustration was given by a particular relation between two room-mates. It was observed in the group therapy that, if somebody asked boy A a question, A kept his mouth shut while B took over and gave the answer. Further analysis showed that in this relationship A reproduced his passivity, to the point of paralysis, in relation to his mother, whereas B's attitude had its roots in a strong rivalry with his father: he therefore seized parental power over his room-mate. The respective infantile problems of these two individuals fitted each other in such a way, that they kept each other in this pathologic situation, preventing further development.

It is mainly due to the experiences of the group therapies that in recent years we pay more attention to the recognition of role distribution in our groups, and to finding techniques to undo the rigid patterns of interaction. To that end meetings were organized, where counsellors and individual therapists discussed this specific problem, under the guidance of the group therapist. The very recognition of a type of interdependent relationship between patients (as boy A and B showed) may already enable the counsellor to liberate them gradually from their narrow interaction pattern. Obviously, counsellors themselves are likely to become involved in the same fixed interaction patterns with the members of their group. During training and supervision hours they learn to recognize this. Their being aware of these transference phenomena may make sure that they adopt a different reaction to the adolescent's behaviour from what the latter expects and tends to force upon them (Schouten[29]).

This survey of our treatment programme shows how individual psychotherapy and the milieu treatment approaches supplement each other to a great extent. While the individual psychotherapy focuses mainly on the development of an 'observing ego' and promotes 'insight' in the defensive nature of the patients' disturbed behaviour, the milieu approaches provide a variety of new emotional experiences in the realm of achievements and relations.

4

Conclusion

It goes without saying that the attempt described above, aimed at integrating individual psychotherapy in a residential centre, asks for an elaborate system of communication within the institution. Psychotherapists in 'Zandwijk' spend more than half their time at meetings. They participate in discussions concerning the practical approach of individuals and groups in the daily life situation. They refrain from reciting the factual incidents brought up in individual sessions with boys, but they do not hesitate to influence decisions on the basis of the specific insights gained during therapeutic hours.

The views presented in this chapter should not be regarded as the fruit of a private intellectual exercise by the authors, but as the result of a close interaction of a team of specialists from different professions: pedagogues, therapists, group-workers, social workers. It was especially S. Hirsch, our group therapist and group-work consultant who—in the course of years—opened our eyes to the impact of institutional life and the dynamics of the group, as they have been discussed in this paper.

Readers may criticize the fact that the authors raise a variety of problems, using a terminology borrowed from completely different frames of reference. The phraseology of classical analysis has been used, as well as concepts belonging to academical psychology and social psychology. This must be attributed to the deplorable situation that residential treatment lacks a well-defined philosophy of its own. In assessing the individual's pathology, we use the model of *intra*-personal conflicts between impulses and defences; when we talk about residential treatment strategy, we think in terms of *inter*-personal interactions. These differences in models of thinking might be the reason why institutions adhere to strategies that have not much bearing on the individual's pathology and its cure. The concept of 'role', as presented in this chapter, by virtue of its intermediate position between the intra- and inter-personal models, might be of value to bridge the gap between the model concerning the individual and the strategy of the institution aimed at changing the individual's way of life.

REFERENCES

1. BETTELHEIM, B. 1950. *Love is not enough.* Glencoe, Illinois: Free Press.
2. BETTELHEIM, B. 1955. *Truants from Life.* Glencoe, Illinois: Free Press.
3. BLANKSTEIN, J. H. 1969. Familientherapie oder das Problem der intrapsychischen im Gegensatz zu der zwischenpersönlichen Dynamik. *Fortschritte der Psychoanalyse.* Jahrbuch, **4.** (In press.)
4. CAUDILL, W. 1958. *The psychiatric hospital as a small society.* Cambridge, Mass.: Harvard University Press.
5. COTTER, HIRSCHBERG, J. and MANDELBAUM, A. 1957. Problems of administration and supervision in an inpatient treatment centre for children. *Bull. Menninger Clinic,* **21,** 208–219.
6. CRAFT, M., STEPHENSON, G. and GRANGER, C. 1964. A controlled trial of authoritarian and self-governing regimes with adolescent psychopaths. *Amer. J. Orthopsychiat.,* **34,** 543–554.
7. DUMONT, J. J. 1969. Theorie, model en strategie: Chapter 8 in *Pedagogisch Mozaïek.* Opstellen aangeboden aan Prof. Dr. J. G. Gielen. Den Bosch, Uitg. Malmberg.
8. EIJER, M. J. 1969. An adventurous activity project for adolescents. In *Scientific Proceedings,* American Psychiatric Association, Washington.
9. ERIKSON, E. H. 1959. Identity and the life cycle. *Psychol. Issues,* **1,** no. 1.
10. FENICHEL, O. 1945. *The psychoanalytic theory of neurosis.* Chapter 17. New York: Norton.
11. FRAIBERG, S. 1955. Some considerations in the introduction to therapy in puberty. *Psychoanalytic study of the child,* **10,** 264–286.
12. FREUD, A. 1958. Adolescence. *Psychoanalytic study of the child,* **13,** 255–278.
13. HIRSCH, S. 1963. Therapeutisch groepswerk met emotioneel gestoorde pubers en adolescenten. *Maandbl. Geest. Volksgezondh.,* **18,** 302–313.
14. JOSSELYN, I. 1950. Treatment of the emotional immature child in an institution framework. *Amer. J. Orthopsychiat.,* **20,** 397–409.
15. KAMP, L. N. J. 1960. Problems of organization andadministration in residential treatment institutions for children. *Int. Child Welf. Rev.,* **24,** no. 9, 1–11.
16. KAMP, L. N. J. 1961. Possibilités et limites du traitement psychiatrique des mineurs en institutions. *A Criança Portuguesa,* **20,** 129–149.
17. KAMP, L. N. J. 1963. Over het contact met ouders in een kinderpsychiatrisch instituut. De Koepel, **17,** 654–661.
18. KAMP, L. N. J. 1969. Entwicklungen in der Kinderpsychotherapie. *Prax. Kinderpsychol.,* **18,** no. 2, 74–76.
19. LEVITA, D. J. DE, 1961. Psychotherapie in de inrichting. *Maandblad voor Kindergeneeskunde,* **29,** 60–74.
20. POLSKY, H. W. 1962. *Cottage Six.* New York: Russell Sage Foundation.
21. REDL, F. 1942. Group emotion and leadership. *Psychiatry,* **5,** no. 4. 573–596.
22. REDL, F. 1949. The phenomenon of contagion and 'shock effect' in group therapy. In *Searchlight on delinquency,* 315–328. Ed. K. R. EISSLER. London: Imago Publ. Co.
23. REDL, F. 1959. The concept of a therapeutic milieu. *Amer. J. Orthopsychiat.,* **29,** 721–736.
24. REDL, F. 1959. The life-space interview. *Amer. J. Orthopsychiat.,* **29,** 1–18.
25. REDL, F. 1966. Disadvantaged—and what else? In Redl: *When we deal with children.* New York: Free Press. London: Collier–Macmillan Ltd.
26. REDL, F. and WINEMAN, D. 1952. *Children who hate.* Glencoe, Illinois: Free Press.

27. REDL, F. and WINEMAN, D. 1952. *Controls from within.* Glencoe, Illinois: Free Press.
28. SCHOUTEN, J. A. M. 1967. *Persoonlijkheidsfactoren en geneigdheid tot delinquentie in de puberteit.* Den Haag. (With a summary in English: Personality factors and delinquency proneness in adolescents.) The Hague: Staatsdrukkerij.
29. SCHOUTEN, J. A. M. 1969. Psychotherapie mit Adoleszenten. Analyse der Uebertragungsphänomene bei Heimbehandlung. *Prax. Kinderpsychol.,* Jahrgang **18**, 233–236.
30. STANTON, A. H. and SCHWARTZ, M. S. 1954. *The Mental Hospital.* New York: Basic Books.
31. WHITE, R. 1963. Ego and reality in psychoanalytic theory. *Psychol. Issues,* **4**, no. 3.

XX

UNIVERSITY PSYCHIATRIC SERVICES IN THE UNITED KINGDOM

ANTHONY RYLE

Director
The University of Sussex Health Service
Brighton, England

1

History

The provision of medical facilities for university students is of relatively recent origin. In Britain, the great majority of Health Services were only set up after the Second World War, and the recognition of the prime importance of psychiatry in these services is still incomplete. In both these respects the best American centres were at least two or three decades in advance and, in general, provisions on the other side of the Atlantic are considerably more lavish than those in Britain. Associated with this fact, special training in student psychiatry is now available in the U.S.A. but not in Britain. On the other hand, American services for the disturbed student tend to be split up, with medical psychiatric and psychological counselling services operating largely independently. The pattern emerging in Britain is usually that of an integrated service with whole-time medical officers, usually with a background in general practice or general medicine, but with a special interest and some training in psychiatry, who either employ psychiatrists part-time in their services, or have a special arrangement for consultations with local National Health Service specialists. To some extent the employment of psychotherapists who are not medically trained is becoming accepted, but on a much smaller scale than in the States. The British arrangement ensures that basic medical care for both physical and emotional problems is given by a doctor acquainted and in contact with the university and its tutors.

Special medical services for students were initially set up to provide a screening and preventive service only, aiming to counter the specific health hazards of the age group which, at that time, were most notably pulmonary tuberculosis. After the introduction of the National Health Service, it was logical to provide general practice care to the student population, most of whom are separated from both family and family doctor. Still later, and, as indicated above, still very unevenly, the services have taken an interest in both the prevention and treatment of the mental health hazards of the age group—an interest which has coincided in Britain with the rapid expansion of student numbers to the present figure of 8 per cent of the age group, and with a growing concern for the loss of investment and the personal cost represented by the illness and dropping out of students from university. Concern with the health of students has also been provoked by a suicide rate three to six times as high as the rate found in those of their age group outside universities (Stengel 1964,[13] Carpenter 1959[3]).

2

Epidemiology

Despite differences in selection procedures, in services provided, and in the criteria used, there is a surprising consistency in the estimates given for the rates of psychiatric disturbance for students in both America and Britain. (Baker,[1] Kidd,[8] Kidd and Caldbeck Meenan [9]). Serious psychiatric disorder affects 1–2 per cent of students during their undergraduate career, while a further 10–15 per cent suffer some emotional or psychiatric disorder of a degree justifying at least some treatment. Serious cases will include psychotic illnesses, both schizophrenia and manic-depressive disorders being found in this age group, and also the more severe late-adolescent identity crises. The milder range will include most of the common personality and neurotic disorders. Psychiatric illness, especially the more serious forms, is more common in the first year at university—evidence that the transition into the institution is the most traumatic experience. This parallels the pattern of breakdown in the armed forces. Examinations, given an exaggerated prominence in some writing about student health, produce numerous minor stress reactions, but seldom provoke a new major psychiatric disorder.

Psychiatric illness is usually reported as being more common in female than male students, repeating here a general epidemiological finding, and the rates in Arts students tend to be higher than in Science students. This last difference is due at least in part to personality differences, present before entry to university. Neuroticism scores, for example, are often found to be significantly different in the two groups, but differences in the type of teaching and in the social experience of Arts and Science students may also play some part.

3

Selection of University Students: Implications for Mental Health

Despite the expansion of British universities, competition for places remains fierce. The provision of grants for those obtaining places has removed the economic bar to higher education, and competition on strictly academic grounds is considerable. In practice, this has come to mean that adequate performance at the 'A' level examination is a necessary qualification for a university place. As competition is a feature of the British educational system from early on, and as emotional disorder is known to be associated with under-achievement, one must assume that those reaching university are, to some degree, positively selected for mental health. However, it seems probable that there are factors working in the opposite direction. For some, academic success may have been achieved at the cost of social restriction and consequent immaturity. For others, the years of compliance to the system may have heightened conflicts about authority and delayed their resolution, and in consequence compulsive acting out of rebellion, or, more often, passive resistance may interfere with the student's ability to make use of his opportunities at university. These tendencies may be heightened by the fact that the parents of high achievers are more likely to be demanding and powerful personalities, so that conflicts over compliance/defiance may have important childhood roots. There is some evidence that students from working-class homes have greater problems in adjusting to university because, as one such student put it, 'The farther I get on here, the farther I move away from there.' Women may also experience more difficulty, at least in some subjects, due to the conflicts between the values and goals of achievement and of femininity. It has been demonstrated that the more feminine girls tend to be rather less successfully academically (Heilbrun [6, 7]).

4

The Psychological Tasks Facing the Student

The transition from adolescent to adult status in our society is accomplished at different rates and through different means in different sections of the population. The route followed by those in higher education is distinct in a number of ways. The adolescent is emotionally and economically dependent upon his family and he usually moves out of this dependence through his experience at work, and through becoming a wage-earner. As he gets older, he spends an increasing proportion of his time with his peer group, and in the end he may move out of the family home for a time, to live alone or at least cut off from relatives—the phase of 'family limbo', which will be ended by his own marriage. In many cases, however, especially for girls, the parental home will not be left until, or even after, marriage. The university student, on the other hand, postpones economic independence to a much later date, certainly throughout his time at school and usually, to some degree, in so far as grants are assessed on parental income, until he graduates. Most students therefore retain inevitably some financial dependence upon their families. Many students will not have lived away from home until they come to university, and hence they have to deal with separation problems on their arrival. Others, on the other hand, who have been at boarding school, may not have resolved fully their relationship with their parents as the adolescent issues of independence and autonomy may have been partially fought out at school, while home has remained an idealised place in which holidays are spent. Whichever kind of school is attended, it is likely that the university student has led a more restricted social life than that of his peers, before he left school, and for those who have been at one-sex boarding schools, experience of the opposite sex may have been very limited.

Entry to university can therefore focus into one move transitions which, for others, occur over a space of time. The student may be faced simultaneously with separation from parents, loss of adult supports of a kind provided in the school system and the challenge of proving his academic worth to the Faculty and of establishing his social capacity and sexual identity and worth with his peers. In moving from an assured place in the hierarchical school society, he finds himself in a situation of total exposure in a great group of competitors of unknown quality all, like himself, under threat, and all coping with the challenge of this society with a range of defensive or aggressive manoeuvres. It is only after the first weeks at university that the defensive postures can be shed and the mutual clingings or exaggerated bravados can be replaced by friendships and by meaningful affiliations to formal and informal groups.

This period of induction is the time of maximum incidence of emotional and psychiatric disorders. In so far as the tasks and pressures are those of transition, of exposure and of self-proof and self-discovery, the concepts of Erikson[4, 5] are of particular relevance in understanding the problems, and the identity crisis and identity diffusion are common presentations of psychological disorder.

Once the transition into university has been accomplished, and of course it is accomplished without grave distress or the need for professional help by the majority of students, the psychological problems are those to do with personal and social relations and with work. Socially, the society of a university offers a wide range of formal possibilities, and an even wider range of informal ones. Most activity, however, takes place in groups made up almost exclusively of fellow-students of similar age. The pressure to conform to the values of this somewhat frenetic society are considerable, even if the values themselves are non-conformist ones, and the search for identity may be diverted by compliance to these pressures or may be manifest by the adoption of a bewildering series of transitory affiliations. While this is going on, the formal requirements of the university must still be met, requirements for attendance at practicals, lectures or tutorials, for the production of written work and for passing tests and examinations. To the degree that a student has already identified with some future career, and to the degree that he can feel that coming to university was his own choice rather than an inevitable stage in his passage through the educational processing machinery, he is likely to be able to meet the reasonable demands of the university without feeling in any way compromised or threatened; but these obligations can echo childhood battles with parents and can easily provoke, in the neurotically pre-disposed student, active protests, passive resistance or frightened retreat. The student who finds himself in opposition to the values of the university may remain in isolation, but many find their way into social groups which support and validate their resistance notably, nowadays, in the drug-taking culture.

At the same time as his social and academic values are being tested and crystallised, the student is also likely to be actively engaged in relationships with the opposite sex, relationships which are often at first little more than a testing out of his own sexuality, but which more and more become experiments in intimacy and relationship. It is rare nowadays for this phase to be postponed to a later age, a fact reflecting both social change and the advance in the age of puberty, and accelerated, no doubt, by the wide availability of effective contraception. Intimate relationships may stabilise and complete the maturation of many, but for some they serve only to reveal the conflicts and immaturities which in less hurried and more chaste ages might have lain dormant until after marriage. Sometimes problems of this sort may be provoked because social pressures have forced an involvement for which the individual was not yet emotionally ready, but much more often it seems that the conflicts would have been manifest inevitably. The treatment of the student who presents with relationship problems may have a better chance of success than the treatment of older married patients, so many of whom have formed a neurotic collusive relationship which stands in the way of any personal change. In this sense, intervention at this stage may represent valuable preventive psychiatry.

To summarise what has been said so far, the economic and emotional independence of the university student is delayed in comparison with others of his age group, and the student has to accomplish the transitions of adolescent into adult through meeting a number of simultaneous abrupt challenges. Problems of independence, problems with authority and problems of identity must be coped with in an environment which offers relatively little adult support or guidance, and which imposes a high level of demand, while the role of student does not provide any very firm guide-line and is in itself essentially transient. Simultaneously to coping with these problems and with the intellectual demands of his course, the student is likely to embark upon intimate relationships which test his capacity to trust others. Though his liability to breakdown is determined by genetic factors and by his family background, the chance of this liability being manifest in disability or illness while he is at university is clearly high.

5

The Clinical Problems of Students

In examining the clinical problems which are likely to preoccupy the psychiatrist working in the university context, a two-fold approach will be offered, looking first at disorders grouped under diagnostic headings and subsequently at various problem issues and situations.

The classification of psychiatric illness is always a vexed issue, and the problems of classification, especially in the sub-classification of neurotic personality disorders, is nowhere more perplexing than in adolescents. The headings of the following sections therefore indicate some unwillingness to be dogmatic in this area.

Schizophrenia, Schizo-affective Disorders and Borderline Psychotic States

In the case of a full-blown and typical schizophrenic illness, there are no considerations which distinguish students from others similarly affected. The most important additional role of the university psychiatrist here, is to give good guidance to the patient and to the university about fitness to return and about the timing of return. There is a common tendency among psychiatrists to recommend return too early. In general, absence of at least a year is desirable after any schizophrenic illness, and the patient's return should then depend upon freedom from any important residual symptoms, although there is no objection to the student who returns still taking drugs. After return, supervision must clearly include careful watch to see that medication is not prematurely discontinued. The chances of successful return will depend very much on the pre-morbid history. Where there has been a slow onset of illness, and a previously markedly disturbed personality, it is unlikely that the student will be fit to return, while the individual with an acute onset of a florid illness has a much better prognosis. Some consideration must be given to the nature of the course being studied, for residual flattening of affect may be more disturbing to the student studying literature than to the chemist, while residual thought disorder may be more critical to the philosopher or mathematician. The implications of depressed or paranoid thinking in the postgraduate with access to powerful chemicals or dangerous apparatus needs serious consideration.

Among the acute psychotic breakdowns of students a number will present with mixed depressive and schizophrenic symptoms. This is particularly true of the illnesses of acute onset in students of reasonable pre-morbid personality. These illnesses often represent the impact of primarily affective disorders upon immature personalities. The prognosis of these cases is therefore better than that of true schizophrenia, and if recurrence occurs, it is likely to be increasingly in the form of an affective rather than a schizophrenic illness.

Occasionally, in the student undergoing what appears to be an acute identity crisis, transient psychotic features may appear. It may be difficult in such cases to determine the point at which the existential ruminations, paradoxical formulations or omnipotent fantasies go beyond the broad limits explored by normal adolescents involved in meeting the emotional and intellectual challenges of university. In many of these cases there seems to be no more than a temporary loosening of ego-structures, and symptoms and behaviour which would indicate the strong probability of psychosis in the older patient may have less grave implications in this group. The psychiatrist is therefore often justified in doing no more than hold a watching brief. It is, of course, possible that some of these cases may prove, in the long run, to suffer from affective disorders.

Affective Psychoses

Serious depressive illness and hypomania are both encountered in the student age group, but the relative frequency of manic or hypomanic presentations is much greater in this age group than in older subjects. Less severe endogenous depressions are relatively common and easily over-looked in this, as in other populations. There are no particular problems in diagnosing the severe cases. Typically, hypomania is tolerated for a surprisingly long time in the student community, and typically the first presentation is through the intervention of tutors or friends rather than through the consultation of the student. Some hypomanic students achieve a quite remarkable range of personal and social commitments in university society. The student with a mild endogenous depression presents more difficulty, for problems of concentration, disturbances of sleep, and particular difficulty in getting up in the morning are very common in students due to other causes. Flattening of affect and restriction of interest, and the absence of the sort of history usually encountered in the neurotic student should arouse suspicion; and in a case of doubt, the use of anti-depressants is clearly justified. These are most likely to be effective in cases of clear onset with definite physiological symptoms. As with other psychiatric disorders, presentation is most frequent in the early stages of the student's career and in some cases the history seems to go back to the last year at school. It is important to distinguish the blankness and futility of the severely schizoid individual from the symptoms of a depressive illness.

Neurotic Reactions

The neurotic reactions of the student, as indicated above, are esentially those associated with the psychological transitions of the age group. The overall psychological task of this student age group is to preserve and develop a sense of personal identity, and the most severe reactions will be those in which this sense is confused or lost, or undergoes a period of acute instability and change. With less acute disturbance in the sense of self, one may still encounter the problems of relationships, including coping with ordinary social relationships, coping with intimacy, testing out of sexual capacity in heterosexual relationships, and coping with exposure to tutors and their demands. Achieving mastery of the subject studied, making personal sense of the role of student and of the incipient career identity, and dealing with the problems of competition and achievement, may all provoke neurotic difficulties in the vulnerable student.

If one accepts some form of psychodynamic model of personality development, difficulties in these areas are to be accounted for in terms of failure to resolve the conflicts of earlier ages, and evidences of earlier stress and suggestions of such failure are indeed to be found in the histories of most psychiatric patients in the age group. It must be borne in mind, however, that the age group is one in which rapid, and at times bewildering, transition is the norm, and transparently neurotic, regressive or disorganised behaviour may be of much less grave significance than would be the case with older patients. It is probably a mistake to give too much weight to the severity of symptoms in arriving at a prognosis. Greater significance needs to be placed upon the level of disorder in terms of the developmental stage from which it is derived. Severe early disturbances of parent–child relationships, marked by schizoid withdrawal or by immature aggressive dependent modes of relating, are not incompatible with academic success; but the personal isolation which some such students achieve for themselves in the university context may lead at least some of them finally to seek help. One such patient described a visit to an aquarium which provided him with an image of his position. He said, 'There was a lobster which seemed to respond when you put your hand over to the glass. It reached out with its feelers over and over again, but all it ever contacted was the glass.' It is my belief that psychotherapy to students of this sort may represent the last chance of 'reaching through the glass', but very few services, and very few sections of the National Health Service, can offer sufficiently intensive or prolonged individual psychotherapy. Group therapy, if available, is often too threatening for such patients to accept. Short of full psychotherapy, some of these students may manage on the basis of support and, for the brighter ones, academic careers may provide a context in which schizoid behaviour is not too maladaptive.

For the less severe neurotic whose problems over dependence, autonomy or sexual identity may be acted out in relation to friends, sexual partners or tutors, relatively brief individual or group psychotherapy should be available. This may have direct survival value in enabling the student to work through problems which might otherwise interfere with academic progress; and more generally, psychotherapy can catalyse change more freely in this age group than in any other.

The Student in Academic Difficulty

About 75 per cent of students entering university graduate on time without experiencing serious academic or emotional difficulty. The remaining 25 per cent will present with psychiatric or emotional problems or experience serious work difficulty of a degree needing additional time or provoking tutorial sanctions. In Britain, 13 per cent of all students drop out before completing the course (U.G.C.[14]).

A proportion of drop-outs and of students in academic difficulty are undermotivated extraverts, or are those who have made genuine errors of career choice. The remainder, probably a majority, have emotional or psychiatric problems of some sort. The nature of the association between psychiatric and emotional and academic difficulty is not a simple one. Obviously severe illness, expecially psychotic breakdown, will block effective work, but such cases are only a small minority of the total number of psychiatrically disordered academic difficulty students. Within a series of such students, in my own experience, there was no evidence of a deficiency of intelligence in the academic difficulty group.[12] Psychiatric symptomatology assessed with the Middlesex Hospital Questionnaire showed that psychiatric patients not in academic difficulty scored highest for neurotic symptomatology, followed by psychiatric patients in academic difficulty, followed by academic difficulty students not classified on clinical grounds as psychiatrically disturbed. Even this last group scored significantly higher than normals for anxiety and depressive symptoms. We see, therefore, within this group of students selected on clinical and academic grounds as being in either emotional or academic difficulty or both, that those with least academic difficulty had most symptoms, and vice versa. What then is the relation of academic difficulty to psychological or psychiatric problems?

The conflicts and failures of motivation underlying neurotic work difficulty can, I believe, be fully understood only on the basis of a psychodynamic diagnosis. The student may present himself or be seen by tutors as lazy or stupid, he may voice philosophical doubts about the meaning of his subject, or political objections to the assumptions of his teachers. He may organise himself with great resource as if to do work, yet succeed with equal resource in setting up diversions and obstacles, or he may present in a number of other ways. The underlying incompatibility between his expressed wish to get a degree and his present mode of behaving can usually be exposed without difficulty. For many, this exposure, coupled with the imposition of adequate reality pressures by tutors, is often all that is required. For others, the present behaviour is a reflection of a neurotic construction of the situation which has roots in the family relationship problems and unresolved conflicts of early childhood. These students need psychotherapy. Provided a student gives permission, psychiatric treatment of this kind of case should be combined with some communication with the student's tutors. Some tutors may be authoritarian towards a student already crippled by anxiety and driven by guilt. Others, more numerous, may, out of false kindness, prolong the student's denial of reality by excusing him from academic requirements and withholding academic discipline. Psychiatrists must clearly protect students incapacitated by illness, and may at times plead for extra time and toleration for the disturbed student. Often, however, the psychiatrist's role will be to block the neurotic student's tendency to provoke collusive responses from his tutors.

The discrimination between different sorts of work difficulty is not always easy. The University Health Service, as well as assessing cases, should devote time and thought to clarifying for tutors the range of problems encountered, and to keeping them in the picture in the case of individual students in difficulty. The psychiatrist should also remain alert to the ways in which aspects of the university society may contribute to the health or sickness of its members.

Examination Reactions

The incidence of minor stress symptoms, insomnia or excessive sleepiness, and of anxiety is not surprisingly higher in the weeks preceding important examinations, but cases of serious psychiatric illness are not particularly prone to present at this time. Treatment of these cases is supportive and pharmacological. Where earlier examinations have produced major crises of evasion or under-performance, investigation of the underlying psychopathology is indicated well in advance of Finals. The meaning of examinations varies, for example, between the ambitious and the lazy, or the obsessional and the extraverted. The neurotic student with problems about exposure or conflicts about success may clearly attach these to the examination system.

Acute panic on the eve of examinations is best treated by firm support, combined if possible with de-sensitisation by means of rehearsal in anticipation, coupled with physical relaxation, as described by Malleson.[11] These students, and those phobic ones who cannot enter, or have to leave examination halls, should be allowed to take their papers elsewhere under medical supervision. If facilities are available for this, very few will fail to complete their papers. These acute reactions tend to occur either in the exceptionally bright student on the brink of a first-class honours degree, or in the weak student on the brink of a fail.

Pregnancy

Between 2 and 3 per cent of women undergraduates become pregnant each year, even in universities where contraceptive advice is easily obtained. In this population neither ignorance nor difficulty in obtaining advice can account for many pregnancies, and pregnant students represent, therefore, an even more neurotic sample than is usually the case in the mothers of unwanted pregnancies. In the majority, unconscious or part conscious motivation had led the girl to take known, though often at the time denied, risks. The origins of this wish to be pregnant are various. Most frequently it is related to fears or doubts about femininity, which are particularly marked in some academic women; but competition with and defiance of the mother and other neurotic mechanisms are often at work. The initial reaction to the pregnancy is usually one of total rejection, and a high proportion of students not referred for termination will organise one for themselves on an illegal or quasi-legal basis.

For the doctor, as always, the decision whether or not to recommend termination is a difficult one. In the first instance it is important to be aware of a tendency to extract a firm opinion at the first interview. There is always conflict and ambivalence about pregnancy, and the first task of the doctor is to help, and even force, the girl to acknowledge both the positive and negative feelings. Where possible, the father should also be seen with the girl, so that his attitude and involvement can be assessed, and if parents are in the picture, they also should be seen, though in my experience they are more likely to press for termination than they are to offer to support the girl through the pregnancy. In a large majority of students the neurotic origins of the pregnancy and the psychological and social consequences of it continuing are such that, in my view, termination is to be recommended. Students as a group are emphatic in rejecting forced marriage, and very reluctant to accept adoption as a good solution for the problem of the unwanted pregnancy, basing their attitudes on values and on evidence which one can respect.

It is clearly desirable and now generally, though not everywhere, true that girls who carry their pregnancies through to term should be allowed to remit and to complete their courses later. It is clearly also desirable that University Health Services should provide counselling on contraception, which should be concerned not only to give the best technical advice but also to show adequate concern for the motivations and feelings of those consulting.

Drugs

Any student wishing to take cannabis can get it, and with a little determination most other illicit drugs are also obtainable (Binnie[2]). Cannabis use is widespread but in the majority of cases does not constitute a psychiatric or academic problem. A few students, however, use cannabis as the alcoholic uses alcohol, repeatedly evading the anxiety or depression which concerns them and blotting out those nasty aspects of reality with which they cannot deal. Such students are liable to fail academically and are at considerable risk of escalation on to harder drugs. Other students, while less dependent on the drug's pharmacological effects, are highly dependent upon the social setting in which it is taken. The drug scene offers a closed supportive group situation and at the same time represents an act of defiance against official authority. It provides therefore a social validation for the drop-outs from official society, and an anti-academic focus for the disturbed failing student.

The other drug of high repute amongst student drug-takers is L.S.D., which combines pharmacological potency with a highly developed myth system, providing a conventionalised set of anti-conventional values. While the incidence of grave psychotic episodes after L.S.D. use is not high, and while some students do seem to gain insight into themselves and their relation to others following L.S.D. 'trips', a disturbing number of students report prolonged abnormal experiences after using the drug.

The psychiatrist, seen as part of the world and university authority system, will see relatively few cannabis or L.S.D. takers, and in general those he sees will not be coming for treatment for the effects of drug-taking, which may often be relatively incidental. A fuller understanding of the phenomena of mass drug use requires an historical anthropological perspective such as that offered by Lidz and Rothenberg.[10]

Amphetamine use, except in small doses for working, is no longer very common among students, but the use of intravenous methyl amphetamine, often combined with heroin, is now being encountered in the hard core drug taker. Students, or more often student drop-outs, represent a significantly high proportion of registered heroin addicts in Britain. Some such registered addicts may be able to continue to work as students, and however much one may fear their contagion of others, the university doctor must clearly observe professional secrecy if such a student is under his care.

6

The Organisation of University Health Services

The majority of University Health Physicians in Britain have a background in general practice, but increasingly those recruited to the field have additional interest and training in psychiatry. Only a few Services employ psychiatrists directly, though in universities with medical schools special arrangements for students are often made.

If psychotherapy is to be provided for the 10 per cent of students who at some time may need it, it is clearly impracticable to provide specialist psychiatric care for all. In any case, the training of psychiatrists is still often deficient in the skill of psychotherapy which is most relevant to work with students. The bulk of treatment will therefore be given by medical officers with additional training, preferably receiving continuing supervision from a psychiatrist trained in psychotherapy. Increasingly, one may also find that non-medical psychotherapists with a background of social work or psychology will be employed for this purpose. Appropriate training for psychotherapists can be obtained through the courses offered by the Tavistock Clinic in Great Britain, but not many places offer such courses at present. I believe that it is appropriate for a university service to employ a psychiatrist who can devote a part of his time to running case seminars and individual supervision of the other doctors, and a part to clinical work.

Pressure of work has led to the increasing use of group psychotherapy in this country. The difficulty of running groups in a university is that members are likely to meet outside the group, but experience has shown that this need not in fact inhibit the work of the group unduly. These groups need careful selection, and should include students with a range of problems. Students in treatment for academic difficulty will often exhibit passive aggressive behaviour and too many of such cases in a group can effectively block it.

Confidentiality and Liaison

Citizens over the age of sixteen have the right to confidentiality in their dealings with doctors. This fact means that the university doctor, even if he desires it, has no right to contact the parents of his patients without their consent. This consent will be withheld by a large proportion of students in psychiatric treatment—a reflection of the views of this age group, and of the disordered families from which most such students come. This, and geographical considerations, would make family therapy impractical. In fact, of all age groups, the late adolescent-early adult would seem to be the one most suited to individually focused psychotherapy, and the psychiatrist or psychotherapist needs above all to preserve his independence from parents and other authorities. This consideration is also of prime importance within the university. Clearly, in clinical work normal professional codes and confidentiality apply, and extra effort is needed to reassure students on this point. Wherever discussion takes place with tutors about individual students, the student's prior consent should be obtained. The psychiatrist in the university will not be immune from the prejudices and myths which are encountered in the world outside, and both students and tutors will suspect him of wrong judgements, incompetence, the creation of disease in the healthy and countless other faults. It is wise to anticipate these criticisms by being available for discussion and by setting up formal channels of communication, but even where this is done, patience and insight will be called for in the face of prejudice. To the extent that the University Health Doctor and psychiatrist are accepted by the university community, there is a chance that they may influence its policies in ways which can diminish unnecessary stress and conflict in the institution, thus having a rare opportunity of preventive psychiatry.

Finally, for the research-minded, the opportunities in university health services should be noted. The combination of clinical work with students with the opportunity to observe the structure and function of the university as an institution is an intriguing one.

REFERENCES

1. BAKER, R. W. 1963. Incidence of psychological disturbance in college students. *J. Am. College Health Ass.*, **13**, 532.
2. BINNIE, H. L. 1969. The attitudes to drugs and drug-takers of students at the University and Colleges of Higher Education in an English midland city. Health Service, University of Leicester.
3. CARPENTER, R. G. 1959. Statistical analysis of suicide and morbidity rates of students. *Brit. J. prev. soc. Med.*, **13**, 163.
4. ERIKSON, E. H. 1950. *Childhood and society.* New York: Norton.
5. ERIKSON, E. H. 1968. *Identity: youth and crisis.* London: Faber & Faber.
6. HEILBRUN, A. B. 1962. Parental identification and college adjustment. *Psychol. Reports*, **10**, 853.
7. HEILBRUN, A. B. 1963. Sex role identity and achievement motivation. *Psychol. Reports*, **12**, 483.
8. KIDD, C. B. 1965. Psychiatric morbidity among students. *Brit. J. prev. soc. Med.*, **19**, 143.
9. KIDD, C. B. and CALDBECK MEENAN, J. 1966. A comparative study of psychiatric morbidity among students of two different universities. *Brit. J. Psychiat.*, **112**, 57.
10. LIDZ, T. and ROTHENBERG, A. 1968. Psychedelism: Dionysus reborn. *Psychiatry*, **31**, (2), 116.
11. MALLESON, N. 1959. Panic and phobia. *Lancet*, **i**, 225.
12. RYLE, A. 1969. The psychology and psychiatry of academic difficulties in students. *Proc. Roy. Soc. Med.*, **62**, 1263.
13. STENGEL, E. 1964. *Suicide and attempted suicide.* Harmondsworth: Penguin.
14. University Grants Committee 1968. *Enquiry into student progress* 1968. London: H.M.S.O.

BIBLIOGRAPHY

B.S.H.A. *The proceedings of the British Student Health Association.* Printed for private circulation within the Association; the secretary of which is Dr K. Finlay, University Health Service, University of Nottingham.
FARNSWORTH, D. L. 1964. *College health administration.* New York: Appleton-Century-Crofts.
FARNSWORTH, D. L. 1966. *Psychiatry, education and the young adult.* Springfield, Illinois: Thomas.
MALLESON, N. 1965. *A handbook on British student health services.* London: Pitman.
Royal College of Physicians, London. *Report of Social and Preventive Medicine Committee.* Sub-committee on the Student Health Service.
RYLE, A. 1969. *Student casualties.* London: Allen Lane, the Penguin Press.
Society for Research in Higher Education, 2 Woburn Square, W.C.1. Various abstracts and reports including: PAYNE, J. A. *Research in student mental health.*

XXI

COMPREHENSIVE COMMUNITY PROGRAMS FOR THE INVESTIGATION AND TREATMENT OF ADOLESCENTS

WILLIAM A. SCHONFELD

M.D.

President, American Society for Adolescent Psychiatry
Assistant Clinical Professor of Psychiatry
Department of Child Psychiatry, College of Physicians and Surgeons
Columbia University, New York
U.S.A.

1

Introduction

It is with some trepidation that I approach the task assigned to me of delineating what I would consider a comprehensive community program for the psycho-social-educational treatment of emotionally disturbed adolescents living at home, and in need of treatment.

The need for more services in this important field has become clear since it is estimated that by 1971, 50 per cent of the total population in the United States will be under 25 years of age. The National Institute of Mental Health statistics[4,104,105,119] reveal that outpatient psychiatric clinics in the United States serve more persons in the 10–19 age group than in any other decade of life. More than one-fourth of all clinic patients are adolescents, many older adolescents are attending college and university mental health clinics and still other adolescents are in private psychotherapy. The recent increase in the inpatient adolescent population is overwhelming, with a 500 per cent increase among boys and 150 per cent increase among girls in the past fifteen years. The National Institute of Mental Health predicts that during the next decade, the present trend continuing, the rate at which young people are hospitalized in state and county mental hospitals will double again. Private psychiatric hospitals and psychiatric services of general hospitals also find their adolescent census increasing markedly. In addition, a large number of youths with emotional disturbances are attending special residential treatment centers, day hospitals and secondary schools.[111,113]

The increase of the hospital population is due not merely to a proportional increase in the emotional disturbances nor even to the increase in the numbers of adolescents in our society, but may be the result of the lack of alternative outpatient clinic facilities in the community.[8,16,21,42,47,77,129]

The waste and inefficiency in our present outpatient treatment services for the adolescent are staggering. Only one-third of the total number of adolescents applying or referred to clinics are offered treatment, while the remainder are evaluated and referred elsewhere, very often without even notifying the primary referring agency. Of the third who are offered treatment, about 40 per cent drop out shortly thereafter. Findings of one survey indicate that long term treatment of adolescents is the exception in general outpatient clinics.[8,104,105] Thus, it is evident that there is a need for a change in the services available to adolescents in outpatient clinics.

Since adolescents are notably difficult to reach and keep in therapy, working with them calls for techniques that are, in many ways, different from those used with adults or children. The adolescent cannot be treated like an adult any more than he can be treated like a child. If he is treated as an adult, he is subjected to responsibilities and a burden on his ego which he often cannot carry. If the treatment he is offered is like that given to a child, it invites fixation at a child's level rather than promoting maturation. Psychiatrists must objectively review their techniques and be willing to accept the changes in management advocated by adolescent psychiatrists.[12,13,18,36,54,55,90,111,114]

Adequate psychiatric care of adolescents requires a comprehensive and integrated community involvement.[31,57] In the United States the trend is toward the organization of comprehensive Community Mental Health Centers.[16,43,94] However, comprehensive psychiatric care for adolescents could also be attained by coordination and integration of the existing local youth-oriented school and recreational facilities, general hospital services, psychiatric services, social agencies and the development of new services as indicated.[21,31,89]

The plans at hand for development of community mental health centers have varying patterns of organization, but the common denominator at the local level must be a program which should include within its framework coordinated services for prevention, treatment and rehabilitation of the mental disorders of all the residents in the catchment area served by the community mental health center. In practice, this would mean the establishment in each community of a general all-purpose outpatient clinic dealing with the whole range of psychiatric problems in children, adolescents, adults and the aged, rather than separate clinics for each category.[43,79]

Senior psychiatrists and qualified members of allied professions would deal with intake, diagnosis and disposition. However, the most recent recommendations of the Joint Commission on Mental Health of Children have advocated the development of family and child neighborhood centers[86,130] to be integrated with the existing comprehensive community and health planning. Such centers could be new and free-standing in some communities, but more likely they would be part of the general hospital and its extramural service related to the work of pediatrics, or they could be in the outreach of neighborhood agencies and attached to community mental health centers; they could be a part of school complexes, but there is no thought of creating an independent system.

A comprehensive program, however, need not imply the end of specialization, either in skills or in service. On the contrary, the generalist and the generalized services will require the collaboration of psychiatrists with special training and experience with adolescents, as consultants in unusual problems of diagnosis, disposition or treatment, as therapists of special cases which overtax the resources of the general outpatient clinic, and as staff indoctrinators.[30,111,114] Since the adequate care of the adolescent is a multidisciplinary problem and not the exclusive prerogative of any one profession, there is need for all disciplines involved to acquire specialized knowledge and skills in assessing and handling the mental health problems of adolescents.[5,9,22,36,90]

However, examination of the programs of the existing centers reveals that inadequate attention is being paid to the ever-growing adolescent segment of our population.[3,41,43] I hope that with the greater understanding of the needs and problems of youth there will develop a more comprehensive program incorporating some of the treatment modalities and services to be discussed.

The community mental health center itself need not be a new building or a new agency, but rather an integrated system of services representing a network of program elements on both inpatient and outpatient levels through which care can be provided to all age groups. One of the specific goals of an effective program would be to provide comprehensive care to an adolescent during all phases of his illness, including prevention, diagnosis, treatment and rehabilitation. A second basic goal is to offer care where and when it is needed. This requires that a range of services be available close to a patient's home, so that he may receive the kind of care that is the most appropriate to his needs. A third basic goal is to provide continuity of care with the opportunity for transfer from one service to another as required throughout his illness. Finally, records and information must be transferred with the patient as he moves from one service in the center to another.[16,122]

Gerald Caplan has presented the major elements for an effective mental health program for adolescents.[21] Ideally, this would be so organized that each adolescent could be handled as an individual with his own idiosyncratic pattern of needs which would be dealt with by a specially tailored combination of program components.

To accomplish this I recommend that comprehensive care on an outpatient level, be dealt with in each community at three levels: the schools, the general community and the community mental health services. For an effective program there is a need for all three levels to be integrated and coordinated. The comprehensive community mental health center, when organized, could serve as the coordinating agency, incorporating total psychiatric service for adolescents administered by an adolescent psychiatrist as part of such a community mental health center.[94]

I shall discuss a variety of treatment modalities and services that are available in different parts of the country, with the realization that any community organizing comprehensive mental health outpatient facilities for adolescents will select those services best fitting its needs and integrate them into a coordinated unit, whether or not it be as part of a comprehensive community mental health center.

2

Within the Schools

Secondary Schools [5, 21, 31, 82, 90, 92, 122]

Schools should play a vital role not only in primary prevention but also in the recognition and even treatment of emotionally disturbed adolescents. Along with early childhood experiences and parental attitudes, wholesome teacher–student relationships and attitudes toward learning, concordance in family and school standards, and academic success are some of the factors which contribute to the healthy emotional development of youth. Although personal experiences are most important, long-range age-appropriate courses in the behavioral sciences may influence the value systems of the youth.

In the case of the emotionally disturbed adolescent, his very presence leaves the school no choice but to deal with him in some way. Ignoring his difficulties, treating him strictly or permissively, overprotecting the student, or pressuring him to learn—these are all ways of dealing with him which may have, according to the individual's needs, either harmful or helpful effects.

There is a need for stronger liaison between the community mental health centers, neighborhood child centers, outpatient psychiatric clinics and the schools in order to develop major new school programs which will provide diagnostic, consultative and direct services to adolescents.[21, 89, 90]

1. Diagnostic, Consultation and Referral Services in Schools

Schoolteachers are the professionals in daily contact with most adolescents. They should be made familiar, through pre-professional and in-service training programs, with the broad categories of disturbances in adolescents, learn how to cope with them within the classroom, and refer the youth possible requiring more specialized care to the school counseling service.

The counseling, or pupil personnel, service should be staffed by school psychologists, a social worker or psychiatrist and guidance counselors. Students should have ready access to these professionals who can appraise the level and nature of possible disturbance, administer appropriate psychological tests, give treatment if indicated and make appropriate referrals outside of the school if necessary.[5,82]

2. Treatment Services in Schools

(a) Counseling and psychotherapy. The school's pupil personnel or counseling service should have available, in addition to remedial reading and speech teachers, a variety of guidance and therapeutic services including individual and group guidance conducted by adequately supervised school personnel.

There are youngsters in need of psychotherapy whose parents would permit them to receive psychotherapy in the school but who, for a multitude or reasons, will not or cannot arrange for such treatment outside of the school. For this group, the community mental health clinic should set up and staff 'satellite' clinics or 'field stations' in the schools which would stress individual psychotherapy, group psychotherapy, psychopharmacology and would coordinate their efforts with the pupil personnel services.[97,114]

(b) Education of disturbed adolescents within the school.[5,92] The problem of dealing with emotionally disturbed children and adolescents is not solely the concern of psychiatrists but is also a problem for the school, not only because emotional disturbances affect learning, creating a high incidence of learning failure but also because whatever happens in school affects the student's development. Although the causes of the emotional stress are often stubbornly rooted in the family milieu, the school can create a therapeutic environment through systematic application of mental health principles within the educational program.

As far as possible, disturbed adolescents should be educated in a normal setting so as to avoid mutual alienation between them and their social milieu. Students who are emotionally disturbed but still well enough to attend a regular school should whenever possible, be spread throughout the system, rather than being concentrated in one class, where they may overburden the tolerance of a teacher and of fellow students. However, they should be brought together in small groups for special classes in group guidance and remedial education.

Disturbed students are likely to present their teacher with a variety of unusual problems in education and management for which the teacher's training and experience do not readily suggest a range of solutions. A school system should provide ways of dealing with this situation by offering both the consultative or supervisory services of mental health specialists and educators with special training in dealing with emotionally disturbed students. Consultations with the school psychiatrist, psychologist or social worker plus sensitivity training can help the teacher and counselor gain effective understanding of the youth's defenses and coping mechanisms. The teacher can be assisted in maintaining professional objectivity, acceptance and tolerance of her students in the face of emotionally disturbing elements in the work situations.[5]

Numerous special programs have been tried in different schools to educate the emotionally disturbed youths and to enhance their adaptations through education. Ungraded classes, remedial education, programmed instruction, small classes, individual instruction and home instruction have all been attempted, using both regular teachers and supervised volunteers.

Some severely disturbed or disturbing adolescents can be maintained in the normal school setting only if a small special class devoted to their needs can be organized within its framework, which these adolescents could attend for varying periods of time depending on their requirements. These special classes would offer remedial education, a course in human relationship through a study of behavioral sciences and group guidance.

The group guidance should be led by teachers and counselors, and the special classes should only be taught by teachers with special training and experience. As the youth improves he may return to his regular classes. The teachers of the special classes should spend part of their time in supervising the progress of their students who have returned to their normal class schedules and in helping the regular teachers improve their skills with disturbed youngsters.

In extreme cases, treatment schools have been advocated. These may be day schools or residential institutions basically education-oriented. In addition to a staff of educators who have special training and experience in teaching emotionally disturbed students, these schools also employ psychologists, psychiatrists and psychiatric social workers who provide individual and group treatment and offer consultation to the teachers on classroom and extra-curricular milieu management problems. The amalgam of educational and psychotherapeutic approaches which characterizes a good treatment school owes much to pioneers like Aichhorn, Redl and Bettelheim.[21]

However, there are numerous schools in which the psychiatric model for treatment of emotionally disturbed youth has been replaced by an educational one. In 'Project Re-Ed' at George Peabody College for Teachers[70] and the 'Educateur' program in France[71] the need for special education is stressed as opposed to psychiatric treatment of the disturbed youth.

Advocates of Re-Education advise us that as a modality of treatment of adolescents it deviates from the medical model by approaching that behavior directly, as an important object of treatment, regardless of the underlying cause. A Re-Ed school is first of all a school, with a treatment program that is educational in orientation and a staff who are essentially teachers. The children are taught 'how to trust, how to have faith in the future and in themselves as well as to read and to do arithmetic. . . .'

They state that Re-Education's emphasis is on 'health rather than illness, on teaching rather than on treatment, on learning rather than on fundamental personality reorganization, on the present and a future rather than on the past, on the operation of the total social system of which the child is a part rather than on intrapsychic processes exclusively'. This may provide an effective as well as a feasible approach to the problems of some emotionally disturbed children, but not to all. For effective treatment there must be a variety of educational and psychiatric approaches to fit the needs of the individual youth.

Many job-training centers are basically treatment schools oriented to train the adolescents to learn a trade, and to work effectively on a variety of jobs.

College Mental Health Services[10,39]

Statistical studies reveal that 10–15 per cent of students attending colleges with mental health clinics seek help from these clinics.[10] Students use college psychiatric services to help them cope with stresses at college rather than for treatment of mental illness.[14,50]

A vast majority of colleges do not have well organized facilities for giving comprehensive mental health services to their students. Often deans or administrative officers are called upon to handle crisis situations, many of which may be outside their areas of competence.

Some colleges have mental health clinics either as separate clinics or as a part of the general health service for students. Other colleges refer their disturbed students to the psychiatric services of the university hospital, to community clinics, state hospital clinics or private psychiatrists in their vicinity. Still others recommend that the student who requires psychiatric care take a medical leave of absence for psychotherapy.

In Boston, Massachusetts, a group of colleges pooled their financial resources and organized the College Center.[117] Full-scale specialized college mental health and treatment services were obtained with a network of liaison psychiatrists assigned to each of the member colleges. In New York City a general hospital organized a special clinic for college students.[60]

3

Within the Community

In the area of primary prevention there is a need by youth for effective recreational and social programs in the community. In order to reduce the duration of mental disorders, diagnostic, consultative and referral services should be readily available to adolescents who feel themselves, or are felt by others, to be disturbed so that attention can be given as early as possible. Adolescents in difficulty often turn for help and guidance to clergymen, family doctors, pediatricians, social workers, police, public health nurses and youth group leaders. Programs of education and consultation similar to those for teachers should be provided to help these key persons improve their effectiveness in offering guidance.[9,16,22]

A community agency such as the Mental Health Association, could serve as the educational arm of the community mental health center. It could set up a variety of programs with the cooperation of religious, parent and community agency groups, to help educate the general public and the professional staffs of community organizations who are directly involved with the management of young people but are not trained in mental health. Such an agency can also be effective in mobilizing citizen cooperation and in setting up pilot projects.

'Youth Advisory Centers', 'Youth Consultation Centers', 'Parent–Youth Workshops' and 'Walk-In Clinics' have been set up in some communities, as part of youth and community organizations, to which adolescents can turn directly for advice on life adjustment problems and crisis intervention.[25,67] These centers include mental health specialists on their staffs who are able to carry out diagnostic investigations, offer brief treatment in a series of three to five sessions, and recommend disposition. It appears that many adolescents who would hesitate to seek assistance within the framework of the school or the usual community mental health service feel free to ask for help in such a setting.

Rehabilitation of disturbed adolescents requires a number of special services which have proved of particular value. These include *sheltered workshops* for ex-patients with chronic residual defects, *supervised industrial placements* for those who can work in normal settings if they and their foremen are given special supervision, and *selective placement*, whereby a skilled attempt is made to find a special niche in some low-demand job for the person with reduced capacities. In an effective rehabilitation program the adolescent would be moved in a graduated manner into occupational situations of progressively increased challenge and burden. At the same time his social mobility would put him in situations demanding increased independence, i.e. from inpatient wards with maximum supervision to those with minimum supervision, and on to transitional institutions such as day hospital, night hospital and week-end hospital, half-way house, and finally home to his family, a foster family or residential hostel.

Those in charge of rehabilitation must also deal with the employers through such organizations as Rotary and other service clubs, the Chamber of Commerce and the trade unions in order to stimulate the provision of an increased range of jobs which are suitable for the rehabilitated adolescents.

Outpatient Facilities of the Community Mental Health Services

In addition to diagnosis and consultation,[75] the psychiatric outpatient center should provide a wide range of treatment modalities fitting the needs of the youth seeking treatment.[31,41,46,90,121] Many youths now in residence could be treated as outpatients if suitable facilities and competent personnel were available.

Adolescents appropriately treated in the outpatient service include those with chronic or acute disorders, major and minor emotional disorders, adolescents with brain damage and retarded youth with emotional problems. The role of the clinic in helping young people cope with psycho-social problems is being studied extensively.[17,34]

I shall first discuss the range of treatment modalities available in outpatient treatment services, then the variety of services which should be developed to allow for the comprehensive psychiatric care of adolescents and their families, and finally the problems of personnel.

4

Treatment Modalities

Individual Psychotherapy[12,13,31,36,46,55,83,114]

The one-to-one relationship of patient and therapist is still the basic modality of psychotherapy. Adolescents in increasing number are being referred to psychiatrists and psychiatric clinics for evaluation and treatment. Since they are notably difficult to reach and to keep in therapy, working with them calls for techniques that are in many ways different from those used with adults or children.[12,13,18,111,115] The fundamental concepts of individual psychotherapy of the adolescent should be carried over to the other treatment modalities.

A question often asked is how intensively can one treat an adolescent through individual psychotherapy. It was thought that the relative weakness of the youth's ego structure mitigated against intense treatment, and it was argued that treatment should focus on removing only those conflicts that impeded growth. However, with improved techniques and experience came the view that the adolescent can and should be treated as intensively as indicated.[12,13,96,112]

Although youths are concerned with their roots in the past and their prospects for the future, their greatest involvement is with the present. Many adolescents resent having to search for insights, or even learning to cope with reality, although both are important for psychotherapy to be effective.

Individual psychotherapy, whether in the clinic or in private practice, should deal mainly with present relationships and concentrate on feelings as well as behavior. Since feelings often result from behavior, adolescents must be helped to do what is realistic, what is responsible and what is right.[45] Therapy, if it is to succeed, must make the youth stop denying reality. The adolescent must be helped to evaluate his own behavior, accept responsibility for it and change it if unrealistic or inappropriate.

Some of the qualities that are especially needed in the psychotherapy of adolescents are engagement, flexibility, tolerance, partiality and willingness on the part of the therapist to play a parent-surrogate role as needed.[111,112,113] Engagement means treating the adolescent as someone who is quite capable of refusing to cooperate with treatment. The task is to get the youth to see his need for treatment from his own point of view and be willing to accept treatment. Many adolescents reject individual psychotherapy because they feel the therapist represents the 'establishment' and the attempt to make him fit into society.

Usually, the psychiatrist has been chosen by the youth's parents, and the patient resents having to confide in someone who he assumes to be a parental ally. All this makes the first visits crucial. The therapist has to convey to the adolescent that he is the one the therapist is directly interested in helping; it is not a matter of his being 'sick' but that he has difficulties which can be worked out if he will think and talk about them. The patient is assured that what he says will be kept confidential and that the therapist will not conspire behind his back with his parents, school or social agencies. Involvement of the patient and the therapist is an essential for successful therapy. There is a need for a completely honest and candid human relationship in which the adolescent, often for the first time in his life, realizes that someone cares enough about him not only to accept him but to help him find fulfillment in life.

The clinic therapist must be sufficiently flexible to adjust to the therapeutic needs of his adolescent patients. Some adolescents express their thoughts freely and will talk about themselves, their peers and their family. Others, particularly the younger adolescents, need an opportunity for activity or play therapy to open the way for discussion. The relationship of the therapist and patient must be active, stimulating and interesting to the youth in order for him to cooperate. Passivity of the therapist, often considered the hallmark of intensive therapy in adults, can have a disorganizing and anxiety-producing effect on the adolescent. However, the therapist must be careful not to be fooled by the adolescent who talks compulsively to avoid facing his feelings and true problems. The therapist must also be tolerant of youth even while he is trying to change his value systems.

Perhaps one of the greatest problems for the therapist is assuming responsibility for curbing the youth's destructive actions. Hendrickson and Holmes[54,55] stress the need for behavior control for intensive treatment and Rinsley[103] regards adolescent acting-out as resistance to treatment. In so doing, one often serves as a parent-surrogate, with the risk of having the patient's negative feelings toward his parents turn toward the therapist. However, it is also true that many adolescents wish to be curbed in their behavior but, unable to accept limitations from a parent, will take it from a therapist with whom the relationship is good. These adolescents want protection, and actually fear their own impulsive behavior as their way of denying their superego.

The acceptance of the therapist as a parent-surrogate is not always a transference response, unless transference is so broadly defined as to include all needed relationships. The adolescent may merely be responding to the maturity of the therapist and seeking guidance. The therapist should be sensitive to his role and should represent stable, empathetic maturity, which offers opportunity for the adolescent's own reality testing.

It should be noted that many adolescents who sense the need of a parent's support accept the therapist as a surrogate parent, always knowing that he can terminate the relationship whenever he wishes. If the emotional tie gets too strong, the restrictions too compelling, or expectations too uncomfortable, he may run away from therapy, either in actuality or emotional decathexis, which the therapist must recognize.

The therapist often, in attempting to win the favour of his adolescent patient or because of overidentification with the youth, will join in condemning the parents, and as a result may mobilize the adolescent's basic loyalty and love for his parents and turn him against the therapist. The psychiatrist should have at least a sympathetic recognition of why the parents are what they are and help the adolescent develop insight and avoid the adolescents' loyalty conflict that may necessitate his escape from the therapeutic situation.

Often the psychiatrist has to work closely with the youth's parents in either concomitant or conjoint family therapy. The young adolescent usually accepts this without questioning, but the older adolescent may initially reject involving his parents, and it becomes necessary for the psychiatrist to convince the adolescent that it is for his welfare. The therapist cannot meet all of the adolescent's needs. When the youth regresses to a dependent phase, he requires the kind of help from his parents that a child requires. Insight alone will not make him wisely independent until his ego is strengthened so that he can be helped to emancipate himself. The adolescent needs to grow out of his childhood, not be freed from it.

When it comes to communication, it is vital to understand that even though the adolescent does verbalize, problems of getting the message across still exist, and it is essential that the therapist be 'tuned in on the youth's wavelength'. Only the psychiatrist with adequate training, interest, experience and empathy with young people can cope with this age group. The problems of communication are often complicated when the psychiatrist mimics the teenager's language and attitudes, when this is contrary to his own personality, in an attempt to win his cooperation.

Group Psychotherapy

Group psychotherapy may be more effective with some adolescents than individual psychotherapy. Adolescents are extremely receptive to group pressure and will often modify their value systems more readily through the influence of their peers than through a relationship only with an adult. The unique power of group therapy is its ability to bring problems out into the open. The members of a group are all equal. The patient is both a participant and a therapist—giving as well as getting support, reassurance, guidance—and his ability to help others increases his self-respect. But the most important single characteristic is the patient's realization that what he thought was unique and shameful is felt by other people.

Depending upon the orientation of the therapist or group leader, the groups vary as to size, composition, the use of a single leader or co-leaders and the degree of spontaneity or direction that is given to the sessions.

Group therapy varies from short-term problem-related counseling to long-term groups which aim at deep-seated character reconstruction. Most therapists focus on every day realities and experiences with the group although a few, such as Slavson and Epstein, report working at a psychoanalytic level.

Some of the group techniques used are:

(*a*) Peer-group psychotherapy at all levels of the community mental health program—clinic, day treatment, inpatient and crisis intervention.[53,112]

(*b*) Problem-oriented groups such as groups of pregnant girls, unwed mothers, cardiac, diabetic or otherwise handicapped adolescents.[44,58,93,107,127]

(*c*) Group guidance at schools.[5]

(*d*) Repressive–inspirational groups, in which the 'have-been-sick' try to help the currently sick. They emphasize building morale through strong group identification. This method has been effective in the treatment of youth who use drugs excessively as well as with chronic alcoholics. Many of these groups use a confrontation approach, in which the patient having the floor is taunted by the others to admit his weakness, to face reality and to promise change, and is held accountable in future sessions. Some of these groups use prolonged marathon sessions in order to break down resistance. These groups (e.g. Synanon, Renaissance, Encounter) usually operate outside of the community mental health service but should be included and adequately supervised.

(*e*) Group intake and evaluation interviews at the clinic to facilitate admission and to give temporary help until individual placement for therapy is made.[126]

(*f*) Groups in which members of several families including the patients and parents are seen together.[29]

(*g*) Group counseling of parents at a single or series of orientation sessions to keep parents informed of their children in therapy.[24]

(*h*) Role-playing techniques: role-playing is the flexible acting out of various types of problems which the patient may frequently have to face in reality, in a permissive group atmosphere. As few as two people can role-play, such as the therapist and the client, but most role-playing is usually in groups where two people act out a situation and the group discusses it.

Since it is free of the tensions and consequences of an actual problem situation, role-playing stimulates the trying out of new alternatives and solutions in life-like situations. This is an effective approach in the treatment of disadvantaged youth who may have difficulty in verbalizing; one should, however, assiduously avoid the theatrical aspects often connected with psychodrama.[101]

Family Therapy[1,2,7,56,83,108,122]

When adolescents are still living emotionally and economically as part of their families, it is often not possible to achieve substantial and permanent change in the youth without family involvement in therapy.

There are three general categories of family therapy used in psychiatric outpatient clinics: (a) collaborative treatment—the more traditional approach of the child guidance clinics, in which the child is seen by one therapist and the parents by the social worker; (b) concomitant, concurrent or parallel family therapy, practised by some therapists when they see different members of the family separately; (c) conjoint family therapy, in which almost all the sessions include all or most of the family members jointly in the same family group session. This has been found most effective, since the adolescent, the normal patient, is often merely the scapegoat and his behavior is a reflection of the family psychopathology which has to be modified before we can anticipate that the youth will improve. Seeing the whole family, on regular sequential weekly sessions, has provided the opportunity to locate more easily those family members who need treatment and is thus a very effective approach in a community-oriented mental health center.

Several modifications of family therapy have been used, including family intake and follow up interviews, family crisis therapy[65,66] and family home therapy.[6,15] Multiple impact family therapy, first reported by MacGregor et al.[76] has been used effectively in Maimonides Hospital in Brooklyn, New York, in their family-centered Mental Health Service for adolescents and young adults.[115] It consists of a single prolonged session of intensive involvement by a multidisciplinary group which is repeated as required at 3- to 6-month intervals.

Family therapy with indigent families may have to be modified, since they are often not interested or are too burdened to be willing to discuss their emotional problems without any tangible gratifications. In these circumstances, groups and clubs are centered initially around activities—whether they be recreational, cooking classes, housing problems or even coffee clubs.[24]

Psychopharmacology[19,32,35]

Although medications are of limited therapeutic value in the treatment of most adolescents there are specific indications for their use, and they should be a part of the therapeutic armamentarium of the psychiatric

R

outpatient clinic. The psychiatrist must develop the skills necessary to utilize medication most effectively in association with psychotherapy. The objectives of psychopharmacological agents are to control impulses, relieve anxiety, encourage patterning and render the patient amenable to significant relationships. Medication in itself does not change established patterns of behavior but is often able to ameliorate symptoms so as to facilitate psychotherapy, education and socialization. Attention must be given at all times to the psychological aspects of the patient–physician relationship which undoubtedly plays as important, if not a more important, role than the medication.

Socio-therapeutic Approaches

The disadvantaged youth especially need a variety of services to help them function in society. Many low-income youth particularly lack 'know-how' with regard to obtaining jobs, work performance, appropriate attitudes, behavior and so on, and much of the training in such programs as HARYOU in New York City has been directed toward this area. In addition, such projects as JOB CORPS require vocationally-oriented psychotherapeutic programs.[73, 74]

Remedial Education [5, 21, 64, 70, 90]

Remedial education may be the function of the community educational facility of the comprehensive mental health clinic. This would be under the supervision of an educational coordinator serving as a liaison between the educational and mental health facilities of a community. The New Orleans Regional Mental Health Center has demonstrated the effectiveness of a school within the outpatient clinic for disturbed youth with learning problems.

5

Patterns of Treatment Services

The chief function of a psychiatric outpatient clinic is to provide services that make it possible for a patient to remain in the community while receiving psychiatric care. In spite of the large numbers of adolescent patients referred for psychiatric outpatient care, very few of the community projects have the spectrum of facilities to provide the wide range of treatment modalities needed by disturbed adolescents.[3, 26, 43, 49, 90, 118, 122, 125]

The concept of the community mental health center, although stressing the mental health needs of the entire community, with its free and reciprocal flow of patients among a variety of facilities will, it is hoped, drastically reduce the waiting lists in outpatient clinics. With the help of an expanded staff, new community facilities and creative methods of dealing with referred patients, the all-purpose, general clinic will ordinarily be able to avoid long delays and arrange for some immediate help for the family needing it.[30, 61] However, there must still be provision made for the long term treatment of adolescents.

The neighborhood health centers for children and youth is another approach recommended by the Joint Commission on Mental Health of Children. These centers would emphasize the total health needs of children and youth including their mental health.[86]

The special needs of the adolescent could be met by either community mental health or neighborhood health centers if the treatment modalities and required patterns of services would be available, either dispersed through the clinic or as an adolescent service within the general clinic. Another approach is the development of separate adolescent psychiatric clinics.

All-purpose Psychiatric Outpatient Clinics[41, 59, 61, 79, 88, 90]

The general, all-purpose or multi-purpose psychiatric clinic would be the largest and key service in the community mental health center. It should be closely integrated with the other services in the community both inpatient and outpatient, and serve as a bridge between these services. Most adolescents would enter the clinic program through the same door as all other patients and be seen by the same intake workers, diagnosticians, and receive individual psychotherapy by the same therapists as the other patients in the general clinic. Some adolescents requiring special treatment would be referred to an adolescent psychiatrist for evaluation and disposition, others for special individual, group or family psychotherapy, placed on medication or referred for some other modality of treatment. In some centers these services would be a part of the all-purpose clinic, but in others there would be a special adolescent service. The important factor in the adequate care of the adolescent is the availability of the treatment modalities that are needed, and psychiatrists trained and interested in this age group.

An adolescent psychiatrist should also be a part of the staff of such an all-purpose clinic and serve as a coordinator of the specialized adolescent services associated with the clinic. He would also be responsible for the training of the mental health personnel in the psychiatric care of the adolescents.

Adolescent Psychiatric Clinics[28, 68, 90]

Special psychiatric clinics for adolescents should be organized in the community mental health centers. The criteria for referral would vary among the centers. Such clinics would be programmed in depth and provide for many of the special needs of adolescents. They would be staffed by adolescent psychiatrists, general and child psychiatrists seeking more experience and training with adolescents and residents. Special clinics for adolescents have been found to be more effective than general clinics, because of the training and orientation of the staff and the fact that the clinic limits its interest to adolescents. Adolescents react more effectively to personnel and services dedicated to their needs.[111,114,121]

The mental health clinics at colleges and the satellite clinics in high schools, previously discussed, are specialized adolescent psychiatric clinics because of their location. The existing adolescent clinics associated with psychiatric institutes, social agencies and general hospitals function as general or specialized psychiatric clinics for adolescents with criteria for admission varying, but determined by an admission clerk or an admission committee.

In some community mental health centers the adolescent psychiatric clinic would be part of an overall adolescent service which would include a day treatment center, group and family psychotherapy and remedial education and the variety of other treatment modalities.

No matter which format is used, the community mental health center or neighborhood health center should have available adolescent psychiatrists to serve as consultants and training supervisors and be available to treat some of the special problem cases.

The adolescent service of the Psychosomatic and Psychiatric Institute of Michael Reese Hospital has a functioning outpatient clinic and day treatment center as well as an inpatient service with a wide range of treatment modalities available for the adolescent patient, and may well serve as a model for this type of program.

Adolescent Health Maintenance Clinics

These general adolescent clinics were the outgrowth of adolescent endocrine or development clinics such as those initiated by the author in the late 1930's[109,110,113] and pediatric group clinics developed through the efforts of such pediatricians as Gallagher,[40] Michelson[81] and Roth.[106] They demonstrated the close interplay between the physical and mental state of teenagers.[113,114] Many clinics for this age group, varying in scope and programs, have been organized in different sections of the country. Some are designed for the general care of adolescents, such as the Adolescent Unit of the Children's Medical Center of Boston[40] and the Comprehensive Care Outpatient Adolescent Clinic at the Jewish Hospital of Brooklyn, New York.[115] Others limit their goals to the management of medical problems, and refer concomitant emotional difficulties to other psychiatric facilities for treatment. In these clinics, pediatricians are usually trained to give the necessary guidance under the supervision of an adolescent psychiatrist. Some integrated clinics, however, such as the Beth Israel Medical Center in New York City[130] use psychiatrists, psychologists, social workers and other professionals trained to work with adolescents to organize a variety of treatment modalities.

Another approach would be through the development of neighborhood health centers which would stress the general health care of the child and adolescent and in this way cope with their emotional needs, as advocated by the Joint Commission on Mental Health of Children. The neighborhood health center could be attached to the pediatric divisions of the general hospitals, servicing the catchment area, with the mental health needs being coordinated through the community mental health center.[86,130]

Either of these approaches could serve the needs of the youth, if provisions are made for their psychiatric care and the required modalities for treatment are available. Until such centers are organized, however, any agency in a community could coordinate the existing youth oriented outpatient psychiatric facilities into an integrated psychiatric service for adolescents. A program in depth with well-trained and motivated personnel is more important than a building to house such a service.

Psychopharmacologic Clinics[32,35]

Because a large number of patients attending outpatient clinics require medication and because of the need to develop a method for systematically evaluating new medications on psychiatric outpatients, a drug clinic could be a part of the total operation of the outpatient clinic to which the few adolescents primarily on medication would be referred.

This type of clinic usually functions very much like a medical clinic held once a week for two hours. Here patients are seen once or twice per month for ten to fifteen minutes by a psychiatrist or a psychiatrically oriented pediatrician or general practitioner. The immediate concern in these interviews is with recent symptoms: hyperactivity, sleep disturbance, anxiety, difficulties in interpersonal relationships, thinking disorder and depression. Besides adjusting the dosage of medication and evaluating toxicity, the physician must also be able to help the patient cope realistically with any problems he may present. The patient should also be able to phone the clinic in case there are any evidences of toxicity.

Partial Hospitalization[21,33,38,63,64,78,87,116,122,124]

Bierer of London and Dzhagaror of Moscow first described partial psychiatric hospitalization in 1937. The day hospital has been the most common form of partial hospitalization.[95] Psychiatric day care is designed for those who do not need twenty-four-hour hospitalization but for whom the usual outpatient therapy is inadequate. It is actually an outpatient day-care service. The patient spends a full day at a special institution or hospital ward and returns home to sleep at night. For the disturbed young adolescent it permits school, in a therapeutic center, and psychotherapy while he still lives at home.

The accelerated rate of growth of day hospitals in the past decade has been remarkable. There is a growing confidence in the suitability of day hospitals for a large group of adolescents now being hospitalized.[116]

The day hospital is more than a substitute for residential care; it is a clinical entity that has specific values of its own. The advantage of day hospitals over residential care centers is that they allow the patient to maintain his ties with his family and community. They are also easier for patients and family to accept than residential care. Yet they allow for more intensive psychosocial and special educational involvement than the usual outpatient treatment.[98] The therapeutic milieu is an important factor in its effectiveness. Such a program is, in effect, among other places, at Los Angeles County General Hospital, California, at Linden Hill in Hawthorne, New York, at Butler Hospital in Providence, Rhode Island, at Michael Reese Hospital in Chicago and at St Elizabeth's Hospital in Washington, D.C.

Some of the institutions and hospitals have used the same facilities twofold by setting up a night hospital for those youth who are able to work or go to school during the day but cannot live with their families at night. This is usually in a hospital setting, where patients come to sleep in the wards at night and partake of the therapeutic program offered by the hospital.[63,116]

Emergency Services[11,20,23,25,44,65,66,85,91,122,123]

There have been a variety of emergency psychiatric services available to adolescents under the descriptive titles of Emergency Services, Short-term Psychotherapy, Walk-in Clinics, Crisis Intervention Clinics, Family Crisis Clinics and Emergency Home Services. The common denominator of these services is the availability of psychotherapeutic consultation without a previous appointment.

These services may be part of the emergency room services of a general hospital, clinic of the community mental health center, neighborhood health center, the psychiatric clinic of a general or psychiatric hospital, or even a youth or community organization. It may be the office of the school psychologist or the social worker in a community agency. They serve as extensions of the outpatient services, and ideally should be available in as close proximity as possible on a twenty-four-hour, seven days-a-week, basis. Some, however, are available only on specific hours, but require no appointments.

Short term psychotherapy consisting at most of five or six sessions is all that these clinics provide. If more treatment is required, the patient is sent to the long-term treatment or all-purpose clinic of the outpatient department. However, Zwerling reports that in the Mental Hygiene Clinic of the Bronx Municipal Hospital Center, New York, only about 10 per cent of all applicants of all ages require such referral.[128]

Crisis intervention is directed at helping the individual avoid regression to the use of maladaptive devices to cope with the crisis and aiding him to capitalize on the growth potential inherent in learning to meet a crisis. Thus well-directed intervention through brief psychotherapy at the appropriate time and place not only can result in a diminution of serious emotional disturbance and recompensation but can also serve as a basis for further emotional development.[84] In addition, crisis intervention can often avoid hospitalization and institutionalization and can frequently save time and effort on the part of mental health professionals.

Crisis intervention therapy does not change long-established patterns of maladaptation or immature behavior. Changes of this magnitude require other approaches to treatment. However, emergency treatment facilities should be expanded as a method of treating psychiatric decompensation.

Another version of crisis intervention service is brief hospitalization such as at the Fort Logan Crisis Intervention Unit, where overnight beds are available in the emergency area of a general hospital [62] while other services like the Connecticut Mental Health Center Emergency Treatment Unit allow a three- to five-day stay.

In a growing number of communities, a suicide-prevention telephone service is being developed on a twenty-four-hour, seven-day-a-week basis.[37]

Foster Homes and Group Homes[27]

Failure in personal relationships is considered to be the most important cause of maladjustment. If the relationships in the home have broken down, it may be necessary to remove the child from the home for more effective treatment. Foster homes or group homes are used as a temporary substitute for the home.

Foster-home placement for maladjusted adolescents or following residential treatment is recognized to be most difficult. It is difficult for adolescents to accept strangers as substitute parents and it is not easy to find foster parents who can tolerate the behavior and have the understanding and maturity necessary to help the youth. Foster homes are of questionable value, but it is considered a possible plan for anxious and unhappy young adolescents, if the home situation is beyond improvement, and if regular visits are made to the foster home by a psychiatric social worker. These adolescents also usually attend an outpatient clinic for psychotherapy. The Southeast Louisiana Hospital in Mandeville, Louisiana, has combined a foster-home project with a day-treatment program.

Hostels, half-way houses and residence clubs are all modifications of the concept of group home facilities and may be a part of a psychiatric hospital or community agency. This type of facility is important for the adequate care of adolescents. It could serve both those discharged from institutions who should not be returned to their families immediately and youths in the community who need a protected and supervised living arrangement away from home, but do not require constant supervision.

These youths go to school or work in the local community, while attending the community psychiatric clinic. They may also have group sessions in the hostel.

Specialized Clinics

Large numbers of clinics have developed with specialized interests such as drop-out clinics, drug-abuse clinics, clinics for unmarried mothers,[44,58,93,127] adolescent cardiacs, adolescent diabetics and several other subgroups of youth. These clinics are doing excellent work, probably more effectively than the general all-purpose clinic, essentially because the staff is oriented, trained and interested in the problem under study.

Psychiatric services for the courts, probation and parole, should also be planned as part of the outpatient clinical facilities of the community.[8] After-care or follow-up clinics for adolescents discharged from psychiatric hospitals are also needed.

Home Care[6,15,22]

Several programs have been developed in which the mental health specialist or public health nurse goes to the homes of multi-problem families to involve them in family therapy.

In addition, the impact of psychiatric knowledge and experience has brought about new emphasis in casework skills and new practices in family and child welfare agencies. Social workers are increasingly concerned with emotional needs and conflicts as well as with environmental and physical stresses. Many agencies maintain programs which are psychiatrically oriented with a psychiatrist as consultant for the staff. Family casework agencies may offer both casework services and psychiatric consultation to the adolescent who needs institutional care, foster-home placement or special group experiences, and to his family.

One of the objectives of a welfare program is to strengthen family relationships and hold the family group together for the sake of the children. Along with psychiatric help, where this is needed, other kinds of support under social welfare auspices are often required.

Special Services for the Indigent[96,100,101,102]

Neighborhood service centers as store-front facilities have been developed in various parts of the country.

Lincoln Hospital Mental Health Service has developed several such centers which are staffed by five or six indigenous non-professional personnel called 'mental health aides'. The center, through the help of the 'expeditor',[52] offers a wide range of services to the residents or the area, giving assistance in problems of housing, welfare, unemployment, school and legal matters. When indicated, the aide will refer the applicant to the center's supervisor, a professional mental health worker, who may, in turn, send the client to the mental health clinic. It is their experience that the use of indigenous non-professionals is an absolute essential for reaching deprived minority groups. The staff is multilingual, and every effort is made to make the atmosphere congenial.[51]

Vocational Guidance, Training and Rehabilitation

Vocational guidance and training of the younger adolescents is essentially the responsibility of the school. The state and federal government vocational advisory and rehabilitation services are helping the older adolescents in close collaboration with the mental health specialist in cases of emotionally disturbed youth, as discussed in the section on services in the community.

Mental disorders in adolescence interfere with the education of the youth and the orderly development of his occupational career. His learning of socially and occupationally required skills is inhibited, and he is removed from the normal channels of communication which usually determine job choice by arousing appropriate interests and providing the opportunity for identification with role models. Once a disturbance has occurred in this complicated process and the adolescent is 'out of step', his return to a normal educational or occupational path becomes very difficult.

There is a need for vocational training facilities which have developed special resources to cope with this program and to work in close collaboration with mental health specialists. Collaboration is best achieved if workers from each system penetrate the other in order to obtain an identification with the other's point of view and learn to appreciate the nature and boundaries of the collaborator's expertness. This means that vocational selection and training personnel should be used as consultants and collaborators in rehabilitation units within the community mental health programs, e.g. in mental hospitals and day-treatment centers; and that psychiatrists, social workers and psychologists should go into the vocational training and rehabilitation institutions in an advisory capacity.

Personnel

There has been a difference of opinion among psychiatrists as to whether adolescents should be treated exclusively by child psychiatrists or by specially trained adolescent psychiatrists, or whether both child and general psychiatrists should accept responsibilities for the treatment of the emotionally disturbed adolescent. This divergence of opinion has been reflected in the organization of both outpatient and inpatient services for adolescents.[3,111,112,114]

It is well known that not all psychiatrists are equipped for or interested in the treatment of adolescents, and only those with special interest and training with this age group manage to do effective work. In addition to training special adolescent psychiatrists, it is hoped that all residents in psychiatry, general as well as child psychiatry, will receive training and supervised experience with adolescents.[4] Psychiatrists who did not have this indoctrination and wish to treat adolescents should acquire on-job experience under supervision.

Separation of adolescent psychiatry as an entity would enhance research, treatment and progress in understanding the particular emotional problems of the teenager. I would recommend that an adolescent psychiatrist be placed in charge of the complete inpatient and outpatient program for adolescents in any community mental health center, with well-qualified mental health personnel working with him. It would be his responsibility to coordinate the work of all the units treating adolescents. The other professionals such as psychologists, social workers, teachers, recreation workers and group leaders dealing with youth in the clinics should also develop the special competence within their specialty required to work effectively with this age group.[120]

Two types of mental health aides have been developed to take care of the special needs of indigent patients. The indigenous non-professionals are selected largely by their demonstration of leadership ability in individual and group situations, and are first trained for three weeks on a full-time basis, and one is then allotted the equivalent of one day a week in conference time. It is felt that because these aides come from the same cultural milieu as the patients, they are more effective in reaching them and helping them. These aides should be differentiated from what Reiff and Riessman called the 'ubiquitous non-professionals', who are middle-class housewives, college students and graduates, trained to serve as clinic and ward aides to relieve the mental health specialists of some of their duties.[69, 99]

6

Summary

Everyone working with youth accepts the fact that adolescence is a reality and represents a crucial stage in the development of an individual as well as in the epidemiological cycle of mental illness. The mental health specialist who is concerned with the preventive aspects of psychiatry should be interested in the individual at a stage in his life cycle when previous identifications are up for review, new ones are being formed and prior to continuing the reproductive stage and transmitting maladaptive patterns to the next generation.

The therapist should take advantage of this situation, since behavior is a continuous dynamic process in which the adaptive functions of one stage become the internalized structure of the next.

All treatment should correlate the intrinsic needs of the adolescent with the available therapeutic resources. The discrepancy between the numbers of adolescents requiring treatment and the availability of professionals and community resources, demands program designs devoted to bridging the gap. With this in mind, outpatient programs for disturbed adolescents require the development of a broad spectrum of coordinated and integrated facilities. This can be achieved through the inclusion of a comprehensive set of program components for prevention, diagnosis, treatment and rehabilitation in each community at three levels—the schools, the general community and the community's psychiatric services.

Numerous ingenious program elements catering to the needs of adolescents are discussed. Each community in setting up a comprehensive mental health program to include adolescents should evaluate its problems, its resources and its personnel, and adopt such of these services as would best fit its situation.

Schools are important components of any comprehensive psychiatric program for adolescents, as they are in the position or encourage the development of normal mental health, to recognize problems early, to involve the troubled youth in individual or group guidance, or to refer him for appropriate psychotherapy either to a school-based mental health clinic or the outpatient clinic in the community.

Community agencies such as the Mental Health Association should provide, in close cooperation with religious, community and parents' groups, a variety of psychiatrically oriented educational programs and workshops for parents for professionals other than mental health specialists. In addition, community based youth social and recreational facilities should be developed.

Outpatient psychiatric facilities for adolescents may be developed within the context of a comprehensive community mental health center, a general psychiatric, a child-guidance or a specialized adolescent clinic. Whichever facility is utilized, there is a need for a variety of treatment modalities including individual, group and family psychotherapy and psychopharmacology. These may be achieved through different treatment services. The all-purpose general psychiatric outpatient clinic is one resource and the specialized adolescent clinic is another; but there is also a need for day hospitals, group homes, walk-in or emergency clinics and other specialized services for adolescents.

For a community mental health program to be effective in the care of adolescents, a staff of mental health specialists, including adolescent psychiatrists with special training and interest in this age group, is essential. A separate adolescent service with adequate staff would enhance the effectiveness of any of the outpatient clinical facilities.

REFERENCES

1. ACKERMAN, N. W. 1961. Emergence of family psychotherapy on the present scene. In *Contemporary psychotherapies*, Ed. M. I. Stein, 228. Glencoe, Illinois: Free Press.
2. ACKERMAN, N. W. 1962. Adolescent problems: a symptom of family disorder. *Fam. Process*, 1, 202.
3. American Psychiatric Association. 1964. *Comprehensive psychiatric programs, a survey of 234 facilities*. Washington, D.C.: Publications Department.
4. American Psychiatric Association. 1967. Position statement on adolescent psychiatry. Committee on psychiatry in childhood and adolescence. *Amer. J. Psychiat.*, 123, 1031.
5. Association of N.Y. State educators of the emotionally disturbed role of the classroom teacher of the emotionally disturbed child. 1966. *Report of the First ANYSEED conference*. Hawthorne Cedar Knolls School, Hawthorne, N.Y. (Mimeo)

6. BEHRENS, M. I. 1967. Brief home visits by the clinic therapist in the treatment of lower-class patients. *Amer. J. Psychiat.*, **124**, 371.
7. BELL, J. E. 1963. A theoretical position for family group therapy. *Fam. Process*, **2**, 1.
8. BERNARD, V. W. and ABBATE, G. M. 1964. Report of the department of hospitals' comm. on psychiatric services for children. New York City Community Mental Health Board (Pub.).
9. BINDMAN, A. J. 1961. *The psychologist as a mental health consultant*. American Psychological Association, New York.
10. BLAIN, G. B. and McARTHUR, C. C. (Eds) 1961. *Emotional problems of the student*. New York: Appleton-Century-Crofts.
11. BLANE, H. T., MULLER, J. J. and CHAFETZ, M. E. 1967. Acute psychiatric services in the general hospital, II. current status of emergency psychiatric services. *Amer. J. Psychiat.*, **124**, 37.
12. BLOS, P. 1962. *On adolescence: a psychoanalytic interpretation*. New York: Free Press.
13. BLOS, P. 1967. Second individuation process of adolescence. *Psychoanalytic study of the child*, **22**, 162. New York: International Universities Press.
14. BOYCE, R. M. and BARNES, D. S. 1966. Psychiatric problems of university students. *Canad. psychiat. Ass. J.*, **11**, 49.
15. BROWN, B. S. 1962. Home visiting by psychiatrists. *Arch. gen. Psychiat.*, **7**, 98.
16. BROWN, B. S. and LEVENSON, A. I. 1966. The expanding vistas of mental health services. *Hosp. Community Psychiat.*, **17**, 33.
17. BROWN, W. N. 1968. Alienated Youth. *Ment. Hyg.*, **52**, 330.
18. BRYT, A. 1966. Modifications of psychoanalysis in the treatment of adolescents. In *Adolescence, dreams and training*, Ed. J. H. Masserman, New York: Grune & Stratton.
19. BURTON, A. 1960. Drugs or psychotherapeutic program for disturbed adolescent boys. *A.M.A. Arch. gen. Psychiat.*, **2**, 5.
20. CAMERON, W. R. 1962. How to set up a community psychiatric emergency service. *Amer. J. publ. Hlth.*, **52**, Suppl. 16.
21. CAPLAN, G. and LEBOVICI, S. (Eds) 1969. *Adolescence: Psychosocial Perspectives*. New York: Basic Books.
22. CAPLAN, G. 1955. The role of the social worker in preventive psychiatry. *Med. Soc. Work*, **4**, 144.
23. CHAFETZ, M. E., BLANE, H. T. and MULLER, J. J. 1966. Acute psychiatric services in the general hospital, I. Implications for psychiatry in emergency admission. *Amer. J. Psychiat.*, **123**, 664.
24. CHILMAN, B. S. and KRAFT, I. 1963. Helping low-income parents—through parent education groups. *Children*, **10**, 127.
25. COLEMAN, J. V. 1968. Research in walk-in psychiatric services in general hospitals. *Amer. J. Psychiat.*, **124**, 1668.
26. COLEMAN, J. V. 1964. Outpatient psychiatry. *Amer. J. Psychiat.*, **120**, 687.
27. DELAGAH, H. C. 1963. Foster-family care following residential treatment: the essentials of planning. *Child Welfare*, **42**, 331.
28. DENEKE, E. 1968. Denmark's first department for adolescent psychiatry. *T. Sygepl.*, **68**, 344.
29. DONNER, J. and GAMSON, A. 1968. Experience with multi-family, time-limited, outpatient groups at a community psychiatric clinic. *Psychiatry*, **31**, 126.
30. EIDUSON, B. J. 1968. The clinic in the year 2000. *Arch. gen. Psychiat.*, **19**, 385.

31. EISENBERG, L. 1960. Emotionally disturbed children and youth. Children and Youth in the 1960s—Survey Papers prepared for the 1960 White House Conference on children and youth. 275.

32. ENGELHARDT, D. M. and FREEDMAN, N. 1965. Maintenance drug therapy: the schizophrenic patient in the community. *Int. Psychiat. Clin.*, **2**, 933.

33. EPPS, R. L., and HANES, L. D. (Eds) 1964. *Day-care of psychiatric patients*, from the National Day Hospital workshop held in Kansas City, Missouri. Springfield, Illinois: Charles C. Thomas.

34. ESTY, G. W. 1967. The prevention of psychosocial disorders of youth: a challenge to mental health, public health and education. *J. Sch. Health.* **37**, 19.

35. EVELOFF, H. H. 1966. Psychopharmacologic agents in child psychiatry. *A.M.A. Arch. gen. Psychiat.*, **14**, 472.

36. FALSTEIN, E. I. and OFFER, D. 1963. Adolescent therapy. In *Prog. Clin. Psych.*, **5**, 60, Eds L. E. Abt and B. F. Riess.

37. FARBEROW, N. L., SCHNEIDMAN, E. S., LITMAN, R. E., WOLD, C. I., HEILIG, S. M. and KRAMER, J. 1966. Suicide prevention around the clock. *Amer. J. Orthopsychiat.*, **36**, 551.

38. FARNDALE, W. A. J. 1961. *The day hospital movement in Great Britain.* Oxford: Pergamon Press.

39. FARNSWORTH, D. L. 1966. *Psychiatry, education and the young adult.* Springfield, Illinois: Charles C. Thomas.

40. GALLAGHER, J. R. 1954. The adolescent unit of the children's medical center. *Children*, **1**, 165.

41. GAYLIN, S. 1968. The adolescent and the mental health center. In *Mental health services for adolescents*, Ed. S. Nichtern, 61.

42. GILBERG, A. 1965. Editorial: *Adolescents in State hospitals: expensive expediency*, **35**, 825.

43. GLASSCOTE, R. M., SANDERS, D. S., FORSTENZER, H. M. and FOLEY, A. R. 1964. *The community mental health center: an analysis of existing models.* Publications Department, American Psychiatric Association, Washington, D.C.

44. GLASSCOTE, R. M., CUMMING, E., HAMMERSLEY, D. W., OZARIN, L. D. and SMITH, L. H. 1966. *The psychiatric emergency—a study of patterns of service.* Washington: APA-NAMH Joint Information Service.

45. GLASSER, W. 1965. *Reality therapy.* New York: Harper & Row.

46. GOULD, R. E. 1965. Suicidal problems in children and adolescents. *Amer. J. Psychother.*, **19**, 228.

47. GRANT, M. Q. and WARREN, M. 1963. Alternates to institutionalization. *Children*, **10**, 147.

48. GREENBLATT, M. 1963. *The prevention of hospitalization: treatment without admission for psychiatric patients.* New York: Grune & Stratton.

49. Group for the advancement of psychiatry. 1968. *Normal adolescence*, 6.

50. HALLECK, S. 1967. Psychiatric treatment of the alienated college student. *Amer. J. Psychiat.*, **124**, 642.

51. HALLOWITZ, E. and RIESSMAN, F. 1967. The role of the indigenous nonprofessional in a community mental health neighborhood service center program. *Amer. J. Orthopsychiat.*, **37**, 4.

52. HANSELL, N., WODARCZK, M., and VISOTSKY, H. M. 1968. Mental health expediter. *Arch. gen. Psychiat.*, **18**, 392.

53. HEACOCK, D. R. 1966. Modification of the standard techniques for out-patient group psychotherapy with delinquent boys. *J. nat. med. Ass.*, **58**, 41.

54. HENDRICKSON, W. J. 1967. Treating adolescents: transference and countertransference problems. *Frontiers Clin. Psychiat.*, **4**, 1.

55. HOLMES, D. J. 1964. *The adolescent in psychotherapy.* Boston: Little, Brown.
56. JACKSON, D. D. and WEAKLAND, J. H. 1961. Conjoint family therapy: some considerations on theory, technique and results. *Psychiatry,* **24,** 30.
57. JORGENSEN, A. 1967. Observations on child and adolescent psychiatric care in Norway. *Sykepleien,* **54,** 430.
58. KAUFMANN, P. N. and DEUTSCH, A. L. 1967. Group therapy for pregnant unwed adolescents in the prenatal clinic of a general hospital. *Int. J. Group Psychother.,* **17,** 309.
59. KNIGHT, J. A. and DAVIS, W. E. 1964. *Manual for the comprehensive community mental health clinic.* Springfield, Illinois: Charles C. Thomas.
60. KOPFF, R. G. and KRAMER, J. 1969. *A college student center: a new concept in community psychiatry,* presented at the American Orthopsychiatric Meeting: New York City.
61. KORNER, H. 1964. Abolishing the waiting list in a mental health center. *Amer. J. Psychiat.,* **120,** 1097.
62. KRAFT, A. M. 1963. Fort Logan Mental Health Center—*Progress Report Feb.* 1963 (Mimeo).
63. KRAMER, B. M. 1962. *Day hospital—a study of partial hospitalization in psychiatry.* New York: Grune & Stratton.
64. LANG, J. L. 1965. Medical-pedagogical outpatient services and day hospitals. *Concours méd.,* **87,** 6361.
65. LANGSLEY, D. G., FAIRBAIRN, R. H. and DE YOUNG, C. D. 1968. Adolescence and family crises. *Canad. psychiat. Ass. J.,* **13,** 125.
66. LANGLSEY, D. G., PITTMAN, F. S., MACHOTKA, P. and FLOMENHAFT, K. 1968. Family crisis therapy—results and implications. *Fam. Process,* **7,** 145.
67. LAUFER, M. 1965. A psychoanalytical approach to work with adolescents. The work of the young people's consultation centre (London) with remarks on diagnosis and technique. *Psychother. Psychosom.,* **13,** 292.
68. LEBOVICI, S. 1965. Out-patient psychiatric services for children and adolescents. *Seminar on Out-Patient Psychiatric Services,* Geneva, September 15–24, 1965. Copenhagen: Regional Office for Europe, World Health Organization.
69. LEIF, H. I. 1966. Sub-professional training in mental health. *Arch. gen. Psychiat.,* **15,** 660.
70. LEWIS, W. W. 1965. *Project re-ed: a pattern of residential treatment for emotionally disturbed children.* George Peabody College for Teachers: Nashville, Tenn. (Mimeo).
71. LINTON, T. E. 1969. The European educateur program for disturbed children. *Amer. J. Orthopsychiat.,* **39,** 125.
72. LION, J. R., BACH-Y-RITA, G. and ERVIN, F. R. 1968. The self-referred violent patient. *J. Amer. med. Ass.,* **205,** 503.
73. LUZZI, M. and GLASSER, B. A. 1966. Adolescent patients join the neighborhood youth corps. *Hosp. Community Psychiat.,* **7,** 172.
74. MACHT, L. B. SCHERL, D. J. and ENGLISH, J. T. 1968. Psychiatric consultation: the job corps experience. *Amer. J. Psychiat.,* **124,** 1092.
75. MANNINO, F. V. 1964. Developing consultation relationships with community agents. *Ment. Hyg.,* **48,** 356.
76. MACGREGOR, R., RITCHIE, A. M., SERRANO, A. C. and SCHUSTER, F. P., JR. 1964. *Multiple impact therapy with families.* New York: McGraw-Hill.
77. McCULLOCH, J. W., HENDERSON, A. S. and PHILIP, A. E. 1966. Psychiatric illness in Edinburgh teenagers. *Scot. med. J.,* **11,** 277.
78. MELTZOFF, J. and BLUMENTHAL, R. L. 1966. *The day-treatment center: principles, application and evaluation.* Springfield, Illinois: Charles C. Thomas.

79. Mental Health Materials Center, Inc. 1966. *Planning program and design for the community mental health center*. New York.
80. MERENDA, P. F. and ROTHNEY, J. W. M. 1958. Evaluating the effects of counseling after eight years. *J. Counsel. Psychol.*, **5**, 163.
81. MICHELSON, J. P., KLEIN, H., DEUTSCH, A. L., KAUFMANN, P. N. and SMITH, C. H. 1965. Comprehensive care in an adolescent clinic. An integrated physical-mental health program. *Clin. Ped.*, **4**, 409.
82. MILLAR, T. P. 1966. Psychiatric consultation with classroom teachers. *J. Amer. Acad. Child. Psychiat.*, **5**, 134.
83. MILLER, D. 1958. Family interaction and adolescent therapy. *Psychiatry*, **122**, 1240.
84. MILLER, L. C. 1959. Short-term therapy with adolescents. *Amer. J. Orthopsychiat.*, **29**, 772.
85. MILLER, W. B. 1968. A psychiatric emergency service and some treatment concepts. *Amer. J. Psychiat.*, **124**, 924.
86. National Association for Mental Health and Joint Commission on Mental Health of Children. 1968. Work Group Reports and Recommendations from the Joint Conference on Childhood Mental Illness, February 21–23. New York City (Mimeo).
87. National Clearing house for Mental Health Information. 1964. *Psychiatric day–night services, a selected biography*. National Institute of Mental Health: Bethesda, Maryland.
88. New York State Department of Mental Hygiene. 1959. *Guide to communities in the establishment and operation of psychiatric clinics*.
89. New York State Planning Committee on Mental Disorders. 1965. Section on mental health—report of the task force on service for children. Report to the Governor. **6**, 45.
90. NICHTERN, S. 1968. *Mental health services for adolescents*. Proceedings of Second Hillside Hospital Conference. New York: Praeger.
91. NORMAND, W., FENSTERHEIM, H., TANNENBAUM, G. and SAGER, G. 1963. The acceptance of the psychiatric walk-in clinic in a highly deprived community. *Amer. J. Psychiat.*, **120**, 533.
92. OLEINICK, M. S. and BAHN, A. K. 1966. Characteristics of adolescent cases receiving psychiatric services and/or school facility services. Presented at the Sixth International Congress of Child Psychiatry, Edinburgh, Scotland.
93. OSOFSKY, H. J., HAGEN, J. H. and WOOD, P. W. 1968. A program for pregnant schoolgirls. Some early results. *Amer. J. Obstet. Gynec.*, **100**, 1020.
94. OZARIN, L. D. and LEVENSON, A. I. 1967. The community mental health centers program in the U.S.: a new system of mental health care. *Soc. Psychiat.*, **2**, 145.
95. PECK, H. B. 1963. The role of the psychiatric day hospital in a community mental health program. *Amer. J. Orthopsychiat.*, **33**, 482.
96. PECK, H. B., ROMAN, M. and KAPLAN, S. R. 1967. Community action programs and the comprehensive mental health center. In *Poverty and mental health*, Eds M. Greenblatt, R. E. Emory and B. C. Glueck, Jr. Am. Psychiat. Assn., Psychiatric Research Report, 21.
97. RABINER, C. J. and HANKOFF, L. D. 1967. Satellite neighbourhood clinics. *Hosp. Community Psychiat.*, **18**, 282.
98. RAFFERTY, F. T. 1961. Day-treatment structure for adolescents. In *Current Psychiatric Therapies*, Ed. J. H. Masserman. New York: Grune & Stratton.
99. REIFF, R. and RIESSMAN, F. 1964. The indigenous non-professional. Nat. Inst. of Labor Education Mental Health Program Report, No. 3.

100. RIESSMAN, F. 1965. New approaches to mental health treatment for low-income people. Social Work Practice. Nat. Congress on Soc. Work. New York: Columbia Univ. Press.

101. RIESSMAN, F. 1965. New approaches to mental health-treatment for labor and low-income groups. A survey report No. 2. Nat. Inst. of Labor Education, New York City.

102. RIESSMAN, F. and HALLOWITZ, E. 1967. The neighborhood service center: an innovation in preventive psychiatry. *Amer. J. Psychiat.*, **123**, 11.

103. RINSLEY, D. B. 1965. *Theory and practice of intensive residential treatment of adolescents*. Fifth Annual Institute of Pennsylvania Hospital Award Lecture in Memory of Edward A. Strecker, M.D. Roche Lab.: Nutley, N.J., 07110.

104. ROSEN, B. M., BAHN, A. K., SHILLOW, R. and BOWER, E. M. 1965. Adolescent patients served in outpatient psychiatric clinics. *Amer. J. publ. Hlth.*, **55**, 1563.

105. ROSEN, B. M., KRAMER, M., REDLICK, R. W. and WILLNER, S. G. 1969. Utilization of psychiatric facilities by children: current status, trends, implications. Nat. Inst. of Mental Health, Office of Program Planning and Evaluation, Biometry Branch (Mimeo).

106. ROTH, A., WEISSMAN, A. and LINDEN, C. 1956. A plan for medical care of adolescents. *Pediatrics*, **18**, 86.

107. ROTMAN, C. B. and GOLBURGH, S. J. 1967. Group counseling mentally retarded adolescents. *Ment. Retard.*, **5**, 13.

108. SATIR, V. 1964. *Conjoint family therapy*. Palo Alto, Calif.: Science and Behavior Books.

109. SCHONFELD, W. A. 1943. Primary and secondary sexual characteristics. *Amer. J. dis. Child.*, **65**, 535.

110. SCHONFELD, W. A. 1951. Pediatrician's role in the management of the personality problems of adolescents. *Amer. J. dis. Child.*, **81**, 762.

111. SCHONFELD, W. A. 1967. Adolescent psychiatry: an appraisal of the adolescent's position in contemporary psychiatry. *A. M. A. Arch. gen. Psychiat.*, **16**, 713.

112. SCHONFELD, W. A. 1968. Reprinted as 'The adolescent in contemporary American psychiatry with critical evaluations by Josselyn, I., Lebovici, S., Masterson, J., Jrs, Staples, H. and Boutourline Young, H.' *Int. J. Psychiat.*, **5**, 470 and **6**, 77.

113. SCHONFELD, W. A. 1969. The body and the body image in adolescents. *Adolescence: psychosocial perspectives*, Eds Caplan G. and Lebovici, S. p. 27. New York: Basic Books.

114. SCHONFELD, W. A. 1969. *Trends in adolescent psychiatry*, Ed. J. H. Masserman. New York: Grune & Stratton.

115. SIEGEL, L. 1966. Prospectus for a program of family centered mental health services for adolescent and young adult patients, 1965–1970 at Maimonides Hospital of Brooklyn, N.Y.

116. SNEDEVIG, J. and AUKEN, K. 1965. Juvenile patients in the day and night hospital 'Montebello', Gentofte. *Nord. psykiat. T.*, **19**, 426.

117. SOLOMON, P., PATCH, V. D., STURROCK, J. D. and WEXLER, D. 1967. A new approach to student mental health in small colleges. A multiple college mental health center. *Amer. J. Psychiat.*, **125**, 658.

118. SONIS, M. 1964. Patterns of child psychiatry. *J. Amer. Acad. Child Psychiat.*, **3**, 9.

119. Statistical Review. 1966. U.S. Dept. of Health, Education and Welfare, Public Health Service. Nat. Inst. of Mental Health—Patients in Mental Institutions. Prepared by Survey and Reports Section, Office of Biometrics, Nat. Inst. of Mental Health.

120. SzUREK, S. A. 1967. The outpatient clinic of the future. Training in thera-
     peutic work with children. In *Langley Porter Child Psychiatry Series*,
     2, 209. Eds S. A. Szurek and I. Berlin. Palo Alto, Calif.: Science and
     Behavior Books.
121. TEICHER, J. D. 1967. A psychiatric unit for adolescents in a general hospital.
     Hosp. Community Psychiat., **18**, 201.
122. U.S. Dept. of Health, Education and Welfare. Five Essential Services of the
     Community Mental Health Center Public Health Service Pub. Nos. 1449,
     1477, 1478, 1578, 1624.
123. WILDER, J. and COLEMAN, M. D. 1963. The walk-in clinic. *Int. J. soc. Psychiat.*,
     9, 192.
124. WILLNER, S. G. and ROSEN, B. M. 1965. A survey of psychiatric day–night
     services in the U.S. Biometry branch, N.I.M.H.
125. WINTER, W. D. and WINTER, L. M. 1968. Clinical experiences with thera-
     peutic camping. *Adolescence*, **3**, 203.
126. WRIGHT, J. J. 1964. Team approach to intake procedure in a community
     mental health clinic. *Public Health Rep.*, **79**, 488.
127. WRIGHT, M. K. 1966. Comprehensive services for adolescent unwed mothers.
     Children, **13**, 171.
128. ZWERLING, I. 1965. Some implications of social psychiatric treatment and
     patient care. Inst. of Penn. Hosp.—Strecker Monograph Series No. 2.
     Pub. by Roche Lab.
129. Anonymous. 1968. Psychiatric care of the adolescent. *Lancet*, **i**, 676.
130. Personal communication.

AUTHOR INDEX

This index covers volumes 1 to 4 of the Modern Perspectives in Psychiatry series, the figure in bold type denoting the volume of the entry.

T

SUBJECT INDEX

This index covers volumes 1, 2, 3 and 4 of the Modern Perspectives in Psychiatry series, the figures in bold type denoting the volume of entry.

Abdominal pain, **1**: 324
Abely-Delmas symptom (*see* Mirror symptom)
Ability
  wastage, **3**: 533
Abortion, **3**: 21, 35, 37
  spontaneous, **3**: 36, 51
  stress, **3**: 29
  threatened, **3**: 43, 45
Accident-proneness, **1**: 350
  emotional stress, **1**: 362
  family, **1**: 361
  incidence, **1**: 352
  personality, **1**: 356, 360
  predisposing factors, **1**: 357
  prevention, **1**: 365
  psychological factors, **1**: 355
  recognition, **1**: 363
  suicide attempts, **1**: 359
  treatment, **1**: 364
Accidents
  monotony, **2**: 272
  sensory deprivation, **2**: 247
Acetylcholinesterase, **2**: 88
Acne
  in adolescence, **4**: 20, 103
Acrocephalosyndactyly, **3**: 33
Acting out
  existential interpretation, **2**: 512
Acute organic psychoses in childhood, **3**: 706–731
  aetiology, **3**: 709–715
  affective disorders, **3**: 728
  behaviour disorders, **3**: 730
  classification, **3**: 716–718
  coma, **3**: 724
  confusional states, **3**: 720
  definition, **3**: 706
  delirium, **3**: 722
  depersonalization, **3**: 725
  disorders of consciousness, **3**: 718
  drowsiness, **3**: 719
  hallucinations, **3**: 726
  hallucinosis, **3**: 726

  illusions, **3**: 726
  oneirism, **3**: 721
  psychomotor disorders, **3**: 729
  psychosensory disorders, **3**: 726
  stuporose state, **3**: 723
  symptomatology, **3**: 716–731
  thought disorders, **3**: 729
  twilight state, **3**: 724
Adaptation
  adolescence, **4**: 39
  of children, **3**: 72
Adaptive maturity
  peptic ulcers, **3**: 485
  promotion of, **3**: 488
Addiction
  drugs (*see* Drug addiction)
  pica and, **3**: 467
Adjustment
  differentials in adolescents, **4**: 165
  goals in adolescents, **4**: 174
Adolescence
  acne, **4**: 20, 103
  adaptation, **4**: 39
  adjustment, **4**: 174
  adjustment differentials, **4**: 165
  age of majority, **4**: 133
  alcoholism, **4**: 296–298
  anorexia nervosa, **1**: 292; **4**: 242, 274–289
  anxiety, **1**: 290; **4**: 106
  arthritis, **4**: 248
  beatniks, **4**: 141
  behaviour disturbances, **1**: 290, 293
  biological development, **4**: 167–168
  bulimia, **4**: 242
  castration anxiety, **4**: 242
  college mental health services, **4**: 489
  colostomy, **4**: 244
  community services, **4**: 483–511
  competition, **4**: 119
  compulsions, **3**: 381
  conduct disorders, **1**: 293
  confabulation, **4**: 123
  conflicts, **4**: 102, 106
  conformist, **4**: 144

Hydrocephalus
  toxoplasmosis, **3**: 24
Hydrochloric acid, **3**: 475
Hydrohypodynamic environment, **2**: 226
Hyperemesis, **3**: 45, 47
Hypertelorism, **3**: 33
Hyperthymic child, **3**: 174
Hyperthyroidism
  adolescents, **4**: 248
Hypno-analysis, **2**: 165
Hypnosis, **2**: xxi, 146
  in animals, **2**: 147, 148
  athletic training, **2**: 178
  autohypnosis, **2**: 271
  classification of phenomena, **2**: 154–186
  collective (*see* Group hypnosis)
  definition, **2**: 146, 147, 151
  experimental, **2**: 152
  form of suggestion, **2**: 153
  group (*see* Group hypnosis)
  history, **2**: 147
  induction, **2**: 149, 152
  learning, **2**: 157
  monotony, **2**: 272
  phylongeny, **2**: 150
  physiological phenomena, **2**: 154, 155, 157, 158, 159, 160, 172–186
  psychoanalysis, **2**: 477
  psychological phenomena, **2**: 154, 155, 156, 157, 161–172
  rapport, **2**: 156
  semantics, **2**: 174
  simultaneous, **2**: 582
  suggestibility, **2**: 585, 586, 587
  symptom substitution, **2**: 586
  trance depth, **2**: 152
Hypnotic drugs, **2**: 215
  adolescent addiction, **4**: 294, 298–300
  memory and, **2**: 109
  prescription statistics, **2**: 207
Hypochondriasis, **2**: 520, 521, 523
Hypogonadism
  adolescents, **4**: 249
Hypopathia, **4**: 333
Hypophyseal insufficiency (*see* Simmond's disease)
Hypothermia
  memory after, **2**: 109
  psychosymptomatology, **3**: 715
Hypotheses
  refutation, **1**: 8
  research, **1**: 8
  selection, **1**: 9
  verification, **1**: 8
Hypoxic encephalopathy, **2**: 114
Hysteresis, **2**: 171
Hysteria, **2**: xxv, 149, 150
  Anna O.'s case, **3**: 293
  conversion symptoms, **2**: 172; **3**: 14; (in adolescents), **1**: 292; **4**: 247

cultural distribution, **2**: 702; **3**: 14
cultural symptomatology, **2**: 704
Dora's case, **3**: 293
existential analysis, **2**: 503
and psychosis, **1**: 484
stammer, **1**: 347
suggestibility test, **2**: 374
treatment, **2**: 366
Hysterical mutism, **1**: 348

Iatrogenic disorders
  in adolescence, **4**: 21
Ideation
  content, **3**: 246
  irrational, **2**: 402
Identification
  sexual, **3**: 303
  social, **3**: 303
Identified patient (*see* Presenting patient)
Identity, **4**: 41–43
  adolescence, **4**: 34, 41–43, 112
  concept, **1**: 246
  conflicts, **4**: 42
  crisis, **4**: 42
  diffusion, **4**: 118, 120
  formation, **4**: 34, 112, 113
  loss, **4**: 122
  negative, **4**: 118, 123
  resistance, **4**: 460
  in schizophrenia, **2**: 398, 402
  search, **4**: 112
  sexual, **3**: 315
  social, **3**: 315; **4**: 129
Identity-formation
  sexual experimentation, **4**: 34
Idioglossia, **1**: 348
Illeostomy, **3**: 507
  clubs, **3**: 520
Illegitimacy
  culture, **3**: 308
  malformations, **3**: 33, 36
  perinatal deaths, **3**: 34, 36
  prematurity, **3**: 34
Illusions, **2**: 335, 336
  déjà vu, **1**: 178; **2**: 335; **4**: 332, 334, 336
  sleep deprivation, **2**: 203
Imagery, **1**: 172
  body image (q.v.)
  emotive, **2**: 565
  déjà vu, **1**: 178; **2**: 335; **4**: 332, 334, 336
  hypnagogic, **1**: 178; **2**: 198, 199, 205, 209, 231, 269, 270
  imaginary companion, **1**: 180
  predominant, **1**: 173
  range, **1**: 174
  strength, **1**: 174
Imagination, **1**: 170
  abstract thinking, **1**: 77
  development, **1**: 68

perceptual, **3**: 531
Piaget's theory, **1**: 59, 80
placebo, **2**: 603, 607
protein formation, **2**: 101
psychogenic retardation, **3**: 537
role of chemical processes, **2**: 89
schizophrenics, **2**: 380, 381
sensory deprivation, **2**: 240
sleep, **2**: 199
sleep deprivation, **2**: 291
studies on, **2**: 92
theory (*see* Learning theory)
therapy, **1**: 154, 155; **2**: 557
uncommitted cortex programming, **2**: 326, 340
visual, **2**: 111
Learning disabilities
social environment, **4**: 177
Learning theorists, **3**: 81
Learning theory, **1**: 104; **2**: 377
child development, **3**: 62
clinical application, **1**: 113; **2**: 557
conditioned inhibition, **1**: 114
conditioning (q.v.)
conduct problems, **1**: 106
desensitisation, **1**: 114
enuresis, treatment of, **1**: 113, 116, 163; **2**: 212, 569
generalization of responses, **1**: 142
intermittent reinforcement, **1**: 141
modification of conduct, **1**: 378
negative practice, **1**: 114
operant conditioning, **1**: 105, 134; **2**: 569
personality problems, **1**: 106
phobias, **1**: 118
reciprocal inhibition, **1**: 128; **2**: 560
school phobia, **1**: 130
shaping, **1**: 143
social reinforcement, **1**: 139
tics, **1**: 115; **2**: 377
Legal controls
dangerous drugs, **4**: 318–319
Leisure, **4**: 137
Leucotomy, **2**: xxiii, 327
dreaming, **2**: 200
Life-space interviews
adolescents, **4**: 436, 437, 446–447, 459
Light stimulation, **2**: 89
Limbic system, **2**: 202
Lipochondrodystrophy, **1**: 507
Local Authorities clinics, **1**: 256
Logical Types, **2**: 404
Lying, **1**: 179, 525
Lyon hypothesis, **2**: 22, 25, 27, 38
LSD (lysergic acid diethylamide) **2**: 266, 273, 274, 275, 278
adolescent addiction, **4**: 312, 318, 480
antidotes, **2**: 279
body image, **2**: 141

chromosomal changes, **2**: 279
clinical use, **2**: 282
comparison with Sernyl, **2**: 302
derealisation syndrome, **4**: 346
effects, **4**: 317
intoxication, **3**: 715
model psychoses, **2**: 279, 301
psychopathological reactions, **2**: 279
psycho-social aspects, **2**: 282
serotonin interaction, **2**: 276
university students, **4**: 480
Lysergic acid diethylamide (*see* LSD)
Lysosome, **2**: 57

Macroglia, **2**: 62
Macropsia, **4**: 335
Macrosomatognosia, **2**: 140
Magnetism, **2**: 147, 148
Malaria therapy, **3**: 613
Mal de mère, **3**: 71
Malformations, **3**: 20–45, 52
illegitimacy, **3**: 33
prenatal influences, **3**: 20–46, 51, 52
Mandala, **2**: 271
Mania, **2**: 425
chronic, **2**: 439
fantastica infantilis, **4**: 385, 387
insomnia, **2**: 208
schizophrenic, **2**: 430, 431
Manic-depressive psychosis, **2**: 6, 439, 440, 444
in adolescence, **4**: 395–398
in childhood, **3**: 652; **4**: 395–398
classification, **4**: 229–230
cyclothymia, **2**: 439; **4**: 230
encephalobaria, **4**: 230
encephalolampsia, **4**: 230
family, **2**: 651
personality development, **2**: 451
psychoanalysis, **2**: 448
suicide, **4**: 398
Manifest patient (*see* Presenting patient)
Marihuana, **2**: 274, 281; **4**: 313 (*see also* Cannabinols)
Marriage
of cousins and schizophrenia, **2**: 11
early and divorce, **4**: 133
Japanese culture, **3**: 350
kibbutz, **3**: 322
monogamy, **3**: 135
plural, **3**: 135
polyandry, **3**: 135
polygyny, **3**: 135
trial, **3**: 299
Marital schism, **3**: 363, 364
Marital skew, **3**: 363
Masturbation, **3**: 236
fantasies, **3**: 211
infantile, **3**: 429
sleep disorders, **3**: 429, 436, 438

Phantom-body, **2**: 133
Phantom limb, **2**: 131, 133–136, 172, 272
  in leprosy, **2**: 134
  after surgery, **2**: 134, 135
  thalidomide babies, **2**: 135
Phenomenology
  in psychiatry, **4**: 216
Phenylketonuria, **1**: 45, 504, 505, 511; **2**:
  14, 626; **3**: 4
  genetic counselling, **1**: 52
Phenylpyruvic oligophrenia (*see* Phenylketonuria)
Phobia, **1**: 113, 118; **2**: 560
  in adolescence, **1**: 291
  aetiology, **1**: 119
  of animals, **3**: 225
  behaviour therapy (q.v.)
  cat, **1**: 158
  confinement, **1**: 121
  extinction, **1**: 158
  imaginal desensitization, **2**: 565
  horse, **3**: 200
  learning theory, applied to children, **1**:
    104–151
  little Hans's case, **3**: 200, 293
  Morita's theory, **2**: 525
  school, **1**: 130, 245, 291, 560
  sleep, **3**: 452
  systematic desensitization, **1**: 118; **2**:
    563, 569, 571, 572
  treatment in children, **1**: 126, 129
Phocomelia, **3**: 50, 51
Photic activation, **3**: 396
Photography symptom, **4**: 340, 341–342
Phrenasthenia, **3**: 594, 598
  progressive, **3**: 592
Physiology
  of adolescence, **4**: 3–27
Piaget's theory, **1**: 58–84, 87, 88, 90, 94, 95,
    98, 188, 213, 214, 376; **2**: 243, 448,
    452, 726
  criticism of, **1**: 78–79
Pica, **3**: 455–469
  addiction and, **3**: 467
  aetiology, **3**: 455
  constitutional factors, **3**: 462
  definition, **3**: 455
  distribution, **3**: 455
  environmental factors, **3**: 462
  incidence, **3**: 455
  maternal deprivation, **3**: 465, 468
  medical evaluation, **3**: 467
  nutritional factors, **3**: 464
  outpatient treatment, **3**: 467
  preventive measures, **3**: 469
  psychiatric study, **3**: 456
  psychodynamic factors, **3**: 464
  psychopathology, **3**: 465
  research study, **3**: 456
Pink spot, **2**: 15, 627

Pinocytic vesicles, **2**: 81
Pinocytosis, **2**: 78
Placebo, **2**: 596
  active, **2**: 611, 612
  age, **2**: 602
  anxiety, **2**: 603
  attitude towards results, **2**: 606
  attitude towards treatment, **2**: 606
  catharsis, **2**: 604
  clinical applications, **2**: 610
  conditioning, **1**: 111; **2**: 603
  defence mechanisms, **2**: 604
  definition, **2**: 598
  direct iatroplacebogenesis, **2**: 605
  double blind procedure, **2**: 612
  effect, **2**: 600, 613
  environmental factors, **2**: 610
  evaluation of therapy, **2**: 611
  faith, **2**: 603
  historical, **2**: 596
  indications for use, **2**: 610
  indirect iatroplacebogenesis, **2**: 608
  inert, **2**: 611
  intelligence, **2**: 602
  learning, **2**: 603, 607
  motivation, **2**: 603
  negative reactors, **2**: 603
  patient–physician relationship, **2**: 600, 605
  personality, **2**: 601
  precautions, **2**: 611
  primitive cultures, **2**: 708, 709
  projective tests, **2**: 602
  psychiatric diagnosis, **2**: 602
  psychological factors, **2**: 610
  sex, **2**: 602
  single-blind procedures, **2**: 611
  situational variables, **2**: 609
  staff attitude, **2**: 609
  suggestion, **2**: 602
  treatment procedure, **2**: 609
  triple-blind procedure, **2**: 612
Planaria
  memory transfer experiment, **2**: 94, 95
Plasma cortisol levels, **2**: 162, 163, 186
Play
  diagnosis, **1**: 277; **2**: 660, 667
  handicapped children, **1**: 213
  interpretation, **3**: 211, 213
  observation, **3**: 215
  practice, **1**: 69
  symbolic, **1**: 69; **3**: 211
  therapy, **1**: 280; **2**: 667
Pleasure principle, **2**: 514
Poliomyelitis
  in pregnancy, **3**: 23
Politics
  adolescents, **4**: 146
Polyandry
  Adelphic, **3**: 135
  incidence, **3**: 135

Vol. 1

MODERN PERSPECTIVES IN CHILD PSYCHIATRY

CONTENTS

Editor's Preface

Vol. 2

MODERN PERSPECTIVES IN WORLD PSYCHIATRY

CONTENTS

Editor's Preface
Introduction *Lord Adrian*, o.m.

PART ONE: SCIENTIFIC

PART TWO: CLINICAL

Vol. 3

MODERN PERSPECTIVES IN INTERNATIONAL CHILD PSYCHIATRY

CONTENTS